MBL Lectures in Biology
Volume 12

MOLECULAR APPROACHES TO PARASITOLOGY

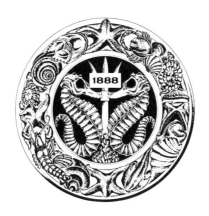

MBL LECTURES IN BIOLOGY

MOLECULAR APPROACHES TO PARASITOLOGY

Editors
John C. Boothroyd
Department of Microbiology and Immunology
Stanford University School of Medicine
Stanford, California

Richard Komuniecki
Department of Biology
University of Toledo
Toledo, Ohio

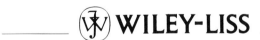

WILEY-LISS

A JOHN WILEY & SONS, INC., PUBLICATION
New York • Chichester • Brisbane • Toronto • Singapore

Address All Inquiries to the Publisher
Wiley-Liss, Inc., 605 Third Avenue, New York, NY 10158-0012

Copyright © 1995 Wiley-Liss, Inc.

Printed in the United States of America

Library of Congress Cataloging-in-Publication Data

Molecular approaches to parasitology / editors, John C. Boothroyd
and Richard Komuniecki.
    p. cm. — (MBL lectures in biology ; 12)
    Includes bibliographical references and index.
    ISBN 0-471-10342-X (hardcover). — ISBN 0-471-10341-1 (pbk.)
    1. Molecular parasitology. I. Boothroyd, John C.
II. Komuniecki, Richard. III. Series: MBL lectures in biology ; v. 12.
    [DNLM: 1. Parasites—physiology. 2. Parasitic Diseases—
immunology. 3. Host-Parasite Relations—physiology. W1 MB999 v.
12 1995 / QX 4 M7175 1995]
    QR201.P27M65 1995
    616.9´6—dc20
    DNLM/DLC   94-41923
    for Library of Congress   CIP

Cover:

Upper left: Late stage of endodyogeny. See Dubremetz, p. 353.

Upper right: Model representing the early stages of the interaction between *T. cruzi* trypomastigotes and mammalian cells. See Andrews, p. 366.

Center left: Model for kDNA replication in vivo. See Englund et al., p. 155.

Center right: Anaphase of the second cleavage division in the two-cell stage of chromatin diminution in *P. univalens*. See Müller, p. 192.

Lower right: Tachyzoites of *T. gondii* shown during intracellular growth within fibroblasts. See Sher, p. 436.

The text of this book is printed on acid-free paper.

Contents

APPENDIX

Contributors

Janet Ajioka, Department of Microbiology and Immunology, University of Tennessee, Memphis, TN 38163 [**269**]

Thomas E. Allen, Department of Biochemistry and Molecular Biology, Oregon Health Sciences University, Portland, OR 97201 [**123**]

Basil Allsopp, Department of Biochemistry, Cambridge University, Cambridge CB2 1QW, England [**43**]

Norma W. Andrews, Cell Biology Department, Yale University School of Medicine, New Haven, CT 06510 [**359**]

Howard Baylis, Department of Biochemistry, Cambridge University, Cambridge CB2 1QW, England [**43**]

Karen L. Bennett, Department of Molecular Biology and Immunology, School of Medicine, University of Missouri, Columbia, MO 65212 [**321**]

Kevin L. Blair, Upjohn Laboratories, The Upjohn Company, Kalamazoo, MI 49001 [**57**]

Tom Blumenthal, Department of Biology, Indiana University, Bloomington, IN 47405 [**281**]

John C. Boothroyd, Department of Microbiology and Immunology, Stanford University School of Medicine, Stanford, CA 94305 [**xv, 211**]

Peter J. Bradley, Department of Microbiolgy and Immunology and Molecular Biology Institute, University of California, Los Angeles, CA 90024 [**399**]

Michael Cappello, Departments of Pediatrics and Epidemiology and Public Health, and Medical Helminthology Laboratory, Yale University School of Medicine, New Haven, CT 06510 [**21**]

Mark Carrington, Department of Biochemistry, Cambridge University, Cambridge CB2 1QW, England [**43**]

Sul-Hee Chung, Department of Microbiology and Immunology, University of Tennessee, Memphis, TN 38163 [**269**]

Jay L. Crary, Department of Microbiology and Immunology, Stanford University School of Medicine, Stanford, CA 94305; present address: Department of Surgery, University of Washington Medical Center, Seattle, WA 98195 [**371**]

Arpita Das, Department of Microbiology and Immunology, Stanford University School of Medicine, Stanford, CA 94305; present address: Seattle Biomedical Research Institute, Seattle, WA 98109 [**371**]

John R. David, Department of Tropical Public Health, Harvard School of Public Health, Boston, MA 02115 [**xiii**]

The numbers in brackets are the opening page numbers of the contributors' articles.

Richard E. Davis, Department of Biology, San Francisco State University, San Francisco, CA 94132 **[299]**

Jean François Dubremetz, Unité 42 INSERM, 59655 Villenueve d'Ascq, France **[345]**

Heidi G. Elmendorf, Department of Microbiology and Immunology, Stanford University School of Medicine, Stanford, CA 94305; present address: Department of Biology, Phillips Academy, Andover, MA 01810 **[371]**

Paul T. Englund, Department of Biological Chemistry, Johns Hopkins Medical School, Baltimore, MD 21205 **[147]**

Jean E. Feagin, Seattle Biomedical Research Institute, Seattle, WA 98109-1651, and Department of Pathobiology, School of Public Health and Community Medicine, University of Washington, Seattle, WA 98195 **[163]**

Martin Ferguson, Departments of Molecular Biophysics and Biochemistry and Genetics, Yale University, New Haven, CT 06510 **[147]**

Fred D. Finkelman, Department of Medicine, F. Edward He'bert School of Medicine of the Uniformed Services University of the Health Sciences, Bethesda, MD 20814 **[467]**

Juliet A. Fuhrman, Department of Biology, Tufts University, Medford, MA 02115 **[77]**

William C. Gause, Department of Microbiology and Immunology, F. Edward He'bert School of Medicine of the Uniformed Services University of the Health Sciences, Bethesda, MD 20814 **[467]**

Timothy G. Geary, Upjohn Laboratories, The Upjohn Company, Kalamazoo, MI 49001 **[57]**

R. Dean Gillespie, Department of Microbiology and Immunology, University of Tennessee, Memphis, TN 38163 **[269]**

Michael E. Gruidl, Department of Molecular Biology and Immunology, School of Medicine, University of Missouri, Columbia, MO 65212 **[321]**

D. Lys Guilbride, Department of Biological Chemistry, Johns Hopkins Medical School, Baltimore, MD 21205 **[147]**

Kasturi Haldar, Department of Microbiology and Immunology, Stanford University School of Medicine, Stanford, CA 94305 **[371]**

Sobha Hariharan, Department of Microbiology and Immunology, University of Tennessee, Memphis, TN 38163 **[269]**

John Hawdon, Departments of Pediatrics and Epidemiology and Public Health, and Medical Helminthology Laboratory, Yale University School of Medicine, New Haven, CT 06510 **[21]**

Norman F.H. Ho, Upjohn Laboratories, The Upjohn Company, Kalamazoo, MI 49001 **[57]**

Peter Hotez, Departments of Pediatrics and Epidemiology and Public Health, and Medical Helminthology Laboratory, Yale University School of Medicine, New Haven, CT 06510 **[21]**

Catharine E. Johnson, Department of Biological Chemistry, Johns Hopkins Medical School, Baltimore, MD 21205 **[147]**

Patricia J. Johnson, Department of Microbiology and Immunology and Molecular Biology Institute, University of California, Los Angeles, CA 90024 **[399]**

Kami Kim, Department of Microbiology and Immunology, Stanford University School of Medicine, Stanford, CA 94305 **[211]**

Patricia R. Komuniecki, Department of Biology, University of Toledo, Toledo, OH 43606 [109]

Richard Komuniecki, Department of Biology, University of Toledo, Toledo, OH 43606 [xv, 109]

Monique A. Kreutzer, Department of Molecular Biology and Immunology, School of Medicine, University of Missouri, Columbia, MO 65212 [321]

Carol J. Lahti, Department of Microbiology and Immunology and Molecular Biology Institute, University of California, Los Angeles, CA 90024 [399]

Sabine Lauer, Department of Microbiology and Immunology, Stanford University School of Medicine, Stanford, CA 94305 [371]

Congjun Li, Department of Biological Chemistry, Johns Hopkins Medical School, Baltimore, MD 21205 [147]

Wen-Lu Li, Department of Microbiology and Immunology, Stanford University School of Medicine, Stanford, CA 94305; present address: Genentech, South San Francisco, CA 94080 [371]

Richard M. Locksley, Departments of Medicine and Microbiology/Immunology, UCSF Medical Center, San Francisco, CA 94143 [455]

Ndavi-Muia Malu, Department of Biochemistry, Cambridge University, Cambridge CB2 1QW, England [43]

John M. Mansfield, Laboratory of Immunology, Department of Animal Health & Biomedical Sciences, University of Wisconsin, Madison, WI 53706 [477]

Fritz Müller, Institute of Zoology, University of Fribourg, Pérolles, CH-1700 Fribourg, Switzerland [191]

Theodore E. Nash, Laboratory of Parasitic Diseases, National Institutes of Health, Bethesda, MD 20892 [31]

Thomas P. Nutman, Laboratory of Parasitic Diseases, National Institutes of Health, Bethesda, MD 20892 [511]

Edward J. Pearce, Department of Microbiology, Immunology, and Parasitology, College of Veterinary Medicine, Cornell University, Ithaca, NY 14853 [497]

David Pérez-Morga, Department of Biological Chemistry, Johns Hopkins Medical School, Baltimore, MD 21205 [147]

S.G. Reed, Infectious Disease Research Institute, Seattle, WA 98109 [443]

Steven L. Reiner, Departments of Medicine and Microbiology/Immunology, UCSF Medical Center, San Francisco, CA 94143 [455]

James P. Richards, Department of Molecular Biology and Immunology, School of Medicine, University of Missouri, Columbia, MO 65212 [321]

Laura J. Rocco, Department of Biological Chemistry, Johns Hopkins Medical School, Baltimore, MD 21205 [147]

Susan P. Rohrer, Merck Research Laboratories, Rahway, NJ 07065 [93]

Deborah L. Roussell, Department of Molecular Biology and Immunology, School of Medicine, University of Missouri, Columbia, MO 65212; present address: Bristol-Myers Squibb, Pharmaceutical Research Institute, Princeton, NJ [321]

James M. Schaeffer, Merck Research Laboratories, Rahway, NJ 07065 [93]

Alan Sher, Laboratory of Parasitic Diseases, National Institute of Allergy and Infectious Diseases, National Institutes of Health, Bethesda, MD 20892 [431]

Yael Shochat, Department of Biochemistry, Cambridge University, Cambridge CB2 1QW, England [43]

David Sibley, Department of Microbiology and Immunology, Stanford University School of Medicine, Stanford, CA 94305; present address: Department of Molecular Microbiology, Washington University School of Medicine, St. Louis, MO [211]

Sandra M. Sims, Upjohn Laboratories, The Upjohn Company, Kalamazoo, MI 49001 [57]

Sarjit Sohal, Department of Biochemistry, Cambridge University, Cambridge CB2 1QW, England [43]

Dominique Soldati, Department of Microbiology and Immunology, Stanford University School of Medicine, Stanford, CA 94305 [211]

Jürg M. Sommer, Department of Pharmaceutical Chemistry, University of California, San Francisco, CA 94143 [413]

John Spieth, Department of Biology, Indiana University, Bloomington, IN 47405 [281]

Kenneth Stuart, Seattle Biomedical Research Institute, Seattle, WA 98109-1651 [243]

John Swindle, Department of Microbiology and Immunology, University of Tennessee, Memphis, TN 38163 [269]

David P. Thompson, Upjohn Laboratories, The Upjohn Company, Kalamazoo, MI 49001 [57]

Al F. Torri, Department of Biological Chemistry, Johns Hopkins Medical School, Baltimore, MD 21205 [147]

Christian Tschudi, Department of Internal Medicine, Yale University School of Medicine, New Haven, CT 06520 [255]

Buddy Ullman, Department of Biochemistry and Molecular Biology, Oregon Health Sciences University, Portland, OR 97201 [123]

Thomas R. Unnasch, Division of Geographic Medicine, Department of Medicine, University of Alabama at Birmingham, Birmingham, AL 35294 [5]

Joseph F. Urban, Jr., Helminthic Diseases Laboratory, Livestock and Poultry Services Institute, Agricultural Research Service, U.S. Department of Agriculture, Beltsville, MD 20705 [467]

Lyle Uyetake, Department of Microbiology and Immunology, Stanford University School of Medicine, Stanford, CA 94305 [371]

Alice L. Wang, Department of Pharmaceutical Chemistry, University of California, San Francisco, CA 94143 [179]

C.C. Wang, Department of Pharmaceutical Chemistry, University of California, San Francisco, CA 94143 [179,413]

Dyann F. Wirth, Department of Tropical Public Health, Harvard School of Public Health, Boston, MA 02115 [227]

Peter A. Zimmerman, Laboratory of Parasitic Diseases, National Institute of Allergy and Infectious Diseases, National Institutes of Health, Bethesda, MD 20892 [5]

Foreword

This volume, *Molecular Approaches to Parasitology*, edited by John C. Boothroyd and Richard Komuniecki, is based on the Biology of Parasitism course, which has been given each summer at the Marine Biological Laboratory (MBL) in Woods Hole, Massachusetts, for the past 14 years. The idea for such a course was born in conversations between and among Drs. Joshua Lederberg, Kenneth Warren, and Anthony Cerami, who, in the late 1970s, considered that the time was ripe to bring the concepts and techniques of molecular biology and modern immunology to the field of parasitology. Indeed, when I began as the first course director in 1980, it would have been difficult to gather a dozen experts in the molecular biology of parasites. By September of 1993, more than three hundred molecular parasitologists attended the three-day annual meeting on the molecular biology of parasites in Woods Hole. Obviously, times have changed.

But back to the beginning. Dr. Paul Gross, then director of the MBL, was excited at the idea of having such a course as part of the MBL summer program. He immediately offered to provide laboratory and classroom space. The funding at different times has come from the Burroughs Wellcome Fund, and the Rockefeller, the Edna McConnell Clark, and the John and Catherine MacArthur Foundations, with fellowships donated by the Special Program for Research and Training in Tropical Diseases (World Bank/UNDP/WHO), the Wellcome Trust, and others.

So far, the course has had 236 students (16 a year for eleven years, 20 for the past three), most of whom were graduate students or postdoctoral fellows, but a considerable number of professors have also participated as students. By inviting laboratory instructors and lecturers who are at the forefront of their fields, the course has continued to engender excitement and enthusiasm in students and instructors alike. Over the years, so many of the students have made the decision to take up study of the biology of parasitism as a career that the course has had a major impact on the field, as was hoped at its initiation.

In 1988, Paul Englund and Alan Sher, then course directors, edited the volume *The Biology of Parasitism: A Molecular and Immunological Approach*. That book reflected the field at the time, emphasizing the molecular biology of antigenic variation in trypanosomes and immunology related to the delineation of antigens required for development of vaccines. Various aspects of cell biology and genetics and global problems of parasitic diseases were also included. Only a few years have passed since the book was published, and from its contents, it is evident that another book is in order.

The chapters in the present volume illustrate the dramatic advances in the field over a very few years. The successful transfection of *Leishmania, Trypanosoma, Toxoplasma,* and *Plasmodium* was a major breakthrough, allowing investigation of a range of new areas in the biology of parasites; this is reflected in the volume. The role of cytokines in immunity to parasites dominates the work on immunology. The new and increased interactions between investigators studying the molecular biology of *Caenorhabditis elegans* and parasitic nematodes is evident in the expansion of nematode molecular biology. The book also covers work in entirely new areas, such as RNA editing, and in general, reflects the major advances of the recent past in understanding cell biology, biochemistry, and pharmacology.

It is difficult, if not impossible, to say that one area of biology is more exciting than another. Study of any area in depth can have tremendous rewards. But the biology of parasitism has some unique features that continue to spark the interest of investigators young and old. Study of animal parasitism presents the investigator with an array of diverse and complex microorganisms (some not so micro). These organisms have developed unique interactions with their hosts, and are often quite promiscuous in their comfort level, able to live happily in insects, invertebrates, and vertebrates. They can also lead the scientist in a merry dance over wide areas of developmental biology, requiring him or her to use sophisticated gene regulation, manipulate microenvironments, puzzle out unique biochemical processes, and define diverse mechanisms of immune evasion. The challenge and excitement of research in this complex area of biology is coupled with our knowledge of the enormous problems such parasites bring to the health of the world's human population. It is easy to see why young investigators come into the field like bears on the trail of a honey tree.

The scientific literature and the work described in this book show us what some of these scientists have already accomplished. Those of us who have had the pleasure of helping these efforts along can only hope that our sponsors, and in a way our masters, will provide the necessary support to take advantage of the rich opportunities at hand.

John R. David
Salvador, Bahia

Preface

Parasitology is an exceptionally broad discipline. It covers organisms that range from the protozoa to helminths and insects. Approaches to the study of these myriad organisms range from the purely molecular to epidemiological or ecological. No single course or book can hope to cover this extraordinary diversity of topics without becoming superficial in the process. As we hope the title suggests, this book focuses on the ways in which molecular tools can be brought to bear on studies of the biology of parasites.

What follows is a compilation of chapters written by people who lectured in the summer course "Biology of Parasitism: Modern Approaches." This is an intensive, nine-week course that has been held for each of the past 14 summers at the Marine Biological Laboratory in Woods Hole, Massachusetts. It is designed for advanced students committed to a research career in the area of parasitology and aims to provide such students with a firm foundation in some of the most powerful and important approaches to the study of parasites. Because of the "wet-lab" nature of the course, formal participation is necessarily limited to a small number of students. Through the writing and publication of this book, we hope to "spread the wealth" by giving a larger number of people access to at least the lecture component of the course.

Some of the chapters will discuss systems that have received relatively little attention at the molecular level. It is hoped that these chapters will inspire others to reexamine these interesting and unexplored organisms. Many chapters will deal with some of the best-studied parasites (e.g., *Trypanosoma* and *Leishmania*). In these cases, stimulating newcomers to study them may not be the goal (the opposite may be more appropriate!); instead, these chapters serve as exciting examples of how particular approaches can be pursued and what riches may await those prepared to take on any of the many parasites that have received only the scantest attention.

The book is divided into six sections: Host–Parasite Interaction, Metabolism and Drug Action, Genomes, Gene Expression and Genetics, Cell Biology, and Immune Response. Each represents a "level of study" or approach taken to understanding something about the detailed biology of parasites. While these six sections represent some of the most exciting work going on in the field today, there are, of course, other important areas that are necessarily touched upon by only one or even a fraction of only one chapter, e.g., population biology, epidemiology, and vector biology. This last omission needs further explanation. The course on which this book is based is specifically designed to complement another annual summer course, sponsored by the MacArthur Foundation, which is entirely on vectors. As a result, our course has relatively little coverage of this topic (not least because finding vector biologists not involved in the other course can be difficult to do!).

The contributing authors were asked to make the chapters as informal as possible, that is, more like a lecture than a formal review. As a result, the reader will not find an exhaustive review of a particular topic. Instead, a more personal discussion of each subject is presented. It is hoped that this somewhat unusual format will prove a valuable complement to the conventional literature. We hope that those just entering the field will benefit from such a presentation more than from a recitation of cold facts.

This book is not meant to duplicate what is to be found in many superb texts. Consequently, the reader will not find much detail on the basic biology of these parasites or clinical details of the diseases they cause discussed in the pages that follow. Instead, we refer them to books such as *Parasitic Diseases* by Katz, Despommier, and Gwadz, *Medical Parasitology* by Markell and Voge, and *Living Together* by Trager, to name but a few of the excellent texts available.

Why has parasitology undergone such an explosion in the past decade? The first reason undoubtedly lies in the emergence of techniques that were equal to the task of dissecting at the molecular level organisms that were both complex and difficult to obtain in the quantities necessary for more conventional analyses. The second reason has been the large number of discoveries that have emerged from studies with these organisms. Many of these discoveries have forced "mainstream" biology to sit up and take notice. The message was clear: the major models for the study of eukaryotic biology are not as representative as once thought and much is to be gained by the study of "lower" eukaryotes. Perhaps the hardest lesson has been that the initially bizarre phenomena discovered in these organisms also exist in "higher" organisms, just not so obviously. These discoveries gave credibility to the field, which resulted in the delving into parasites by persons who would not otherwise have judged them worthy. And, finally, there has been a growing sense among many scientists that they have a responsibility to apply the recently developed and enormously powerful technologies to serious pathogens that have long been neglected.

The expectation is that, sooner or later, breakthroughs will be made that will result in the means to control parasitic diseases. This may not come tomorrow, it may not come next year, but it will surely happen within our lifetimes, and ultimately the knowledge that it will happen is what motivates many in this most exciting field.

John C. Boothroyd
Richard Komuniecki

Acknowledgments

We wish to acknowledge the support of many without whom the course, and hence this book, would not have happened. First, of course, are the lecturers themselves, who give their time and energy each year. What follows is a chance sampling of the speakers from only one summer. It must be emphasized that we have made an effort to enlist different speakers each year to keep the course vibrant and to spread the benefit that comes from lecturing in it to as many individuals as possible.

In addition to the lecturers, we must also acknowledge all those directly involved with the teaching of the labs: the course assistants, the teaching assistants, and the faculty. The enthusiasm and dedication of all these individuals are the key ingredients that make or break a course such as this. We could not have asked for any finer people or scientists with whom to work.

We thank the foundations that have provided the major financial support. Through their generosity, we were able to invite an outstanding array of speakers, provide substantial financial aid to the students, and expose them to the most powerful technologies. Major support has come from the MacArthur Foundation, the Burroughs Wellcome Fund, and the Edna McConnell Clark Foundation, with additional support from the Wellcome Trust, the American Society of Cell Biology, and the Zeiss Foundation. Many companies have also generously provided us with the free loan of equipment and gifts of reagents that, again, enable us to expose students to the latest and greatest. Noteworthy among these are Aminco, Beckman, Becton-Dickinson, BTX, Cambridge Tech., Eppendorf, Hoeffer, IAC, IBI, Jouan, Labline, Leica, New England Biolabs, Perkin Elmer, Pharmacia, Promega, RMC, Shandon, Stratagene, and Zeiss.

The staff at the Marine Biological Laboratory, too many to name, have provided not only efficient and competent support, but they have done so with grace and good humor. Their professionalism and tolerance of frequently missed deadlines and other faux pas are enormously appreciated.

Last, but not least, are the students themselves, for they are the people for whom the money is provided, the equipment loaned, the reagents sent, the protocols written, and the lectures delivered. Their commitment, energy, stamina, and insatiable thirst for knowledge make teaching the course all worthwhile. A keener and more able collection of students does not exist, and we look forward to following their success in the belief that the course played a part.

HOST–PARASITE INTERACTION

Preface

The six chapters in the first section discuss the interaction of host and parasite, with an emphasis on adaptations by the parasite to life in the cells or tissues of its host (adaptations by the host are dealt with in the final section of the book, "Immune Response").

The first chapter in this section, by Unnasch and Zimmerman, is a discussion of how DNA sequences can be used to help classify parasitic organisms. What has this to do with the host–parasite interaction? A great deal is the answer. In addition to describing in very clear terms the methodologies used, Unnasch and Zimmerman initiate the reader into the subject of co-evolution of host and parasite. Such co-evolution has obvious and dramatic implications for the host–parasite interaction and will undoubtedly influence our thinking of how change in one can result in a compensating change in the other or how physical isolation of the host can sometimes result in genetic isolation of the parasite. This is but one of the many important roles systematics has to play in modern parasitology.

In the next chapter, Hotez and colleagues describe some of the adaptations of hookworms to their parasitic lifestyle, particularly the role of parasite enzymes in inviasion, the role of proteases and anticoagulants in feeding, and the importance of arrested larval development to transmission.

For extracellular parasitic protozoa, a well-known strategy to ensure a chronic infection (and thus increase chances of transmission) is to change continually the antigenic nature of the infecting population. While most in parasitology are now well familiar with the phenomenon of antigenic variation in African trypanosomes, the emerging story with *Giardia* is an equally important and interesting variation on this theme. The chapter by Ted Nash relates recent progress in this exciting field.

Intracellular parasites face particular challenges in terms of "host–parasite interaction." The section on Cell Biology includes several chapters on the detailed physical processes involved in invasion and intracellular life, but, in this section, Carrington and colleagues describe how *Theileria* stimulates each infected host cell (lymphocytes) to reproduce to enable the parasite population to expand without the need for repeated invasion and exit of new host cells.

Tim Geary and his colleagues at UpJohn take a close look at a tremendously understudied area, the nematode surface, and synthesize recent results

3

and ideas on how these surfaces are involved in life in a host. The authors stress that a thorough understanding of cuticular permeability and the maintenance of turgor pressure are critical not only as potential sites for chemotherapy but also for any rational insight into drug delivery in these parasites.

Juliet Fuhrman closes this section with her chapter on chitinases from both protozoa and helminthic parasites. Among the functions proposed for these molecules in microfilaria is a role in the interaction of the parasite with the insect gut. This is an important area of research that may ultimately lead to strategies for blocking transmission of some parasites. It must also be remembered that the distinction being made when talking of a human as "host" and insect as "vector" is not always biologically justifiable and thus possible adaptations of the parasite to the insect "host" is a critical aspect of the "host–parasite" interaction.

Molecular Approaches to Parasitology, pages 5–20

Systematics: Questions and Approaches for the Molecular Parasitologist

Thomas R. Unnasch and Peter A. Zimmerman

Division of Geographic Medicine, Department of Medicine, University of Alabama at Birmingham, Birmingham, Alabama 35294 (T.R.U.); Laboratory of Parasitic Diseases, National Institute of Allergy and Infectious Diseases, National Institutes of Health, Bethesda, Maryland 20892 (P.A.Z.)

INTRODUCTION

Systematics is the study of how different organisms are related to one another. By determining such a relationship, or phylogeny, it is possible to infer how the different groups studied have evolved throughout time. Until recently, much of the information used to derive phylogenies has been primarily based on morphological characteristics. Systematics has therefore been more the territory of anatomists and zoologists rather than of molecular biologists. However, the recent development of a variety of molecular methods based primarily on the polymerase chain reaction (PCR) has made it possible to apply molecular methods to answer systematic questions. The goal of this chapter is to approach the study of systematics from the perspective of a molecular parasitologist.

Parasitic organisms have several features that make them particularly appropriate to study from an evolutionary point of view. For example, many human parasites cannot be cultured *in vitro*, and no suitable animal hosts have been found in which these organisms can be easily propagated. In such a case, it is necessary to use related parasites that may be cultured in an animal system as models for the human parasite. Systematics may be used to identify the animal parasite that is most closely related to the human pathogen, allowing the most relevant animal model system to be identified. A second application of systematics to the study of parasites arises from the fact that many of the parasites that we study occur in widely separated areas throughout the world. Use of techniques that are able to distinguish parasite populations may be used to develop relationships among parasite populations separated by large distances. Such information may be used to shed some insight into how parasites have been introduced into regions where they are now endemic.

A final application of systematics has to do with the question of how the host–parasite relationship has affected the evolution of the parasite. The close relationship of a parasite and its host has led to the theory of co-evolution. This theory states that, due to the intimate association of a parasite with it's host, it may be expected that the parasite may evolve in parallel with its host. This is due to the fact that any force affecting the host species may also have an effect on the host's parasites.

Brooks (1979) has suggested that co-evolution of a parasite and its host has both a microevolutionary and a macroevolutionary component. The microevolutionary component, which has been called *co-accommodation* (Brooks, 1979), represents all of the mechanisms that the parasite uses to adjust to life in the host and, conversely, the adjustments that the host makes in response to having to live with the parasite. Some examples of adjustments that the parasite might make to life in the host include the development of methods of evading the host's immune response, such as the process of antigenic variation seen in the African trypanosomes. Another such example might be the general and parasite-specific immunosuppression seen in infections with the filarial parasites. Sometimes, the parasite may take this process further, actually using the host's immune mechanisms to its own advantage. An example of this might be the use of tumor necrosis factor by *Schistosoma mansoni* as a stimulatory factor for egg production in the adult female (Amiri et al., 1992).

All of the mechanisms used by the parasite to adapt to life within its host of course come with some cost. This cost is the fact that, as the parasite becomes ever more adapted to it's host, it is becoming ever more specialized for life within that particular host, which may be thought of as an ecological niche. Thus, by adapting to living so closely with the host, the parasite is essentially enclosing itself in a gilded cage. Once this happens, whatever happens to the host population also affects the parasite population that the host is carrying. For example, if a host population becomes reproductively isolated, the parasites carried by that host population, stuck as they are with the host, will also become isolated. This leads to the macroevolutionary aspect of co-evolution, deemed *co-speciation* (Brooks, 1979). This theory suggests that any event that results in the development of a new species in the host (a process termed *speciation*) will also result in pressure on the parasite population also to undergo a speciation event. Thus, the theory of co-evolution predicts that speciation events in the host should be matched by corresponding speciation events in the parasite populations that the host carries. Therefore, evolution in the parasite should parallel evolution in the host.

To begin to study relationships among groups of organisms, it is first necessary to develop some measure of how closely related the organisms are to one another. Traditionally, the process used has been to identify characteristics that vary within the group of organisms to be studied and to use these differences to construct a phylogeny. Often morphological characteristics or biochemical differences (such as alloenzyme differences) were used for this purpose. However, such traits are only reflections of differences in the genotype of the organisms studied. For this reason, direct examination of the genotype of an organism, either by DNA sequence data or by some other means, has an inherent theoretical appeal. In addition, the development of PCR primer sets for a variety of conserved genes has made it possible to develop DNA sequence data from a large number of different organisms in a short period of time.

The use of DNA sequence data has a second practical advantage, because different types of sequences appear to evolve at different rates. This allows one to choose the DNA sequence one is examining to match the question one is posing. For example, if one is interested in looking at groups of organisms that have diverged over a long period of time, it is best to choose relatively invariant sequences for analysis. One common choice for such studies has been the sequence of the small subunit rRNA genes, which appear to contain relatively slowly evolving domains. For example, Sogin and his colleagues (1989) have used small subunit rRNA sequences to show that *Giardia lamblia* separated very early from the evolutionary branches that have led to the prokaryote and eukaryote kingdoms. In a similar manner, the same sequence has been used to demonstrate that the malaria parasite and other apicomplexa have diverged from the other eukaryotes before the evolution of multicellular organisms [Gunderson et al., 1986]. In contrast, if one is looking for differences that occur over a shorter evolutionary time period, one may choose sequences that evolve more rapidly. A common choice for such studies are mitochondrially encoded sequences. Because different regions of the mitochondrial genome appear to accumulate mutations at varying rates, it is often possible to use these sequences to develop phylogenies of both distantly and closely related organisms (Kocher et al., 1989).

Finally, for studies involving populations within a single species or genus, it is important to use sequences that evolve quite rapidly. The DNA sequences most commonly used in such studies are repeated sequences. The neutral mutation theory (Kimura, 1983) predicts that, because such sequences represent non coding DNA, they should evolve at a more rapid rate than sequences that code for proteins. In fact, as we discuss later, it is clear that mutations in such sequences do not occur completely freely; change in these sequences is under some constraint. Despite this, experience has shown that these sequences are capable of distinguishing closely related populations and species.

Perhaps the most powerful method for detecting differences in closely related organisms is based on the use of dispersed repeated sequences. This is a PCR-based method known as *random amplification of polymorphic DNA,* (RAPD). This method uses randomly chosen PCR primers 10 bp in length for the amplification of genomic DNA. For reasons that are poorly understood, this results in the amplification of specific DNA fragments, that often appear to vary in size within and between closely related species. The presence or absence of a particular amplification fragment may then be used as a character to construct a phylogeny for the organisms under study.

Thus, the use of DNA sequences has many advantages for the development of phylogenies. These include the fact that, by using DNA sequence data, one approaches the basis for species diversity as closely as possible. A second advantage is that because sequences evolve at different rates, it is possible to tailor one's choice of DNA sequence to represent a "molecular calendar," a "molecular clock," or a "molecular stopwatch." A final advantage is that DNA sequence data are a totally objective form of data and thus not subject to biases that may be introduced by the researcher. However, there are some caveats that should be respected when one is planning to use DNA sequence data to construct phylogenies (Welsh and McClelland, 1990). Perhaps the most important of these is that a DNA sequence represents a single gene present in the organism studied. By examining a single gene, one is therefore looking at a very small portion of the information that goes into making an organism what it is. Phylogenies based on DNA sequence data are thus really only "gene trees." The implicit assumption made in using DNA sequence data is that the evolution of the gene must be representative of the evolution of the organism as a whole, and therefore the "gene tree" is really equivalent to the "species tree." This may or may not be the case. For example, in organisms using sexual reproduction, the mitochondrial genome is generally inherited strictly from the maternal parent. This means it is not subject to the reassortment pressures that exist for nuclear genes, which code for most of the genes that make an organism what it is. For this reason, it is often best to develop phylogenies based on several different DNA sequences, if possible. By doing this, one is testing the hypothesis that the evolutionary pattern deduced from a given sequence is indeed representative of the evolution in the organism as a whole.

With the advent of PCR, the collection of DNA sequence data necessary for building a phylogeny has become relatively simple. However, once the data have been obtained, it is necessary to use them to construct a phylogeny. There are several different methods currently in use for constructing phylogenies, and unfortunately none of the methods is universally agreed upon as the best. In many cases, the choice of method may be made based on how the phylogeny is to be used. It is often useful to develop phylogenies using several different approaches in the hope that these approaches will prove to be mutually reinforcing.

The methods used to develop phylogenies may be loosely classified into two categories; numerical methods and character state methods. Numerical methods are perhaps the easiest to use and to understand. Such methods are based on the approach of first developing a numerical measure of the differences between two DNA sequences and then using these values to develop a phylogeny. Numerical methods therefore involve two steps. The first step is to use some method to measure the difference between two sequences. This will lead to the production of a distance matrix, whose values may then be used to construct the phylogeny. There are several methods that may be used to construct the necessary distance matrix. Perhaps the simplest method of determining the distance between two sequences is simply to determine the percentage difference between them by counting the total number of differences and dividing by the total number of bases analyzed. This approach, although simple minded, is often sufficient to develop a distance matrix in cases in which the total divergence between two sequences is relatively low. However, as the distance between two different sequences becomes relatively large (say, greater than 10%), two factors come into play that serve to distort the results produced by this method. The first is that the number of mutations begins to approach saturation. The second problem is that back mutations, or double mutations that result in no net change at a given position (e.g., A to G and then G back to A) begin to become more frequent. It is therefore necessary to adjust the distance measure to take these factors into account. The simplest method to accomplish this is only to consider mutations that occur relatively infrequently. For example in some cases, the third codon positions in a protein coding sequence may be eliminated from the distance calculation, since the first and second codon positions generally change more slowly than do the bases in the third position. A similar approach is to translate the DNA sequence into a putative protein sequence and to use the translated sequence to construct the distance matrix. A third approach, applicable to both coding and non coding sequences, is to count only the number of transversion mutations (purine to pyrimidine or pyrimidine to purine), ignoring the more common transition mutations (purine to purine or pyrimidine to pyrimidine).

In addition to the simple approaches described above, two mathematical methods are commonly used to derive distances from DNA sequence data. Both of these methods take the possibility of mutational saturation and the possibility of back mutation into account. Jukes and Cantor's one parameter method (1969) is derived upon the assumption that all types of mutations are equally probable, while Kimura's two parameter method (1980) allows for differences in the rates of transitions and transversions. Either of these methods is preferable to the simple methods described above when the amount of overall divergence between the sequences to be analyzed is relatively large.

The second step in the development of a phylogeny when one is using a distance method is the actual development of a tree representing the phylogeny from the distance data. The simplest approach to accomplishing this is known as the *unweighted pair group method with arithmetic mean,* (UPGMA) (Sokal and Michener, 1958). This method first identifies the two most closely related groups, or taxa, in the analysis. This is taken to be the pair of taxa that has the smallest distance between them. These two taxa are then considered as the most terminal branches of the tree, and the two taxa are connected by a branch point (or node) located halfway between them. The two most closely related taxa are then considered as a single taxon, and the taxon most closely related to the group is then identified. The process is repeated until all taxa have been included in the tree. As an example, consider the following hypothetical distance matrix:

Taxon	B	C	D
A	0.2	0.9	0.35
B			0.25
C			1.0

We first note that taxa A and B have the smallest distance between them, and thus are the most closely related. Therefore, we place the initial node of the tree half way between them and make the branch lengths to each taxon equal to half the total distance:

A an B are then considered as a single taxon, and the next most closely related taxon is chosen. As we can see in the table, taxon D is the most closely related to the group A plus B. We therefore take the mean of the distances AD and BD as the distance from the group A+B and taxon D. This is (0.25 + 0.35)/2 = 0.3. We then place a node halfway between the AB group and D, with the branch lengths corresponding to half the distance between AB and D. Thus the total length of each branch must be (0.3)/2 = 0.15. Since the length of the terminal branches to A and B are each 0.1 unit in length, and the total branch length from the AB group to the node connecting the AB group to D is 0.15, the distance from the node connecting A and B to the node connecting the AB group to D must be 0.15 minus 0.10 = 0.05. We thus add a new branch to the tree as follows:

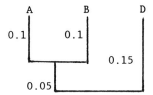

Finally, we treat A, B, and D as a single group. Doing this, the overall mean distance from the group ABD and C is (AC + BC + CD)/3 = (0.9 + 1.2 + 1.0)/3 = 1.03. We place the node at half this distance, or at 0.515. Our completed tree is thus:

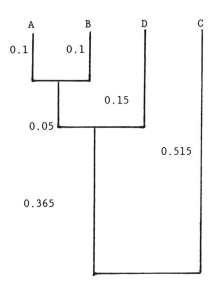

The UPGMA method works well if the rate of evolution is fairly constant throughout all of the taxa in the tree. This is because UPGMA makes this assumption implicitly, by placing the nodes at a point equidistant from the taxa in question, resulting in equal branch lengths from each internal node. If the rate of evolution is not equal in all branches, UPGMA will give a distorted version of the tree and may in some cases result in the development of an incorrect tree. Two somewhat more sophisticated methods, essentially based on UPGMA, known as the *transformed distance method* (Klotz et al, 1979) and the *neighbor joining method* (Saitou and Nei, 1987), have been developed that do not require the assumption of equal rates of evolution in all branches. These methods use a designated outgroup, which is a taxon known by other means to be more distantly related to the taxa under study than these taxa are to each other. Distances derived from each internal taxon to the outgroup are then used to correct for differences in rates of evolution among the taxa in question. For more details concerning these methods, see (Li and Grauer, 1991).

Character state methods are based on Ockham's razor, the scientific maxim that the simplest explanation is most likely to be the correct one. Thus, the method constructs a phylogeny by examining the data and trying to find the tree that requires the minimum number of changes, or mutational events, that explain the data adequately. The most common character state method currently in use is called *maximum parsimony*. This is the method that the popular computer algorithm PAUP (Swofford, 1990) and the DNAPARS subroutine of PHYLIP (Felsenstein, 1990) use in constructing phylogenies.

Maximum parsimony relies upon what are called *informative sites* when using DNA sequence data. An informative site is one that favors one phylogeny over another. For example, consider a hypothetical sequence for four taxa:

POSITION	I	II	III	IV	V	VI
TAXON 1	A	A	G	C	T	T
2	A	A	A	C	T	T
3	A	A	C	T	C	T
4	A	G	T	T	A	T

Positions I and VI are the same for all for taxa and thus clearly are not informative. In the same way, we assume that all the taxa are different when we begin the analysis, and position III, which merely confirms the fact that all are different, is also not informative. In the same way, at position II, taxon 4 differs from the rest of the taxa by having a G instead of an A. This only tells us that 4 is different from the rest of the other taxa, which we have already assumed. Thus, the site is not informative. Position V, somewhat surprisingly, is also not informative. This is because an informative site must favor one particular phylogeny over another. Three different phylogenies may be constructed to explain the history of the changes that have occurred at position 5:

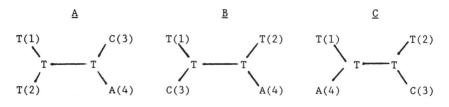

Note that all of these trees require two mutations to explain the data, and thus the data do not favor one tree over another. Thus, the data at position V are not informative. In contrast, at position IV, again three trees may be made to explain the data:

In this case, phylogeny A requires only one mutation to explain the data, while the other phylogenies require two mutations. Therefore, the data favor phylogeny A, and this site is informative. From the example above, it is clear that an informative site is one where a difference is detected in the taxa being analyzed. Furthermore, each of the different nucleotides present at an informative site must be present in at least two of the taxa.

As mentioned above, neither the numerical method nor the character state method is favored in every situation. Both methods lose some of the information contained in the data during the course of the analysis. For example, the numerical methods, by distilling the differences between sequences down to a single number, lose all of the positional data contained in the sequence. Thus, the numerical method does not care if an informative site in a sequence clearly favors one particular phylogeny; it considers all changes to be equal and will count them this way. In contrast, maximum parsimony methods rely solely upon positional data and analyze only those sites deemed informative by the method. They will therefore ignore some information, such as that found in positions II and V of the example above. It is therefore often useful, if possible, to use both numerical and character state methods to analyze sequence data, since the approaches are mutually reinforcing.

Once one has developed a phylogeny, it is important to know how robust that phylogeny really is. In other words, is the phylogeny chosen really much better supported by the data than are the other possible phylogenies that may have been developed in its place? There have been many attempts to develop methods to answer this question, (Felsenstein, 1988), and no one method is completely agreed upon. Perhaps the most commonly used method, however, is known as the bootstrap. This method relies upon a protocol of sampling with replacement to test the robustness of a phylogeny. This is done by first identifying the number of data points in the starting set, and then using the starting data set to construct a number of artificial data sets which are the same size as the starting set. For example, let us say that a given data set consists of 20 informative sites. The bootstrap will select one of these 20 sites at random from the starting data set and make a copy of the data contained at that site into a file containing the artificial data set. It returns that particular point to the starting data set, and repeats this process 20 times. At the end of 20 replications, the algorithm has produced an artificial data set drawn from the original data set, which, as in the original data set, contains 20 informative sites. However, this artificial data set is not identical to the original data set, since it will most likely contain duplicates of some of the informative sites found in the original data set and lack some of the sites found in the original data set. The algorithm then determines the best phylogeny from the artificial data set and saves it. The process is repeated a number of times, and the artificially developed trees are then compared. The algorithm then scores the number of times a given branch was found in the trees developed from the artificial data sets. Branches that occur a high percentage of the time in the artificially constructed data sets are strongly supported by the data.

As described above, there are at least three types of questions of interest to parasitologists that one may address using systematic methods: 1) questions concerning the relationship of various animal parasites to their human counterparts, 2) biogeographic questions concerning the origin and relationship of various parasite populations, and 3) questions concerning the co-evolution of parasites and their hosts. DNA sequence data have been used to address these questions in a variety of host–parasite systems. Two examples will be given in the following paragraphs.

The question of the relationship of various human parasites to similar animal parasites may be of use in deciding which animal parasites are the most appropriate to use as model systems. For example, Waters [1991 and his colleagues constructed a phylogeny for various rodent, avian, and human malaria species, using DNA sequence data derived from the small subunit rRNA. Surprisingly, they found that *Plasmodium falciparum*, the most malignant form of human malaria, was more closely related to the avian malarias than to the other human malarias or to the primate and rodent malarias. This result suggests that *P. falciparum* may have originally arisen from an avian progenitor that somehow became adapted to life in humans. The results also suggest that for some studies avian malarias may be more appropriate models than are the rodent or primate malarias.

DNA sequence based systematic studies have also been used to determine the relationship between various populations of parasites. For example, our laboratory had previously demonstrated that DNA probes based on a tandemly repeated DNA sequence designated 0–150 were capable of distinguishing the forest- and savanna-dwelling strains of *Onchocerca volvulus* in West Africa (Erttman et al,. 1987,1990; Zimmerman et al., 1992). The 0–150 family was found to be present in approximately 2,000 copies per haploid genome, and was restricted to parasites of the genus *Onchocerca*. Furthermore, DNA sequence analysis of PCR products produced from the 0–150 family could be used rationally to design new DNA probes with predicted specificities (Zimmerman et al., 1993). Taken together, these results suggested that the 0–150 family might be useful as an "evolutionary stopwatch" to investigate the relationship of different populations of the parasite. To accomplish this, we cloned and sequenced a large number of individual PCR products derived from the 0–150 repeat family. When the sequence data were examined, it became clear that there was some constraint on the variation that occurred in the 0–150 family. An example of this is shown in Figure 1. The sequence data for 20 individual repeats (Fig. 1A) have been transformed into a geometric symbolic format (Fig. 1B). When this was done, it was clear that the individual repeat sequences could be arranged into clusters (Fig. 1C). Within each of these clusters, the repeats appeared to be identical, or nearly identical. This is an example of concerted evolution, which has been seen in repeated sequence families in a variety of other organisms. In such repeated families, variation appears to be constrained, through mechanisms that are as yet not completely understood. This constraint results in the formation of distinct families, or clusters of sequence types, which occur as identical or nearly identical copies in the genome.

The fact that repeated sequences are subject to concerted evolution has important practical implications for their use as a phylogenetic marker. If variability in such sequences was completely unconstrained, it would be possible for each individual example of the repeat family to evolve independently. Thus, in the case of the 0–150 family, each of the 2,000 copies of the sequence could conceivably be unique. This would mean that it would be necessary to sequence all of the examples of the repeat in order to gain an understanding of the composition of the repeat family, which is obviously an impossible task. However, since these sequences are subject to concerted evolution, there are not 2,000 unique examples of the repeat, but only 4 to 6 sequence types that are repeated over and over in the genome. It is thus possible to gain an understanding of the structure of the repeat population by determining the DNA sequence of a relatively limited number of individual repeats.

To use repeated sequences as a phylogenetic tool, it was necessary to develop new methods of analyzing the sequence data. This is due to the fact that, in all of the methods described above, a single DNA sequence is taken to represent the taxon to be studied. Any variability of that DNA sequence within the taxon is ignored by simply constructing a consensus sequence to represent the taxon as a whole. In the case of the repeated sequences, it was obviously not appropriate to ignore the internal variability. It was thus necessary to develop a method that would take this internal variability into account. To ac-

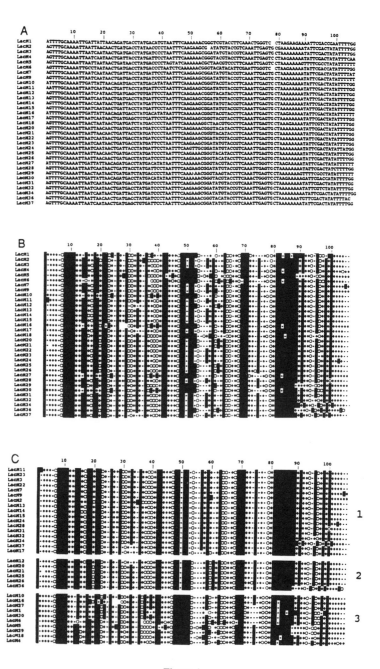

Figure 1.

complish this we adapted to this problem randomization methods recently developed in statistics. This allowed us to determine if two repeated sequence families were indeed statistically different while continuing to take the internal variation within each repeat population into account.

The question that we first addressed using this model was that of the origin of onchocerciasis in the New World. Onchocerciasis is endemic throughout much of sub-Saharan Africa, and also occurs in several isolated foci in the New World. The origin of these New World foci has been obscure. Biochemical differences in the parasite populations in the two hemispheres (Yarzabal et al., 1983), together with the inability of American parasites to develop in African blackflies (Duke et al., 1966), have suggested that American and African *O. volvulus* populations have been isolated for a long period of time. In contrast, inefficient transmission of American *O. volvulus* by American blackflies (WHO Expert Committee on Onchocerciasis, 1987), together with cytotaxonomic similarities between American and African parasites (Hirai et al., 1987), has supported the argument that parasite populations on these two widely separated continents became isolated from one another within recent evolutionary history. If some ancient event was responsible for introduction of African *O. volvulus* into the Americas, it would be expected that the American isolates would be more closely related to each other than to any of the African isolates. This is because the geographic separation of the American and African parasite gene pools would allow unique differences to evolve in 0–150 between the parasite populations on the two different continents. In contrast, if *O. volvulus* was recently introduced into the Americas, it might be expected that an American isolate would be closely related to its African ancestor. These two competing models are summarized in Figure 2. In Figure 2A–C, the New World isolates are closely related to an African ancestor, supporting the hypothesis of a recent introduction of onchocerciasis into the New World. In contrast, the model in Figure 2D shows that the American isolates are distantly related to the African parasites, supporting the hypothesis of an ancient introduction.

When the 0–150 sequence data were analyzed using the method described above, it was found that, as expected, the 0–150 populations found in the forest and savanna strains of the parasite were indeed statistically different from one another ($P = 0.033$). In contrast, the New World isolates were found

---

Fig. 1. Clustering of members of the 0–150 repeat family: (**A**): DNA sequence of 33 examples of the 0–150 isolated and cloned from the Liberian rainforest isolate of *O. volvulus*. Cloning and DNA sequence analysis were performed as previously described (Zimmerman et al., 1993). (**B**): DNA sequence data in diamond A transformed into a symbolic format. Closed rectangle, A; closed square, G; open circle, C; closed diamond, T. (**C**): Sequences are rearranged into the clusters described in the text.

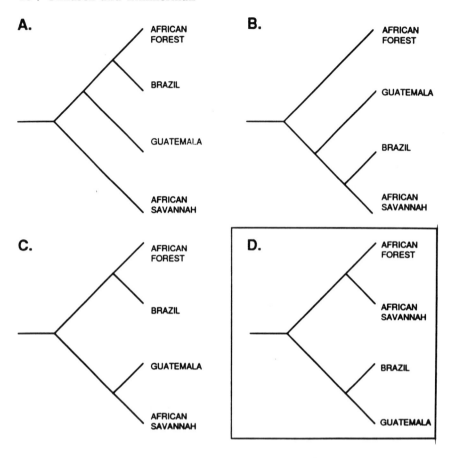

Fig. 2. Hypothetical phylogenies supporting hypothesis of ancient versus recent introductions of *O. volvulus* into the New World. (**A–C**): Possible phylogenies supporting a recent introduction of *O. volvulus* into the New World. (**D**): Phylogeny supporting an ancient introduction in *O. volvulus* into the New World.

to be indistinguishable from the African savanna isolates ($P > 0.5$). This finding was equivalent to the model shown in Figure 2B, which supported the hypothesis of a recent introduction of onchocerciasis into the New World. If it is true that onchocerciasis was introduced recently into the New World, it should be possible to correlate this introduction to a historical event. Perhaps the most frequent interchange between Africa and the New World was the trade in African slaves that existed in the 16th through 19th centuries. Interestingly, 19th century medical records from Rio de Janeiro suggest that Africans with symptoms consistent with onchocerciasis were seen by physicians in this city, which was one of the most significant Portuguese slave ports in

Brazil (Karasch, 1987). Because slaves imported into the Caribbean Islands and Latin America originated from both the forest and savannah of Africa, it is perhaps surprising that parasite samples obtained from New World specimens are so closely related to *O. volvulus* from the African savannah. However, the African savannah is considered by many historians to have been the primary source of slaves imported into the New World during the peak of the slave trade during the 18th and 19th centuries (Davidson, 1961). The fact that African savannah and American *O. volvulus* populations are indistinguishable, together with the fact that the majority of the slaves imported into the Americas originated from savannah regions thus argues that onchocerciasis was introduced into the New World as a result of the trade in African slaves.

The development of PCR-based methods for rapid DNA sequence analysis has revolutionized systematics in the past 4 years. In the discussion presented above, we hope that we have demonstrated that these methods may be useful in answering a number of questions of interest to parasitologists. Because of this fact, it is likely that systematics based on DNA sequence data will be become an increasingly important tool for parasitologists in the future.

REFERENCES

Amiri P, Locksley RM, Parslow TG, Sadick M, Rector E, Ritter D, McKerrow JH (1992): Tumor necrosis factor α restores granulomas and induces parasite egg-laying in schistosome-infected SCID mice. Nature 356:604–607.

Brooks DR (1979): Testing the context and extent of host-parasite coevolution. Syst Zool 28:299–307.

Davidson B (1961): Black Mother. London: Victor Gollancz, Ltd.

Duke BOL, Lewis DJ, Moore PJ (1966): *Onchocerca-Simulium* complexes I. Transmission of forest and Sudan-Savannah strains of *Onchocerca volvulus*, from Cameroon, by *Simulium damnosum* from various West African bioclimatic Zones. Ann Trop Med Parasitol 60:318–336.

Erttmann KD, Meredith SEO, Greene BM, Unnasch TR (1990): Isolation and characterization of form specific DNA sequences of *O. volvulus*. Acta Leidensia 59:253–260.

Erttmann KD, Unnasch TR, Greene BM, Albiez EJ, Boateng J, Denke AM, Ferraroni JJ, Karam M, Schulz-Key H, Williams PN (1987): A DNA sequence specific for forest form *Onchocerca volvulus*. Nature 327:415–417.

Felsenstein J (1988): Phylogenies from molecular sequences: Inferences and reliability. Annu Rev Genet 22:521–565.

Felsenstein J (1990): PHYLIP Phylogeny Inference Package, Version 3.3. Department of Genetics, SK50. Seattle, WA: University of Washington.

Gunderson JH, McCutchan TF, Sogin ML (1986): Sequence of the small subunit ribosomal RNA gene expressed in the bloodstream stages of *Plasmodiun berghei*: Evolutionary Implications. J Protozool 33:525–529.

Hirai H, Tada I, Takahashi H, Nwoke EB, Ufomadu GO (1987): Chromosomes of *Onchocerca volvulus* (Spirurida: Onchocercidae): A comparative study between Nigeria and Guatemala. J Helminthol 61:43–46.

Jukes TH, Cantor CR (1969): Evolution of Protein Molecules. In H.N. Munro (ed): Mammalian Protein Metabolism. New York: Academic Press pp 21–132.

Karasch MC (1987): Slave Life in Rio de Janeiro: 1808–1850. Princeton, NJ: Princeton University Press.

Kimura M (1983): The Neutral Theory of Molecular Evolution. Cambridge: Cambridge University Press.

Kimura M (1980): A simple method for estimating evolutionary rates of base substitutions through comparative studies of nucleotide sequences. J Mol Evol 16:111–120.

Klotz LC, Komar N, Blanken RL, Mitchell RM (1979): Calculation of evolutionary trees from sequence data. Proc Natl Acad Sci USA 76:4516–4520.

Kocher TD, Thomas WK, Meyer A, Edwards SV, Paabo S, Villablanca FX, Wilson AC (1989): Dynamics of mitochondrial DNA evolution in animals: Amplification and sequencing with conserved primers. Proc Natl Acad Sci USA 86:6196–6200.

Li W, Graur D (1991): Fundamentals of Molecular Evolution. Sunderland, MA: Sinauer Associates.

Saitou N, Nei M (1987): The neighbor joining method: A new method for reconstructing phylogenetic trees. Mol Biol Evol 4:406–425.

Sogin ML, Gunderson JH, Elwood HJ, Slonso RA, Peatte DA (1989): Phylogenetic meaning of the kingdom concept: An unusual ribosomal RNA from *Giardia lamblia*. Science 243:75–80.

Sokal RR, Michener CD (1958): A statistical method for evaluating systematic relationships. Univ Kansas Sci Bull 28:1409–1438.

Swofford DL (1990): PAUP. Version 3.0. Champaign: Illinois Natural History Survey.

Waters AP, Higgins DG, McCutchan TF (1991): *Plasmodium falciparum* appears to have arisen as a result of lateral transfer between avian and human hosts. Proc Natl Acad Sci USA 88:3140–3144.

Welsh J, McClelland M (1990): Fingerprinting genomes using PCR with arbitrary primers. Nucleic Acids Res 18:7213–7218.

WHO Expert Committee on Onchocerciasis (1987): Third Report. WHO Tech Rep 752. Geneva: World Health Organization.

Yarzabal L, Petralanda I, Arango M, Lobo L, Botto C (1983): Acid phosphatase patterns in microfilariae of *Onchocerca volvulus s.l.* from the Upper Orinoco Basin, Venezuela. Tropenmed. Parasitol 34:109–112.

Zimmerman PA, Dadzie KY, De Sole G, Remme J, Soumbey Alley E, Unnasch TR (1992): *Onchocerca volvulus* DNA Probe Classification Correlates with Epidemiological Patterns of Blindness. J Infect Dis 165:964–968.

Zimmerman PA, Toe L, Unnasch TR (1993): Design of *Onchocerca* DNA probes based upon analysis of a repeated sequence family. Mol Biochem Parasitol 58:259–269.

Molecular Approaches to Parasitology, pages 21–29
© 1995 Wiley-Liss, Inc.

Molecular Mechanisms of Invasion by *Ancylostoma* Hookworms

Peter Hotez, John Hawdon, and Michael Cappello

Departments of Pediatrics and Epidemiology and Public Health, and Medical Helminthology Laboratory, Yale University School of Medicine, New Haven, Connecticut 06510

INTRODUCTION

Human hookworm infection is a major cause (possibly the leading cause) of iron-deficiency anemia in the tropics, affecting up to 1 billion people. The anemia of hookworm disease results directly from blood loss caused by adult worms as they lacerate capillaries in the lamina propria of the small intestine and ingest the extravasated blood. The development of hypochromic microcytic anemia from intestinal blood loss is highly dependent on the daily iron intake and iron reserves of the host. Two populations, namely, women of child-bearing age and young children, are particularly vulnerable to the effects of hookworm iron deficiency.

Women of child-bearing age have increased iron requirements that are not usually met by dietary intake in most developing countries. The exacerbation of iron deficiency caused by hookworm infection during pregnancy has a detrimental effect on the fetus. Iron-deficiency anemia has been linked to placental ischemia and fetal growth retardation (Rusia et al., 1988). Moreover, in experimental animal models, *Ancylostoma* infection causes female reproductive alterations by affecting the hypophyseal–gonadal axis, resulting in inhibition of ovarian function and arrest of follicular development (Gupta et al., 1992).

Young children develop growth failure as well as attention deficit and intellectual impairment directly as a consequence of hookworm-induced iron deficiency (Hotez, 1989). These defects are permanent when iron deficiency develops during infancy (Lozoff et al., 1991). In many rural areas of the developing world, hookworm anemia is the single major cause of intellectual and physical growth retardation of children. An infantile form of hookworm attributable only to the species *Ancylostoma duodenale* has been described from endemic areas. Infantile ancylostomiasis is a major cause of

TABLE 1. Major Invasion Factors Identified From *Ancylostoma* Hookworms

Stage	Macromolecule	Molecular weight (kD)	Postulated Function
L3	Hyaluronidase	49	Tissue invasion
L3	Metalloprotease	68–90	Reactivation/invasion
L3	Metalloprotease	38–50	Reactivation/invasion
Adult	Hyaluronidase	66	Tissue invasion
Adult	Xa/Tf Inhibitor	8	Anticlotting

neonatal morbidity and mortality in tropical developing countries and the most significant helminthiasis of neonates (Hotez, 1989). In highly endemic areas, such as in the rural villages of West Bengal, India, or in the Shangdong province of northern China, these infants can present within 3 months of birth with clinical features of profound hookworm anemia. An infant with *Ancylostoma duodenale* infection will present with a very pale complexion, melena, diarrhea, and failure to thrive (Sen-hai and Wei-xia, 1990). In many cases, their circulating hemoglobin concentrations will range between 3 and 5 g %; i.e., they are virtually exsanguinated by parasitism! The mortality is as high as 6.0% (Sen-hai and Wei-xia, 1990). However, even infants with less dramatic anemia are at risk for long-lasting developmental disadvantage as determined by tests of mental and motor functioning at school entry (Hotez, 1989).

Despite the overwhelming global importance of human ancylostomiasis, little is known about the mechanisms of invasion by the parasite at the molecular level. In our laboratory, we have been studying the biochemistry of natural products produced by the parasite in order to invade the host and have identified and isolated a number of these macromolecules (Table 1). This chapter summarizes our progress on the major macromolecules associated with parasite invasion and outlines our plans to evaluate them as potential vaccine candidates.

HOOKWORM HYDROLASES AND THEIR ROLE IN TISSUE INVASION

We have identified two major classes of hydrolytic enzymes (hyaluronidase and metalloprotease) released by larval and adult stages of *Ancylostoma* spp. in vitro.

Hyaluronidase

The glycosaminoglycan hyaluronic acid is an abundant structural component of the connective tissue interstitial matrix. In the skin, hyaluronic acid is a major component of the epidermis, where it is a ligand for the hyaluronic acid receptor CD 44 (Green and Underhill, 1988), and the dermis, where it comprises the ground matrix. Hyaluronic acid is also a major component in the lamina propria of the gastrointestinal tract; its concentration there has been estimated to be 0.5 mg/ml of interstitial fluid (Reed et al., 1992).

Hyaluronidases, enzymes that disaggregate and depolymerize the mucopolysaccharide, were among the first virulence factors to be identified from invasive microorganisms and snake venoms (Duran-Reynals, 1933). In the early literature they were referred to as *spreading factor*, in reference to their ability to facilitate the dissemination of india ink and other diffusible dyes through the skin (Duran-Reynals, 1933). Early studies also determined that a hyaluronidase activity is present in some species of invasive intestinal protozoa, such as *Entamoeba histolytica* and *Balantidium coli* (Brading, 1953; Tempelis and Lysenko, 1957).

Despite their probable importance in skin and intestinal invasion, the study of this class of hydrolytic enzymes has lagged far behind research being carried out on proteases. No reported studies have extended the early findings of spreading factors from endoparasitic helminths, such as those released by cercariae of *Schistosoma mansoni* (Levine et al., 1948; Stirwalt and Evans, 1952) and some other helminth larvae (Lewart and Lee, 1957).

By using a sensitive assay that relies on the ability of the dye Stains-all, to bind to intact hyaluronic acid and other glycosaminoglycans, we have found that infective larvae (L3) of *Ancylostoma* spp. release a hyaluronidase in vitro (Hotez et al., 1992). Based on enzyme zymogram assays that incorporate hyaluronic acid into SDS-polyacrylamide gels, the major larval hyaluronidase migrates with an apparent M_r of 49,000 (Hotez et al., 1992).

A predominant hyaluronidase activity with an apparent M_r of 66,000 is also present in both soluble extracts and secretory products from the adult stage of *A. caninum* (Hotez et al., 1993a). Both larval and adult hookworm hyaluronidases have a pH optimum in the neutral range. There are a number of possibilities to explain why both larval and adult hookworms secrete a hyaluronidase. As mentioned above, hyaluronic acid is a major structural component of both the skin and gut lamina propria. In the former, hyaluronic acid may serve as a bridging molecule that links the keratinocytes in the epidermis, which may be broken during host entry by the parasite. Indeed, we found that *A. braziliense*, the cause of cutaneous larva migrans, has the greatest hyaluronidase activity of the larval hookworm species tested (Hotez et al., 1992). Moreover, both larval and adult hookworms of the genus *Ancylostoma* invade the intestinal mucosa, a process that would also be facilitated by hyaluronidase release.

Consistent with the notion that the hyaluronidase may function in gastrointestinal mucosal entry, we have recently determined that infective larvae of the "sushi parasite" *Anisakis simplex* also release a hyaluronidase having an M_r of 40,000 (Hotez et al., 1994). Interestingly, the pH optimum of this enzyme is approximately 4.0, consistent with the ability of this parasite to invade the mucosa of the stomach. Isolation and chemical characterization of the major hyaluronidases from these invasive nematodes are in progress.

Metalloprotease

Two proteases having apparent M_rs of 68,000 and 38,000, respectively, on SDS-gelatin gels are also present in soluble extracts of the infective larval stage of *Ancylostoma* (Hotez et al., 1990). Both protease activities are abolished in the presence of *o*-phenanthroline, suggesting that they belong to the zinc metalloprotease class. The proteases will degrade some connective tissue macromolecules in vitro, such as fibronectin, but will not degrade basement membrane components such as laminin, elastin, or native collagen. This has suggested to us that these enzymes may have a role other than tissue invasion (see the following section).

HOOKWORM ANTICOAGULANT

The adult hookworm causes intestinal blood loss by directly attaching to the intestine and digesting the plug of intestinal mucosa contained within its buccal capsule. During this process intestinal capillaries of the lamina propria are lacerated, and the extravasated blood is either ingested by the fastened worm or leaks at the site of parasite attachment. It has been postulated for nearly a century that the hookworm secretes an anticlotting agent to facilitate feeding and promote host blood loss (Loeb and Fleisher, 1910). Over the past 30 years, various investigators have identified the presence of both a major anticoagulant and an antiplatelet aggregating agent in soluble extracts of adult worms (Spellman and Nossel, 1971; Carroll et al., 1984; Eiff, 1966; Hotez and Cerami, 1983), although the process remains poorly understood at the molecular level.

Recently, we identified a low-molecular-weight soluble peptide from *A. caninum* that blocks two procoagulants in the clotting cascade: Factor Xa and the tissue factor complex (Cappello et al., 1993). Primary amino acid sequencing of the isolated anticoagulant shows that the peptide is a unique serine protease inhibitor, which is characterized by slow, tight binding inhibition of its target enzymes.

Recently, a second PCR product was obtained (using the corresponding oligonucleotides as primers in a polymerase chain reaction with cDNA from an adult *A. caninum* library), which showed extensive homology to mammalian tissue factor pathway inhibitor (mTFPI). mTFPI is a globular protein with three domains that also block the activity of Factors Xa and

VIIa/tissue factor complex (Rappaport, 1991). Thus, we believe that the hookworm anticoagulant will prove to be the first invertebrate-derived TFPI.

In addition to the anticoagulant, we have also identified a bioactivity from *A. caninum* that blocks ADP-induced platelet aggregation. Studies are underway to attempt to ascribe this activity to an apyrase, an ATP diphosphohydrolase present in the saliva of many hematophagous arthropods (Ribeiro, 1987).

MOLECULAR MECHANISMS OF HOOKWORM LARVAL ARREST AND REACTIVATION

Human ancylostomiasis, caused by the hookworm *A. duodenale*, is the most clinically significant parasitic infection affecting neonates in developing countries. The route by which neonates become infected with hookworm larvae differs considerably from the routes of infection that are traditionally published in most medical parasitology textbooks. A typical published hookworm life cycle will show that humans become infected when the third-stage hookworm larva penetrates skin. This entry is followed by larval migration through the venous circulation and lungs before entry into the intestine. In fact, this classic route of percutaneous entry is only one of several pathways of entry for an infective hookworm larva. The human hookworm *A. duodenale*, for instance, is also orally infective, and ingestion of third-stage larvae may be a predominant mode of transmission (Leiby et al., 1987). Furthermore, a large body of evidence indicates that hookworm larvae do not always continue development to the adult blood-feeding stage immediately upon host entry. Instead, infective hookworm larvae can remain in a developmentally arrested stage in the tissues for several months (Schad, 1991). One of the major conditions in which hookworm larvae will remain arrested in their development is during pregnancy. Evidence suggests that the neonatal or infantile form of ancylostomiasis results from vertical transmission of larvae that underwent reactivation from developmental growth arrest (sometimes referred to as *hypobiosis*) in the maternal tissues (Schad, 1991). When females are infected with hookworm larvae, a proportion of the infecting dose enters hypobiosis in the muscles (Little et al., 1983), where they remain developmentally arrested until parturition. In response to the hormonal fluxes that develop prior to parturition, a population of arrested larvae is mobilized to enter the mammary glands and resume development. A variety of animal and human hookworm larval species have the capacity to pass by this route to offspring. The term *amphiparatenesis* has been used to describe vertical transmission of a previously hypobiotic parasite to a neonate (Schoop, 1991).

In humans, amphiparatenesis has been described for *A. duodenale* but not for the other major hookworm species of humans, *Necator americanus*. This explains the frequent observation that neonatal and infantile hookworm infection occurs only in areas where *A. duodenale* infection is prevalent (Schad, 1990). Evidence for lactogenic transmission of *A. duodenale* infection to neonates has been found in China, India, Japan, and Africa (Schad, 1990).

Despite the importance of amphiparatenesis in the life history of hookworms and its role in neonatal infection, essentially nothing is known about its biochemical basis. A more complete understanding of the factors that induce hypobiosis, and the host signals that trigger reactivation of arrested stages, would allow the design of rational intervention strategies that take hypobiotic stages into consideration. For example, hypobiotic larvae could be manipulated either to remain arrested in the tissues indefinitely, where they are harmless to the host, or to resume development at the time of treatment, thereby making them vulnerable to an anthelminthic drug.

The third-stage infective hookworm larva of the genus *Ancylostoma* is a developmentally arrested stage and is the stage that remains hypobiotic in the host. We and others have noted that the L3 of hookworms resemble the so-called dauer (German for *enduring*) larval stage of the free-living nematode *Caenorhabditis elegans* (Riddle et al., 1981; Hotez et al., 1993). We have used this similarity as a basis for comparison and ultimately as a paradigm for the molecular elucidation of arrested development in hookworms as well as other nematodes that arrest as third-stage larvae (Hotez et al., 1993). As we have pointed out previously, when humans are infected with third-stage hookworm larvae they are infected with dauer-like larvae, which can remain in the arrested state for months before resuming development (Hotez et al., 1993). This situation would presumably occur during pregnancy.

One approach that we have taken to validate the comparison between dauer larvae of *C. elegans* and infective hookworm larvae is to try to use heterologous probes corresponding to the dauer-forming (*daf*) genes of the former. Our other major approach is to use an in vitro system for looking at the reactivation of developmentally arrested hookworm larvae (Hawdon and Schad, 1990). Observing that one of the early behaviors exhibited by arrested larvae upon reactivation is resumption of esophageal pumping and feeding, Hawdon and Schad (1991) were able to assay for reactivation by measuring the ingestion of a fluoresceinated dye when the larvae were placed in tissue culture medium under stimulatory conditions (37°C, 5% CO_2). Using this assay, they determined that certain ligands will stimulate the resumption of hookworm larval development (Hawdon and Schad, 1991; Hawdon et al., 1992), including muscarinic agonists (Tissenbaum et al., 1993). The latter is also stimulatory for the resumption of *C. elegans* dauer development (Tissenbaum et al., 1993).

Recently, we made the observation that during reactivation the stimulated third-stage hookworm larvae release a zinc metalloprotease (see Metalloprotease, above) into the tissue culture medium (Hawdon et al., 1992). Moreover, by inhibiting the metalloprotease with the zinc chelating agent o-phenanthroline, the reactivation of larvae can be inhibited; reactivation can be subsequently rescued by titration with zinc. A possible explanation for this observation is that the metalloprotease functions to degrade the electron-dense plug that occludes the buccal capsule of the parasite. The initial event in the resumption of feeding might be the breakdown of the plug by the parasite enzyme. The observation that specific inhibition of the hookworm larval zinc metalloprotease can prevent reactivation suggests that we now have a biochemical approach to examine the recovery from larval arrest. Moreover, it allows us to test our hypothesis that larval reactivation and therefore vertical transmission can be prevented in vivo by inhibiting the hookworm metalloprotease. Recently, a second larval activation factor has been cloned and sequenced.

CONCLUSION

We have identified several candidate molecules from *Ancylostoma* hookworms that appear to have importance in parasite invasion. Over 50 years ago Asa Chandler proposed that neutralizing antibodies elicited against parasite enzymes could diminish the morbidity associated with a parasitic infection (Hotez et al., 1987). We feel that we are now in a position to test this hypothesis. Studies are underway to immunize experimental animals with the hookworm-derived natural products outlined in Table 1. Our goal will be to inhibit, for example, hookworm-associated blood loss by eliciting an immune response to the anticoagulant, or tissue invasion by an immune response to the hyaluronidase and/or protease. The antiprotease response will also be evaluated for its ability to prevent the reactivation of arrested larvae in situ.

ACKNOWLEDGMENTS

We thank Drs. G.A. Schad and F.F. Richards for their advice and encouragement. P.H. is a Medical Science Scholar of the Culpeper Foundation and is further supported by NIH grant 1R29-AI32726-01Al and by a March of Dimes Clinical Research Grant. J.H. and M.C. are recipients of a USPHS National Research Service Award from the NIH.

REFERENCES

Bradin JL (1953): Studies on the production of hyaluronidase by *Entamoeba histolytica*. Exp Parasitol 2:230–235.

Cappello M, Clyne LP, McPhedran P, Hotez PJ (1993): *Ancylostoma* Factor Xa inhibitor: Partial purification and its identification as a major hookworm-derived anticoagulant in vitro. J Infect Dis 167:1474–1477.

Carroll SM, Howse DJ, Grove DI (1984): The anticoagulant effects of the hookworm,

Ancylostoma ceylanicum: Observations on human and dog blood in vitro and infected dogs in vivo. Thromb Haemost 51:222–227.

Duran-Reynals F (1993): Studies on a certain spreading factor existing in bacteria and its significance for bacterial invasiveness. J Exp Med 58:161–181.

Eiff JA (1966): Nature of an anticoagulant from the cephalic glands of *Ancylostoma caninum*. J Parasitol 52:833–843.

Green SJ, Underhill CB (1988): Hyaluronate appears to be covalently linked to the cell surface. J Cell Physiol 134:376–386.

Gupta S, Srivastava JK, Malaviya B, Katiyar JC (1992): *Ancylostoma ceylanicum* infection in female hamsters: An observation on altered reproductive function. Exp Mol Pathol 57:1–7.

Hawdon JM, Schad GA (1990): Serum-stimulated feeding in vitro by third-stage infective larvae of the canine hookworm *Ancylostoma caninum*. J Parasitol 76:394–398.

Hawdon JM, Schad GA (1991): Albumin and a dialyzable serum factor stimulate feeding in vitro by third-stage larvae of the canine hookworm *Ancylostoma caninum*. J Parasitol 77:587–591.

Hawdon JM, Volk SW, Pritchard DI, Schad GA (1992): Resumption of feeding in vitro by hookworm third-stage larvae: A comparative study. J Parasitol 78:1036–1040.

Hawdon JM, Perregaux M, Hotez PJ (1993): Protease release coincides with reactivation of developmentally arrested hookworm larvae (abstract). International *C. elegans* Meeting.

Hotez PJ, Cerami A (1983): Secretion of a proteolytic anticoagulant by *Ancylostoma* hookworms. J Exp Med 157:1594–1603.

Hotez PJ, Le Trang N, Cerami A (1987): Hookworm antigens: The potential for vaccination. Parasitol Today 3:247–249.

Hotez PJ (1989): Hookworm disease in children. Pediatr Infec Dis J 8:516–520.

Hotez PJ, Haggerty J, Hawdon J, Milstone L, Gamble HR, Schad GA, Richards FF (1990): Infective *Ancylostoma* hookworm larval metalloproteases and their possible functions in tissue invasion and ecdysis. Infect Immun 58:3883–3892.

Hotez PJ, Narasimhan S, Haggerty J, Milstone L, Bhopale V, Schad GA, Richards FF (1992): Hyaluronidase from *Ancylostoma* hookworm larvae and its function as a virulence factor in cutaneous larva migrans. Infect Immun 60:1018–1023.

Hotez P, Hawdon J, Schad GA (1993): Hookworm larval infectivity, arrest and amphiparatenesis: The *Caenorhabditis elegans* Daf-c paradigm. Parasitol Today 9:23–26.

Hotez P, Cappello M, Hawdon J, Beckers C, Sakanari J (1994): Hyaluronidases of the gastrointestinal invasive nematodes *Ancyclostoma caninum* and *Anisakis simplex*: Possible functions in the pathogenesis of human zoonoses. J Infect Dis 170 (in press).

Leiby DA, El Naggar HMS, Schad GA (1987): Thirty generations of *Ancylostoma duodenale* in laboratory-reared beagles. J Parasitol 73:844–848.

Levine MD, Garzoli RF, Kuntz RE, Killough JH (1948): On the demonstration of hyaluronidase in cercariae of *Schistosoma mansoni*. J Parasitol 34:158–161.

Lewert RM, Lee C-L (1957): Studies on the presence of muco-polysaccharidase in penetrating helminth larvae. J Infec Dis 100:287–294.

Little MD, Halsey NA, Cline BL, Katz SP (1983): *Ancylostoma* larva in a muscle fiber of a man following cutaneous larva migrans. Am J Trop Med Hyg 32:1285–1288.

Loeb L, Fleisher MS (1910): The influence of extracts of *Anchylostoma caninum* on the coagulation of the blood and on hemolysis. J Infect Dis 7:625–631.

Lozoff B, Jimenez E, Wolf AW (1991): Long-term developmental outcome of infants with iron deficiency. N. Engl J Med 325:687–694.

Rappaport SI (1991): The extrinsic pathway inhibitor: A regulator of tissue factor-dependent blood coagulation. Thromb Haemost 66:6–15.

Reed RK, Townsley MI, Laurent TC, Taylor AE (1992): Hyaluronan flux from cat intestine: changes with lymph flow. Am J Physiol 262 (Heart Circ Physiol 31): H457–H462.

Ribeiro JMC (1987): Role of saliva in blood-feeding by arthropods. Ann Rev Entomol 32:463–478.

Riddle DL, Swanson MM, Albert PS (1981): Interacting genes in nematode dauer larva formation. Nature 290:668–671.

Rusia U, Bhatia A, Kapoor S, Madan N, Nair V, Sood SK (1988): Placental morphology and histochemistry in iron deficiency anemia. Indian J Med Res 87:468.

Schad GA (1990): Hypobiosis and related phenomena in hookworm infection. In Schad GA, Warren KS, (eds): Hookworm Disease, Current Status and New Directions London: Taylor & Francis, pp. 71–88.

Schad GA (1991): Hooked on hookworms, twenty-five years of attachment. J Parasitol 77:177–186.

Sen-hai Y, Wei-xia S (1990): Hookworm infection and disease in China. In: Schad GA, Warren KS (eds); Hookworm Disease, Current Status and New Direction. London: Taylor & Francis, pp. 44–54.

Shoop WL (1991): Vertical transmission of helminths: Hypobiosis and amphiparatenesis. Parasitol Today 7:51–53.

Spellman GG, Nossel HL (1971): Anticoagulant activity of dog hookworm. Am J Physiol 23:1046–1053.

Stirwalt MA, Evans AS (1952): Demonstration of an enzymatic factor in cercariae of *Schistosoma mansoni* by the streptococcal decapsulation test. J Infect Dis 91:191–197.

Tempelis CH, Lysenko MG (1957): The production of hyaluornidase by *Balantidium coli*. Exp Parasitol 6:31–36.

Tissenbaum HA, Hawdon J, Perregaux M, Hotez P, Ruvkun G (1993): The neuropharmacology of dauer recovery in *C. elegans* and *Ancylostoma caninum* (abstract). International *C. elegans* Meeting.

Molecular Approaches to Parasitology, pages 31–42

Antigenic Variation in *Giardia lamblia*

Theodore E. Nash

Laboratory of Parasitic Diseases, National Institutes of Health, Bethesda, Maryland 20892

INTRODUCTION

Giardia lamblia is an important intestinal parasite of humans and other animals. *Giardia* infections are almost universal in many developing countries and are among the most common parasitic infections in developed regions (Mata, 1978). In the United States, contamination of drinking water has led to massive water-borne epidemics (Juranek, 1979). Infections are also frequent in day care centers (Black et al., 1977) and among travelers (Brodsky et al., 1974), homosexuals (Schemerin et al., 1978), immigrants, institutionalized persons, and backpackers (Barbour et al., 1976)—and wherever persons are exposed to fecal contamination. Disease manifestations vary from none to fulminant diarrhea and malabsorption. The reasons for variability in disease and infectivity are unknown.

Interest in *G. lamblia* has increased for a number of reasons. First, the ability to maintain *Giardia* axenically in culture and the development of animal models have allowed the study of previously unapproachable questions. Second, evidence suggests that the parasite is one of the earliest branching eukaryotes (Sogin et al., 1989); how *Giardia* differs from higher eukaryotes and the mechanisms it employs to survive can give insight into eukaryote evolution and an understanding of critical differences that may provide chemotherapeutic or immunologic targets. Third, the parasite has unique characteristics of interest. For instance, *Giardia* has two nuclei that appear similar. It has been suggested that the activities of both are the same (Kabnick and Peattie, 1990), and, if so, it is unknown how their activities are coordinated. *Giardia* also undergoes surface antigenic variation (Nash, 1990). The molecular mechanisms involved, the nature of the variant-specific surface proteins (VSP), and the biological relevance are areas of increasing interest.

THE PARASITE

G. lamblia is a heterogenous group of related organisms (Nash, 1992). Differences have been noted in restriction fragment length polymorphisms (RFLP)

(Nash et al., 1985), isoenzymes (Korman et al., 1986; Meloni et al., 1988), pulse field gel patterns (Adam et al., 1988b), antigenic makeup (Smith et al., 1982), rDNA sequences (Weiss et al., 1992), DNA sequence of homologous genes (Murtagh et al., 1992), virus susceptibility (Miller et al., 1988), excretory–secretory products (Nash and Keister, 1985), isoelectric focusing (Isaac-Renton et al., 1988), VSP expression (Nash et al., 1990b), and VSP repertoires (Nash et al., 1990b). Despite the large degree of heterogeneity, organisms fall into related groups even though the criteria for grouping include a number of apparently unrelated features such as VSP repertoires, rDNA sequence divergence, and the presence of specific genes (Nash and Mowatt, 1992a). We analyzed 29 separate isolates and were able to divide them into three major groups (Table 1) (see Nash, 1992). Others using isoenzyme analysis found three to four groups (Andrews et al., 1989). How these two methods of grouping relate to one another is not known. The ease of differentiating isolates using a number of unrelated characteristics and methods is consistent with a relatively large degree of divergence among groups.

The biological relevance of isolate diversity is unclear. However, isolates differ in infectivity to humans (Nash, 1987) and other animals, course of infection, ability to induce immunity (Aggarwal and Nash, 1987), VSP expression in vivo (Nash, 1992; Nash et al., 1990c; Gottstein et al., 1990), and often in their in vitro growth characteristics (T.E. Nash, unpublished observations).

A large number of mammalian species harbor *Giardia* morphologically identical to those found in humans. One explanation for the large degree of diversity among *Giardia* isolates in humans is that animals may serve as reservoirs for human infection. There is indirect evidence to support this idea, as beavers have been implicated in water-borne epidemics (Juranek, 1979). Although studies are limited, no specific isolate or grouping has been associated with a particular animal (Nash et al., 1985; Jonckheere et al., 1990), but this may be due to cross-infections. These could be so common among hosts that detection of a specific host–*Giardia* association would be difficult. *Giardia* isolated from one species can sometimes infect other species, but the extent of this is unknown. The DNA sequences of the triosephosphate isomerase genes of two different *Giardia* isolates differed by 19% (M.R. Mowatt, T.C. Howard, and T.E. Nash manuscript in preparation). If the rate of sequence change is similar to that of other organisms, these isolates diverged more than 100 million years ago (Creighton, 1984) and were subsequently reintroduced into humans.

ANTIGENIC VARIATION

Giardia also undergoes surface antigenic variation (Nash et al., 1988; Adam et al., 1988a; Bruderer et al., 1993). One of a family of related cysteine-rich proteins covers the entire surface and flagella of the parasite (Fig. 1) (Nash et al., 1988; Pimenta et al., 1991). The original VSP may be lost spontaneously during routine culture and replaced by another antigenically distinct VSP. The rate of appearance of new epitopes is both isolate and epitope dependent (Nash et al., 1990a). For the WB isolate, rates were about 1 in every 12 generations for two epitopes and about 1 in every 13 generations for a third epitope. Rates were significantly faster, about once in every 6.5 generations for the one epitope studied in the H7 clone of isolate GS (Nash et al., 1990a). A particular isolate can express a restricted set of epitopes or VSPs characteristic of its lineage (Nash, 1992; Nash et al., 1990b). Expression of some VSPs are mutually exclusive between *Giardia* groups, and in most instances *Giardia* unable to express a particular VSP lack the gene coding for that VSP (Nash, 1992; Nash et al., 1990b; Nash and Mowatt, 1992a).

Although the biological importance of antigenic variation is unknown, the parasite's ability to alter its surface could profoundly affect the host–parasite relationship. Assuming that VSPs are an essential target of immunity, the ability of the parasite to escape the hosts' immune responses could depend on the rates of appearance of other VSPs and the number of different VSPs trophozoites can present to the host. For instance, isolates that express and present all their VSPs to a host within a short period of time will exhaust their supply of novel epitopes. The host will be able to respond to all trophozoites, and the parasite should not be able to escape the immune response further. In contrast, a parasite able to express new epitopes, occasionally over time, may lengthen the duration of infection.

Nonimmunological selection may also be important. Clones expressing certain VSPs are variably susceptible to digestion by the intestinal enzymes trypsin and α-chymotrypsin (Nash et al., 1991). The ability of the parasite to adapt readily to its environment may expand its range of hosts or may allow the parasite's survival in different regions of the intestines. If this is true, certain VSPs will be biologically selected or favored over others in a specific host or environment.

PROPERTIES OF VSPS

VSPs are a family of unique cysteine-rich proteins (Fig. 2) (Nash, 1992; Adam et al., 1988a; Gillin et al., 1990; Mowatt et al., 1991; Nash and Mowatt, 1992b; Ey et al., 1993). The sequences of six have been published, and parts of others are known (Adam et al., 1988a; Gillin et al., 1990; Nash et al., 1990a; Nash and Mowatt, 1992b; Ey et al., 1993). Although they vary in molecular weight from 35 to 200 kD, they share a number of features (Nash, 1992). First, VSPs are cysteine rich and contain between 11% and 12% cysteine, which commonly appear as CXXC motifs. The last 33 C-terminal amino acids are well conserved and are hydro-

TABLE 1. Grouping and Summary of 29 Different Isolate Features From Humans and Animals[a]

Isolate	Group	mAb6E7	mAb5C1	mAb3F6	mAbG10	VSPA6	VSPH7	VSP1267	C4	Giardin	RNA
WB	I	+	+	+	o	E+	o	E	o	23	—
LT	I	+	+	+	o	S+	ND	E	o	23	ND
Isr	I	+	+	+	o	S+	o	E	o	23	—
Be2	I	+	+	+	o	S+	o	E	o	23	—
CAT	I	+	+	+	o	S+	o	E	o	23	—
RS	I	+	+	+	o	E+	o	E	o	23	ND
P-1	II	+	+	+	o	S+	o	E	o	23	ND
G2M	ND	+	+	+	o	S+	ND	E	o	23	—
Dan	II	+	+	+	o	E+	ND	E	o	23	ND
GP	II	+	+	+	o	S+	ND	E	o	23	—
G3M	ND	+	+	+	o	S+	ND	E	o	23	—
E2	ND	+	o	o	o	P+	ND	P	o	23	=
N	II	o	o	+	o	P+	ND	P	o	23	=
Ac	-	o	o	+	o	P+	ND	P	o	23	ND
DH	II	o	o	+	o	P+	ND	P	o	23	=
JH	II	o	o	+	o	P+	o	ND	o	23	=
Sug	ND	o	o	+	o	o	ND	?	o	ND	ND
AB	II	o	o	+	o	P+	ND	P	o	ND	=
Nat	ND	ND	ND	ND	ND	P+	ND	ND	o	ND	ND
Andi	ND	o	o	o	o	P+	ND	P	o	23	ND
Mar	ND	o	o	o	o	P+	ND	P	o	23	ND
Erin	ND	o	o	+	o	P+	ND	P	o	?	ND

G1M	ND	O	O	O	ND	O	O	+	4	≡
PM	ND	O	O	O	ND	O	O	+	4	ND
Be1	≡	O	O	O	ND	O	O	+	ND	≡
E9	ND	O	O	O	O	O	O	+	4	≡
E4	ND	O	O	O	ND	O	O	+	4	=
GS	≡	O	O	O	+	O	+	+	4	≡
CM	≡	O	O	O	+	O	+	+	4	≡

[a]The features analyzed are shown across the top of the table, and the isolates studies are shown in the first column at the far left. A full explanation of the features and isolates are reviewed by Nash (1992) and Nash and Mowatt (1992a).
+, Presence of the feature; and 0, absence of the feature; ND, not done; ?, results were not interpretable; group, the initial classification (Nash et al., 1985); columns 3–6, presence or absence of the epitopes recognized by the named monoclonal antibody (mAb); columns 7–9, hybridization to VSP-specific internal fragments or oligonucleotides to the DNA of the various isolates (Nash et al., 1990b; Nash and Mowatt, 1992a); E, a banding pattern identical to isolate WB; S, a banding pattern similar to WB showing some bands in common; P, the presence of dissimilar bands compared with WB; C4, presence or absence of GS-like C4 gene; Giardin, the size of fragment in Kb after digestion of genomic DNA with EcoR1 and probed with a β_1-giardin (Nash and Mowatt, 1992a); and RNA, common sequence changes in the 19S rDNA (Weiss et al., 1992).

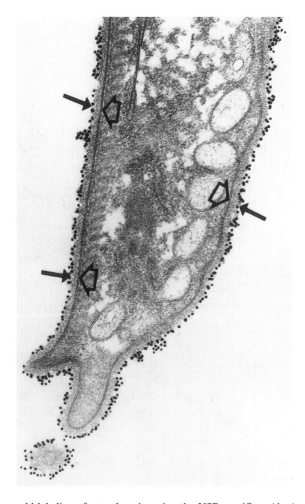

Fig. 1.   Immunogold labeling of a trophozoite using the VSP-specific mAb. An 18 nm cell coat (closed arrows) covers the entire parasite. The large arrow indicates the plasma membrane. (Reproduced from Pimenta et al., 1991, with permission of the publisher.)

phobic except for the terminal pentapeptide, which is hydrophilic. Some VSPs contain repetitive units that in part account for the varying and sometimes high molecular weights (Mowatt et al., 1994). Analysis of a family of VSPs expressing an epitope found in one repetitive unit showed that they varied mostly, but not exclusively, in the number of repeating units. The N-terminal region is hydrophobic, not well conserved among VSPs, and most likely serves as a signal peptide.

ALIGNMENT OF C-X-X-C MOTIFS OF VSPs FROM THE
3' TERMINAL MOTIFF

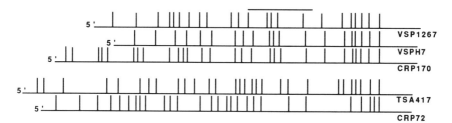

Fig. 2. Comparison of the alignments of CXXC motifs in different VSPs. The horizontal line on top of VSP1267 signifies the region of the metal-binding domain. The spacing is relatively conserved at the distal two-thirds of some of the VSPs. (Reproduced from Nash and Mowatt, 1993, with permission of the publisher.)

A unique Zn^{2+} finger-like metal-binding motif has recently been identified in five of six VSPs (Nash, 1992). The motif $CX_2CX_{5-11}CX_{2-3}CX_{10-14}$-$CX_2CHX_2CX_{7-8}CX_2CX\ CX_{15-16}CX_{2-3}CX_{7-8}CX_{2-4}CX_9CX_2C$ has similarities to two families of Zn^{2+}-binding proteins containing the LIM or Ring finger motifs (Nash and Mowatt, 1993). The one VSP lacking this motif contains a similar sequence but has a glycine substituted for the essential histidine. Two recent studies show that VSPs bind Zn^{2+} as well as other metals in a manner similar to other ZN^{2+}-finger proteins (Nash and Mowatt, 1993; Zhang et al., 1993). However, fusion proteins containing other regions of one VSP also bound Zn^{2+}, which indicates that multiple potential metal-binding sites are present (Nash and Mowatt, 1993). Most likely, these consist of $CXXCX_nCXXC$ motifs (Nash and Mowatt, 1993); intervening numbers of amino acids of 13, 19, and 20 are known metal-binding motifs, and these as well as others with varying n's most likely bind Zn^{2+} (Berg, 1990). Analysis of the metal content of *Giardia* trophozoites showed a large amount of Zn^{2+}, almost 1 mM (Nash and Mowatt, 1993), which is consistent with the presence of Zn^{2+} in VSPs. The surface location of proteins containing this type of zinc-binding motif is unique and suggests novel, but as yet undefined, mechanisms of host–parasite interactions. All LIM or Ring finger-containing proteins are intracellular and function in the regulation of transcription, and many bind DNA (Berg, 1990). If VSPs have similar roles, they must enter a cell relatively intact, find their way to the nucleus, and bind DNA or other transcription-regulating proteins, which would then result in a particular biological effect. Another possible host–parasite interaction might be preferential binding of Zn^{2+} by VSPs, thereby depriving the host of Zn^{2+}. Zn^{2+} nutritional deficiency is a frequent problem in areas where giardiasis is common (Udomkesmalee et al., 1992). Alternatively, Zn^{2+}, which is an essential cofactor of important intestinal enzymes such as carboxypeptidases, may be bound preferentially and sequestered by VSPs causing malabsorption, a known consequence of giardiasis (Mills et al., 1967).

Because the spatial arrangements of CXXC motifs was potentially important for metal binding, the spacing in various VSPs was analyzed. When aligned from the C-terminal end, the placement of CXXC motifs was well conserved for about two-thirds the length of the protein among a subset of VSPs (Fig. 2) (Nash and Mowatt, 1993). This suggests conservation of structure despite antigenic diversity among VSPs, a finding similar to VSGs (variant surface glycoproteins) in trypanosomas (Blum et al., 1993).

The benefit(s) of VSPs to *Giardia* are not known. Aley and Gillin (1994), as well as ourselves (T.E. Nash et al., unpublished observations), have been unable to detect free sulfhydryl groups in VSPs on the surface of trophozoites. They may be bound, hidden, or perhaps complexed with Zn^{2+}. VSPs may sequester potential toxic metal ions such as Cu^{2+} and thereby prevent oxygen-mediated toxicity, protect the trophozoite from intestinal proteases, or interact with intestinal mucins in some special way. The paucity of carbohydrates on the surface of *Giardia* may allow the trophozoite to associate easily with intestinal mucins.

As mentioned earlier, epitopes, and presumably VSPs, are reexpressed predictably in vitro, suggesting the presence of a repertoire of VSPs. The size of the repertoires was estimated in two ways. In one, the rate of appearance of particular VSPs in vitro was compared with the rate of appearance of all VSPs (Nash et al., 1990a). In the other, the intensity of hybridization to genomic DNA was compared using a conserved 3´ oligonucleotide and a VSP-specific oligonucleotide. Both estimates suggested relatively low numbers of VSP repertories, with a median value of between 20.5 and 184.5 VSPs for the former and between 130 and 150 VSPs for the latter. Additional calculations indicated four gene copies for each VSP, so 30–40 unique genes are estimated to be present (Nash and Mowatt, 1993).

ANTIGENIC VARIATION IN THE INFECTED HOST

Because antigenic variation was initially described as an in vitro phenomenon, it was essential to determine if antigenic variation occurred in vivo. Antigenic variation of *Giardia* occurs in infected humans (Nash et al., 1990c) and gerbils and in neonatal as well as in adult mice infections (Byrd et al., 1994). In humans experimentally infected with clone GS/H7, the initial epitope remained unchanged until day 14, after which there was a gradual loss of the original VSP and replacement with a mixture of other VSPs by day 22 (Nash et al., 1990c). Similar results were seen in mice and gerbils, the change being faster in gerbils (Gottstein et al., 1990; Aggarwal and Nash, 1988). In adult mice infected with GS/H7, VSP loss was followed by a marked diminution in the numbers of *Giardia* in the intestine at 2 weeks and apparent self-cure at 3 weeks (Byrd et al., 1994). However, small numbers of *Giardia*, undetected by microscopic assessment of intestinal contents, were detected by culture up to several months after inoculation in some mouse strains (Byrd et al., 1994). Cyclical changes in the number of parasites in the intestines of mice or gerbils have not been detected, although the nature of the VSPs expressed in the small number of surviving parasites after 3 weeks is difficult to examine and therefore has not been studied adequately. Gerbils most likely harbor small numbers of trophozoites following apparent self-cure, as in adult mice, because immunosuppression with steroids leads to recurrences (Lewis et al., 1987).

Immune mechanisms are involved in antigenic variation in vivo. Adult (Byrd et al., 1994) and neonatal SCID mice (Gottstein and Nash, 1991) do not undergo the usual decrease in the numbers of intestinal trophozoites seen in immunocompetent mice and maintain the original expressed epitope. In contrast, neonatal nude mice are similar to immunocompetent mice and replace the initially expressed epitope (Gottstein and Nash, 1991). Since nude mice have a competent humoral system, but lack a cellular immune system, humoral responses appear to be required for loss of the original epitope.

MOLECULAR MECHANISMS

Mechanisms involved in antigenic variation are unknown. Analysis of the genes of VSPs expressed in parent and progeny do not reveal likely rearrangements. The ability of isolates to reexpress epitopes and most likely VSPs predictably suggests the presence of a set of relatively stable VSPs, one of which is somehow selected for expression. Stable transcripts of specific VSP genes are found in organisms expressing that VSP and are absent from organisms not expressing that particular VSP (Adam et al., 1988b; Mowatt et al., 1991). Expression-linked copies have not been identified. Transcriptional control mechanisms seem likely. Comparison of cDNA and genomic DNA of one VSP, vsp1267, has not revealed differences within the genes (Mowatt et al., 1991). In the genome, two identical genes are arranged tail to tail (Mowatt et al., 1991). Two specific genes have also been seen for another VSP, vspH7, but the genomic arrangement apparently differs from that mentioned above (T.E. Nash and M.R. Mowatt, unpublished observations).

Giardia is a unique parasite that on the one hand makes it inherently interesting and, on the other, difficult to understand. It is a parasite whose importance and interest are only now becoming recognized.

REFERENCES

Adam RD, Aggarwal A, Lal AA, De la Cruz VF, McCutchan T, Nash TH (1988a): Antigenic variation of a cysteine-rich protein in *Giardia lamblia*. J Exp Med 167:109–118.

Adam RD, Nash TE, Wellems TE (1988b): The *Giardia lamblia* trophozoite contains sets of closely related chromosomes. Nucleic Acids Res 16:4555–4567.

Aggarwal A, Nash TE (1987): Comparison of two antigenically distinct *Giardia lamblia* isolates in gerbils. Am J Trop Med Hyg 36:325–332.

Aggarwal A, Nash TE (1988): Antigenic variation of *Giardia lamblia* in vivo. Infect Immun 56:1420–1423.

Aley SB, Gillin FD (1993): Post-translational processing and status of exposed cysteine residues in TSA 417, a variable surface antigen. Exp Parasitol 77:295–305.

Andrews RH, Adams M, Boreham PFL, Mayrhofer G, Meloni BP (1989): *Giardia intestinalis*: Electrophoretic evidence for a species complex. Int J Parasitol 19:183–190.

Barbour A, Nichols CR, Fukushima T (1976): An outbreak of giardiasis in a group of campers. Am J Trop Med Hyg 25:384–389.

Berg JM (1990): Zinc fingers and other metal-binding domains. J Biol Chem 265:6513–6516.

Black RE, Dykes AC, Sinclair SP, Wells JG (1977): Giardiasis in day-care centers: Evidence of person-to-person transmission. Pediatrics 360:486–491.

Blum ML, Down JA, Gurnett AM, Carrington M, Turner MJ, Wiley DC (1993): A structural motif in the variant surface glycoproteins of *Trypanosoma brucei*. Nature 362:603.

Brodsky RE, Spencer HC, Schultz MG (1974): Giardiasis in American travelers to the Soviet Union. J Infect Dis 130:319–323.

Bruderer T, Papanastasiou P, Castro R, Kohler P (1993): Variant cysteine-rich surface proteins of *Giardia* isolates from human and animal sources. Infect Immun 61:2937–2944.

Byrd LG, Conrad JT, Nash TE (1994): *Giardia lamblia* infections in adult mice. Infect Immun 62:3583–3585.

Creighton TE (1984): Proteins: Structures and Molecular Principles. New York: W.H. Freeman and Co.

Ey PL, Khanna K, Manning PA, Mayrhofer G (1993): A gene encoding a 69-kilodalton major surface protein of *Giardia intestinalis* trophozoites. Mol Biochem Parasitol 58:247–258.

Gillin FD, Hagblom P, Harwood J, Aley SB, Reiner DS, McCaffery M, So M, Guiney DG (1990): Isolation and expression of the gene for a major surface protein of *Giardia lamblia*. Proc Natl Acad Sci USA 87:4463–4467.

Gottstein B, Harriman GR, Conrad JT, Nash TE (1990): Antigenic variation in *Giardia lamblia*: Cellular and humoral immune response in a mouse model. Parasite Immunol 12:659–673.

Gottstein B, Nash TE (1991): Antigenic variation in *Giardia lamblia*: Infection of congenitally athymic nude and *scid* mice. Parasite Immunol 12:659–673.

Gottstein B, Nash TE (1991): Antigenic variation in *Giardia lamblia*: Infection of congenitally athymic nude and *scid* mice. Parasite Immunol 13:649–659.

Isaac-Renton JL, Byrne SK, Prameya R (1988): Isoelectric focusing of ten strains of *Giardia duodenalis*. 74:1054–1056.

Jonckheere JFD, Majewska AC, Kasprzak W (1990): *Giardia* isolates from primates and rodents display the same molecular polymorphism as human isolates. Mol Biochem Parasitol 39:23–28.

Juranek D (1979): Waterborne giardiasis. In Jukubowski W, Hoff JC (eds): Waterborne Transmission of Giardiasis. Washington, DC: U.S. Environmental Protection Agency, pp 150–163.

Kabnick KS, Peattie DA (1990): In situ analyses reveal that the two nuclei of *Giardia lamblia* are equivalent. J Cell Sci 95:353–360.

Korman SEH, LeBlancq SM, Spira DT, El On J, Reifen RM, Deckelbaum RJ (1986): *Giardia lamblia*: Identification of different strains from man. Z Parasitenkd 72:173–180.

Lewis PD Jr, Belosevic M, Faubert GM, Curthoys L, MacLean JD (1987): Cortisone-induced recrudescence of *Giardia lamblia* infections in gerbils. Am J Trop Med Hyg 36:33–40.

Mata LJ (1978): The Children of Santa María Cauqué: A Prospective Field Study of Health and Growth. Cambridge, MA: MIT Press.

Meloni BP, Lymbery AJ, Thompson RCA (1988): Isoenzyme electrophoresis of 30 isolates of *Giardia* from humans and felines. Am J Trop Med Hyg 38:65–73.

Miller RL, Wang AL, Wang CC (1988): Identification of *Giardia lamblia* isolates susceptible and resistant to infection by the double-stranded RNA virus. Exp Parasitol 66:118–123.

Mills CF, Quarterman J, Williams RB, Dalgarno AC (1967): The effects of zinc deficiency in pancreatic carboxypeptidase activity and protein digestion and absorption in the rat. Biochem J 102:712–718.

Mowatt MR, Nguyen BY, Conrad JT, Adam RD, Nash TE (1994): Size heterogeneity among antigenically related *Giardia lamblia* variant-specific surface proteins is due to differences in tandem repeat copy number. Infect Immun 62:1213–1218.

Mowatt MR, Aggarwal A, Nash TE (1991): Carboxyl-terminal sequence conservation among variant-specific surface proteins of *Giardia lamblia*.Mol Biochem Parasitol 49:215–228.

Murtagh JJ Jr, Mowatt MR, Chii-Ming L, Lee FJS, Mishima K, Nash TE, Moss J, Vaughan M (1992): Guanine nucleotide-binding proteins in the intestinal parasite *Giardia lamblia*. J Biol Chem 267:9654–9662.

Nash T (1992): Surface antigen variability and variation in *Giardia lamblia*. Parasitol Today 8:229–234.

Nash TE, Keister DB (1985): Differences in excretory–secretory products and surface antigens among 19 isolates of *Giardia*. J Infect Dis 152:1166–1171.

Nash TE, McCutchan T, Keister D, Dame JB, Conrad JD, Gillin FD (1985): Restriction-endonuclease analysis of DNA from 15 *Giardia* isolates obtained from humans and animals. J Infect Dis 152:64–73.

Nash TE, Herrington DA, Losonsky GA, Levine MM (1987): Experimental human infections with *Giardia lamblia*. J Infect Dis 146:974–984.

Nash TE, Aggarwal A, Adam RD, Conrad JT, Merritt JW Jr (1988): Antigenic variation in *Giardia lamblia*. J Immunol 141:636–641.

Nash TE, Banks SM, Alling DW, Merritt JW Jr, Conrad JT (1990a): Frequency of variant antigens in *Giardia lamblia*. Exp Parasitol 71:415–421.

Nash TE, Conrad JT, Merritt JW Jr (1990b): Variant specific epitopes of *Giardia lamblia*. Mol Biochem Parasitol 42:125–132.

Nash TE, Herrington DA, Levine MM, Conrad JT, Merritt JW Jr (1990c): Antigenic variation of *Giardia lamblia* in experimental human infections. J Immunol 144:4362–4369.

Nash TE, Merritt JW Jr, Conrad JT (1991): Isolate and epitope variability in susceptibility of *Giardia lamblia* to intestinal proteases. Infect Immun 59:1334–1340.

Nash TE, Mowatt MR (1992a): Identification and characterization of a *Giardia lamblia* group-specific gene. Exp Parasitol 75:369–378.

Nash TE, Mowatt MR (1992b): Characterization of a *Giardia lamblia* variant-specific surface protein (VSP) gene from isolate GS/M and estimation of the VSP gene repertoire size. Mol Biochem Parasitol 51:219–228.

Nash TE, Mowatt MR (1993): Variant-specific surface proteins of *Giardia lamblia* are zinc-binding proteins. Proc Natl Acad Sci USA 90:5489–5493.

Pimenta PFP, da Silva PP, Nash T (1991): Variant surface antigens of *Giardia lamblia* are associated with the presence of a thick cell coat: Thin section and label fracture immunocytochemistry survey. Infect Immun 59:3989–3996.

Schemerin MJ, Jones C, Klein H (1978): Giardiasis: Association with homosexuality. Ann Intern Med 88:801–803.

Smith PD, Gillin FD, Kaushal NA, Nash TE (1982): Antigenic analysis of *Giardia lamblia* from Afghanistan, Puerto Rico, Ecuador, and Oregon. Infect Immun 36:714–719.

Sogin ML, Gunderson JH, Elwood HJ, Alonso RA, Peattie DA (1989): Phylogenetic meaning of the kingdom concept: An unusual ribosomal RNA from *Giardia lamblia*. Science 243:75–77.

Udomkesmalee E, Dhanamitta S, Sirisinha S, Charoenkiatkul S, Kramer TR, Smith JC Jr (1992): Effect of vitamin A and zinc supplementation on the nutriture of children in northeast Thailand. Am J Clin Nutr 56:50–57.

Weiss JB, van Keulen H, Nash TE (1992): Classification of subgroups of *Giardia lamblia* based upon ribosomal RNA gene sequence using the polymerase chain reaction. Mol Biochem Parasitol 54:73–86.

Zhang Y-Y, Aley SB, Stanley SL Jr, Gillin FD (1993): Cysteine-dependent zinc binding by membrane proteins of *Giardia lamblia*. Infect Immun 61:520–524.

Molecular Approaches to Parasitology, pages 43–56
© 1995 Wiley-Liss, Inc.

Lymphoproliferation Caused by *Theileria parva* and *Theileria annulata*

Mark Carrington, Basil Allsopp, Howard Baylis, Ndavi-Muia Malu, Yael Shochat, and Sarjit Sohal

Department of Biochemistry, Cambridge University, Cambridge CB2 1QW, England

INTRODUCTION

The objective of this chapter is to discuss some of the results obtained in investigating the biology of *Theileria parva* and *Theileria annulata*. The one thing that everyone remembers about these species of *Theileria* is the unique parasite-induced clonal proliferation of host lymphocytes, and, after an introduction to the parasite, the chapter focuses on this. The discussion is presented from a personal perspective and is not meant in any way to be a systematic review; the ideas presented should be treated as hypotheses that can hopefully be tested. The potential for using *Theileria* as a model intracellular parasite will perhaps become apparent in this chapter.

DISEASE AND LIFE CYCLE

In many protozoal parasitic diseases it is probable that the parasite persists at very low levels in a subset of a population and only becomes debilitating or pathogenic under unusual circumstances. A more patent infection can arise through immune suppression of the host, acquisition of virulence by the parasite, or transmission to a new, previously unexposed, host population or species. East Coast fever (ECF) of domestic cattle is a prime example of the last. *T. parva,* the causal agent of ECF, is a parasite of the wild buffalo in sub-Saharan Africa, and in most circumstances it persists in the wild host without any severely debilitating effects. When transmitted to newly imported cattle, through a feeding tick, the parasite proliferates very rapidly, causing ECF that has a greater than 90% incidence of mortality unless treated. ECF is second only to trypanosomiasis in economic importance for cattle rearing in East Africa. The same effect can be seen with a second species, *Theileria annulata,* which causes tropical theileriosis in cattle and domestic buffalo in North Africa, the whole of southern Asia, and the extreme south of Europe. In Asia the mortality rate for European cattle (*Bos taurus*) is roughly 50%, 10 times higher than the indigenous Boran cattle (*Bos indicus*). In both diseases imported cattle become less susceptible to the disease after a few generations and tend to carry a persistent low-level infection, but still do not have the tolerance of indigenous breeds.

The genus *Theileria* is a member of the phylum Apicomplexa, along with other well known parasitic genera such as *Plasmodium, Eimeria,* and *Babesia.* The life cycle starts when an infected tick takes a blood meal, resulting in the introduction of sporozoites into the host bloodstream. The vector for *T. parva* is usually *Rhipicephalus appendiculatus* and for *T. annulata* is *Hyalomma* sp. The sporozoite is nonmotile, and the initial binding to the lymphocyte occurs through a passive process, though the subsequent entry into the cell is active. Once inside the cell the sporozoite discharges its secretory organelles; the surrounding membrane of host origin is dissipated so that the parasite is free in the host cytoplasm but becomes bound to the host microtubule array (Shaw et al., 1991).

The specificity of invasion of host cell types appears to be at the level of the initial recognition, as the sporozoite does not bind to macrophages, granulocytes, or fibroblasts (Shaw et al., 1991). The ligand–receptor interaction involved in the recognition remains a mystery; however, the antigens recognized by monoclonal antibodies (mAbs) that prevent sporozoite host binding are known: the MHC class I molecules and β_2-microglobulin on the host cell surface (Shaw et al., 1991) and transmission-blocking mAbs that recognize a polypeptide on *T. annulata* sporozoites that contains peptide repeats similar to those found in elastin (Hall et al., 1992). This finding raised hopes that the polypeptide was a ligand for the elastin receptor, but a direct demonstration of a ligand–receptor interaction involving the elastin repeats has not been forthcoming and a homologous polypeptide from *T. parva* recognized by a transmission-blocking mAb lacks the repeats (Nene et al., 1992). At first it can seem strange that mAbs that block recognition do not actually bind the receptor or ligand but transmission can be blocked in other ways and there are precedents from *Plasmodium* (discussed by Shaw et al., 1991). Thus, although the ligand–receptor pair(s) have yet to be characterized, the binding of the sporozoite defines which cells are invaded. In vitro B or T cells, but not monocytes, can be infected by *T. parva,* although in vivo most parasitized cells recovered from an animal are of T-cell origin. *T. annulata* infects B cells and monocytes, but not T cells, and both are recovered from infected animals (Spooner et al., 1989).

Once a lymphocyte is infected a most remarkable change occurs: the sporozoite starts growing and forms a syncytial macroschizont with between 10 and 20 nuclei, and then the host lymphocyte undergoes clonal expansion.

Thus, as the host cell grows and divides the parasite grows and divides with it (Hulliger et al., 1964). At a later stage the number of nuclei in the schizont greatly increases to more than 100; each nucleus is then cellularized to form individual merozoites (merogony). These are released on host cell rupture to invade erythrocytes in which they differentiate to piroplasms. Piroplasms have been observed undergoing binary fission, but this occurs to a very limited extent and there are rarely more than three or four piroplasma per erythrocyte. ECF is characterized by an uncontrolled lymphoproliferation, whereas anemia caused by a high piroplasm burden is more typical of tropical theileriosis.

On ingestion by a tick, the piroplasm is released and differentiates to form gametes, the formation of microgametes involving further nuclear division and subsequent cellularization (gamogony). A microgamete and macrogamete fuse to form a zygote, which enters a gut epithelial cell and emerges, during a molt, into the hemolymph as a kinete. The kinete migrates and enters an E cell of a type III acinus in the salivary gland. It undergoes nuclear division and subsequent cellularization to produce large numbers of sporozoites (sporogony), which are released into the saliva.

The clonal expansion of infected lymphocytes grabs the attention of most people, especially as when transferred to culture the lymphocytes are immortalized. This fascinating ability of the parasite tends to overshadow a second unusual feature: The *Theileria* cell undergoes an increase in cell number by a range of mechanisms—by binary fission as a piroplasm in erythrocytes, and by cell division of a syncytium as a schizont and merogony in bovine lymphocytes, gamogony in the tick gut, and sporogony in a tick salivary gland cell. In the first two mechanisms cell division follows nuclear division but in merogony, gamogeny, or sporogony growth by occurs by several rounds of nuclear division that occur without conventional cell division and are followed by cellularization of the individual nuclei. The linkage between nuclear division and cell division is developmentally regulated. For example, a sporozoite with a single nucleus becomes a syncytial macroschizont with 10–20 nuclei, then, after a period in which nuclear division is linked to schizont division, a change occurs so that the nuclear number increases to more than 100 followed by the cellularization of each nucleus to form merozoites (merogony).

It has been possible to investigate the merogony both in vitro and in vivo. In selected *T. annulata*–infected cell lines it is possible to induce merogony by elevating the temperature to 41°C for more than 2 days (up to 2 days the effect of the elevated temperature being reversible), with the percentage of cells staining positive with a merozoite-specific mAb increasing up to 7 days at 41°C (Shiels et al., 1992). The increase in the number of nuclei in the schizont is accompanied by an increase in size; although difficult to measure, it is probable that the number of nuclei per unit volume of cytoplasm remains constant. If it is assumed that nuclear division in the parasite is triggered when the cytoplasmic volume per nucleus exceeds a certain value, then blocking host cell cycling would allow continued growth of the parasite with an automatic increase in nuclear number. Schizont division would also have to be blocked, but this would occur if it were dependent on host cell cycling. There is some circumstantial evidence for this model, as specific disruption of host microtubules with colchicine, blocking host cell cycling, leads to an increased number of parasite nuclei (to a mean of 115 from 18 after 48 hours) (Hulliger et al., 1964).

How could the parasite achieve this? There are two possibilities: either by producing a specific factor that inhibits host cell events or by no longer providing the stimulation for lymphoproliferation provided previously. The latter is possibly favored as the simpler model. If this is indeed what is happening, then the switch to merogony in culture may be the best approach to identifying the factor(s) causing the previous lymphoproliferation.

Once merogony has begun, the syncytium is left with the problem of how to pack each of the 100 or more nuclei in its own bit of cytoplasm with the complete set of organelles. The process starts with the migration of the nuclei to the periphery of the cytoplasm so that part of the nuclear envelope becomes associated with the cell membrane. The rhoptries originate from the smooth endoplasmic reticulum, move toward the nuclei, and often lie adjacent to the spindle pole body embedded in the nuclear membrane. The mitochondria also become associated with the nucleus on the side opposite the cell membrane. The nucleus "collects" the necessary organelles at the syncytial surface and then buds off to form an individual merozoite (Figs. 9, 10 in Shaw and Tilney (1992).

CLONAL EXPANSION OF INFECTED LYMPHOCYTES

Clonal expansion¯of infected lymphocytes is the unique feature of the *Theileria* life cycle and has attracted much interest, as both the behavior of lymphocytes and control of cell cycle are beginning to be understood. We first present the data and then discuss whether a coherent picture emerges.

An attractive model for the proliferation of T cells infected with *T. parva* was an autocrine cycle in which the cells secreted interleukin-2 (IL-2), which stimulated them to divide and produce more IL-2, and so on (Dobbelaere et al., 1988a). In a wonderfully thorough set of papers (Heussler et al., 1992, and references therein) it has been shown that most but not all *Theileria*-infected cell lines constitutively express IL-2 mRNA, albeit at very low levels in some lines, and that most also express the high-affinity IL-2 receptor. Exogenous IL-2 increases the rate of growth, indicating that the signal transduction pathway is present. Cyclosporin A and anti-IL-2 antibody both reduced the growth rate by up to 50%, the exact amount depending on the cell line used, but neither stopped the growth of the cells as might be expected if the proliferation was solely IL-2 dependent.

It has been found that *T. parva* infected T-cell lines in culture secrete interferon-γ (IFN-γ) to high levels: 4–20 ng/ml, one to five times the levels secreted by concanavalin A blasts (Malu, 1992). When a high-affinity IgM mAb that inactivates IFN-γ in a viral killing assay was used to deplete the secreted IFN-γ the cells stopped growing; however, the neutralization had no effect on growth of an infected B-cell line that also secreted IFN-γ (Malu, 1992). The secretion of IFN-γ could also be detected in the serum of an infected animal: elevated serum IFN-γ appeared 10 days after initiating the infection and coincided with the appearance of patently infected cells in the efferent lymph (Malu, 1992).

Any line of *Theileria*-infected cells does not grow if seeded at less than a certain density. This can overcome by adding IL-2 in most cases and by irradiated or glutaraldehyde-fixed cells in all cases. The latter reflects a requirement for cell–cell contact for growth (Dobbelaere et al., 1988b).

Once infected with *T. parva* or *T. annulata,* lymphocytes do not retain their preinfection phenotype and do not go down any fixed pathway of differentiation. The majority of B cells infected with *T. parva* or *T. annulata* cease expression of surface immunoglobulin; the response of T cells to *T. parva* infection is even more variable. It is possible to detect BoCD4$^-$BoCD8$^-$, BoCD4$^+$BoCD8$^-$, BoCD4$^-$BoCD8$^+$, and BoCD4$^+$BoCD8$^+$ cells in a clonally derived population after a period in culture. Other T-cell–derived lines are much more stable and present a majority of cells with a single phenotype (Dobbelaere et al., 1990).

To try and synthesize these events into a unified scheme it is necessary to make two assumptions. 1) There is a single mechanism used by both *T. parva* and *T. annulata* to stimulate host cell cycling regardless of the starting phenotype of that cell. This mechanism involves the activation at a point in a common signal transduction pathway in the host cell, as yet unknown, resulting in the onset of cell division. 2) As part of the immune system, lymphocytes have, present or readily inducible, at least one other signal transduction pathway to stimulate cell division and one to end cell division, and these pathways may vary for different preinfection lymphocyte types.

It could then be proposed that the observed stimulation of growth in many *T. parva*–infected lines by exogenously added IL-2 is due to the (hyper)activation of a second growth-stimulatory pathway so that two pathways are operating at once—the pathway stimulated by the parasite and the IL-2 pathway. The reduction in growth rate caused by treatment with cyclosporine or anti-IL-2 could be due to the inhibition of one of these pathways. Different *Theileria*-infected cell lines are stimulated to different extents by IL-2 (Dobbelaere et al., 1990). This could be due to the amount of endogenous IL-2, IL-2 receptor, and transduction components synthesized per cell and to the percentage of cells in the culture synthesizing them.

The observation that growth is inhibited either by the depletion of secreted IFN-γ with a mAb or by reducing cell–cell contact could be explained if these events trigger a growth-inhibitory pathway and this pathway overrides the parasite stimulatory growth pathway. The T-cell–derived lines that stop dividing on IFN-γ depletion have the inhibitory pathway; the B-cell–derived line, which is unaffected by IFN-γ-depletion, does not have all the components of the pathway.

As it appears that infected cells do not follow a single developmental pathway, infected cells in vivo and especially in culture are in competition with one another, and those with a more rapid rate of division will predominate. This may be reflected in the observation that most T cells infected with *T. parva* use an IL-2 autocrine loop that results in a decreased cell cycle time, and thus such cells predominate in the culture (and in vivo?). There are some predictions possible from this model. The phenotypes present in a culture derived directly from an infected animal may decrease over a period of time as the more rapidly dividing cells predominate. This, of course, would only be applicable to cells that develop a reasonably stable phenotype.

It should be possible to order a hierarchy of pathways. For example, IL-2 can override the block caused by cell dilution, but could it also overcome the block caused by IFN-γ depletion? In essence, the model proposes that *Theileria*-infected cells are still susceptible to some of the controls exerted on normal lymphocytes, but the stimulatory and inhibitory pathways present depend on the initial cell type infected and to a degree on chance epigenetic changes and selection in vivo and during culture.

A more direct approach to finding components of signal transduction pathways stimulated in *Theileria*-infected cell lines has been taken in the demonstration that six *T. parva*– and one *T. annulata*–infected lines have elevated levels of casein kinase II (ole-MoiYoi et al., 1993). It is difficult to know whether this is a result or a cause of the parasite-induced proliferation; however, as signal transduction pathways in mammalian cells are currently being elucidated, it defines one such pathway operating in *Theileria*-infected cells. When this observation is coupled with the finding that the *T. parva* casein kinase II α-subunit gene encodes a polypeptide with a signal sequence (ole-MoiYoi et al., 1992), then the exciting possibility is that the elevated levels are due to enzyme secreted from the parasite but the elevated levels of casein kinase II are inhibited by antiserum raised against the bovine enzyme (ole-MoiYoi et al., 1993). In the context of the model proposed for the role of cytokines in the parasite-induced lymphoproliferation, it would be interesting to know the effects of cyclosporine on casein kinase II activity.

The approaches described above all suffer from the difficulty of having to separate the cause of host cell proliferation from the effects resulting from that proliferation. It is difficult to think of any experiments that address the problem directly. One approach is to take one step back in the hope of later being able to take two steps forward and look at communication between an intracellular parasite and host cell at a more general level. *Theileria*-infected lymphocytes provide an excellent model system for investigating this, as 99% of the cells in any culture are infected and the parasite gives the host cell an obvious phenotype—proliferation. In addition, the infected cells are readily maintained in culture, each liter of culture yielding more than 1×10^9 growing infected cells. The most likely molecule used to communicate between host and parasite is a polypeptide; the interaction can occur in either the host cell, which includes the parasite cell surface, as the schizont lies free in the host cytoplasm or within the *Theileria* cell.

How can polypeptides that are exported from or imported into the parasite be identified? When the infected cells are radiolabeled with [^{35}S]methionine the vast majority (95%) of the radiolabel is incorporated into polypeptides of host origin, as would be expected (the parasite is 1/4 the diameter of the host cell and thus 1/64 the volume). However, schizonts can be purified from the host cells after radiolabeling (Sugimoto et al., 1988). On electrophoretic analysis this provides a pattern of the polypeptides present in, or on the surface of, the schizont, whether of parasite or host origin. It is possible to visualize the polypeptides synthesized in the parasite by pretreating the cells with the plant toxin ricin before labeling with [^{35}S]methionine. Ricin is an AB dimer, the A and B subunits are disulfide linked, and the B subunit binds to a cell surface; its function is to introduce the A subunit into the cell cytoplasm, which then catalytically inactivates the ribosomes. In this process the two subunits become separated. Because the two subunits separate, the toxin can only cross one membrane so that the ribosomes in the host cell compartment are inactivated but those in the parasite are not. Mitochondrial protein synthesis can be eliminated with chloramphenicol. Thus on electrophoretic analysis of polypeptides radiolabeled after ricin pretreatment, and in the presence of chloramphenicol, a pattern representing protein synthesis by the parasite is obtained whatever the final cellular location of the polypeptides. A comparison of the patterns obtained from purified schizonts and ricin-treated cells allows the identification of imported and exported polypeptides (Fig. 1). When this theory is put into practice, apparently imported and exported polypeptides can be seen even with one-dimensional electrophoretic analysis (Fig. 2). This assay provides a basis for the identification of imported and exported polypeptides through cloning and analysis of cDNA. In addition, it provides

On [35S]-methionine pulse labelling:

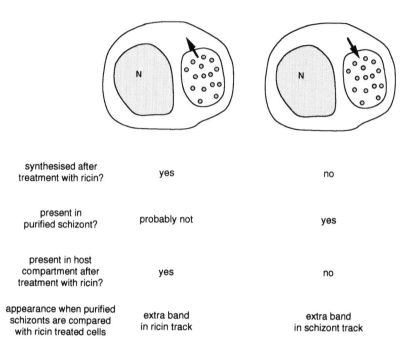

synthesised after treatment with ricin?	yes	no
present in purified schizont?	probably not	yes
present in host compartment after treatment with ricin?	yes	no
appearance when purified schizonts are compared with ricin treated cells	extra band in ricin track	extra band in schizont track

Fig. 1. How to identify polypeptides exported from and imported into an intracellular schizont, with *T. parva* as an example.

a method for the more detailed targeting of polypeptides for further analysis. Examples include the following. 1) The cellular localization of proteins exported from the parasite can be analyzed by [35S]methionine labeling after pretreatment with ricin followed by the fractionation of the host cell. In the case of *Theileria*-infected cells it would be interesting to know if any exported polypeptides were targeted to the host cell nucleus. 2) Interactions on the surface of the schizont could be visualized by comparing the electrophoretic patterns of [35S]methionine-radiolabeled polypeptides in membranes isolated from purified schizonts labeled with and without ricin pretreatment; host proteins attached to the surface of the schizont would be unlabeled in the ricin-pretreated preparation.

These methods are generally applicable to most intracellular parasites, although the analysis of the location of exported proteins may be more complicated when the parasite lies within a vacuole. In addition to the work on *T.*

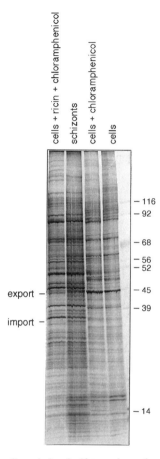

Fig. 2.   Autoradiograph of a sodium dodecylsulfate–polyacrylamide gel showing a comparison of polypeptides found in purified schizonts and those synthesized after pretreatment of the *T. parva*–infected cells with ricin. Cells + Ricin + chloramphenicol: Cells were pretreated with ricin prior to labeling with [^{35}S]methionine in the presence of chloramphenicol; the sample contains total protein from infected lymphocytes. Schizonts: Infected cells were labeled with [^{35}S]methionine, and then schizonts were purified, so the sample contains total schizont protein. Cells (+ chloramphenicol): Infected lymphocytes were labeled with [^{35}S]-methionine with or without chloramphenicol. The sample contains total protein from the infected lymphocytes. The clearest candidate imported and exported polypeptides are indicated. Equal counts were loaded for each sample; pretreatment with ricin reduces the incorporation by 90%–95%.

parva, it has been used to visualize the protein synthesis by *Eimeria tenella* in avian epithelial cells (A. Gurnett and M. Carrington, unpublished results). In this case, sporozoites are used to infect a layer of cells. Only 5% of the cells subsequently support development of the parasite through to merozoites. Pretreatment with ricin prior to metabolic labeling with [^{35}S]methionine results in all of the host protein synthesis being eliminated and, after electrophoretic analysis, a clear pattern of parasite protein synthesis. This has allowed the visualization of the changes in protein synthesis in a developmental series from sporozoite to merozoite. The relative ease of working with *Theileria*-infected cells has allowed the development of a method that can be applied to a range of parasites and pathogens from *Trypanosoma cruzi* and *Leishmania* to *Listeria.*

Although the method above provides an assay for the isolation of cDNAs encoding imported and exported polypeptides, assigning a function to these is dependent on the possibility of homology to known polypeptides but also on an accurate description of the phenotype of the infected cell. Thus, for example, in *Theileria*-infected cells, the interdependency of events in the host and parasite cell cycles have to be described. The use of colchicine described above shows that nuclear division in the parasite is not dependent on host nuclear division and that parasite cell division is probably dependent on the integrity of the host microtubule array. The experiments to study the events of the cell cycle and their interdependency are relatively simple. For example, the observation that a histogram of the number of nuclei per schizont yields a distribution with a single peak indicates that the nuclear division of the parasite occurs very late in the host cell cycle (Irvin et al., 1982). The basic cell cycle of the host and parasite was described some time ago based on [^{3}H]thymidine incorporation (Fig. 3) (Irvin et al., 1982). The essential features are that the host cell has a typical cycle for a proliferating cell and the parasite stays in G1 for most of the cycle and goes into S phase and mitosis as the host cell enters mitosis. Thus the host and parasite S phases are out of synchrony but nuclear division and cell division occur in synchrony. This ensures that the parasite is divided into each daughter cell (Shaw et al., 1991; Irvin et al., 1982).

Since this original description of the cycle, reagents have been developed that allow a more precise description of the phenotype of the infected cell. A cDNA encoding a *T. parva* schizont surface protein has been expressed and used to raise an antiserum that can help to visualize the schizont via immunofluorescence microscopy (Baylis et al., 1993). If this is used in conjunction with a stain to visualize DNA, then the morphology of the schizont during host cell mitosis can be determined. The heterogeneity of *Theileria*-infected cells for cell surface markers has been discussed above. The results from visualizing the schizont show that there is also a heterogeneity in the size of the schizont that varies by much more than can be accounted for by growth during the cell cycle and probably is caused by unequal cell division of the parasite. A result of this heterogeneity is that in some experiments it is a mistake to treat a culture as a uniform population and it is necessary to design experiments in which the response of individual cells is measured, not the response of the culture as a whole. Figure 4 shows a number of micrographs that illustrate cells in which the host and/or the schizont is going through cell division. Figure 4a,b shows events previously described (Shaw et al., 1991). The schizont is aligned with the spindle by metaphase, and the two cells go through cell division together. In many of such metaphase cells the schizont has two protrusions, possibly pointing toward the host centrioles although this has to be confirmed by immunofluorescence. Cells in which the schizont is undergoing, or has undergone, cell division out of synchrony with the host cell are also readily visible. Illustrated also in Figure 4 are host cells in metaphase, telophase, and interphase in which the two daughter schizont cells are still joined by a thin thread of cytoplasm. The conclusion is that schizont division can occur independently of host cell division, most frequently in the earlier stages of mitosis but sometimes in interphase. A prediction from this is that it should be possible to find interphase cells with two schizonts, as shown in Figure 4f. There is an increasing frequency of schizont division from interphase (late G2?) through to host cell division. It

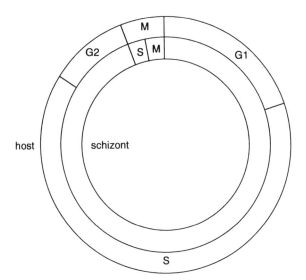

Fig. 3.   The cell cycles of the host lymphocyte and schizont, based on a 20 hour cycle. (Reproduced from Irvin et al., 1982, with permission of the publisher.)

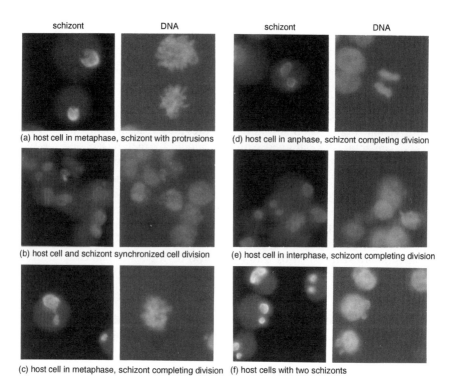

Fig. 4. Dividing schizonts visualized with an antiserum raised against a schizont surface polypeptide and a fluorescein-tagged second antibody. DNA was visualized using Hoechst 33342. Cells were fixed in suspension, stained, and mounted in wells and thus have not been compressed against the slide. The different intensities of staining of the schizont is the result of two different dilutions of antiserum being used. The cells are 12–15 μm diameter on average. For bovine cells, 2n = 60; and most of the chromosomes have their centromere near a telomere so the metaphase plates look very jumbled. It is possible that the top cell in a is 4n. **a,b:** The schizont is aligned with the spindle by metaphase, and the two cells go through cell division together. **c:** Metaphase. **d:** Telophase. **e:** Interphase. **f:** Interphase cells with two schizonts.

would be interesting to know if any schizont division occurs before host cell centriole duplication and separation. The use of this kind of analysis is that if host centriole duplication is necessary before schizont division then a clearly defined host event has been linked to a parasite event. The host event must be communicated to the parasite and a target for communication has been defined.

Prerequisites for schizont division are DNA replication and nuclear division. This could be analyzed by visualizing DNA replication with 5-bromouracil incorporation and immunofluorescence and at the same time visualizing the host centriole(s), also by immunofluorescence. This experiment is important because if the communication between host and parasite is to be fully understood then the first event in the parasite triggered by a host event has to be defined. Thus, a possible model is that host centriole replication must occur before DNA replication is initiated in the parasite. There is only a little circumstantial evidence for this model, but it is consistent with all the observations.

Why is there variability in the timing of schizont division within the host cell cycle? By extrapolating from other eukaryotes it is a relatively safe assumption that all the nuclei in a schizont undergo synchronous S-phase and nuclear division as they share a common cytoplasm. The variability in timing must be due to variability either in the time taken to complete the necessary events after the trigger, either in host or parasite, or in the time taken to receive the information that the trigger event has occurred. One model that is attractive is that the time taken for the trigger to reach the schizont is proportional to the distance between the centriole and the point of attachment of the schizont to the host microtubule array; but that is enough wild speculation.

This work has been aimed at linking host and parasite events that are more amenable to analysis than how the parasite causes the host cell to proliferate in the first place. The question that remains is which events in the host cell cycle are dependent on the completion of events in the schizont cycle. This information is not as accessible due to the absence of inhibitors that specifically affect the parasite and not the host.

CONCLUSION

Trying to elucidate what goes on between an intracellular parasite and its host cell is not a choice for the faint-hearted. However, in the case of *Theileria*-infected lymphocytes, the next few years could see substantial advances as great progress is being made in understanding the control of lymphocyte proliferation and the mechanisms of cell cycle control.

ACKNOWLEDGMENTS

Work in the authors' laboratory has been funded by The Jowett Fund, The British Council, and The Overseas Development Administration.

REFERENCES

Baylis H, Allsopp B, Hall R, Carrington M (1993): Characterization of a glutamine and proline rich (QP) protein from *Theileria parva*. Mol Biochem Parasitol 61:171–178.
Dobbelaere DAE, Coquerelle TM, Roditi IJ, Eichhorn M, Williams RO (1988a): *Theileria*

parva infection induces autocrine growth of bovine lymphocytes. Proc Natl Acad Sci USA 85:4730–4736.

Dobbelaere DAE, Roditi IJ, Coquerelle TM, Eichhorn M, Kelke C, Williams RO (1988b): Lymphocytes infected with *Theileria parva* require both cell–cell contact and growth factor to proliferate. Eur J Immunol 21:89–95.

Dobbelaere DAE, Prospero TD, Roditi IJ, Kelke C, Baumann I, Eichhorn M, Williams RO, Ahmed JS, Baldwin CL, Clevers H, Morrison WI (1990): Expression of Tac antigen component of bovine interleukin-2 receptor in different leukocyte populations infected with *Theileria parva* or *Theileria annulata*. Infect Immun 58:3847–3855.

Hall R, Hunt P, Carrington M, Simmons D, Williamson S, Mecham R, Tait A (1992): Mimicry of elastin repetitive motifs by *Theileria annulata* sporozoite surface antigen. Mol Biochem Parasitol 53:105–112.

Heussler VT, Eichhorn M, Reeves R, Magnuson NS, Williams RO, Dobbelaere DAE (1992): Constitutive IL-2 mRNA expression in lymphocytes infected with the intracellular parasite *Theileria parva*. J Immunol 149:562–567.

Hulliger L, Wilde JKH, Brown CGD, Turner L (1964): Mode of multiplication of *Theileria* in cultures of bovine lymphocytic cells. Nature 203:728–730.

Irvin AD, Ocama JGR, Spooner PR (1982): Cycle of bovine lymphoblastoid cell parasitized by *Theileria parva*. Res Vet Sci 33:298–304.

Malu NM (1992): The role of γ-interferon in *Theileria parva* induced lymphoproliferation. PhD thesis, University of Cambridge, Cambridge, England.

Nene V, Iams KP, Gobright E, Musoke AJ (1992): Characterisation of the gene encoding a candidate vaccine antigen of *Theileria parva* sporozoites. Mol Biochem Parasitol 51:105–112.

ole-MoiYoi OK, Sugimoto C, Conrad PA, Macklin MD (1992): Cloning and characterization of the casein kinase IIα subunit gene from the lymphocyte transforming intracellular protozoan parasite *Therileria parva*. Biochemistry 31:6193–6202.

ole-MoiYoi OK, Brown WC, Iams KP, Nayar A, Tsukamoto T, Macklin MD (1993): Evidence for the induction of casein kinase II in bovine lymphocytes transformed by the intracellular protozoan parasite *Theileria parva*. EMBO J 12:1621–1631.

Shaw MK, Tilney LG, Musoke AJ (1991): The entry of theileria parva sporozoites into bovine lymphocytes: Evidence for MHC class I involvement. J Cell Biol 113:87–101.

Shaw MK, Tilney LG (1992): How individual cells develop from a syncitium: Merogony in *Theileria parva* (Apicomplexa). J Cell Sci 101:109–123.

Shiels B, Kinnaird J, McKellar S, Dickson J, Ben Miled L, Melrose R, Brown D, Tait A (1992): Disruption of synchrony between parasite growth and host cell division is a determinant of differentiation to the merozoite in *Theileria annulata*. J Cell Sci 101:99–107.

Spooner RL, Innes EA, Glass EJ, Brown CGD (1989): *Theileria annulata* and *T. parva* infect and transform different bovine mononuclear cells. Immunology 66:284–288.

Sugimoto C, Conrad PA, Ito S, Brown WC, Grab DJ (1988): Isolation of *Theileria parva* schizonts from infected lymphoblastoid cells. Acta Tropica 45:203–216.

Molecular Approaches to Parasitology, pages 57–76
© 1995 Wiley-Liss, Inc.

Biological Functions of Nematode Surfaces

Timothy G. Geary, Kevin L. Blair, Norman F.H. Ho, Sandra M. Sims, and David P. Thompson

Upjohn Laboratories, The Upjohn Company, Kalamazoo, Michigan 49001

INTRODUCTION

The sweeping advance of modern biology, propelled by ever more elegant nucleic acid–based technology, has unfortunately left in its wake some topics of substantial importance. Insufficiently well developed for the useful application of molecular biology techniques, they languish in relative and increasing obscurity. Experimental questions cannot be phrased in ways that make molecular techniques sensible, and data cannot be fully and correctly interpreted unless enough is known about the biology of the system under investigation. One example is the nematode surface. While something is known about the biochemistry of the cuticle and a few immunogenic proteins (and the genes that encode them) have been characterized, little can be stated with certainty about the biological functions of this tissue.

Nematode surfaces of interest include the cuticle–hypodermis complex and the tissues involved in ingestion and digestion (esophagus, pharynx, gut); these represent the major interfaces between the nematode and its environment. Functions that we associate with these surfaces include the formation and maintenance of a permeability barrier and structural support; nutrient and waste product transport; and the generation of transmural hydrostatic (turgor) pressure and electrochemical gradients. Several recent books provide excellent reviews of the structure of the tissues of interest (Wharton, 1986; Wright, 1987; Kennedy, 1991; Bird and Bird, 1991).

The temptation to generalize about nematodes must be resisted. Most studies on the biology of these organisms have used a single species. The field has been both blessed and cursed by the availability of the free-living nematode *Caenorhabditis elegans* and large parasitic species of the genus *Ascaris* (*A. suum* and *A. lumbricoides*). Most work on the function of worm surfaces has been carried out on one or the other of these nematodes, each of which has certain advantages. For *C. elegans,* it is the depth of knowledge available on anatomy, development, genetics, and molecular biology; for the *Ascaris* species, it is the large size. Unfortunately, there has been a tendency to extrapolate from experiments done on these species to nematodes in general. Rarely, though, have similar studies been done on more than one organism simultaneously or sequentially. What we do know is that various aspects of surface biology unite nematodes, while other areas distinguish them. The reader should be continuously wary of the tendency to unwarranted generalizations that plagues reviews such as this.

This discussion is restricted largely to the adult stages of nematodes that parasitize mammals, reflecting the experimental interests of the authors. We have chosen to focus on a few areas of nematode surface biology that present unusual research challenges and unresolved, basic questions about the physiology of these organisms.

PERMEABILITY BARRIER PROPERTIES OF NEMATODE SURFACES

Our interest in the biology of worm surfaces arose from a pragmatic question related to drug design for improved anthelminthic delivery: How do drugs get into nematodes? Two obvious routes are oral ingestion and transcuticular diffusion or uptake; we were uncertain if either was a more important route for anthelminthic absorption by parasites. Studies in the literature indicated that nutrient absorption across the cuticle was likely to be of great importance to filarial parasites (Howells, 1980), but the situation is less clear for nematodes that parasitize the gastrointestinal (GI) tract (see Pappas and Read, 1975; Thompson and Geary, 1994, for review) and free-living worms. Studies on diffusion of anthelminthics and other solutes across the cuticle have generally demonstrated that permeation does occur (Hobson, 1948; Trim, 1949; Hollis, 1961; Howells, 1980; Fetterer, 1986; Court et al., 1988), but the relative importance of the two available routes was rarely measured (see, however, Verhoeven et al., 1980). Using isolated cuticles and intact specimens of *A. suum*, we were able to demonstrate that organic solutes diffuse across the surface of this parasite in a way that can be mathematically defined (Ho et al., 1990) and that this route was fare more important than oral ingestion (Ho et al., 1992). The latter studies were done with parasites ligated to close the mouth and anus. Similar studies have also been done in other GI parasites, including *Haemonchus contortus* and *Trichostrongylus colubriformis,* using ivermectin to paralyze the pharynx and thus prevent oral ingestion (Avery and Horvitz, 1990; Geary et al., 1993). Transcuticular diffusion in these three species seems to be quantitatively similar when rates of transport are expressed per unit surface area (Thompson et al., 1993). Although ivermectin paralyzes the pharynx of *C. elegans* (Avery and Horvitz, 1990), potentially enabling one to conduct similar experiments with this organism, its small size has thus far precluded attempts to obtain accurate data on permeation. However, experiments with levamisole demonstrated that breeching the cuticle greatly increased the potency and speed of action of this compound, suggesting that transcuticular diffusion controls its activity (Lewis et al., 1980). The apparent lack of function of the gut in some adult filariae strongly suggests that transcuticular permeation is the route of entry of solutes in these animals.

The accumulated data show that transcuticular diffusion is the major route of entry for non-nutrient, nonelectrolyte solutes in nematodes. This is likely to be true for all species. The data obtained from *A. suum* were used to delineate the biophysical characteristics of the transport process (Ho et al., 1990, 1992). Permeability barriers include the aqueous environment of the cuticle structure and a lipid layer that in *A. suum* is the boundary layer between the cuticle and hypodermis (which we have termed the *hypocuticle*; see Fig. 1). These barriers operate in series. Anatomical pores are not apparent in the cuticle of GI parasites (Martin et al., 1987), but functional pores are present. This term describes the fact that the cross-linked protein fibers that constitute the various layers of the cuticle are hydrated and that tortuous channels exist for the passage of solutes through this structure. The average radius of these channels

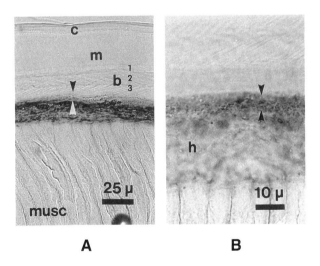

A   **B**

Fig. 1.   Sections of the body wall of adult *A. suum* stained with osmium. **B** is a close-up of the area denoted by arrows in **A**. The osmiophilic (lipidic) layer seen between the muscle (musc) and cuticle (top of both panels) is the hypodermis. The basal layers (b 1–3) of the cuticle are clearly evident in A. The area between the arrows in each panel represents the boundary between the hypodermis and the cuticle; we have termed this the *hypocuticle*. It represents the major lipidic barrier to transcuticular solute diffusion in this species.

was calculated to be about 1.5 nm (Ho et al., 1992). Molecular size thus restricts entry of large compounds (ivermectin, with radius = 0.6 nm, approaches the limit). Passage through the aqueous channels is further influenced by charge; the electrochemical force provided by fixed negative charges (probably sulfate groups) on cuticular proteins (Murrell et al., 1983) propels cations and retards anions. However, the major barrier for most solutes is the lipid layer (Ho et al., 1992).

When adjusted for surface area, the kinetics of permeation of solutes into intact parasites were very similar to the kinetics of diffusion through isolated patches of cuticle (Ho et al., 1992). However, some discrepancies were noted between the two systems for weak acids and weak bases. One would predict that the pH of the medium, by defining the ratio of charged to uncharged species of the permeant, would determine the rate of diffusion of the substance through the rate-controlling lipidic barrier of the cuticle. Instead, we found that changes in external pH influenced the rate of uptake of these solutes to a much lower extent than expected in intact nematodes (Sims et al., 1992). This discrepancy arises because living worms maintain a strongly buffered environment in the aqueous spaces of the cuticle structure. Thus, the ratio of charged to uncharged species of a weak acid or weak base will be controlled not by the external medium, but by the pH microenvironment in the cuticle. The pH of this compartment is around 5.0 in several parasitic species (Sims et al., 1992; unpublished observations). This value is due to the accumulation of organic acid end products of carbohydrate metabolism (which vary in presence and proportion among different species), including lactate, acetate, propionate, butyrate, 2-methylbutyrate, and 2-methylvalerate. The pK_a values for these molecules are generally about 5.0; they buffer aqueous solutions strongly in that range. Organic acids are present in the cuticle water because they are excreted across this surface (Sims et al., 1992; unpublished observations), as discussed in detail below. As shown in Figure 2, the rate of appearance of organic acids and concomitant change in pH in the medium surrounding *A. suum* in culture are identical in control animals and in worms whose mouth and anus are ligated. Similar results are observed for adult *H. contortus* in the presence of ivermectin, which paralyzes the pharynx (Sims et al., unpublished observations). Finally, we have found in preliminary experiments that isolated patches of *A. suum* body wall in two-cell diffusion chambers transport organic acids across the cuticle at a reasonably high rate. These data suggest that the nematode surface is the primary site for organic acid excretion, contrary to the findings of Harpur (1969), who postulated that fecal excretion was the primary route of exit of organic acids from this parasite.

Why all parasitic nematodes make organic acids as the end products of carbohydrate metabolism is a long-standing puzzle; even the filariae, which live in oxygenated tissues, follow this pattern (see Bryant, 1993). Having been

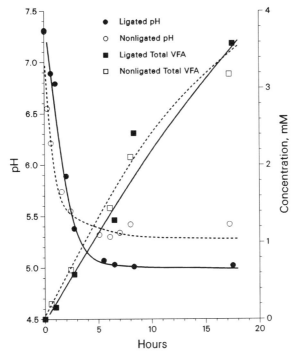

Fig. 2. Results of a typical experiment comparing organic acid excretion and pH changes in ligated versus nonligated adult *A. suum.* The rate of change in pH is nearly identical in the two groups, as is the rate of appearance of organic acids in the medium. Summation of a large series of such experiments showed that the rate of change and final plateau of pH was not significantly different in the two groups (see Sims et al., 1992).

made, they must be eliminated to avoid poisoning the metabolic pathway that creates them. In that sense, the excretion of organic acids is not different from the exhalation of carbon dioxide in mammals. There is precedent for the coupling of organic acid transport to energy generation in *Escherichia coli* (Konings, 1985). Whether a similar situation exists in nematodes is unknown.

It is not possible to study the physiology of organic acid excretion in nematodes through the genetics of *C. elegans,* as it appears that this free-living worm excretes primarily carbon dioxide and glycerol. Interestingly, under similar conditions the free-living species *Panagrellus redivivus* excretes organic acids (lactate, acetate, propionate; Butterworth and Barrett, 1985; our unpublished results). Why these two organisms differ in this regard is not clear. To return to the topic that began this discussion, one must realize that the uptake of weak acid or weak base drugs may be different in the "model" nematode *C. elegans* than in parasitic species. It is also apparent that an understanding of organic acid transport can best be achieved by physiological studies in parasites.

PHYSIOLOGY OF TRANSMURAL ORGANIC ACID EXCRETION IN NEMATODES

Though considerable information exists about energy-generating pathways in nematodes, particularly for *Ascaris,* less is known about the sites at which the organic acid end products of carbohydrate metabolism are excreted or the mechanisms that underlie this process. A second, perhaps more intriguing question is why nematodes maintain high levels of organic acid end products within both their cells and the pseudocoelomic fluid that fills their body cavity.

In *A. suum,* the concentration of the combined organic acid end products of carbohydrate metabolism is maintained at 60–80 mM in both muscle cells and hypodermis, while the concentration in pseudocoelomic fluid is 20–40 mM higher (Sims et al., 1992; and unpublished observations); these concentrations are much higher than those found in vertebrate tissues. The relative concentrations of individual organic acids in the various compartments (muscle, hypodermis, pseudocoelom) are constant and mirror the concentrations that accumulate in the external medium.

The pH of pseudocoelomic fluid in *A. suum* is typically in the range of 6.5–6.8, and intracellular pH (measured in muscle and hypodermis using pH-sensitive microelectrodes) is maintained at 6.8–7.0 (our unpublished observations). Since pK_a values for most of the organic acids excreted by *A. suum* are in the range of 4.8–5.0, less than 1% of these end products will exist within the parasite in the protonated (i.e., uncharged, lipid-permeable) form. Thus, passive diffusion of uncharged acids across hypodermal membranes probably contributes little to the overall excretion capacity of the hypodermis. Our studies indicate that less than 5% of the organic acids excreted by *A. suum* during in vitro incubations can be accounted for solely on the basis of passive diffusion (unpublished observations). The concept that passive diffusion plays a small role in organic acid excretion by nematodes is further supported by the fact that the relative concentrations of the organic acids between tissues, the pseudocoelomic fluid, and the external medium is constant. If passive diffusion was important, the higher lipid–water partition coefficients that characterize the higher molecular weight organic acids would greatly favor their excretion, but this is clearly not the case (Sims et al., 1994).

Recent studies in Martin's laboratory (see Dixon and Martin, 1993) demonstrate the existence of an anion channel in nematode membranes that could provide an energetically efficient pathway for organic acid excretion. This channel, which has been partially characterized using isolated patches of *A.*

suum muscle membrane and single-channel voltage-clamp recordings, is selective for anions and conducts Cl⁻ and each of the organic acids excreted by *A. suum*. The existence of a 30–40 mV electrical potential (inside negative) across the plasma membrane of *A. suum* muscle cells provides an outward-directed driving force for organic anion conductance. Although a –40 mV electrical potential also exists across the body wall of *A. suum* (Pax et al., 1994), it is not known if channels that conduct organic anions are also present in hypodermal membranes, where they could provide a pathway for excretion. Furthermore, the studies of Martin et al. demonstrate that conductance across this channel is inversely related to the Stoke's radius of the anion. Therefore, this mechanism would lead to differential accumulation of the larger organic anions. Again, the excretion kinetic data for *A. suum* are not consistent with this (Sims et al., 1994). Too little is known, however, about the biophysical properties of this channel or other channels in nematodes to conclude that they are unimportant for organic acid excretion. It is likely that recent advances in the molecular pharmacology of ion channels will be extended to parasites, providing useful paradigms for the discovery of agents that selectively affect channels such as the one described by Martin and colleagues.

In vertebrates, organic acid end products of carbohydrate metabolism are transported across plasma membranes by specific carrier molecules. These proteins have not been studied in nematodes, but their existence may be inferred from the preceding observations. Studies to characterize organic acid transport systems in vertebrates have capitalized on the fact that they are generally coupled with either H^+ or Na^+ transport and can be selectively inhibited by agents such as the cinnamates or the benzenesulfonates or by altering gradients for Na^+, K^+, or choline. Use of these approaches in studies with intact nematodes is made difficult by the cuticle, which limits access, particularly of inorganic ions and charged organic molecules, to the outward-facing membrane of the hypodermis. Application of these approaches, however, should be possible using isolated body wall preparations (Thompson et al., 1993; Pax et al., 1994) and patches of hypodermal membrane prepared using variations of the protocol developed for recording ion channel activity in muscle membrane (Dixon and Martin, 1993).

Many questions remain to be answered. Is transport of all organic acids mediated by a single protein, or is there a family of transporters with selective affinity for different organic acids? Kinetic studies show that excretion of organic acids occurs at twice the rate of proton excretion in intact *A. suum* (Sims et al., 1993). What is the counterion used in the transport of the other half of the organic acids? Organic acid excretion occurs at a constant rate in the face of vastly differing pH (proton) gradients (Sims et al., 1993; see Fig. 3). How are tissue protons dumped in the face of an external pH of 3.25?

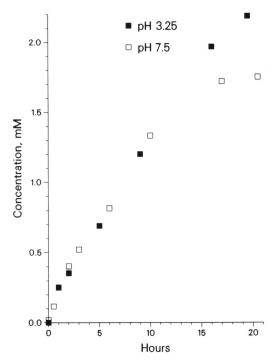

Fig. 3. Excretion kinetics of organic acids by adult *A. suum* into medium initially buffered at pH 7.5 or 3.25. Depicted are results of a typical experiment demonstrating that the transmural proton gradient does not influence the rate of appearance of organic acids in the medium. The rates of excretion of total organic acids are essentially identical: 90 ($\pm$30) nmol/cm^2 hour at pH 7.5 and 60 ($\pm$ 20) nmol/cm^2 hour at pH 3.25 (see Sims et al., 1992, 1994).

Solving these puzzles could open a new arena for drug discovery, since drugs that block the transport of organic acids should have selective effects on nematodes and would poison them. If multiple transporters exist, however, the ability of nematodes to shift metabolism to a different end product might defeat this strategy. Nonetheless, more basic research on the physiology and biochemistry of organic acid transport is clearly warranted.

It may be more difficult to determine why nematodes maintain high levels of organic acids within their cells and pseudocoelom than to delineate the mechanisms involved in their excretion. The possibility that they serve a role in osmoregulation is discussed in the next section. It does not appear that organic acids are used directly to regulate internal pH in nematodes, as the rate of excretion for each acid by *A. suum* is insensitive to external pH over the range of 3.25–7.5 (Sims et al., 1994), and these acids possess little buffering capacity at physiological pH. However, as discussed earlier, the transmural excretion of organic acids and protons maintains a microenvironmental pH of about 5 within the aqueous pores of the cuticle. This may buffer fluids that come in contact with the limiting membrane of nematodes and explain why they are able to tolerate wide fluctuations in external pH during in vitro incubations. There is, in fact, no information about how nematodes regulate pH within their cells or across their body wall. In vertebrates and most other eukaryotes, cytosolic pH is maintained by a Na^+/H^+ antiporter (at pH <7.0) and an HCO_3^-/Cl^- exchanger (at pH >7.0). Our preliminary studies using intact specimens and isolated segments of *A. suum* exposed to drugs or altered media that inhibit these transport processes in vertebrates have yielded essentially negative results, suggesting that proton extrusion across plasma membranes in nematodes may be mediated by novel mechanisms.

It is possible that organic acids are used to maintain electrochemical gradients in nematodes that are essential for other cell functions, such as membrane excitability. In *A. suum,* for instance, the resting potentials across muscle and hypodermal membranes and the transmural potential across the body wall are only weakly sensitive to the concentrations of inorganic ions in the medium (del Castillo et al., 1964; Pax et al., 1994). This condition is unlike that found in most vertebrate preparations, where membrane potential is usually controlled by selective permeability to K^+. Recent studies demonstrate that the transmural potential in *A. suum* is more sensitive to some small organic anions (with high levels of external acetate or butyrate leading to increased polarization) than to Na^+, K^+, or Cl^-, even though the collagen barrier of the cuticle is far more permeable to the inorganic ions. When acetate or butyrate is replaced by Cl^- or gluconate (an impermeable anion), the transmural potential becomes markedly yet reversibly depolarized (Pax et al., 1994).

Perhaps the organic acids are simply substrates for ATP synthesis, accounting for their apparent ability to maintain a more polarized state across the body wall. Indeed, pseudocoelomic fluid from *A. suum* maintained in high acetate medium contains higher levels of this anion, as well as its condensation product, 2-methylbutyrate, than parasites maintained in medium in which Cl^- is substituted for acetate (Sims et al., 1994). However, energy charge and the total organic acid excretion rate by intact *A. suum* is not affected by this substitution (Sims et al., 1994), suggesting that the exogenous organic acids do not influence metabolism. The simplest explanation consistent with these observations is that acetic (or butyric) acid diffuses into the parasite along its concentration gradient. Once inside it dissociates, and the protons it carries are excreted at a rate that exceeds excretion of the acetate (or butyrate) anion. This would contribute to the more polarized transmural potential recorded. Central to this hypothesis is the existence of a microclimate pH at the cuticle–hypodermis interface in *A. suum,* which would promote inward diffusion of the uncharged organic acids by ensuring relatively high levels of the proton-ated form of the molecule at that site.

TURGOR PRESSURE

Anyone who has nicked or cut a living nematode has witnessed the some-times explosive evisceration that accompanies a breech in the cuticle. This seems to be generally true; we have witnessed it for a variety of parasitic and free-living species. This simple observation indicates that the internal cham-ber of nematodes is under a considerable pressure gradient compared with the external medium. Indeed, this gradient has been measured at 70 mmHg at rest in *A. suum* (Harris and Crofton, 1957; our unpublished observations), with surges to 225 mmHg during motion. Why worms maintain a turgor pressure can be reasonably well argued; how they do so is another matter.

Nematodes are unusual for animals of a similar cylindrical shape in that they have only longitudinal muscles. Coupled with circular muscles, as in schistosomes and earthworms, longitudinal muscles provide an adequate means of locomotion. On their own, however, no net motion is possible unless the force of contraction of the muscle fiber can be made to work against a lever of some kind. In vertebrates, the lever is provided by bones. Nematodes have solved the problem differently: The turgor pressure generates a semirigid in-ternal hydrostatic skeleton that can antagonize the contraction of the longitu-dinal muscles, permitting work (=motion) to occur. The efficiency of the system is enhanced by the quasielastic nature of the cuticle. Change in length of a body region due to contraction of the local ensemble of muscles must be bal-anced by expansion elsewhere, since the system is closed. In this regard, as Wharton (1986) notes, the hydrostatic skeleton acts like the fluid in a hydraulic brake, transmitting pressure increases from local muscle contractions to other parts of the body. The resulting expansion is in length, not in diameter; this provides the antagonistic force against which the longitudinal muscles contract.

The reader is directed to the accounts by Harris and Crofton (1957), O'Grady (1983) and Wharton (1986) for a more thorough explanation of the biophysics of nematode movement and of the particular anatomical features of the cuticle that account for it. Here, our attention will shift to the question of how a hy-drostatic pressure gradient is maintained across the nematode surface.

A hydrostatic pressure gradient depends on the selective retention of water on one side of a barrier. Water flows across the cuticle structure of nematodes (Hobson et al., 1952; Marks et al., 1968; Ho et al., 1990), and nematodes seem to be able to osmoregulate to some degree (see Wright and Newall, 1980). The turgor pressure gradient also responds to variations in external osmolar-ity (R.A. Pax et al., unpublished observations). For instance, the internal pres-sure of adult *A. suum* increases dramatically when the animal is placed in very

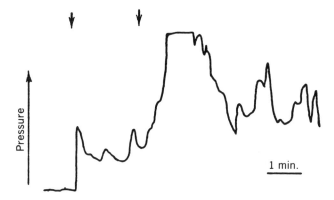

Fig. 4. Osmotically induced changes in turgor pressure in an adult *Ascaris suum* in culture. The tracing represents pressure measured in arbitrary units; the time scale is given at the bottom right. The first arrow denotes the moment when the microelectrode equipped with a pressure transducer penetrated into the pseudocoelomic cavity of an adult female *A. suum*. At the second arrow, the medium was changed from isosmotic with saline to a medium that was reduced in osmolarity by 80%. The internal pressure surge was back to essentially baseline levels within 3 minutes. (Courtesy of R.A. Pax.)

hypotonic saline. However, internal pressure returns to the previous level after a few minutes (Fig. 4). It thus appears that the influx of water is reversed by some adjustment in internal osmolarity.

The turgor pressure may thus be maintained in the face of varying osmolarity in the external environment. Adult filarial parasites have the luxury of dwelling in tissue or fluid compartments of the host, which vary little in osmolarity. The situation for gut parasites is less obvious. Lumen dwellers face the onslaught of intestinal contents, which, depending on time since feeding and rate of fluid secretion (consider, for example, diarrhea), face solutions of quite variable osmolarity. Parasites that live more closely apposed to the mucous layer may be in a more constant osmotic environment, but we are unaware of direct measurements in parasitized animals that would settle the question.

One can, however, determine the osmolarity of standard pig intestinal fluid. Compared with it, the pseudocoelomic fluid of *A. suum* is hypotonic (Hobson et al., 1952). Here is the unsolved riddle: Both the osmotic and pressure gradients work in the same direction, tending to force water out of the pseudocoelom and into the external medium. Yet the animals retain an internal–external hydrostatic gradient even though the cuticle is permeable to water. How this is accomplished remains an open question and an excellent topic for basic research in parasite physiology.

Many invertebrates, especially marine organisms, regulate internal osmolarity in the face of varying external conditions (see Kinne, 1993). They do so by excreting three different kinds of compounds: polyhydric alcohols (sorbitol, glycerol), urea or trimethylamines, or various amino acids. We do not yet know if nematodes use any of these as osmotic balancers or use some other osmolyte to maintain internal homeostasis. One likely candidate might be the organic acids, which are present at high concentrations in the pseudocoelomic fluid of *A. suum*. However, we have found that these concentrations do not change dramatically when parasites are placed in distilled water for up to several hours, and thus other candidates must be sought. Identifying the substance(s) used by nematodes in osmoregulation might lead to a better understanding of the mechanism(s) that maintain turgor pressure. It is worth noting that cylindrical tubes of *A. suum* and *Dirofilaria immitis* adults formed from the midbody region minus the gut and ovaries can, when clamped and sealed, generate a hydrostatic pressure gradient (R.A. Pax et al., unpublished observations). This preparation could prove useful for the experimental analysis of the gradient.

Understanding the physiology of water in nematodes is a prelude to identifying key biochemical events that are responsible for the maintenance of turgor pressure. In turn, knowledge of the biochemistry can be used in targeted drug discovery programs. Drugs that block the regulation of turgor pressure would be of great interest as anthelmintics, because deflating worms should lead to their evacuation from the GI tract. Adult filariae of the species *Onchocerca volvulus* may also be susceptible. It is thought that these parasites acquire nutrients transcuticularly from the small blood vessels that closely surround them (see Smith et al., 1988). Adult females are intricately intertwined in the nodule and probably move very rarely in situ. How are nutrients acquired locally transported throughout the 0.5 m length of a (large) female? One can observe a tremendous mixing current in the pseudocoelomic fluid of living specimens of *O. volvulus* still in place in a nodule (J.F. Williams, personal communication). It is tempting to speculate that this motion arises from coordinated local fluctuations in turgor pressure. If so, blockade of the mechanisms responsible could effectively starve the parasite.

HOW DOES THE CUTICLE GROW?

Nematodes develop through a series of molts in which the old cuticle is shed after a new cuticle is elaborated beneath it. This process has been characterized (at least structurally) in several species. The molecular biology of molting is only beginning to be studied; a large number of collagen genes has been cloned from *C. elegans* and some parasitic species. The stage-specific expression of collagen genes can be tied to some of the molts (see Cox et al.,

1989; Cox, 1990; Kingston, 1991; our unpublished observations), though we are far from understanding the regulation of molting at a genetic level.

Our interest lies elsewhere. After the last larval molt, parasitic nematodes continue to grow. In *A. suum,* the larvae are <10 mm in length after the last molt. Mature females can reach 40 cm (Soulsby, 1982). In *H. contortus,* the growth is less spectacular, but still reaches a doubling in length or more (Conder et al., 1992). In addition to the expansion in length (and width), the cuticle also gets thicker as worms mature. For *Brugia pahangi,* it has been proposed that this increase in cuticle volume is achieved by simple expansion of a folded, densely packed cuticular network present in the last larval stage (Howells and Blainey, 1983). However, it is difficult to see how such a mechanism can account for the enormous increases in size that characterize parasites such as *A. suum* and *O. volvulus* following the last molt. Given the complex, layered organization of the cuticle, how does it enlarge in a coordinated fashion along with the somatic tissue of the worm?

In some respects, the bacterial cell wall is a model for the cuticle of nematodes. It is highly cross-linked, has a complex organization, and is assembled outside of the cytoplasm. The bacterial cell wall grows as the bacterium enlarges. New components are assembled into the existing structure at a specific site on the surface. Surface-associated enzymes (autolysins) clip apart the framework to allow new material to be added and cross-linked at this growth point. Growth of the nematode cuticle would be easy to understand if a similar engineering strategy was employed. However, there is no anatomical evidence for a specialized region of the cuticle responsible for synthesis of new material and no evidence of a growth furrow, like that seen in bacteria, in this tissue.

Instead, the cuticle must expand by the insertion of new proteins at multiple points along its undersurface (coming out from the hypodermis). It is difficult to imagine how the new protein molecules are successfully transported to and inserted in the existing scaffolding in a coordinated manner. There are no data about hydrolytic enzymes that open the cuticular network to allow the insertion of new components. The proteins of the cuticle are linked by various means, including sulfhydryl linkages and covalent cross-links through tyrosine residues; the latter include a typical dityrosine linkage and a more unusual isotrityrosine complex (Fujimoto et al., 1981). The enzymology involved in the formation of tyrosine cross-links is only now being investigated (see Fetterer et al., 1993). Transglutaminases may also play a role in stabilizing the structure of the cuticle proteins. Inhibitors of transglutaminases block development of several parasitic species and also have toxic effects on adults (Lustigman, 1993). However, these adulticidal effects are not accompanied by morphological changes consistent with disruption of cuticle integrity, and it is possible that the toxicity is due to drug effects in other aspects of parasite metabolism.

Studies on *C. elegans* have led to the identification of genes for several kinds of cuticle proteins. In general, this free-living nematode is a good model for cuticle structure and function in parasitic species (Politz and Philipp, 1992). However, unlike *A. suum, C. elegans* grows only a little after the last molt (Wilson, 1976). The events that underlie cuticle expansion may thus be difficult to explore in this organism. It is worth pointing out that characterization of mutant *C. elegans* has identified a number of genes that affect the morphology of the cuticle (Park and Horvitz, 1986). One family, termed *bli* (for *blister*), results in the formation of fluid-filled bubbles between the basal and cortical layers of the cuticle. Recent work indicates that the gene encoded by *bli-4* may play a role in the processing or assembly of cuticle components in the adult (Peters et al., 1991). Further work on this and other genes in *C. elegans,* and the identification of homologous genes in parasites, may greatly enhance our understanding of cuticle synthesis as adult nematodes grow.

It appears that at least some nematodes release surface proteins into the environment, suggesting that cuticle components are synthesized and replaced as they are lost (see Philipp and Rumjaneck, 1984; Selkirk, 1991; Politz and Philipp, 1992). The pathway through which newly synthesized cuticle proteins (antigens) reach the surface has not been conclusively identified. It is still not certain that this phenomenon occurs in all nematodes, but further studies may nonetheless reveal a common route for newly synthesized proteins to enter the cuticle matrix, whether for assembly or release.

The β-lactam antibiotics (the penicillins and cephalosporins) act by blocking bacterial cell wall synthesis. Disruption of the bacterial cell wall is lethal only when the bacteria are exposed to hypo- or hyperosmotic conditions; the cell membrane is too fragile to protect the cell from osmotic lysis. We have already seen that a considerable inside–outside hydrostatic pressure gradient is maintained by nematodes. Mechanical breech of the cuticle leads to the dramatic appearance of internal materials in the external medium. Understanding the biochemical processes that underlie the remodeling and synthesis of the cuticle in adult nematodes should identify interesting targets for new drugs. Blockade of the coordinated expansion of the cuticle as the worm grows should lead to death by explosion; such a mechanism would likely be macrofilaricidal as well. Realizing this possibility rests on the basic research required to elucidate the physiology and biochemistry of cuticle assembly in adult worms.

DRUGS AND NEMATODE SURFACES

Three major classes of anthelmintic drugs are currently dominant. Levamisole (and related compounds, like pyrantel and morantel) act as agonists at the nicotinic acetylcholine receptor on nematode somatic muscle. Paralysis of the musculature leads to expulsion of the worm, at least from the GI tract (see Geary et al., 1993, for review). Even though a considerable amount if known about the biochemical pharmacology of the other two classes (avermectins and benzimidazoles), we cannot yet say with certainty how they cause the elimination of parasites from the treated host (or, for that matter, how they lead to the demise of *C. elegans* on a plate of *E. coli*). It is possible that both classes of drugs act by interfering with the functions of surface tissues. The surfaces of interest are the pharynx and gut, which play an important role for at least some nematodes in feeding and nutrient transport, respectively.

The avermectins open Cl⁻ channels in parasitic nematodes and other invertebrates. Exactly which Cl⁻ channel is the target of these drugs has not yet been resolved. Early work focused on channels associated with the GABA receptors that mediate inhibitory synaptic transmission in nematodes, but these are not likely to be the real target (see Geary et al., 1993). The problem is that the avermectins are not particularly potent at paralyzing nematodes, at least in comparison with the concentrations needed to impair viability. In fact, it is reasonably difficult to detect ivermectin-induced paralysis in parasites such as *H. contortus* by eye (though it can be seen when motility is assessed electronically) (Geary et al., 1993).

Avery and Horvitz (1990) identified another potential target for these drugs in *C. elegans,* and we found similar results in *H. contortus* (Geary et al., 1993). Pharyngeal pumping and ingestion are inhibited by ivermectin concentrations up to 100-fold lower than those needed to impair motility. The uptake and metabolism of glucose, and tissue ATP levels, were unaffected by ivermectin concentrations that paralyzed the pharynx of *H. contortus.* We interpreted these data to mean that glucose enters this parasite across the cuticle, at least in culture. However, since the life span of *H. contortus* in vitro is quite limited, we suspect that additional nutritional factors must be acquired from the host for viability and that these are obtained by oral ingestion. Blockade of feeding induced by ivermectin is a plausible explanation of the drug's ability to clear parasites in vivo. It also may explain the lack of activity of drugs of this class against adult filariae; these parasites seem to have limited gut function and probably obtain essential nutrients via transcuticular absorption. The unimportance of pharyngeal function in these organisms may be why the avermectins have little activity against them.

The benzimidazoles present an interesting pharmacological problem: We have a very clear idea of their mechanism of anthelmintic action, but they have almost no detectable effects (at relevant concentrations) on parasitic nematodes maintained in culture, and we cannot easily explain how they get rid of worms from a host. An enormous amount of biochemical, pharmacological, and genetic evidence supports the hypothesis that the benzimidazoles bind to tubulin and depolymerize the network of microtubules that is essential for the function and replication of all eukaryotic cells (see Lacey, 1988, for review). However, as noted, parasitic nematodes do not seem to be bothered much by these drugs in culture. Inhibition of the secretion of acetylcholinesterase by the benzimidazoles has been noted (Watts et al., 1982), but this effect is not clearly related to the elimination of parasites in vivo.

Effects of these drugs on a worm surface may provide a solution to this dilemma. The earliest morphological effect of a typical benzimidazole (mebendazole) following treatment of infected animals is the disappearance of the microtubular network in parasite intestinal cells (Borgers and De Nollin, 1975; Borgers et al., 1975). Mebendazole is concentrated in nematode gut tissue following exposure of worms to radiolabeled drug in culture (Kohler and Bachmann, 1981). We have found that other solutes, including benzimidazoles, are also concentrated in the gut of A. suum following in vitro exposure, even in parasites tightly ligated at the head and tail (Ho et al., 1992; our unpublished observations).

These observations may be related to data recently obtained from C. elegans. Many organisms express proteins that are structurally (and probably functionally) related to proteins originally identified in tumor cells resistant to many anticancer drugs. This mdr (for multiple drug resistance) phenotype is often due to the overexpression or mutation of large glycoproteins (P-glycoproteins) that pump out drugs and other substances from cells. A family of P-glycoprotein genes is present in C. elegans (Lincke et al., 1992); we have found a similar family in H. contortus (Sangster et al., 1993). At least two of the mdr genes of C. elegans are expressed only in the gut (Lincke et al., 1993).

If the mdr genes of parasitic nematodes are also expressed in the gut, a mechanism is evident to explain the action of the benzimidazoles. Presumably, the P-glycoproteins in nematodes act to pump compounds from the pseudocoelomic fluid into the gut lumen and thus out into the environment. The exceptional concentration of drugs and other solutes in the gut following exposure in culture could be due to this pumping action. The microtubule disruption evident in the gut cells would be due to the high concentration of drug present in this compartment.

The consequences of disruption of the gut microtubular system should be a cessation of nutrient transport into the pseudocoelomic fluid; indeed, there is evidence that mebendazole inhibits the uptake of small nutrients by A. suum (Van den Bossche and De Nollin, 1973). The result in vivo would be starvation and eventual elimination of GI parasites. A similar effect would be expected for C. elegans browsing on E. coli. However, as for ivermectin, disruption of ingestion or digestion would not be expected to have much effect on adult filariae, which acquire nutrients by transcuticular uptake. Like ivermectin, the benzimidazoles have little efficacy as macrofilaricides. While pharmacokinetic inadequacies have been invoked to explain this lack of activity, it may instead be the case that the action of these drugs on adult filariae has no deleterious consequences. Again, the lack of activity of the benzimidazoles against other parasites in vitro can be explained by the fact that oral ingestion of nutrients does not contribute to survival under these conditions.

The idea that gut microtubules are the target of benzimidazole anthelmintics is not new (Kohler and Bachmann, 1981). The recent discovery of gut-specific P-glycoprotein expression in *C. elegans* provides a pharmacodynamic basis for the hypothesis. It is intriguing to think that the primary actions of two of the three major anthelmintic classes are directed against surface functions of nematodes. Further work is needed to verify or refute this possibility. The distribution and function of P-glycoproteins in parasites and the physiological consequences of exposure to the benzimidazoles and avermectins are excellent topics for research. It is intriguing to speculate that functions of the cuticular surface are equally susceptible to selective drug interdiction and that learning more about them will improve our chances of finding new drugs.

ACKNOWLEDGMENTS

We are grateful to our collaborators and colleagues who participated in the research described in this review and who continue to assist in the work. They include Ron Klein, Steve Nelson, George Conder, Craig Barsuhn, and Jeff Day (The Upjohn Company); John Oaks (University of Wisconsin); Ray Fetterer, Delores Hill, Linda Mansfield, and Ray Gamble (USDA-ARS, Helminthic Diseases Laboratory, Beltsville, MD); Lisa Vanover (SmithKline Beecham Animal Health); and Ralph Pax, Jeff Williams, Mark Huntington, Charles Mackenzie, and Jim Bennett (Michigan State University).

REFERENCES

Avery L, Horvitz HR (1990): Effects of starvation and neuroactive drugs on feeding in *Caenorhabditis elegans*. J Exp Zool 253:263–270.

Bird AF, Bird J (1991): The Structure of Nematodes, 2nd ed. San Diego: Academic Press.

Borgers M, De Nollin S (1975): Ultrastructural changes in *Ascaris suum* intestine after mebendazole treatment in vivo. J Parasitol 61:110–122.

Borgers M, De Nollin S, De Brabander M, Thienpont D (1975): Influence of the anthelmintic mebendazole on microtubules and intracellular organelle movement in nematode intestinal cells. Am J Vet Res 36:1153–1166.

Bryant C (1993): Organic acid excretion by helminths. Parasitol Today 9:58–60.

Butterworth PE, Barrett J (1985): Anaerobic metabolism in the free-living nematode *Panagrellus redivivus*. Physiol Zool 58:9–17.

Conder GA, Johnson SS, Hall AD, Fleming MW, Mills MD, Guimond PM (1992): Growth and development of *Haemonchus contortus* in birds, *Meriones unguiculatus*. J Parasitol 78:492–497.

Court JP, Murgatroyd RC, Livingstone D, Rahr E (1988): Physicochemical characteristics of non-electrolytes and their uptake by *Brugia pahangi* and *Dipetalonema viteae*. Mol Biochem Parasitol 27:101–108.

Cox GN (1990): Molecular biology of the cuticle collagen gene families of *Caenorhabditis elegans* and *Haemonchus contortus*. Acta Trop 47:269–281.

Cox GN, Fields C, Kramer JM, Rosenzweig B, Hirsh D (1989): Sequence comparisons of developmentally regulated collagen genes of *Caenorhabditis elegans*. Gene 76:331–344.

del Castillo J, de Mello WC, Morales T (1964): Influence of some ions on the membrane potential of *Ascaris* muscle. J Gen Physiol 48:129–140.

Dixon DM, Martin RJ (1993): Patch-clamp and chloride channels on *Ascaris suum*. Parasitol Today 9:341–344.

Fetterer RH (1986): Transcuticular solute movement in parasitic nematodes: Relationship between non-polar solute transport and partition coefficient. Comp Biochem Physiol 84A:461–466.

Fetterer RH, Rhoads ML, Urban JF Jr (1993): Synthesis of tyrosine-derived cross-links in *Ascaris suum* cuticular proteins. J Parasitol 79:160–166.

Fujimoto D, Hortiuchi K, Hirama M (1981): Isotrityrosine, a new crosslinking amino acid isolated from *Ascaris* cuticle. Biochem Biophys Res Commun 99:637–643.

Geary TG, Sims SM, Thomas EM, Vanover L, Davis JP, Winterrowd CA, Klein RD, Ho NFH, Thompson DP (1993): *Haemonchus contortus*: Ivermectin-induced paralysis of the pharynx. Exp Parasitol 77:88–96.

Harpur RP (1969): The nematode intestine and organic acid excretion: Volatile acids in *Ascaris lumbricoides* faeces. Comp Biochem Physiol 28:865–875.

Harris JE, Crofton HD (1957): Structure and function in the nematodes: Internal pressure and cuticular structure in *Ascaris*. J Exp Zool 34:116–130.

Ho NFH, Geary TG, Barsuhn CL, Sims SM, Thompson DP (1992): Mechanistic studies in the transcuticular delivery of antiparasitic drugs II: Ex vivo/in vitro correlation of solute transport by *Ascaris suum*. Mol Biochem Parasitol 52:1–14.

Ho NFH, Geary TG, Raub TJ, Barsuhn CL, Thompson DP (1990): Biophysical transport properties of the cuticle of *Ascaris suum*. Mol Biochem Parasitol 41:153–166.

Hobson AD (1948): The physiology and cultivation in artificial medium of nematodes parasitic in the alimentary tract of animals. Parasitology 38:183–227.

Hobson AD, Stephenson W, Beadle LC (1952): Studies on the physiology of *Ascaris lumbricoides*. I. The relation of the total osmotic pressure, conductivity and chloride content of the body fluid to that of the external environment. J Exp Biol 29:1–21.

Hollis JP (1961): Nematode reactions to coal-tar dyes. Nematologica 6:315–325.

Howells RE (1980): Filariae: Dynamics of the surface. In H. Van den Bossche (ed): The Host-Invader Interplay. Amsterdam: Elsevier/North-Holland, pp 69–84.

Howells RE, Blainey LJ (1983): The moulting process and the phenomenon of intermoult growth in the filarial nematode *Brugia pahangi*. Parasitology 87:493–505.

Kennedy MW (ed) (1991): Parasitic Nematodes—Antigens, Membranes and Genes. London: Taylor and Francis.

Kingston IB (1991): Collagen genes in *Ascaris*. In M.W. Kennedy (ed): Parasitic Nematodes—Antigens, Membranes and Genes. London: Taylor and Francis, pp 66–83.

Kinne RKH (1993): The role of organic osmolytes in osmoregulation: From bacteria to mammals. J Exp Zool 265:346–355.

Kohler P, Bachmann R (1981): Intestinal tubulin as possible target for the chemotherapeutic action of mebendazole in parasitic nematodes. Mol Biochem Pharmacol 4:325–336.

Konings WN (1985): Generation of metabolic energy by end-product efflux. Trends Biochem Sci 10:317–319.

Lacey E (1988): The role of the cytoskeletal protein, tubulin, in the mode of action and mechanism of drug resistance to benzimidazoles. Int J Parasitol 18:885–936.

Lewis JA, Wu C-H, Levine JH, Berg H (1980): Levamisole-resistant mutants of the nematode *Caenorhabditis elegans* appear to lack pharmacological acetylcholine receptors. Neuroscience 5:967–989.

Lincke CR, The I, van Groenigen M, Borst P (1992): The P-glycoprotein family of *Caenorhabditis elegans*—cloning and characterization of genomic and complementary DNA sequences. J Mol Biol 228:701–711.

Lincke CR, Broeks A, The I, Plasterk RHA, Borst P (1993): The expression of two P-glycoprotein (*pgp*) genes in transgenic *Caenorhabditis elegans* is confined to intestinal cells. EMBO J 12:1615–1620.

Lustigman S (1993): Molting, enzymes and new targets for chemotherapy of *Onchocerca volvulus*. Parasitol Today 9:294–297.

Marks CF, Thomason IJ, Castro CE (1968): Dynamics of the permeation of nematodes by water, nematocides and other substances. Exp Parasitol 22:321–327.

Martin RE, Foster LA, Kester AS, Donahue MJ (1987): *Ascaris lumbricoides suum:* Morphological characterization of apparent cuticular pores by ionic permeability and electron microscopy. Exp Parasitol 63:329–336.

Murrell KD, Graham CE, McGreevy M (1983): *Strongyloides ratti* and *Trichinella spiralis:* Net charge of epicuticle. Exp Parasitol 55:331–339.

O'Grady RT (1983): Cuticular changes and structural dynamics in the fourth-stage larvae and adults of *Ascaris suum* Goeze, 1782 (Nematoda: Ascaridoidea) developing in swine. Can J Zool 61:1293–1303.

Pappas PW, Read CP (1975): Membrane transport in helminth parasites: A review. Exp Parasitol 37:469–530.

Park EC, Horvitz HR (1986): Mutations with dominant effects on the behavior and morphology of the nematode *Caenorhabditis elegans*. Genetics 113:821–852.

Pax RA, Geary TG, Bennett JL, Thompson DP (1994): *Ascaris suum*: Characterization of transmural and hypodermal potentials. Exp Parasitol (in press).

Peters K, McDowall J, Rose AM (1991): Mutations in the *bli*-4 (*I*) locus of *Caenorhabditis elegans* disrupt both adult cuticle and early larval development. Genetics 129:95–102.

Philipp M, Rumjaneck FD (1984): Antigenic and dynamic properties of helminth surface structures. Mol Biochem Parasitol 10:245–268.

Politz SM, Philipp M (1992): *Caenorhabditis elegans* as a model for parasitic nematodes: A focus on the cuticle. Parasitol Today 8:6–12.

Sangster NJ, Klein RD, Geary TG (1993): A P-glycoprotein gene family from *Haemonchus contortus*. J Cell Biochem 17C:119.

Selkirk ME (1991): Structure and biosynthesis of cuticular proteins of lymphatic filarial parasites. In M.W. Kennedy (ed): Parasitic Nematodes—Antigens, Membranes and Genes. London: Taylor and Francis, pp. 27–45.

Sims SM, Ho NFH, Magas LT, Geary TG, Barsuhn CL, Thompson DP (1994): Biophysical model of the transcuticular excretion kinetics of organic acids, cuticle pH and buffer capacity in gastrointestinal nematodes. J Drug Target 2:1–8.

Sims SM, Magas LT, Barsuhn CL, Ho NFH, Geary TG, Thompson DP (1992) Mechanisms of microenvironmental pH regulation in the cuticle of *Ascaris suum*. Mol Biochem Parsitol 53:135–148.

Smith RJ, Cotter TP, Williams JF, Guderian RH (1988): Vascular perfusion of *Onchocerca volvulus* nodules. Trop Med Parasitol 39:418–421.

Soulsby EJL (1982): Helminths, Arthropods and Protozoa of Domesticated Animals, 7th ed. Philadelphia: Lea & Febiger.

Thompson DP, Geary TG (1994): Helminth surfaces. In J.J. Marr, M. Muller (eds): Biochemistry of Parasitic Organisms and Its Molecular Foundations. London: Academic Press (in press).

Thompson DP, Ho NFH, Sims SM, Geary TG (1993): Mechanistic approaches to quantitate anthelmintic absorption by gastrointestinal nematodes. Parasitol Today 9:31–35.

Trim AR (1949): The kinetics of the penetration of some representative anthelmintics and related compounds into *Ascaris lumbricoides* var. *suis*. Parasitology 39:281–290.

Van den Bossche H, De Nollin S (1973): Effects of mebendazole on the absorption of low molecular weight nutrients by *Ascaris suum*. Int J Parasitol 3:401–407.

Verhoeven HLE, Willemsens G, Van den Bossche H (1980): Uptake and distribution of levamisole in *Ascaris suum*. In H. Van den Bossche (ed): The Host–Invader Interplay. Amsterdam: Elsevier/North-Holland, pp. 573–579.

Watts SDM, Rapson EB, Atkins AM, Lee DL (1982): Inhibition of acetylcholinesterase secretion from *Nippostrongylus brasiliensis* by benzimidazole anthelmintics. Biochem Pharmacol 31:3035–3040.

Wharton DA (1986): A Functional Biology of Nematodes. Baltimore: The Johns Hopkins University Press.

Wilson PAG (1976): Nematode growth patterns and the moulting cycle: The population growth profile. J Zool 179:135–151.

Wright DJ, Newall DR (1980): Osmotic and ionic regulation in nematodes. In B.M. Zuckerman (ed): Nematodes as Biological Models, vol 2. New York: Academic Press, pp. 143–164.

Wright KA (1987): The nematode's cuticle—its surface and the epidermis: Function, homology, analogy—a current consensus. J Parasitol 73:1077–1083.

Molecular Approaches to Parasitology, pages 77–87
© 1995 Wiley-Liss, Inc.

Filariasis: The Role of Chitinase in Larval Development and Transmission

Juliet A. Fuhrman

Department of Biology, Tufts University, Medford, Massachusetts 02155

INTRODUCTION

Filarial nematodes include many species of great medical and veterinary significance. Human filarial infections currently number over 100 million worldwide. Yet, relatively little is known about this major class of parasite and how its members interact with both host and vector. In this chapter, recent results on filarial chitinases are reviewed and their possible role in the interaction of host and parasite discussed.

THE PARASITES

The vast majority of human filarial infections are lymphatic, caused by *Brugia malayi, B. timori,* and *Wuchereria bancrofti.* These infections can lead to elephantiasis and tropical pulmonary eosinophilia. *Onchocerca volvulus,* a skin-dwelling parasite, is the causative agent of "river blindness" and sowdah (dermatitis). *Loa loa,* the eyeworm, causes pronounced allergic inflammation and Calabar swellings. Filarial parasites of animals include several *Onchocerca* spp. and *Dirofilaria immitis,* the dog heartworm.

All filarial parasites are transmitted between vertebrate hosts and arthropod vectors. Within the vertebrate, adult worms produce first-stage larvae through sexual reproduction. These first-stage larvae, known as *microfilariae,* can circulate in the blood (the case for *Brugia* spp., *W. bancrofti,* and *D. immitis*) or migrate through the tissues (the case for *Onchocerca* spp.) of the infected host. The biting arthropod vector must ingest these microfilariae during feeding for continuation of the life cycle.

Filariae can be divided into two groups according to their pattern of embryogenesis: One group produces sheathed microfilariae, and the second group produces unsheathed microfilariae. The former group is exemplified by *Brugia* spp., *W. bancrofti,* and *L. loa.* Examples of the latter group are *D. immitis* and *Onchocerca* spp.

Ellis et al. (1978) and Rogers et al. (1976) have studied the intrauterine development of both kinds of microfilariae. Sheathed microfilariae appear to stretch their eggshell membranes as the larval body develops within, so that later stages of the embryo are elongated rather than round. This elongation continues until birth, at which point the developed larva is no longer folded up within the eggshell, but is fully stretched out and filariform. The remnant of the eggshell that surrounds each larva is now an elongated, extracuticular structure, known as the *sheath*. In contrast, unsheathed microfilariae develop in a different way within the gravid female. The eggshell surrounding the developing larva does not elongate with the growing larva. Instead, the larval body remains tightly curled within the shell until just before birth. At that time, there is an apparent hatching, which releases the larva from the eggshell. The unsheathed microfilaria subsequently emerges from the female. Thus, the two classes of filariae use very different processes during embryogenesis and produce first-stage larvae that differ dramatically at their outermost surface.

Within the arthropod, the microfilariae follow a species-specific pattern of migration and development that is just as complex as the vertebrate portion of their life cycle. The parasites enter the vector's midgut with the bloodmeal, but then migrate to various tissues that serve as their ultimate site for development (see Lavoipierre, 1958, for a comprehensive review). Most species of microfilariae escape from the vector's midgut by penetrating directly through the single epithelial layer that lines this section of the gut tract. In both mosquitoes and black flies, this escape probably occurs before completion of the peritrophic membrane. Once out of the midgut, the microfilariae find their way to various tissues in a species-dependent manner. For *Brugia* spp., *W. bancrofti,* and *Onchocerca* spp., the final destination is the thoracic flight muscles, but other species of filariae develop in the fat body (*L. loa*) or the parenchyma (*L. carinii*). In contrast to those species that penetrate the midgut wall, some species escape through the open end of the Malpighian tubules at the posterior of the gut and develop within the tubules. *D. immitis* is one example of this developmental pattern. Two molts are achieved within these sites, and the resulting third-stage larvae must finally migrate to the insect's mouthparts for delivery to a vertebrate host during a subsequent bloodmeal.

The control of filarial infection and pathogenesis in the vertebrate host has proven a daunting task. As integrated strategies for parasite control gain favor, the significance of the invertebrate phase of the parasite's life cycle becomes apparent. Studies of transmission-blocking immunity in protozoal infections such as malaria (Carter and Chen, 1976; Gwadz, 1976, for example) have led the way in clarifying parasite–vector interactions, and many of the same principles are being investigated in filariasis.

To date, most studies of parasite–vector interactions in filariasis have detailed the physiology and genetics of the insect that determine vector competence. Laboratory-derived strains of *Aedes aegypti* demonstrate a single, sex-linked gene that controls susceptibility to *W. bancrofti, B. malayi,* and *B. pahangi* (MacDonald and Ramachandran, 1965). Yet in the more natural vector group, *A. scutellaris,* inheritance of susceptibility is more complex, with no evidence for a single determining locus (Meek and MacDonald, 1982).

Attributes of the parasite critical to infection are only now being determined. This research is hampered primarily by the absence of genetic markers and mutant strains that could be used to understand the gene products critical to these processes. For this reason, comparison of the developmental pathways among the filarial species may prove helpful in understanding the individual molecules used during migration and infection in the arthropod vector.

IDENTIFICATION OF TWO DEVELOPMENTALLY REGULATED ANTIGENS

Our studies of parasite–vector interactions began with the identification of two antigens, p70 and p75, in the microfilariae of *B. malayi* (Fuhrman et al., 1987). These antigens were defined originally by a monoclonal antibody called *MF1*. Using the MF1 antibody in Western blots, we were able to show that p70 and p75 are not expressed by microfilariae that have recently been shed by adult females. The two molecules appear only after the microfilariae have developed for several days within the vertebrate host. Thus, their expression is developmentally regulated within the first larval stage. In addition, their appearance coincides temporally with the onset of infectivity of microfilariae for the mosquito. Microfilariae that have recently been shed by adult females cannot escape from the mosquito midgut and do not develop to third-stage larvae (deHollanda et al., 1982; Fuhrman et al., 1987). After "maturing" for several days in the vertebrate host, however, the microfilariae become functional with regard to infecting the mosquito.

CLONING THE P70 cDNA

This correlation between expression of p70/p75 and the onset of microfilarial infectivity for the mosquito led to our further analysis of these developmentally regulated proteins. The full sequence of p70 was elucidated at the cDNA level (Fuhrman et al., 1992). As shown for other messages in *Brugia* spp., the p70 message contains the 22 nt spliced leader sequence at its 5′ terminus (Fig. 1). In addition, a 22 amino acid signal peptide is encoded upstream from the known N-terminus of the mature protein (as determined by amino acid sequencing for both p70 and p75). From peptide sequencing of the native proteins, no differences could be found between p70 and p75 over the first two-thirds of the proteins, but several difference peaks could be observed (though not sequenced) from chromatograms of tryptic peptides.

Figure 1.

P70 AND P75 ARE CHITINASES

Several regions of the p70 sequence show significant similarity with sequences of known bacterial and yeast chitinases. Therefore, the microfilarial proteins were tested for chitin-degrading activity using a substrate gel format, wherein chitin is cast in a polyacrylamide gel prior to electrophoresis of the samples (Trudel and Asselin, 1989). Chitinase activity in microfilarial extracts comigrates with p70 and p75 in one-dimensional SDS gels and copurifies with p70 and p75 in ion-exchange chromatography (Fuhrman et al., 1992). Thus, we concluded that p70 and p75 are isoforms of microfilarial chitinase.

The regions of sequence similarity with bacterial and yeast chitinases are confined to the N-terminal two-thirds of the microfilarial proteins, suggesting that p70 and p75 may consist of at least two separate structural domains. Precedents for this come from chitinases described in other organisms, which contain separate catalytic domains followed by C-terminal tails that serve to localize the enzyme to some physiologic substrate (Watanabe et al., 1990; Kuranda and Robbins, 1991). Chitinase activity is retained when these localization domains are removed from the intact molecules. We hoped that, if we could define separate domains within the microfilarial chitinase, we could investigate the function or binding specificity of the C-terminal noncatalytic domain. Affinity studies with this region of the molecule could point to the physiologic substrate for the enzyme or its target molecule during the parasite's development.

Protease digestion of native proteins has been used as a tool to investigate domain structure. The classic example of this technique is the production of Fab and Fc fragments from intact antibodies by cleavage with papain (Porter, 1959). We attempted to excise a catalytic domain from intact p70 and p75 using Glu-C protease. The protease was insolubilized on agarose beads to facilitate its removal from the parasite-derived reaction products. With increasing time of digestion, a 43 kD product is generated by the action of Glu-C protease on purified p70/75 (Fig. 2A, lanes 1–4). The 43 kD fragment is specific to the combination of protease and p70/75 and does not appear in replicate incubations of protease alone (Fig. 2A, lanes 6–9) or purified starting material alone (Fig. 2A, lanes 11–14). The 43 kD fragment shows chitin-degrading activity in substrate gels (Fig. 2B). N-terminal sequence analysis of

Fig. 1. Nucleotide and amino acid sequence for the MF1 antigen. The consensus polyadenylation signal is underlined. Lower case letters on the amino acid line represent the predicted signal peptide. The N-terminal sequence derived from the combined p70 and p75 is underlined with dashes. Peptides sequenced from native p75 are shaded, and peptides sequenced from native p70 are boxed. A triangle marks the peptide unique to p75 tryptic profile.

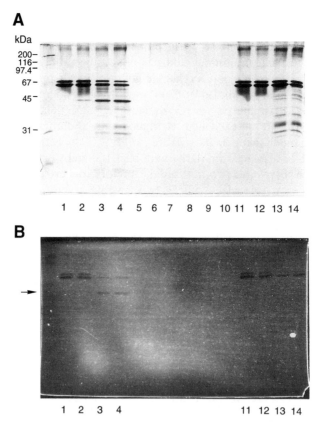

Fig. 2. Glu-C digestion of native p70/75: Purified native p70/75 was digested under nondenaturing conditions with Glu-C agarose, and digestion products were analyzed by electrophoresis following removal of the protease beads by centrifugation. Digestion products from each time point were split and analyzed on both silver-stained gels (**A**) and substrate (chitin-containing) gels (**B**). Digestion times were 0 hours (lanes 1, 6, and 11); 2 hours (lanes 2, 7, and 12); 18 hours (lanes 3, 8, and 13), and 24 hours (lanes 4, 9, and 14). Incubations included p70/75 and Glu-C agarose (lanes 1–4), Glu-C agarose alone (lanes 6–9), and p70/75 alone (lanes 11–14), all at 37°C in PBS.

this fragment demonstrates its identity with the N-terminal sequence of intact p70 and p75. Thus the N-terminal two-thirds of the isozymes forms an enzymatic domain that retains chitin-degrading activity when cleaved from the rest of the molecule.

Unfortunately, no peptides representing the C-terminal fragment could be isolated from the digestion products. This could result from the preponderance of Glu and Asp residues in this section of the protein sequence—perhaps the C-terminal region is completely degraded under these conditions. This has hampered our ability to map conclusively the boundary of the catalytic domain and to isolate the remainder of the molecule for affinity studies. These studies will require the use of different proteases or the production of recombinant fragments.

FUNCTION OF THE MICROFILARIAL CHITINASE

What is the role of microfilarial chitinase in the life cycle of this parasite? Several suggestions stem from studies on other arthropod-borne pathogens. The insect-invasive stages of both malaria and leishmania have been shown to produce chitinase. In malaria, this chitinase has been suggested as a mechanism by which the oocyst can penetrate the peritrophic membrane surrounding the infective bloodmeal (Huber et al., 1991). In leishmania-infected sandflies, it has been proposed that chitinase degrades the pericardial lining, resulting in regurgitation of the bloodmeal (Schlein et al., 1991, 1992). Thus, there is precedence for parasite chitinases degrading structures in the insect vector to potentiate infection or transmission. Microfilarial chitinase could act in this way, though it is not clear what structural barriers might be degraded.

A second possible mode of action for this enzyme is suggested from studies of trypanosome infections in tsetse flies (Maudlin and Welburn, 1987, 1988; Welburn and Maudlin, 1991). Chitinase activity derived from rickettsia-like endosymbionts in the tsetse gut has been postulated to generate oligosaccharide inhibitors of defensive agglutinins. These defensive agglutinins presumably act to prevent the trypanosomes from infecting the fly, but this natural immunity is abrogated by the endosymbiont-generated oligosaccharides. This complex three-party system explains the correlation between endosymbiont infection in the tsetse gut and susceptibility to trypanosome infection. Flies that have been cured of their endosymbionts are refractory to trypanosome infection. A similar mechanism could exist in the mosquito–microfilaria system, but as yet mosquito midgut agglutinins are poorly characterized, and the possibility that such lectins could block microfilarial development has not been tested.

A third possible role for the microfilarial chitinase could involve the microfilarial sheath, a structure shown to bind lectins specific for oligomers of $\beta 1 \rightarrow 4$-linked N-acetylglucosamine (Furman and Ash, 1983; Kaushal et al., 1984; Devaney, 1985; Fuhrman and Piessens, 1985). Since the microfilariae must escape from their sheaths as part of their development in the insect, this exsheathment, and subsequent infection, could depend on enzymatic degradation.

We are using a comparative approach to study these possibilities and to discern the role(s) of chitinase during filarial transmission. This entails an

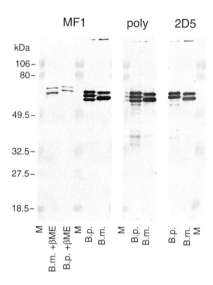

Fig. 3. Chitinase isozymes in brugian microfilariae. Total extracts of microfilariae from *B. malayi* (Bm) or *B. pahangi* (Bp) were Western blotted with two monoclonal antibodies (MF1 and 2D5) or polyclonal mouse antisera raised to gel-purified p70/75. Samples were electrophoresed in the absence or presence (+βME) of mercaptoethanol.

examination of other species to correlate the presence of chitinase activity with particular aspects of filarial development.

For instance, *B. pahangi*, a parasite very closely related to *B. malayi* but not infective to humans, expresses a family of three chitinase isozymes that are closely related to p70/75. The *B. pahangi* isozymes, referred to here as p69, p73, and p76, can be detected by their cross-reactivity with monoclonal and polyclonal antibodies specific for p70/75 (Fig. 3). N-terminal sequence analysis of the purified proteins indicates extensive sequence similarity with the *B. malayi* isozymes (Table 1).

Enzymatic activity of these chitinases was analyzed using oligosaccharide conjugates of 4-methylumbelliferone (4-MU) as substrates. Chitinases have been classified according to their relative exo- and endo-activities, with endochitinases defined as those enzymes that will cleave anywhere within the

TABLE 1. AN-Terminal Sequences of Brugian Chitinase Isozymes

BM p70/75	YVRGCYYTNWAQYRDGEGKFLPGNIPNGLCTHILYAFAKVDEL....
Bp p69	YVRGCYYTNWAQYRDGEGKFLPENIPNGLCTHILYAFAK-
Bp p73	YVRGCYY-
Bp p76	YVRGCYY-

TABLE 2. Cleavage of 4-Methylumbelliferyl (4-MU) Oligosaccharides by Microfilarial Chitinases

Enzyme	Rate[a] of formation of 4-MU from (nmol/min/mg)		
	4-MU disaccharide	4MU-trisaccharide	Ratio (Tri/di)
B. malayi, crude extract	1.92	30.6	16
Purified p70/75	55.2	950	17
B. pahangi, crude extract	1.80	32.0	18
Purified p69/73/76	6.60	95.4	14
D. immitis, crude extract	ND[b]	ND[b]	

[a]Initial rates measured in 50 mM PO_4 buffer, pH 6.5, at 37°C; substrates at 10 µM (disaccharide) and 5µM (trisaccharide)
[b]ND, not detectable.

chain of poly-$\beta 1 \rightarrow 4$-linked N-acetylglucosamine and exochitinases defined as those enzymes that cleave disaccharide units processively from the nonreducing end of the chitin chain (Robbins et al., 1988). While 4-MU-N,N-diacetylchitobioside can be cleaved by either endo- or exochitinase to yield a fluorescent product, 4-MU-N,N,N-triacetylchitotrioside will only yield a fluorescent product upon digestion by an endochitinase. The relative degradative activities of the B. malayi and B. pahangi chitinases on the disaccharide and trisaccharide substrates are presented in Table 2. Clearly, the isozymes from both species of parasite demonstrate functional similarity.

Chitinase activity could not be detected in the microfilariae of D. immitis (Table 2). Both brugian and D. immitis microfilariae circulate in the bloodstreams of infected hosts. Therefore, this disparity may indicate that the brugian chitinase is not inherent to the blood-borne life style in the vertebrate, but rather has to do with either the property of being sheathed or the particular developmental pathway the microfilariae follow within the mosquito. As mentioned previously, the microfilariae of D. immitis do not penetrate through the mosquito midgut or traverse the hemocoel; nor do they have a sheath. Chitinase activity is readily detectable in the adult female of D. immitis and may therefore be involved in embryogenesis or hatching, but we failed to detect this activity in the microfilariae.

CONCLUSION

We have characterized a family of chitinase isozymes from the microfilariae of two brugian parasites. This family consists of five closely related glycoproteins that display endochitinase activity, as measured by the cleavage of 4MU-N,N,N-triacetylchitotriose. In B. malayi microfilariae, this activity appears during development coincident with the onset of microfilarial infectivity for the mosquito vector. No such activity could be detected in microfilariae of *D. immitis*, which differ in structure and development from the brugian larvae. Thus, these molecules offer a well-characterized set of targets to test the possibility of controlling filariasis by interfering with parasite transmission in the insect vector.

REFERENCES

Carter R, Chen DH (1976): Malaria transmission blocked by immunisation with gametes of the malaria parasite. Nature 263:57–60.

de Hollanda JC, Denham DA, et al. (1982): The infectivity of microfilariae of *Brugia pahangi* of different ages to *Aedes aegypti*. J Helminthol 56:155–157.

Devaney E (1985): Lectin-binding characteristics of *Brugia pahangi* microfilariae. Trop Med Parasitol 36:25–28.

Ellis DS, Rogers R, et al. (1978): Intrauterine development of the microfilariae of *Dipetalonema viteae*. J Helminthol 52:7–10.

Fuhrman JA, Piessens WF (1985): Chitin synthesis and sheath morphogenesis in *Brugia malayi* microfilariae. Mol Biochem Parasitol 17:93–104.

Fuhrman JA, Urioste S, et al. (1987): Functional and antigenic maturation of *Brugia malayi* microfilariae. Am J Trop Med Hyg 36:70–74.

Fuhrman JA, Lane W, et al. (1992): Transmission-blocking antibodies recognize microfilarial chitinase in brugian lymphatic filariasis. Proc Natl Acad Sci USA 89:1548–1552.

Furman A, Ash LR (1983): Analysis of *Brugia pahangi* microfilariae surface carbohydrates: Comparison of the binding of a panel of fluoresceinated lectins to mature in vivo–derived and immature in utero–derived microfilariae. Acta Tropica 40:45–51.

Gwadz RW (1976): Malaria: Successful immunisation against sexual stages of *Plasmodium gallinaceum*. Science 193:1150–1151.

Huber M, Cabib E, et al. (1991): Malaria parasite chitinase and penetration of the mosquito peritrophic membrane. Proc Natl Acad Sci USA 88:2807–2810.

Kaushal NA, Simpson AJG, et al. (1984): *Brugia malayi:* Stage-specific expression of carbohydrates containing *N*-acetylglucosamine on the sheathed surface of microfilariae. Exp Parasitol 58:182–187.

Kuranda MJ, Robbins PW (1991): Chitinase is required for cell separation during growth of *Saccharomyces cerevisiae*. J Biol Chem 266:19758–19767.

Lavoipierre MMJ (1958): Studies on the host-parasite relationships of filarial nematodes and their arthropod hosts II. The arthropod as a host to the nematode. Ann Trop Med Parasitol 52:326–345.

MacDonald WW, Ramachandran CP (1965): The influence of the gene fm on the susceptibility of *Aedes aegypti* to seven strains of *Brugia, Wuchereria,* and *Dirofilaria*. Ann Trop Med Parasitol 59:64–73.

Maudlin I, Welburn SC (1987): Lectin mediated establishment of midgut infections of *Trypanosoma congolense* and *Trypanosoma brucei* in *Glossina moristans*. Trop Med Parasitol 38:167–170.

Maudlin I, Welburn SC (1988): Tsetse immunity and the transmission of trypanosomiasis. Parasitol Today 4:109–111.

Meek SR, MacDonald WW (1982): Studies on the inheritance of susceptibility to infection with *B. pahangi* and *W. bancrofti* in the *Aedes scutellaris* group of mosquitoes. Ann Trop Med Parasitol 76:347–354.

Porter RR (1959): The hydrolysis of rabbit γ-globulin and antibodies with crystalline papain. Biochem J 73:119.

Robbins PW, Albright C, et al. (1988): Cloning and expression of *Streptomyces plicatus* chitinase (chitinase-63) in *Escherichia coli*. J Biol Chem 263:443–447.

Rogers R, Ellis DS, et al. (1976): Studies with *Brugia pahangi:* Intrauterine development of the microfilaria and a comparison with other filarial species. J Helminthol 50:251–257.

Schlein Y, Jacobson RL, et al. (1991): Chitinase secreted by *Leishmania* functions in the sandfly vector. Proc R Soc Biol 245:121–126.

Schlein Y, Jacobson RL, et al. (1992): *Leishmania* infections damage the feeding meçhanism of the sandfly vector and implement parasite transmission by bite. Proc Natl Acad Sci USA 89:9944–9948.

Trudel J, Asselin A (1989): Detection of chitinase activity after polyacrylamide gel electrophoresis. Anal Biochem 178:362–366.

Watanabe T, Suzuki K, et al. (1990): Gene cloning of chitinase A1 from *Bacillus circulans* WL-12 revealed its evolutionary relationship to *Serratia* chitinase and to the type III homology units of fibronectin. J Biol Chem 265:15659–15665.

Welburn SC, Maudlin I (1991): Rickettsia-like organisms, puparial temperature and susceptibility to trypanosome infection in *Glossina moristans*. Parasitology 102:201–206.

METABOLISM AND DRUG ACTION

Preface

There are two general routes to get new drugs for treating infectious diseases. The first involves random screening of crude compounds in the hope of finding one that shows the desired properties. One of the most recent, spectacular successes using this approach is the discovery of the avermectin class of compounds, which have a broad spectrum of activity against nematodes. The chapter by Sue Rohrer and Jim Schaeffer retells the story of the discovery of this drug and describes recent data on its mode of action.

The second approach is to make educated guesses about potential targets, characterize those targets in detail, and then design drugs that might be expected to interfere with them. The chapter by the Komunieckis shows the initial stages of such an approach: the elucidation of novel metabolic processes in the parasites, in this case the changes that occur during the switch from aerobic to anaerobic metabolism in *Ascaris*. In the third chapter of this section, Buddy Ullman and Tom Allen present a case in which a novel target has been identified and characterized (hypoxanthine-guanine phosphoribosyltransferase), and they describe initial efforts to exploit differences between host and parasite in the design of new drugs.

Molecular Approaches to Parasitology, pages 93–107
© 1995 Wiley-Liss, Inc.

Ivermectin

Susan P. Rohrer and James M. Schaeffer

Merck Research Laboratories, Rahway, New Jersey 07065

INTRODUCTION

Avermectins are a family of macrocyclic lactones discovered and developed as anthelmintic agents at the Merck Research Laboratories in the middle to late 1970s (Burg et al., 1979; Egerton et al., 1979). They are natural fermentation products synthesized by the soil bacterium, *Streptomyces avermitilis*. The avermectin-producing organism was initially isolated from a soil sample collected in Japan as part of a collaborative agreement between the Merck Research Laboratories and the Kitasato Institute in Tokyo (Burg and Stapley, 1989). The potent anthelmintic activity of the test sample was detected by incorporating the fermentation broth into the diet of mice that had been experimentally infected with the intestinal nematode *Heligmosomoides polygyrus* (*Nematospiroides dubius*) and then monitoring for fecal egg output and presence of worms in the gut as an indication of efficacy. This screen, like many *in vivo* screens, allowed for simultaneous assessment of the compound's efficacy, oral activity and bioavailability, and absence of toxic side effects. Subsequent investigations revealed that this class of compounds also possessed potent insecticidal activity (Ostlind et al., 1979; Putter et al., 1981) but lacked antibacterial or antifungal properties.

GENERAL CHARACTERISTICS OF THE AVERMECTINS

Avermectin nomenclature is based on the biosynthetic variations that occur at the C-5 and the C-22,23 positions and at the C-25 side chain (Fig. 1). The C-5 hydroxy-substituted avermectin analogs (B series) are generally more potent anthelmintic agents than the C-5 methoxy derivatives (A series). In addition to the naturally occurring compounds, a large number of biologically active, semisynthetic analogs have been described in the patent literature (Fisher and Mrozik, 1989). Ivermectin (22,23-dihydroavermectin B_{1a}), a semisynthetic avermectin analog (Chabala et al., 1980), was introduced commercially in 1981 and rapidly became the drug of choice for treating a broad spectrum of

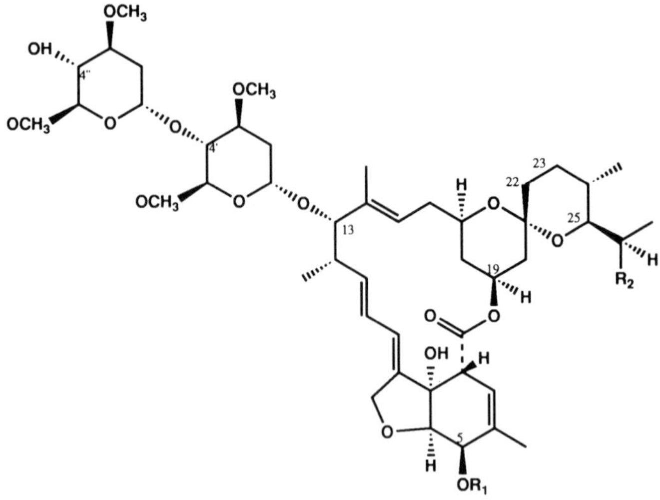

Fig. 1. Naturally occurring avermectins and ivermectin.

Avermectin	R_1	R_2	C_{22}-C_{23}
(1) A_{1a}	CH_3	C_2H_5	CH≏CH
(2) A_{1b}	CH_3	CH_3	CH≏CH
(3) B_{1a}	H	C_2H_5	CH≏CH
(4) B_{1b}	H	CH_3	CH≏CH
(5) A_{2a}	CH_3	C_2H_5	CH_2-CH(OH)
(6) A_{2b}	CH_3	CH_3	CH_2-CH(OH)
(7) B_{2a}	H	C_2H_5	CH_2-CH(OH)
(8) B_{2b}	H	CH_3	CH_2-CH(OH)
(9) Ivermectin	H	C_2H_5	CH_2-CH_2

conditions caused by nematode and arthropod parasites (for review see Campbell, 1985, 1993). Abamectin (avermectin B_{1a}), developed for use as an insecticide in crop protection programs, was introduced in 1985 (Lasota and Dybas, 1991).

Although there is limited need for an antiparasitic drug for human health applications in industrialized nations, the need does exist in many third world nations that are still plagued with a high incidence of parasitic diseases affecting humans. Ivermectin was shown to be effective in the treatment and prevention of human onchocerciasis in West Africa and in Central and South America. A single annual oral dose of ivermectin (Mectizan), administered at 200 µg/kg is sufficient to control microfilaremia and prevent both the dermal and ocular pathologies associated with the infection (Greene et al., 1985; Lariviere et al., 1985; Taylor et al., 1986). Since the half-life of the drug in humans is on the order of hours, the need for only a single dose per year has lead to speculation that avermectins may have a secondary action on the host immune system (Schulz-Key et al., 1992); however, there are no substantive data supporting this hypothesis. It is more likely that 1 year efficacy represents the length of time required for the adult worms to recover and reinitiate production of microfilariae. Mectizan treatment of infected individuals has not produced the severe side effects observed in response to treatment with diethylcarbamazine, and consequently the World Health Organization has initiated a wide spread distribution program for Mectizan in parts of West and Central Africa for the treatment and prevention of human onchocerciasis. The subject of ivermectin use in humans was recently reviewed by Campbell (1991).

Figure 2 graphically presents a list of anthelmintic agents that have been used commercially over the past 50 years as a function of their efficacy. It is apparent that each newly introduced product has been more potent than it's predecessor. Considering the correlation between the relative potencies of anthelmintics shown in Figure 2 and the year of their introduction it appears that ivermectin was discovered 20 years sooner than would have been predicted by the historical trend. Noteworthy for their extraordinary potency against a broad spectrum of endoparasites, the avermectins have proven to be extremely nontoxic to mammals. These features together contribute to the superior therapeutic index displayed by the avermectins over previously dis-

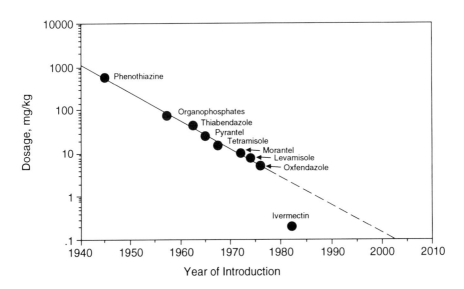

Fig. 2.   Anthelmintics through the ages. (Based on original data borrowed from Campbell, 1986.)

covered anthelmintics. They are also the first widely used anthelmintic agents that are natural fermentation products. Therefore mass production of ivermectin and abamectin could be carried out economically without requiring extensive and costly synthetic chemical processes.

Except for thiabendazole and oxfendazole, which disrupt microtubule assembly (Lacey, 1990), all the compounds shown in Figure 2 are drugs that act on the neuromuscular system of the worm. The organophosphates affect acetylcholinesterase (Knowles and Casida, 1966), pyrantel and morantel are cholinergic agonists (Eyre, 1970; Forbes, 1972), and levamisole and tetramisole act at nicotinic acetylcholine receptors (Lewis et al., 1980). Judging by anthelmintic drugs that have actually been developed and marketed commercially, the worm's neuromuscular system seems an excellent target for chemotherapy. Since the avermectins were so much more potent than all of these other compounds, the discovery generated much interest in their mode of action and whether they too were affecting nematode neuromuscular transmission.

MECHANISM OF ACTION

Initial studies on the mode of action of ivermectin suggested that the biological activity was mediated via an interaction with a ligand-gated chloride channel. The sensitivity of this chloride channel to picrotoxin led to the speculation that ivermectin interacts with GABA-gated chloride channels (Kass et al., 1980). The work of Duce and Scott (1985) and of Zufall et al. (1989) supported the hypothesis that avermectins modulate a chloride channel; however, their results demonstrated that GABA-insensitive cells were responding to ivermectin (for review, see Arena, 1994). Recent work in our group has shown that the *Caenorhabditis elegans* ivermectin-sensitive chloride channel is blocked by picrotoxin but does not respond to GABA. These results support the hypothesis that ivermectin affects a non-GABA-gated chloride channel (Arena et al., 1991).

A major objective in our laboratory has been to isolate and characterize the nematode-specific ivermectin channel from the free-living nematode *C. elegans*. First among the many reasons for selecting this as our model system is the fact that *C. elegans* is sensitive to all known anthelmintic agents. The ease with which the organism can be maintained in the laboratory and the feasibility of culturing massive quantities of worms for large-scale experiments were additional reasons for choosing *C. elegans* over parasitic nematodes. We recently developed a protocol for reproducible cultivation of *C. elegans* worms in 150 liter bioreactors (Gbewonyo et al., 1994). Routine large-scale preparations yielding 500 gm quantities of worms have facilitated much of the biochemistry and molecular biology to be described (Cully and Paress, 1991; Arena et al., 1991, 1992; Rohrer et al., 1992). In addition, the neuromuscular system of *C. elegans* has been well characterized developmentally, biochemically, and physiologically (Chalfie and White, 1988), and the neuronal cytoarchitecture is similar to that of parasitic nematodes (Johnson and Stretton, 1980; Stretton et al., 1985).

C. elegans has become the "*Escherichia coli*" of metazoan organisms due to the availability of a variety of techniques for genetic manipulation. Generation and characterization of mutant phenotypes (Brenner, 1974) and restoration of normal phenotypes by gene transformation (Fire, 1986; Fire et al., 1990) afford one the opportunity to test the functional importance of individual genes once they are cloned; and, since the entire genome of the organism has been cloned in yeast artificial chromosomes (YACs) and cosmids (Coulson et al., 1986, 1988), it is possible to determine the chromosomal location of a gene and to characterize genomic copies of any cDNA clone of interest.

Specific high-affinity ivermectin-binding sites have been identified and thoroughly characterized in membrane preparations isolated from *C. elegans* (Schaeffer and Haines, 1989). The affinities of a series of avermectin analogs for this binding site were determined and compared with the biological activity of each compound in a *C. elegans* motility assay. The strong correlation between the binding affinity and biological activity demonstrated the physiological significance of this binding site. The receptor-binding assay has been used as a simple method for evaluation of a large number of avermectin analogs.

High-affinity ivermectin-binding sites also have been identified in the parasitic nematode *Haemonchus contortus* (Fig. 3). The question of target site involvement in the development of resistance to ivermectin was addressed by comparing ivermectin-sensitive and ivermectin-resistant worms. Membranes were prepared from L3 larvae of both the wild-type susceptible worms and the ivermectin-resistant worms. Both tissue preparations exhibited high-affinity avermectin-binding sites, and the number of sites per milligram of protein was the same, indicating that resistance in this particular strain was not due to a change in the affinity of the receptor for the ligand or in the number of receptors present on the membranes. This experiment also demonstrated that the membrane receptor from a parasitic target organism was nearly identical to the *C. elegans* membrane receptor with respect to affinity for ivermectin (K_d) and receptor density or number of binding sites per milligram of membrane protein (B_{max}). We have used the same-receptor binding assay with minor modifications to examine tissues from a variety of arthropods and nematodes and have demonstrated its utility for conducting comparative biochemical and pharmacological experiments (Rohrer et al., 1994a).

Crude *C. elegans* membrane preparations have been useful for characterizing many aspects of the interaction of ivermectin with the nematode-binding site. However, purification and cloning of the nematode receptor could lead to a more precise understanding of the mechanism of action and facilitate the establishment of new mechanism-based screens for identification of novel

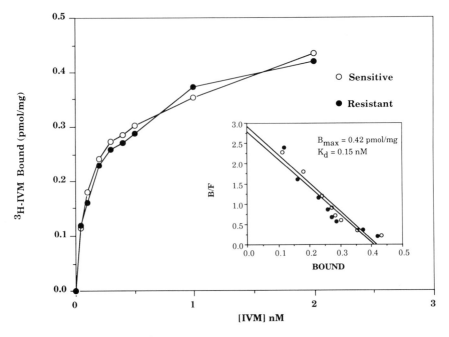

Fig. 3. [³H]ivermectin binding to *H. contortus* membranes. Membranes were prepared from L3 larvae of wild-type and ivermectin-resistant organisms. The assay was performed with 150 µg of membrane protein in 1 ml of 0.05 M Hepes (pH 7.4). [³H]ivermectin at concentrations ranging from 0.05 to 2 nM was incubated with tissue for 1 hour at room temperature. Samples were then filtered over Whatman GF/B filters and washed with 0.5% Triton X-100. (Reproduced from Rohrer et al., 1994b, with permission of the publisher.)

compounds that interact with the same ion channel protein. Because of the inherent difficulties associated with isolation and cloning of ion channel proteins, two independent approaches toward obtaining the *C. elegans* ivermectin-sensitive chloride channel were taken.

BIOCHEMICAL IDENTIFICATION AND ISOLATION OF THE INVERMECTIN RECEPTOR

The purification of the invertebrate ivermectin receptor was facilitated by the use of an azido-AVM analog as a photoaffinity probe (Rohrer et al., 1992). The compound shown in Figure 4 was synthesized (Meinke et al., 1992) and found to be biologically active in the *C. elegans* motility assay as well as in the *C. elegans* ivermectin binding assay in spite of the addition of the large substituent at the 4″ position. The ivermectin receptor was solubilized from *C. elegans* membranes with Triton X-100 and then exposed to the photoaffinity

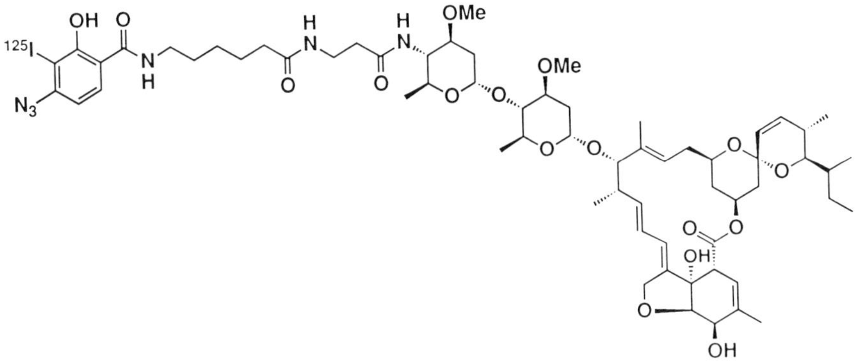

Fig. 4.   Azido-AVM was synthesized from a 4″ amino derivative (Meinke et al., 1992). Biological activity was confirmed in both the *C. elegans* motility assay and in the *C. elegans* [³H]ivermectin binding assay.

probe at room temperature in the dark. After a 1 hour incubation, dextran-coated, activated charcoal was added to adsorb any of the [^{125}I]azido-AVM not bound by high affinity to the receptor.

The affinity ligand was cross-linked to the receptor by exposure of the sample to ultraviolet (UV) light and the result analyzed by autoradiography of an SDS-PAGE gel (Fig. 5). Three *C. elegans* proteins with molecular weights of 53, 47, and 8 kD were radiolabeled. Increasing concentrations of unlabeled ivermectin (lanes 2–5) resulted in elimination of the affinity labeling pattern. The low concentrations of ivermectin required to block the labeling pattern suggested that all three proteins were associated with the high-affinity drug-binding site. It is unknown whether the three labeled proteins represent nonidentical subunits of a multisubunit receptor, metabolic breakdown products of a larger precursor, or tissue-specific forms of the receptor. The scheme for purification of all the proteins associated with this binding site is outlined in Figure 6.

Purification of the photoaffinity labeled *C. elegans* proteins has been accomplished using a monoclonal antibody against avermectin B$_{1a}$ to capture the [^{125}I]azido-AVM–labeled proteins (Rohrer et al., 1994c). The antibody was purified by ammonium sulfate precipitation and Protein A Sepharose chromatography before coupling it to CNBr Sepharose beads. After UV cross-linking, the crude mixture of Triton X-100–soluble *C. elegans* membrane proteins was partially purified under denaturing conditions on a Sephacryl S-300 gel filtration column. Pooled fractions containing the 53 and 47 kD affinity labeled proteins are shown in lane 1 of Figure 7. Lane 2 shows the same protein sample after incubation with and removal of the anti-AVM Sepharose beads.

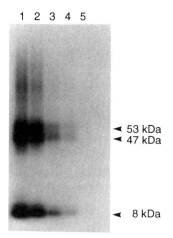

Fig. 5. Photoaffinity labeling of the *C. elegans* avermectin binding site. Autoradiography of a 5–20% polyacrylamide gel showed that three proteins with molecular weights of 53, 47, and 8 kD were associated with the high-affinity binding site. Each lane contained 200 mg of Triton X-100–soluble membrane protein. *C. elegans* proteins were labeled with [^{125}I]azido-AVM in the absence of unlabeled ivermectin (lane 1) or in the presence of of 0.2, 0.8, 2, or 20 nM ivermectin (lanes 2–5). (From Rohrer et al., 1992.)

The anti-AVM Sepharose beads specifically bound all of the [^{125}I]azido-AVM–labeled receptor protein and left behind the unrelated proteins visible by Coomassie blue staining. The receptor proteins were eluted from the anti-AVM Sepharose beads with SDS-PAGE gel loading buffer (lane 4).

The insect receptor from *Drosophila melanogaster* has been studied using the same approach. The [^{3}H]ivermectin-binding assay indicated that membranes isolated from heads contained a high-affinity avermectin-binding site ($K_d = 0.2$ nM). The number of binding sites per milligram of protein was 10-fold greater than what was observed for homogenates of *C. elegans*. Due to the increased concentration of high-affinity binding sites associated with this tissue, the *Drosophila* receptor was pursued in order to obtain pure receptor in sufficient quantities for amino acid sequencing. Photoaffinity labeling of the *Drosophila* head membranes resulted in identification of an apparent doublet in the 45 kD size range (Fig. 8). Labeling was blocked by ivermectin at low concentrations, indicating that these two proteins are part of the high-affinity drug-binding site. A biologically inactive avermectin analog (3,4,8,9,10,11,22,23-octahydroavermectin B$_{1a}$), did not block the labeling pattern, consistent with the interpretation that the two proteins at 45 kD were specific labeling products. As with the *C. elegans* ivermectin receptor, the anti-AVM monoclonal antibody was used to capture affinity-labeled *Drosophila* proteins after partial purification by gel filtration chromatography under denaturing conditions.

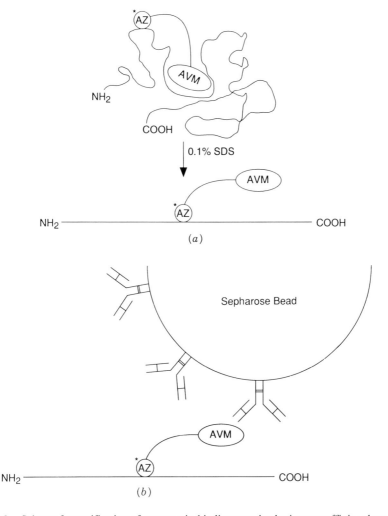

Fig. 6. Scheme for purification of avermectin-binding proteins by immunoaffinity chromatography. Photoaffinity labeled avermectin-binding proteins from *C. elegans* and *Drosophila*
were purified according to this scheme. After the affinity labeling step, the crude protein mixture was denatured by boiling in the presence of SDS and dithiothreitol and then partially
purified over a Sephacryl S-300 gel filtration column. Fractions containing the photoaffinity
labeled proteins were pooled and dialyzed and then incubated with anti-AVM Sepharose
beads in order to facilitate capture of the receptor proteins via the covalently linked
avermectin ligand. (From Rohrer et al., 1994c.)

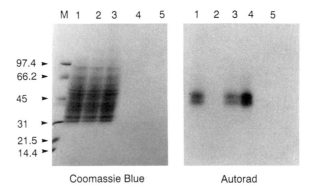

Fig. 7. Immunoprecipitation of the photoaffinity labeled AVM binding proteins from *C. elegans*. The anti-AVM monoclonal antibody was coupled to CNBr Sepharose. Aliquots of the partially purified *C. elegans* protein mixture containing both the 53 and the 47 kD labeled proteins were incubated with 100 ml aliquots of the anti-AVM beads. The 53 and 47 kD labeled proteins present in the untreated control (lane 1) were eliminated from the supernatant by virtue of their binding interaction with the anti-AVM Sepharose beads. The purified receptor proteins were recovered from the anti-AVM beads by elution with 5% SDS in 50 mM Tris, pH 6.8 (lane 4). Lane 3 served as the negative control for this experiment. A purified murine IgG1 with no specificity for avermectin was coupled to CNBr Sepharose. This reagent did not bind the affinity labeled *C. elegans* proteins. (From Rohrer et al., 1994c.)

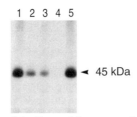

Fig. 8. Photoaffinity labeling of the *Drosophila* avermectin binding proteins. Autoradiography of a 5–20% gradient gel showed affinity labeled proteins with molecular weights of approximately 45 kD. The affinity labeled product appeared to be a doublet (lane 1). In the presence of increasing concentrations of unlabeled ivermectin (0.1, 1, and 10 nM in lanes 2–4 respectively) the labeling pattern was progressively blocked, indicating that the 45 kD doublet was associated with the high-affinity site. The inactive analog octahydro avermectin added at a concentration of 1 nM did not block labeling (lane 5), indicating specificity of the labeling result shown in lane 1. (From Rohrer et al., 1994a.)

ELECTROPHYSIOLOGY AND PHARMACOLOGY OF THE IVERMECTIN RECEPTOR

The tough cuticle and small size of neuronal cell bodies precluded the use of standard electrophysiological techniques for the characterization of the *C. elegans* ivermectin channel in whole worm preparations. Therefore, the *Xenopus* oocyte system was explored as a surrogate for expression of the *C. elegans* ivermectin gated channel. This approach consisted of isolating mRNA from *C. elegans* and injecting it into *Xenopus* oocytes, allowing the protein translational and processing machinery of the oocyte to express a functional ion channel from the nematode mRNA (Arena et al., 1991, 1992; Arena, 1994). Application of ivermectin to *C. elegans* mRNA-injected oocytes caused opening of chloride channels present on the oocyte surface. Water-injected or -uninjected *Xenopus* oocytes served as negative controls and displayed no such responses. The opening of channels by ivermectin was irreversible and consistent with tight binding of the ligand to the channel protein previously observed with the [³H]ivermectin binding assay and *C. elegans* membranes (Arena et al., 1991; Schaeffer and Haines, 1989).

The avermectin-sensitive chloride current expressed in *C. elegans* mRNA-injected oocytes was not responsive to GABA or to glycine but could be activated by application of glutamate. The amplitude of channel opening by coapplication of ivermectin and glutamate was the same as the response observed with maximal concentrations of either glutamate or ivermectin alone, suggesting that the two compounds were interacting with the same chloride ion channel. Opening of the channel by glutamate or ivermectin could be inhibited by high concentrations of picrotoxin.

The critical experiment for understanding the interaction of ivermectin with this glutamate gated chloride channel was performed by first subjecting *C. elegans* mRNA-injected oocytes to a submaximal concentration of glutamate (Arena et al., 1992). The glutamate was washed out of the bath, and then ivermectin was added at a concentration insufficient for eliciting a response (10 nM). Subsequent coapplication of glutamate and ivermectin resulted in a sixfold increase in the response to glutamate. The interpretation of this result was that low concentrations of ivermectin could potentiate the interaction of glutamate with its receptor-binding site. Therefore it appears that ivermectin at high concentrations (>10 nM) directly opens the channel whereas ivermectin at low concentrations (<10 nM) potentiates channel opening by glutamate. Glutamate has no effect on [³H]ivermectin binding, suggesting that glutamate and ivermectin act at separate and distinct sites on the same channel (Fig. 9).

The avermectins are highly selective for invertebrate chloride ion channels and only interact with vertebrate receptors at high concentrations. They appear to act on a GABA gated chloride channel in vertebrate brain as shown in

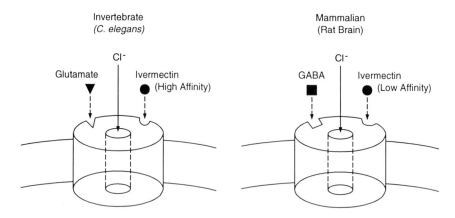

Fig. 9. Simplified schematic representation of the invertebrate and vertebrate chloride ion channels under avermectin control.

Figure 9. Since avermectins do not readily cross the blood–brain barrier, only very low concentrations ever come in contact with vertebrate receptors. The combination of lower affinity and compartmentalization of host receptors may account for the low incidence of host toxicity with this class of compounds.

CONCLUSION

The *Xenopus* oocyte expression system is currently being used as a functional assay for direct cloning of the *C. elegans* ivermectin-sensitive chloride channel. Purification of the photoaffinity labeled *Drosophila* avermectin-binding proteins has been scaled up in order to facilitate recovery of sequenceable amounts of pure protein. Therefore, cloning of the nematode and insect receptors appears imminent. The native configuration and conformation of the ion channel, localization of the receptor in nematode and insect tissue preparations, cloning of homologous ion channel protein genes from parasitic nematodes and arthropods, and developmental regulation of the expression of this gene constitute a partial list of the studies that will be performed once the gene is cloned.

The next major challenge lies in testing the hypothesis that cloning of the target will facilitate the discovery of new chemical entities. The avermectin gated chloride channel is likely to be similar to other ion channel proteins known to possess multiple discrete drug-binding sites. Mammalian GABA receptors, for example, have separate nonoverlapping binding sites for GABA, benzodiazepines, barbiturates, cyclodienes, avermectin and picrotoxin, any one of which can interfere with normal channel function. Identification of novel compounds that modulate the invertebrate avermectin-sensitive chloride channel could provide new leads for anthelmintic drug development. If additional drug-binding sites exist on the nematode and insect avermectin-sensitive chloride channels, functionally based assays designed around the cloned receptors should result in their elucidation and lead to the discovery of nonavermectin agonists for these unique invertebrate ion channels.

ACKNOWLEDGMENTS

Many people at Merck were involved in the work that has been presented. Ed Hayes, Ethel Jacobson, and Elizabeth Birzin were key players in the affinity labeling and purification experiments. Doris Cully and Joe Arena, with assistance from Philip Paress and Ken Liu, carried out the characterization of the *C. elegans* receptor expressed in *Xenopus* oocytes. Helmut Mrozik, Peter Meinke, and Tom Shih provided chemistry support for the projects described here and synthesized numerous other avermectin analogues. Kodzo Gbewonyo, Leonard Lister, and Bruce Burgess provided *C. elegans* tissue from large-scale preparations at the fermentation plant. Scott Costa was responsible for rearing the large quantities of *Drosophila* flies needed for receptor purification. Clint Eary and Wes Shoop supplied the *H. contortus* larvae used in the [^{3}H]ivermectin-binding assay. We would also like to acknowledge the support of Merv Turner, Roy Smith, and Mike Fisher.

REFERENCES

Arena JP, Liu KK, Paress PS, Cully DF (1991): Avermectin-sensitive chloride currents induced by *Caenorhabditis elegans* RNA in *Xenopus* oocytes. Mol Pharmacol 40:368–374.

Arena JP, Liu KK, Paress PS, Schaeffer JM, Cully DF (1992): Expression of a glutamate-activated chloride current in *Xenopus* oocytes injected with *Caenorhabditis elegans* RNA: evidence for modulation by avermectin. Mol Brain Res 15: 339–348.

Arena JP (1994): Expression of *Caenorhabditis elegans* mRNA in *Xenopus* oocytes: A model system to study the mechanism of action of avermectins. Parasitol Today 10:35–37.

Brenner S (1974): The genetics of *C. elegans*. Genetics 77:71-94.

Burg RW, Miller BM, Baker EE, Birnbaum J., Currie SA, Hartman R, Kong YL, Monaghan RL, Olson G, Putter I, Tunac JB, Wallick H, Stapley EO, Oiwa R, Omura S (1979): Avermectins, new family of potent anthelmintic agents: Producing organism and fermentation. Antimicrob Agents Chemother 15:361–367.

Burg RW, Stapley EO (1989): Isolation and characterization of the producing organism. In W.C. Campbell (ed): Ivermectin and Abamectin. New York: Springer-Verlag, pp. 24–32.

Campbell WC (1985): Ivermectin: an update. Parasitol Today 1:10–16.

Campbell WC (1986): Historical introduction. In W.C. Campbell, R.S. Rew (eds): Chemotherapy of Parasitic Diseases. New York: Plenum Press, pp. 3–21.

Campbell WC (1991): Ivermectin as an antiparasitic agent for use in humans. Annu Rev Microbiol 45:445–474.

Campbell WC (1993): Ivermectin, an antiparasitic agent. Medicinal Res Rev 13:61–79.

106 / Rohrer and Schaeffer

Chabala JC, Mrozik H, Tolman RL, Eskola P, Lusi A, Peterson LH, Woods MF, Fisher MH (1980): Ivermectin, a new broad-spectrum antiparasitic agent. J Med Chem 23: 1134–1136.
Chalfie M, White J (1988): The nervous system. In W.B. Wood (ed): The Nematode *Caenorhabditis elegans*. NY: Cold Spring Harbor Laboratory, pp. 337–391.
Coulson A, Sulston J, Brenner S, Karn J (1986): Toward a physical map of the genome of the nematode *Caenorhabditis elegans*. Proc Natl Acad Sci USA 83:7821–7825.
Coulson A, Waterston R, Kiff J, Sulston J, Kohara Y (1988): Genome linking with yeast artificial chromosomes. Nature 335:184–186.
Cully DF, Paress PS (1991): Solubilization and characterization of a high affinity ivermectin binding site from *Caenorhabditis elegans*. Mol Pharmacol 40:326–332.
Duce IR, Scott RH (1985): Actions of dihydroavermectin B_{1a} on insect muscle. Br J Pharmac 85:395–401.
Egerton JR, Ostlind DA, Blair LS, Eary CH, Suhayda D, Cifelli S, Riek RF, Campbell WC (1979): Avermectins, new family of potent anthelmintic agents: efficacy of the B_{1a} component. Antimicrob Agents Chemother 15:372–378.
Eyre P (1970): Some pharmacodynamic effects of the nematocides: Methyridine, tetramisole and pyrantel. J Pharm Pharmacol 22:26–36.
Fire A (1986): Integrative transformation of *C. elegans*. EMBO J 5:2673–2680.
Fire A, Harrison SW, Dixon D (1990): A modular set of LacZ fusion vectors for studying gene expression in *C. elegans*. Gene 93:189–198.
Fisher MH, Mrozik H (1989): Chemistry. In W.C. Campbell (ed): Ivermectin and Abamectin. New York: Springer-Verlag, pp. 1–23.
Forbes L (1972): Toxicological and pharmacological relations between levamisole, pyrantel and diethylcarbamazine and their significance in helminth chemotherapy. Southeast Asian J Trop Med Publ Health 3:235–241.
Gbewonyo K, Rohrer SP, Lister L, Burgess B, Cully D, Buckland B (1994): Large scale cultivation of the free living nematode *Caenorhabditis elegans*. Biotechnology 12:51–54.
Greene BM, Taylor HR, Cupp EW, Murphy RP, White AT, Aziz MA, Schulz-Key H, D'Anna SA, Newland HS, Goldschmidt, LP, Auer C, Hanson AP, Freeman SV, Reber EW, Williams PN (1985): Comparison of ivermectin and diethylcarbamazine in the treatment of onchocerciasis. N Engl J Med 313:33–138.
Johnson CD, Stretton AOW (1980): Neural control of locomotion in *Ascaris*: Anatomy, electrophysiology, and biochemistry. In B.M. Zuckerman (ed): Nematodes as Biological Models. New York: Academic Press, pp. 159–195.
Kass IS, Wang CC, Walrond JP, Stretton AOW (1980): Avermectin B_{1a}: A paralyzing anthelmintic that affects interneurons and inhibitory motor-neurons in *Ascaris*. Proc Nat Acad Sci USA 77:6211–6215.
Knowles CO, Casida JE (1966): Mode of action of organophosphate anthelmintics. Cholinesterase inhibition in *Ascaris lumbricoides*. J Agric Food Chem 14:566–572.
Lacey E (1990): Mode of action of benzimidazoles. Parasitol Today 6:112–115.
Lariviere M, Aziz MA, Weimann D, Ginoux J, Gaxotte P, Vinotain P, Brauvae B, Derouin F, Schulz-Key H, Barret D, Sarfati C. (1985): Double-blind study of ivermectin and diethylcarbamazine in African onchocerciasis patients with ocular involvement. Lancet 2:174–177.
Lasota JA, Dybas RA (1991): Avermectins, a novel class of compounds: Implications for use in arthropod pest control. Annu Rev Entomol 36:91–117.
Lewis J, Wu C, Levine J, Berg H (1980): Levamisole resistant mutants of the nematode *Caenorhabditis elegans* appears to lack pharmacological acetylcholine receptors. Neuroscience 5:967–989.

Meinke PT, Rohrer SP, Hayes EC, Schaeffer JM, Fisher MH, Mrozik H (1992): Affinity probes for the avermectin binding proteins. J Medicinal Chem 35:3879–3884.

Ostlind DA, Cifelli S, Lang R (1979): Insecticidal activity of the antiparasitic avermectins. Vet Rec 105:168.

Putter I, MacConnell JG, Preiser FA, Haidri AA, Ristich SS, Dybas RA (1981): Avermectins: Novel insecticides, acaricides and nematicides from a soil microorganism. Experientia 37:963–964.

Rohrer SP, Meinke PT, Hayes EC, Mrozik H, Schaeffer JM (1992): Photoaffinity labeling of avermectin binding sites from *Caenorhabditis elegans* and *Drosophila melanogaster*. Proc Natl Acad Sci USA 89:4168–4172.

Rohrer SP, Birzin E, Costa S, Arena JP, Hayes EC, Schaeffer JM (1993a): Avermectin binding sites from *Drosophila melanogaster* and *Schistocerca americana*. Biochem J (submitted for publication).

Rohrer SP, Birzin E, Eary C, Schaeffer JM, Shoop W (1993c): Ivermectin binding sites in sensitive and resistant *Haemonchus contortus*. J Parasitol (submitted for publication).

Rohrer SP, Jacobson EB, Hayes EC, Birzin E, Schaeffer JM (1993b): Immunoaffinity purification of avermectin binding proteins from *Caenorhabditis elegans* and *Drosophila melanogaster*. Anal Biochem (submitted for publication).

Rohrer SP, Birzin ET, Costa SD, Arena JP, Hayes EC, Schaeffer JM (1994a): Identification of neuron-specific ivermectin binding sites in *Drosophila melanogaster* and *Schistocerca americana*. Insect Biochemistry and Molecular Biology (in press).

Rohrer SP, Birzin ET, Eary CH, Schaeffer JM, Shoop WL (1994b): Ivermectin binding sites in sensitive and resistant *Haemonchus contortus*. J Parasitol 80:493–497.

Rohrer SP, Jacobson EB, Hayes EC, Birzin ET, Schaeffer JM (1994c): Immuno-affinity purification of avermectin binding proteins from *Caenorhabditis elegans* and *Drosophila melanogaster*. Biochem J (in press).

Schaeffer JM, Haines HW (1989): Avermectin binding in *Caenorhabditis elegans*: A two-state model for the avermectin binding site. Biochem Pharmacol 38:2329–2338.

Schulz-Key H, Soboslay PT, Hoffman WH (1992): Ivermectin-facilitated immunity. Parasitol Today 8:152–153.

Stretton AOW, Davis RE, Angstadt JD, Donmoyer JE, Johnson CD (1985): Neural control of behavior in *Ascaris*. Trends Neurosci 8:294–300.

Taylor HR, Murphy RP, Newland HS, White AT, D'Anna SA, Keyvan-Larijani E, Aziz MA, Cupp EW, Greene BM (1986): Comparison of the treatment of ocular onchocerciasis with ivermectin and diethylcarbamazine. Arch Opthalmol 104:863–870.

Zufall F, Franke C, Hatt H (1989): The insecticide avermectin B_{1a} activates a chloride channel in crayfish muscle membrane. J Exp Biol 142:191–205.

Molecular Approaches to Parasitology, pages 109–121
© 1995 Wiley-Liss, Inc.

Aerobic–Anaerobic Transitions in Energy Metabolism During the Development of the Parasitic Nematode *Ascaris suum*

Richard Komuniecki and Patricia R. Komuniecki

Department of Biology, University of Toledo, Toledo, Ohio 43606

INTRODUCTION

Most parasitic helminths exhibit marked aerobic–anaerobic transitions during their development, with adults possessing varying abilities to generate energy anaerobically even in the presence of oxygen (Komuniecki and Harris, 1994; Tielens and van den Bergh, 1993; Kohler, 1991). The parasitic nematode *Ascaris suum* is probably the best studied and, because of its large size and microaerobic habitat, the most anaerobic of these helminths (Komuniecki and Harris, 1994; Kita, 1992). In this chapter, we discuss changes in mitochondrial function as the parasite switches from aerobic to anaerobic metabolism. The reader is referred to the chapter by Müller for relevant details of the biology of *Ascaris*.

Mitochondria from early ascarid larval stages contain a functional tricarboxylic acid cycle (TCA) cycle and are cyanide (CN) sensitive. In contrast, mitochondria from later larval stages and adult body wall muscle are CN insensitive and use unsaturated organic acids, such as fumarate and 2-methyl branched-chain enoyl CoAs, instead of oxygen as terminal electron acceptors. The pathway of anaerobic carbohydrate dissimulation in adult ascarid muscle mitochondria has been well characterized and is summarized in Figure 1. It results in the accumulation of a complex mixture of reduced organic acids, including acetate, propionate, succinate, and the branched-chain fatty acids (BFA) 2-methylbutyrate and 2-methylvalerate as the major end products of carbohydrate metabolism. In fact, BFA levels may reach 100 mM and rival Cl^- as the most abundant anions in the perienteric fluid (Sims et al., 1992).

These anaerobic organelles generate energy through both substrate-level

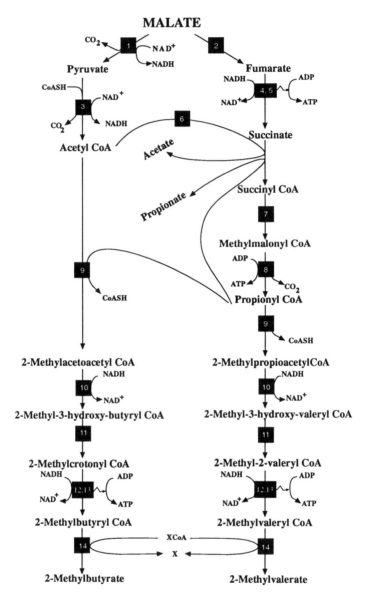

Fig. 1. Enzymes involved in malate metabolism in mitochondria from *Ascaris suum* body wall muscle. The numbers in the boxes represent the following enzymes: 1, malic enzyme, Allen and Harris (1981); 2, fumarase, Payne et al. (1979); 3, pyruvate dehydrogenase complex, Komuniecki et al. (1979), Thissen et al. (1986); 4, 5, succinate-CoQ reductase (complex II, fumarate reductase), Kita et al. (1988), Takamiya et al. (1984, 1986); 6, acyl CoA transferase, McLaughlin et al. (1986); 7, methylmalonyl mutase, Han et al. (1984); 8, methylmalonyl

phosphorylations, coupled to the decarboxylation of methylmalonyl CoA, and site 1 electron-transport–associated phosphorylations, coupled to the NADH-dependent reductions of fumarate and 2-methyl branched-chain enoyl CoAs (Kita, 1992). An outline of electron transport in mitochondria from adult body wall muscle is presented in Figure 2. Surprisingly, the magnitude of the proton gradient in these anaerobic organelles appears to be similar to that reported for aerobic mitochondria, even though they appear to contain only a single site of proton translocation (Chojnicki et al., 1987). Adult ascarid muscle mitochondria appear to be designed exclusively for the generation of energy in the absence of oxygen. They contain no functional TCA cycle, no β-oxidation, and no urea cycle, and amino acid metabolism is very limited. Both the mitochondrial matrix and membrane-bound enzymes involved in these novel anaerobic pathways are quite abundant, and each has been purified to homogeneity and at least partially characterized (Fig. 1).

Surprisingly, the properties of these enzymes generally are quite similar to those reported for the corresponding enzymes from aerobic tissues except for those specific properties that have been under the intense selective pressures associated with the exploitation of microaerobic habitats. For example, although the amino acid sequence of the 2-methyl branched-chain enoyl CoA reductase is over 60% identical to the human medium chain acyl CoA dehydrogenase, it has a different substrate specificity, regulatory properties, and reactivity with oxygen, and physiologically catalyzes a reaction opposite to that of the mammalian enzyme (Komuniecki et al., 1985; Duran et al., 1993). For this reason, these ascarid enzymes should serve as excellent comparative models for the establishment of structure–function relationships within these enzyme families.

Even though much is known about the pathway and enzymes of anaerobic energy generation, little is known about the timing or regulation of this process. How different are the enzymes in ascarid mitochondria from aerobic and anaerobic stages? Are only a few key enzymes modified, or is the transition accompanied by a wholesale substitution of anaerobic and aerobic specific isozymes? What role does oxygen play in metabolism by anaerobic muscle mitochondria? When do the switches from aerobic to anaerobic and anaerobic to aerobic occur? What factors trigger these switches?

---

decarboxylase, Saz and Pietrzak (1980); 9, propionyl CoA condensing enzyme, Suarez de Mata et al. (1991); 10, 2-methyl acetoacetate CoA reductase, Suarez de Mata et al. (1983); 11, 2-Methyl-3-oxo-acyl CoA hydratase; 12, electron transfer flavoprotein, Komuniecki et al. (1989); 13, 2-methyl branched chain enoyl CoA reductase, Komuniecki et al. (1985); 14, acyl CoA transferase, Saz and deBruyn (1987).

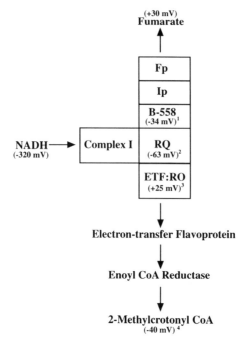

Fig. 2.   Pathway of NADH-dependent 2-methyl branched-chain enoyl CoA reduction in muscle mitochondria of adult *Ascaris suum*. F_p, flavoprotein of fumarate reductase (Kita, 1992); I_p, iron-sulfur flavoprotein of fumarate reductase (Kita, 1992). Source of redox potentials: 1 and 2, Kita et al. (1990); 3, Ma et al. (1993); 4, Lenn et al. (1990). (Reproduced from Ma et al., 1993, with permission of the publisher.)

HOW DIFFERENT ARE THE ENZYMES IN MITOCHONDRIA FROM AEROBIC AND ANAEROBIC ASCARID STAGES?

It is clear that a number of different strategies have been operative in the evolution of the adult ascarid muscle mitochondria for functioning in a microaerobic environment. These are summarized in Table 1. Some enzymatic activities that are nonessential to the functioning of anaerobic pathways have been deleted or reduced to very low levels. These include citrate synthase, aconitase, isocitrate dehydrogenase, α-ketoglutarate dehydrogenase, and re-duced cytochrome c oxidase. Complex III (reduced ubiquinone:cytochrome c oxidoreductase) is still present, but at greatly reduced levels, although it appears to play no significant role in electron transport (Takamiya et al., 1993). Perhaps its recently identified role in the processing of proteins imported into the mitochondrial matrix accounts for its partial retention (Braun et al., 1992)? In contrast, some enzymes are tremendously overexpressed in accord with

TABLE 1. Modifications of Classic Aerobic Mitochondria for Anaerobic Energy Generation in Body Wall Muscle of the Adult Parasitic Nematode *Ascaris suum*

Deletion or reduction of nonessential activities
  Ubiquinone
  Complex III (ubiquinone:cytochrome *c* oxidoreductase)
  Reduced cytochrome *c* oxidase
  Citrate synthase, aconitase, isocitrate dehydrogenase, α-ketoglutarate dehydrogenase
Overexpression of key enzymes
  Pyruvate dehydrogenase complex (PDC)
  Complex II (succinate:ubiquinone oxidoreductase)
  ETF:rhodoquinone oxidoreductase (ETF:RO)
  2-Methyl branched-chain enoyl CoA reductase
Altered kinetics
  Apparent K_ms for pyruvate and CoA of the PDC
  Fumarate stimulation of malic enzyme
  E_ms of the *b* cytochrome of complex II and the iron-sulfur and flavin centers of ETF:RO
Expression of novel components
  Rhodoquinone
  Protein Y of PDC
Expression of anaerobic-specific isozymes
  E1α subunit of PDC
  2-Methyl branched-chain enoyl CoA reductase
  ?

their new function in anaerobic pathways and are found at specific activities up to 10-fold greater than those present in the corresponding aerobic organelles. These include the pyruvate dehydrogenase complex (PDC), which is more abundant in adult ascarid mitochondria than in any other mitochondria studied; complex II (succinate:ubiquinone oxidoreductase), which functions as a fumarate reductase; and key enzymes involved in the formation of BFAs, such as the ETF:rhodoquinone oxidoreductase (ETF:RO) and the 2-methyl branched chain enoyl CoA reductase. Finally, anaerobic mitochondria contain some novel components that do not appear to be found in the corresponding aerobic organelles. For example, rhodoquinone ($E_m = -63$ mV) replaces ubiquinone ($E_m = +110$ mV) in anaerobic electron-transport chains. Rhodoquinone's much more negative midpoint potential facilitates electron transfer from NADH to either fumarate or enoyl CoAs. In fact, rhodoquinone appears to be essential if significant rates of fumarate reduction are to be achieved, and it is found in all helminths capable of significant rates of succinate formation (Kita, 1992; Kita et al., 1990). Protein Y of the PDC also appears to be much more abundant in anaerobic muscle mitochondria and may play a role in the regulation of PDH_a kinase activity (Komuniecki et al., 1992).

In addition to being overexpressed, many of the enzymes present in the adult ascarid muscle mitochondria have properties that differ significantly from those reported for similar enzymes from aerobic mitochondria and that appear to be modified to function under the reducing conditions present in the anaerobic ascarid organelle. For example, many of the kinetic properties of the ascarid PDC are significantly different from those reported for mammalian PDCs. For example, the apparent K_ms for both pyruvate and CoA are substantially altered and are probably important in the inhibition of PDH_a kinase activity and the maintenance of low intramitochondrial CoA levels, respectively (Thissen et al., 1986; Thissen and Komuniecki, 1988). Reduced levels of free CoA greatly facilitate the reversal of β-oxidation observed during the switch to anaerobic pathways. Similarly, both the PDC and its associated kinase are much less sensitive to elevated NADH:NAD$^+$ ratios (Thissen et al., 1986). Other enzymes also exhibit altered regulatory properties. For example, stimulation of ascarid malic enzyme by fumarate plays an important role in regulating malate dismutation (Landsperger et al., 1978). Finally, the E_ms of the *b* cytochrome of complex II and the iron-sulfur and flavin centers of the ETF:rhodoquinone oxidoreductase appear to be poised to function efficiently in a more reduced environment (Hata-Tanaka et al., 1988; Kita et al., 1988; Ma et al., 1993).

While it is clear that many of the properties of the enzymes present in adult ascarid muscle mitochondria differ from their counterparts in mammalian mitochondria, there is little direct evidence for the existence of anaerobic-specific isozymes, since few of these enzymes have also been characterized in aerobic ascarid stages. Takamiya et al. (1993) demonstrated that the ratio of apparent K_m values for fumarate and succinate in complex II changed from 0.79 to 0.04 in membranes isolated from aerobic larval and anaerobic adult muscle mitochondria, respectively, and suggested the existence of stage-specific isozymes that favored fumarate reduction in the adult muscle mitochondria. More directly, we have recently demonstrated the existence of two distinct α-pyruvate dehydrogenase (E1α) subunits in *A. suum* that are designed to function in either aerobic or anaerobic environments (Johnson et al., 1992). E1α subunits from mammalian PDCs contain three distinct phosphorylation sites, and inactivation of the PDC is associated almost exclusively with the phosphorylation of site 1. Phosphorylation of the additional sites "locks" the complex in an inactive state, since they appear to be the preferred sites for the PDH_b phosphatase. Not surprisingly, phosphorylation and inactivation of the PDC in anaerobic muscle mitochondria is modified (Thissen and Komuniecki, 1988; Komuniecki and Thissen, 1989). The elevated NADH:NAD$^+$ ratios found in adult muscle mitochondria stimulate PDH_a kinase activity and have the potential to inactivate the PDC at a time when maximal carbon flux is needed to maintain energy generation during the switch to less energy efficient anaerobic pathways. The E1α subunit isolated from adult muscle contains only two phosphorylation sites, and phosphorylation of both sites is required for complete inactivation, effectively maintaining at least a portion of the PDC in the active state. This altered regulation coupled with the overexpression of the PDC and its reduced sensitivity to elevated $NADH:NAD^+$ ratios maintains the PDC in an active state in the reduced, microaerobic environment encountered in the porcine gut. cDNAs for both E1α subunits have been cloned and sequenced (Johnson et al., 1992). They are 85% identical but differ in the number of phosphorylation sites. One contains the two phosphorylation sites identified in the PDC from adult muscle by direct sequencing of tryptic phosphopeptides and is associated with the modified phosphorylation and inactivation described above. The other contains the three phosphorylation sites found in PDCs from aerobic organisms. Most importantly, Northern blotting indicates that the mRNA coding for the E1α with two phosphorylation sites is specific for anaerobic muscle. These results are the first report of physiologically significant aerobic- and anaerobic-specific isozymes in any parasitic helminth. Similar results indicate that the 2-methyl branched-chain enoyl CoA reductase also is anaerobic muscle specific and developmentally regulated (Duran et al., 1993). As mentioned above, this enzyme is similar in many respects to acyl CoA dehydrogenases from aerobic organisms but operates in the opposite direction in anaerobic mitochondria during the final step in the synthesis of branched-chain fatty acids. Over 50% of the fatty acids in "egg" triglycerides are 2-methyl branched-chain derivatives and are converted to carbohydrate during aerobic development by the action of the glyoxylate cycle and β-oxidation (Saz and Lescure, 1966). Therefore, distinct aerobic- and anaerobic-specific enzymes must be present to account for the oxidation of BFA in aerobic larvae and its synthesis in adult muscle. Taken together, these results suggest that the conversion from aerobic to anaerobic metabolism is accompanied by significant changes in the mitochondrial polypeptide composition.

WHAT ROLE DOES OXYGEN PLAY IN METABOLISM BY ADULT MUSCLE MITOCHONDRIA?

All adult parasitic helminths generate a portion of their energy anaerobically but have varying degrees of aerobic capacity. Small nematodes, such as *Nippostrongylus braziliensis,* which lie close to the mucosa where oxygen tensions are high, are largely aerobic, while large nematodes, such as *A. suum,* probably represent the anaerobic extreme (Kita, 1992; Paget et al., 1987). All helminth mitochondria will take up oxygen if it is available, and this has led to postulation of a variety of branched electron-transport pathways, which include both CN-sensitive and CN-insensitive terminal oxidases. The presence of these different terminal oxidases has been inferred from results with different inhibitors but, to date, no CN-insensitive terminal oxidase has been purified from any helminth mitochondria. It is clear that adult *A. suum* muscle mitochondria lack significant reduced cytochrome *c* oxidase activity and that oxygen uptake results almost exclusively in the formation of hydrogen peroxide (Kita, 1992; Kohler, 1985). In fact, there is no compelling evidence for the existence of a physiological terminal oxidase in these mitochondria. To the contrary, the existing evidence suggests that peroxide formation results from the interaction of oxygen directly with a number of the reduced flavoproteins functioning physiologically in anaerobic pathways. Many of these flavins appear to be more reactive with oxygen than their aerobic counterparts and, at least in the case of the ETF:RO, would be expected to be almost fully reduced under physiological conditions given the midpoint potentials of rhodoquinone, the iron-sulfur and flavin components of the ETF:RO, and the 2-methyl branched-chain enoyl CoA/acyl CoA couple (R. Komuniecki et al., 1985; Ma et al., 1993). In addition, both malonate, an inhibitor of the fumarate reductase, and antisera to the ETF:RO significantly inhibit peroxide formation in submitochondrial particles incubated with NADH (Komuniecki, unpublished data). While the mechanism of this inhibition is unclear, it implicates the involvement of these flavoproteins in peroxide formation and further supports the notion that these organelles lack a specific terminal oxidase.

TRANSITION FROM AEROBIC TO ANAEROBIC METABOLISM

Ascarid second-stage larvae (L2) contain a functional TCA cycle and significant cytochrome oxidase activity and are aerobic (Saz et al., 1968; Barrett, 1976). Third-stage larvae (L3) isolated directly from rabbit lungs also are aerobic and CN-sensitive, but after 3 days in culture molt to fourth-stage larvae (L4) and begin to produce the BFA characteristic of the anaerobic pathways of the adult (Komuniecki and Vanover, 1987; Vanover-Dettling and Komuniecki, 1989). Surprisingly, freshly isolated L3, in contrast to L2, also contain most of the enzymes necessary for BFA formation from malate. For example, the 2-methyl branched-chain acyl CoA dehydrogenase and its mRNA are absent from L2 but are found at significant levels in L3 (Duran et al., 1993). Whether aerobic- and anaerobic-specific enzymes are found in the same mitochondria or compartmentalized into different mitochondria or different muscle cells is unclear at present. In general, nematodes exhibit cell constancy, and growth is accompanied by little increase in cell number. It is of interest to note that in *A. suum* the switch from aerobic to anaerobic energy metabolisms is accompanied by an enormous proliferation of body wall muscle cells, which increase in number from 600 to about 21×10^3 during the development of the L4 (O'Grady, 1984). Whether these cell divisions, which are a specific adaptation to the large size of *A. suum,* represent the proliferation of anaerobic-specific muscle cells and whether a limited number of aerobic muscle cells persist in the adult remain to be determined. The preparation of high titer specific antisera to many of the anerobic-specific proteins should facilitate immunocytochemical approaches to answer these questions. A number of other intriguing questions also remain unanswered. For example, even though the L3 contain most of the enzymes of anaerobic metabolism, they are still CN-sensitive and do not make BFA. What additional development is necessary for the transition to anaerobiosis? What enzymatic machinery is involved in rhodoquinone biosynthesis, and how is it regulated? In addition, little is known about the physiological factors triggering the transition to anaerobic pathways. An elevation of the pCO_2 is important, but a reduction in oxygen tension does not appear to be essential (Komuniecki and Vanover, 1987; Vanover-Dettling and Komuniecki, 1989).

TRANSITION FROM ANAEROBIC TO AEROBIC METABOLISM

Much less is known about the transition from anaerobic to aerobic metabolism that occurs in the embryo ("egg") after it leaves the host. The embryonation process is oxygen dependent and after 22 days at 25°C results in the development of an infective, aerobic L2 within the egg shell (Barrett, 1976). Unembryonated eggs have low levels of rhodoquinone and cytochrome oxidase activity, and development to the L2 is accompanied by a 2,000-fold increase in cytochrome oxidase activity and substantial synthesis of ubiquinone (Takamiya et al., 1993). Both processes are potentially interesting and warrant further study. For example, cytochrome oxidase is a mosaic of subunits coded for by both mitochondrial and nuclear genomes, but the regulation of its synthesis or the potential existence of some of these subunits in the unembryonated "egg" is unknown. Recently, we demonstrated that sperm, and apparently oocyte, mitochondria contain greatly elevated levels of the TCA cycle enzymes, although these organelles still generate energy anaerobically and lack significant cytochrome oxidase activity (Komuniecki et al., 1993). For example, the specific activities of citrate synthase and isocitrate dehydrogenase are over 100-fold greater in sperm mitochondria than adult muscle mitochondria and, in fact, are higher than activities reported from some aerobic mitochondria. Since these mitochondria do not have an operational TCA cycle, it is tempting to speculate that these enzymes have been synthesized for use later during the embryonation process. The function of sperm mitochondria during fertilization in *A. suum* is unclear but is potentially different from that observed in other organisms. *A. suum* sperm are ameboid and relatively large and contain about 100 mitochondria (Burghardt and Foor, 1978; Sepsenwol et al., 1989). In contrast to the situation in vertebrates, ascarid sperm mitochondria represent a potentially major contribution to the mitochondrial pools of the oocyte that contains about 1,000 mitochondria prior to fertilization. However, little is known about the functioning of either sperm or oocyte mitochondria in the early embryo or the potential persistence or inheritance of sperm mitochondria during *A. suum* development. Interestingly, by the four-cell stage, about 40% of ascarid embryonic DNA is mitochondrial, and it is estimated that about 25×10^3 mitochondria are present (Tobler and Gut, 1974; Cleavinger et al., 1989). This suggests that mitochondrial biogenesis is rapid in early embryos, even though they appear to be largely transcriptionally inactive, and lends support for the potential importance of preformed proteins. However, the number of mitochondria present in the four-cell stage may need to be examined more directly since the estimates of mitochondrial number do not appear to consider the estimate of eight DNA molecules per fertilized egg mitochondria calculated by Rodrick et al. (1977).

CONCLUSION

The enzymatic changes associated with the aerobic–anaerobic transition in developing *A. suum* larvae have been defined, and most of the enzymes crucial for the operation of these pathways in the adult have been purified and characterized. In contrast, virtually nothing is known about the factors regulating these events or the underlying molecular or genetic mechanisms governing mitochondrial biogenesis during these respiratory transitions. This situation should change rapidly now that the problem can be defined in molecular terms. In addition, as discussed in detail in the chapter by Gruidl et al., the development of a transformation system in the free-living nematode *Caenorhabditis elegans,* the dramatic progress made in sequencing its genome, and the development of an in vitro transcription system from 32-cell ascarid "eggs" should provide additional tools for the study of transcriptional regulation in parasitic nematodes (Grant, 1992; Maroney et al., 1990).

REFERENCES

Allen BL, Harris BG (1981): Purification of malic enzyme from *Ascaris suum* using NAD+-agarose. Mol Biochem Parasitol 2:367–372.
Barrett J (1976): Intermediary metabolism in *Ascaris* eggs. In H. Van den Bossche (ed): Biochemistry of Parasites and Host–Parasite Relationships. Amsterdam: Elsevier, pp. 117–123.
Braun H, Emmermann M, Kruft VV, Smitz UK (1992): The general mitochondrial processing peptidase from potato is an integral part of cytochrome *c* reductase of the respiratory chain. EMBO J 11:3219–3227.
Burghardt RC, Foor WE (1978): Membrane fusion during spermiogenesis in *Ascaris.* J Ultrastruct Res 62:190–202.
Chojnicki K, Dudzinska M, Wolanska P, Michejda J (1987): Membrane potential in mitochondria of *Ascaris.* Acta Parasitol Pol 32:67–78.
Cleavinger PJ, McDowell JW, Bennet K (1989): Transcription in nematodes: Early *Ascaris* embryos are transcriptionally active. Dev Biol 133:600–604.

Duran E, Komuniecki R, Komuniecki PR, Wheelock MJ, Klingbeil MM, Ma Y-C, Johnson K (1993): Characterization of cDNA clones for the 2-methyl branched chain enoyl CoA reductase from *Ascaris suum*. J Biol Chem 268:22391–22396.

Grant WN (1992): Transformation of *Caenorhabditis elegans* with genes from parasitic nematodes. Parasitol Today 8:344–346.

Han Y, Bratt JM, Hogenkamp HPC (1984): Purification and characterization of methylmalonyl-CoA mutase from *Ascaris lumbricoides*. Comp Biochem Physiol 78B:41–45.

Hata-Tanaka A, Kita K, Furushima R, Oya H, Itoh S (1988): ESR studies on iron-sulfur clusters of complex II in *Ascaris suum* mitochondria, which exhibits strong fumarate reductase activity. FEBS Lett 242:183–186.

Johnson KR, Komuniecki R, Sun Y, Wheelock MJ (1992): Characterization of cDNA clones for the alpha subunit of pyruvate dehydrogenase from *Ascaris suum*. Mol Biochem Parasitol 51:37–47.

Kita K (1992): Electron-transfer complex of mitochondria in *Ascaris suum*. Parasitol Today 8:155–159.

Kita K, Takamiya S, Furushima R, Ma Y, Suzuki H, Ozawa T, Oya H (1988): Electron transfer complexes of *Ascaris suum* muscle mitochondria. III. Composition and fumarate reductase activity of complex II. Biochim Biophys Acta 935:130–140.

Kita K, Takamiya S, Furushima R, Suzuki H, Ozawa T, Oya H (1990): Indispensability of rhodoquinone in the NADH-fumarate reductase system of *Ascaris muscle* mitochondria. In G. Lenaz, O. Barnabei, A. Rabbi, M. Battino (eds): Highlights in Ubiquinone Research. London: Taylor and Francis, pp. 174–177.

Kohler P (1985): The strategies of energy-conservation in helminths. Mol Biochem Parasitol 17:1–18.

Kohler P (1991): Energy metabolism in helminths. In AJ Woakes, MK Greishaber, CR Bridges (eds): Physiological Strategies for Gas Exchange and Metabolism. Cambridge: Cambridge University Press, pp. 15–34.

Komuniecki PR, Johnson J, Kamhawi M, Komuniecki R (1993): Mitochondrial heterogeneity in the parasitic nematode, *Ascaris suum*. Exp Parasitol 76:424–437.

Komuniecki PR, Vanover L (1987): Biochemical changes during the aerobic–anaerobic transition in *Ascaris suum* larvae. Mol Biochem Parasitol 22:241–248.

Komuniecki R, Fekete S, Thissen J (1985): Purification and characterization of the 2-methyl-branched chain acyl CoA dehydrogenase, an enzyme involved in the enoyl CoA reduction in anaerobic mitochondria of the nematode: *Ascaris suum*. J Biol Chem 260:4770–4777.

Komuniecki R, Harris B (1995): Helminth carbohydrate metabolism. In J Marr, M Mueller (eds): Parasite Biochemistry and Molecular Biology. New York: Academic Press (in press).

Komuniecki R, Komuniecki PR, Saz HJ (1979): Purification and properties of the *Ascaris* pyruvate dehydrogenase complex. Biochim Biophys Acta 571:1–11.

Komuniecki R, McCrury J, Thissen J, Rubin N (1989): Electron-transfer flavoprotein from anaerobic *Ascaris suum* mitochondria and its role in NADH-dependent 2-methyl branched-chain enoyl CoA reduction. Biochim Biophys Acta 975:127–131.

Komuniecki R, Rhee R, Bhat D, Duran E, Sidawy E, Song H (1992): The pyruvate dehydrogenase complex from the parasitic nematode *Ascaris suum*: Novel subunit composition and domain structure of the dihydrolipoyl tranacetylase component. Arch Biochem Biophys 196:115–121.

Komuniecki R, Thissen J (1989): The pyruvate dehydrogenase complex from the parasitic nematode, *Ascaris suum*: Stoichiometry of phosphorylation and inactivation. Ann NY Acad Sci 573:175–182.

Landsperger WJ, Fodge DW, Harris BG (1978): Kinetic and isotope-partitioning studies on the NAD$^+$ malic enzyme from *Ascaris suum*. J Biol Chem 253:1868–1873.

Lenn ND, Stankovich MT, Liu H (1990): Regulation of the redox potential of general acyl-CoA dehydrogenase by substrate binding. Biochemistry 29:3709–3715.

Ma Y-C, Funk M, Dunham WR, Komuniecki R (1993): Purification and characterization of electron-transfer flavoprotein: rhodoquinone oxidoreductase from anaerobic mitochondria of the adult parasitic nematode, *Ascaris suum*. J Biol Chem 268:20360–20365.

Maroney PA, Hannon GJ, Nielsen TW (1990): Transcription and cap trimethylation of a nematode spliced leader RNA in a cell-free system. Proc Natl Acad Sci USA 87:709–713.

McLaughlin GL, Saz HJ, deBruyn BS (1986): Purification and properties of an acyl CoA transferase from *Ascaris suum* muscle mitochondria. Comp Biochem Physiol 83B:523–527.

O'Grady RT (1984): Changes in the somatic musculature of the fourth-stage larvae of *Ascaris suum* Goetze, 1782 (Nematoda: Ascaridoidea). Parasitology 88:141–151.

Paget TA, Fry M, Lloyd D (1987): Effects of inhibitors on the oxygen kinetics of *Nippostrongylus braziliensis*. Mol Biochem Parasitol 22:125–133.

Payne DM, Powley DG, Harris BG (1979): Purification, characterization and presumptive role of fumarase in the energy metabolism of *Ascaris suum*. J Parasitol 65:833–841.

Rodrick GE, Carter CE, Woodcock CLF, Fairbairn D (1977): *Ascaris suum:* Mitochondrial DNA in fertilized eggs and adult body muscle. Exp Parasitol 42:150–156.

Saz HJ, deBruyn BS (1987): Separation and function of two acyl CoA transferases from *Ascaris lumbricoides* mitochondria. J Exp Zool 242:241–245.

Saz HJ, Lescure OL (1966): Interrelationships between the carbohydrate and lipid metabolism of *Ascaris lumbricoides* eggs and adult stages. Comp Biochem Physiol 18:845–857.

Saz HJ, Lescure OL, Bueding E (1968): Biochemical observations of *Ascaris suum* lung-stage larvae. J Parasitol 54:457–461.

Saz HJ, Pietrzak SM (1980): Phosphorylation associated with succinate decarboxylation to propionate in *Ascaris* mitochondria. Arch Biochem Biophys 202:399–404.

Sepsenwol S, Ris H, Roberts TM (1989): A unique cytoskeleton associated with crawling in the amoeboid sperm of the nematode, *Ascaris suum*. J Cell Biol 108:55–66.

Sims SM, Magas LT, Barshun CL, Ho NFH, Geary T, Thompson DP (1992): Mechanisms of microenvironmental pH regulation in the cuticle of *Ascaris suum*. Mol Biochem Parasitol 53:135–148.

Suarez de Mata Z, Arevalo J, Saz HJ (1991): Propionyl-CoA condensing enzyme from *Ascaris* muscle mitochondria II. Coenzyme A modulation. Arch Biochem Biophys 258:166–171.

Suarez de Mata Z, Zarranz ME, Lizardo R, Saz HJ (1983): 2-methylacetoacetyl coenzyme A reductase from *Ascaris* muscle: Purification and properties. Arch Biochem Biophys 226:84–93.

Takamiya S, Furushima R, Oya H (1984): Electron transfer complexes of *Ascaris suum* muscle mitochondria. I. Characterization of NADH-cytochrome *c* reductase (complex I–III), with special reference to cytochrome localization. Mol Biochem Parasitol 13:121–134.

Takamiya S, Furushima R, Oya H (1986): Electron-transfer complexes of *Ascaris suum* muscle mitochondria. II. Succinate coenzyme Q reductase (complex II) associated with substrate-reduceable cytochrome b_{558}. Biochim Biophys Acta 848:99–107.

Takamiya S, Kita K, Wang H, Weinstein P, Hiraishi A, Oya H, Aoki T (1993): Developmental changes in the respiratory chain of *Ascaris* mitochondria. Biochim Biophys Acta 1141:65–74.

Thissen J, Desai S, McCartney P, Komuniecki R (1986): Improved purification of the pyruvate dehydrogenase complex from *Ascaris suum* body wall muscle and characterization of PDH kinase activity. Mol Biochem Parasitol 21:129–138.

Thissen J, Komuniecki R (1988): Phosphorylation and inactivation of the pyruvate dehydrogenase from the anaerobic parasitic nematode, *Ascaris suum:* Stoichiometry, and amino acid sequence around the phosphorylation sites. J Biol Chem 263:19092–19097.

Tielens AGM, van den Bergh SG (1993): Aerobic and anaerobic energy metabolism in the life cycle of parasitic helminths. In PW Hochachka, PL Lutz, T Sick, M Rosenthal, G van den Thillert (eds): Surviving Hypoxia—Mechanisms of Control and Adaptation. Ann Arbor, MI: CRC Press, pp. 19–40.

Tobler H, Gut C (1974): Mitochondrial DNA from 4-cell stages of *Ascaris lumbricoides.* J Cell Sci 16:593–601.

Vanover-Dettling L, Komuniecki PR (1989): Effect of gas phase on carbohydrate metabolism of *Ascaris suum* larvae. Mol Biochem Parasitol 36:29–40.

Molecular Approaches to Parasitology, pages 123–141
© 1995 Wiley-Liss, Inc.

Hypoxanthine-Guanine Phosphoribosyltransferase in Trypanosomatids: A Rational Target for Antiparasitic Chemotherapy

Buddy Ullman and Thomas E. Allen

Department of Biochemistry and Molecular Biology, Oregon Health Sciences University, Portland, Oregon 97201

INTRODUCTION

Parasitic protozoa cause a plethora of devastating and often fatal diseases in humans and their domestic animals. Due to the virtual absence of effective vaccines, chemotherapy often offers the only line of defense in the treatment and control of diseases of parasitic origin. The contemporary arsenal of drugs that are used to treat parasitic diseases is far from ideal, however, and the need for more efficacious and improved therapies is acute. In this chapter, we describe recent results on hypoxanthine–guanine phosphoribosyltransferase and its potential as a target for antiparasitic chemotherapy.

CURRENT STATE OF PARASITE CHEMOTHERAPY

Currently available drugs are often moderately to severely toxic, exhibit mutagenic and carcinogenic properties in appropriate test systems, and require protracted therapy with multiple drug administrations. Most of these antiparasitic agents were either discovered or designed empirically, and the lack of absolute selectivity of many of these compounds for the parasite biochemical machinery is presumably based on the lack of target specificity between parasite and host. Furthermore, many parasitic diseases lack satisfactory remedies altogether, and for those diseases such as malaria in which previously reliable drugs have been accessible, drug resistance has materialized as a devastating impediment to treatment. This dramatic emergence of drug resistance and therapeutic failure, in addition to the intrinsic toxicity of many antiparasitic agents, has exacerbated the necessity for more selective and effective therapeutic and prophylactic antiparasitic agents. Unfortunately, as most parasitic diseases are localized mainly in the tropical and subtropical regions of the world, most pharmaceutical companies and governmental agencies anticipate little financial reward in the search for new antiparasitic compounds, and, as a consequence, the search for new drugs is a limited priority.

The establishment of an effective parasite-specific therapeutic regimen for the treatment of any parasitic disease depends on a fundamental understanding of the various metabolic pathways of the cell. The rational design of chemotherapeutic protocols based on biochemical differences between the infectious agent and host cells has been a goal of scientists for decades. Such fundamental metabolic discrepancies form the basis of many antibacterial remedies, such as the ability of penicillin and its derivatives to interfere with bacterial cell wall biosynthesis. Such rational underpinnings also exist for certain antineoplastic regimens, such as leucovorin rescue of methotrexate toxicity or leucovorin enhancement of 5-fluorouracil efficacy. Due to the vast phylogenetic distance that separates mammals and parasitic protozoa, one might expect a high probability of unmasking therapeutically exploitable biochemical or metabolic differences between the parasite and the host in order to treat or prevent disease.

Unfortunately, our knowledge about the basic biochemistry and metabolic pathways of parasites that might eventually prove amenable to chemotherapeutic intervention has progressed slowly for a number of reasons, including limited financial resources, lack of scientific familiarity with third world diseases, occasional difficulties in parasite cultivation, and general lack of excitement within the scientific community for pharmacological investigations. However, fundamental structural, molecular, and metabolic differences between parasite and host do exist, and exploitation of these discrepancies is a mechanism by which selective and rational antiparasitic chemotherapies could be formulated (Fairlamb, 1989; Wang, 1984). For instance, parasites of several genera possess unique intracellular organelles, such as the kinetoplast, the glycosome, and the hydrogenosome. Parasites of the Trypanosomatidae family perform an assortment of molecular oddities not found in mammalian systems, including *trans*-splicing, RNA editing, the synthesis of polycistronic mRNAs, and the amplification of small extrachromosomal elements. Finally, novel metabolic pathways in parasitic protozoa provide the most promising avenue for antiparasitic therapy. The sequestration of glycolysis and electron transport in unique organelles, differences in polyamine and thiol metabolism, e.g., trypanothione, and in nucleotide and folate biosynthetic pathways are perhaps the best characterized of the metabolic pathways that are discrepant between parasite and mammalian host.

PURINE AND PYRIMIDINE METABOLISM IN PARASITIC PROTOZOA

Perhaps the most striking metabolic disparity between parasites and human cells is the pathway by which the two groups generate purine nucleotides. Whereas mammalian cells can synthesize the purine ring *de novo* from ribose-5-phosphate, all of the parasitic protozoa studied to date, including *Plasmodia* (Walsh and Sherman, 1968), *Trypanosoma* (Berens et al., 1981; Fish et al., 1982), *Leishmania* (Marr et al., 1978), *Toxoplasma* (Schwartzman and Pfefferkorn, 1982), *Giardia* (Wang and Aldritt, 1983), *Eimeria* (Wang and Simashkevich, 1981), *Entamoeba* (Boonlayangoor, et al., 1980), and *Trichomonas* (Miller and Linstead, 1983), are auxotrophic for purines (Table 1). To scavenge host purines for their own use, each genus of parasite has evolved a unique series of purine salvage enzymes that enable them to scavenge host purines. The purine auxotrophy and the constitution of the purine salvage systems in these parasites have been demonstrated experimentally by the composition requirements for growth in defined culture media and by radiolabeled precursor and purine incorporation studies. The unusual nature of this purine auxotrophy in parasitic protozoa is bolstered by the fact that this purine biosynthetic pathway is remarkably conserved throughout evolution and consists of the same linear progression of 10 catalytic reactions that produce inosine 5´-monophosphate (IMP) from phosphoribosylpyrophosphate (PRPP), amino acids, and one-carbon compounds. Whether parasitic protozoa lack one, several, or all of the enzymes involved in IMP biosynthesis has not been ascertained. Once IMP, the first purine nucleotide of the de novo pathway, is synthesized, the pathway branches, and IMP is converted either to adenylate or guanylate nucleotides. The branchpoint enzymes are found in most parasitic protozoa with the exception of *G. lamblia* (Wang and Aldritt, 1983), *E. histolytica* (Boonlayangoor, et al., 1980), and *T. vaginalis* (Miller and Linstead, 1983).

TABLE 1. Genera or Species of Parasitic Protozoa in Which Auxotrophy for Purines, Pyrimidines, or Deoxyribonucleosides Has Been Established

Purine	Pyrimidine	Deoxynucleoside
Leishmania	*Giardia*	*Giardia*
Plasmodia	*Trichomonas*	*Trichomonas*
Toxoplasma	*Tritrichomonas*	
Trichomonas		
Giardia		
Trypanosoma cruzi		
Trypanosoma brucei		
Eimeria		
Entamoeba		

In contrast to the universal auxotrophy for purines, most parasitic protozoa are prototrophic for pyrimidines and synthesize pyrimidine nucleotides by a pathway similar to that found in higher eukaryotes. A notable and unique feature of the pyrimidine pathway in many parasitic protozoa is the bifunctional dihydrofolate reductase/thymidylate synthase polypeptide that catalyzes the synthesis of thymidylate nucleotides for DNA synthesis (Garrett et al., 1984). Dihydrofolate reductase and thymidylate synthase are biochemically distinct proteins in mammalian cells. Although the general rule for parasitic protozoa is purine auxotrophy and pyrimidine prototrophy, there are exceptions. *T. vaginalis* (Hill et al., 1981) and *G. lamblia* (Lindmark and Jarroll, 1982) are both incapable of synthesizing pyrimidines, as well as purines (Table 1). Moreover, *T. vaginalis* (Wang and Cheng, 1984) and *G. lamblia* (Baum et al., 1989) are obligatory scavengers of deoxyribonucleosides, suggesting that they lack a functional ribonucleotide reductase activity, or at least a ribonucleotide reductase that lacks the broad substrate specificity of its mammalian counterpart (Table 1).

Although mammalian cells manifest a complement of purine salvage enzymes, the purine salvage system of each parasite is unique and differs significantly from its counterpart in the mammalian host. Thus, the purine salvage system, at least in the abstract, affords an opportunity for identifying specific targets within the parasite that might be amenable to therapeutic manipulation. The precise nature of the purine salvage pathway systems varies considerably among the various parasitic protozoa and probably evolved as a response to the diverse environmental milieus in which the parasites reside. For instance, *T. vaginalis* (Hill et al., 1981) and *E. histolytica* (Lo and Wang, 1985) convert purine bases through the nucleoside to the nucleotide level, thereby bypassing the necessity of phosphoribosyltransferases, enzymes that are critical for purine salvage in most parasites. *G. lamblia* funnels purines into adenine and guanine followed by phosphoribosylation to the nucleotide level (Wang and Simashkevich, 1981). Neither *T. vaginalis* (Hill et al., 1981), *E. histolytica* (Lo and Wang, 1985), nor *G. lamblia* (Wang and Aldritt, 1983) interconvert adenylate and guanylate nucleotides, another unusual feature. *Plasmodia* (Walsh and Sherman, 1968), *Trypanosoma* (Berens et al., 1981; Fish et al., 1982), *Leishmania* (Marr et al., 1978), *Toxoplasma* (Schwartzman and Pfefferkorn, 1982), and *Eimeria* (Wang and Simashkevich, 1981) rely largely on phosphoribosyltransferase activities for purine salvage and express the enzymatic machinery to convert IMP to both AMP and GMP. Currently, it is the purine salvage pathways of *Trypanosoma* and *Leishmania* that offer the most promise for chemotherapy in that a number of lead compounds with antitrypanosomal and antileishmanial activity that are activated by the purine enzymatic machinery have been identified and one, allopurinol, has been exploited clinically.

PURINE METABOLISM IN TRYPANOSOMA AND LEISHMANIA

The purine salvage pathway of *Trypanosoma* and *Leishmania* is cursorily presented in Figure 1. The major sources of host purines to which these parasites have access are adenylate and guanylate nucleotides and inosine and hypoxanthine. Several cell surface phosphatases and nucleotidases that dephosphorylate nucleotides have been characterized in *L. donovani* (Dwyer and Gottlieb, 1984), and extracellular nucleosides and nucleobases can be imported into the parasite by a variety of facilitated diffusion mechanisms (Aronow et al., 1987). The translocated host purines can then be efficiently converted to the nucleotide level by a myriad of different enzymatic activities.

Purine-metabolizing enzymes that have been identified in trypanosomatids include phosphoribosyltransferases, nucleosidases, a nucleoside phosphotransferase, adenosine phosphorylase, adenosine kinase, and adenine deaminase, although not all activities are expressed in both *Trypanosoma* and

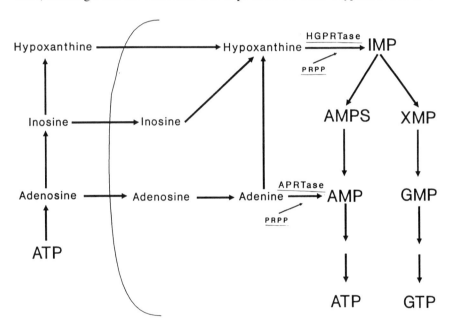

Fig. 1.   The purine salvage pathway of *Trypanosoma* and *Leishmania*. The purine metabolic pathway in trypanosomatids is cursorily outlined to the right of the curved line. The production of salvageable purines in mammalian cells is indicated to the left of the curved line. In mammalian cells ATP is dephosphorylated to adenosine, deaminated to inosine, and phosphorylyzed to hypoxanthine. Trypanosomatids can transport any of the dephosphorylated purines. All of the indicated catalytic reactions have been found in all stages of *T. brucei*, *T. cruzi*, and *L. donovani* except the conversion of adenine to hypoxanthine, which is catalyzed by adenine deaminase and is found only in the promastigote stage of *L. donovani*.

Leishmania or in all life stages of the parasite (Hammond and Gutteridge, 1984). Metabolic flux studies measuring rates of radiolabeled purine incorporation indicated that *Leishmania* promastigotes funnel adenine via adenine deaminase and inosine via a nucleosidase into hypoxanthine, which implies that hypoxanthine–guanine phosphoribosyltransferase (HGPRT) plays a critical role in the salvage of all purine bases (Marr et al., 1978; LaFon et al., 1982). The prominence of HGPRT in purine salvage by *Leishmania* promastigotes was corroborated by mutational analyses in *L. donovani* genetically deficient in some component of purine salvage (Iovannisci et al., 1984). Purine metabolism in *Leishmania* amastigotes, however, differs somewhat from that in promastigotes. Amastigotes lack adenine deaminase, suggesting that adenine is directly phosphoribosylated and, therefore, that adenine phosphoribosyltransferase (APRT), as well as HGPRT, plays a central nutritional function in the mammalian stage of the parasite (Looker et al., 1983). Thus, HGPRT and APRT are both important purine salvage enzymes in *Leishmania*.

Moreover, the provision of the PRPP substrate for purine base phosphoribosylation by HGPRT and APRT should not be overlooked. PRPP synthetase, the enzyme that catalyzes PRPP synthesis, is just as essential as the two phosphoribosyltransferases to purine salvage in *Leishmania* and other parasites that phosphoribosylate purines. Adenine deaminase is also absent in both *Trypanosoma cruzi* and *Trypanosoma brucei* (Hammond and Gutteridge, 1984). Otherwise, the complement of purine salvage enzymes in the pathogenic *Trypanosoma* appears similar to that in *Leishmania* (Hammond and Gutteridge, 1984). All the biochemical, kinetic, and genetic data on purine salvage in *Trypanosoma* and *Leishmania*, however, do not indicate which routes are critical to the purine salvage process when parasites induce disease in the mammalian host. The precise delineation of the relative importance of specific enzymes to purine salvage by intact parasites can now begin to be addressed, at least in *Leishmania* and *T. cruzi*, by appropriate gene knockout technology.

Pyrazolopyrimidines

The unique features of the purine salvage system of *Leishmania* and *Trypanosoma* cause a selective susceptibility to the cytotoxic effects of several pyrazolopyrimidine analogs of the naturally occurring purines hypoxanthine and inosine (Marr and Berens, 1983; Ullman, 1984). Examples of antileishmanial and antitrypanosomal pyrazolopyrimidines that are selectively metabolized by trypanosomatids include allopurinol (HPP), allopurinol ribonucleoside (HPPR), 4-thiopurinol, 4-thiopurinol ribonucleoside, and formycin B. These pathogenic protozoa are capable of efficient conversion of the pyrazolopyrimidines to the nucleotide level. The pyrazolopyrimidine metabolites, which are isomers of inosine monophosphate, are subsequently aminated and incorporated as the adenylate analog into RNA. Mammalian cells are incapable of these metabolic transformations. The sulfur containing pyrazolopyrimidines, however, are neither aminated nor incorporated into nucleic acids.

Each of the pyrazolopyrimidines has been tested extensively against *Leishmania*, *T. cruzi*, and *T. brucei* and is effective against some, but not necessarily all, parasite stages. For instance, HPP, the most extensively tested of the pyrazolopyrimidines and an isomer of hypoxanthine, is effective against all insect vector and mammalian forms of *T. cruzi* and *Leishmania*, but is quite ineffectual against *T. brucei* infections in mice (Fairlamb et al., 1992). HPP, a drug that is extensively employed in the treatment of hyperuricemia and gout in humans, has been tested against both leishmaniasis (Martinez and Marr, 1992) and Chagas' disease (Gallerano et al., 1990). Encouragingly, HPP did demonstrate significant therapeutic efficacy in patients with either cutaneous leishmaniasis or chronic Chagas disease, although sporadic adverse reactions and occasional therapeutic failures are observed. Thus, the pyrazolopyrimidines are lead compounds in the rational design of therapeutic agents that exploit the unique enzymatic machinery for salvaging host purines in the genera *Leishmania* and *Trypanosoma*.

The metabolic activation of HPP is initiated by the HGPRT enzyme in *Leishmania*, *T. cruzi*, and *T. brucei* (Marr and Berens, 1983; Ullman, 1984). *L. donovani* and *L. braziliensis* promastigotes are capable of accumulating millimolar concentrations of HPP as the allopurinol ribonucleoside 5´-monophosphate (HPPR-MP). Approximately 10% of the HPPR-MP is subsequently aminated to the adenylate derivative by the sequential actions of adenylosuccinate synthetase and adenylosuccinate lyase. Conversely, mammalian cells accumulate only minuscule amounts of HPPR-MP and none of the aminopyrazolopyrimidine derivatives, which can account for the disparate toxicities of both HPP and HPPR toward trypanosomatids and humans. The differential metabolism of HPP in *Leishmania* and human cells can be attributed to the considerably greater amount of HGPRT activity in the parasite and to the fact that the pyrazolopyrimidine is a more efficient substrate for the parasite enzyme by at least one order of magnitude (Marr and Berens, 1983; Ullman, 1984). The inability of mammalian cells to accumulate aminopyrazolopyrimidines can be ascribed to the failure of the mammalian adenylosuccinate synthetase, unlike the parasite enzyme, to recognize HPPR-MP as a substrate. In humans, 60% of ingested HPP is converted to oxipurinol, a suicide substrate of the liver xanthine oxidase, an enzyme that is lacking in trypanosomatids, whereas the remainder is excreted either unchanged or as the ribonucleoside. The differential metabolism of HPP in trypanosomatids and human cells is compared in Figure 2. The fundamental peculiarity in the

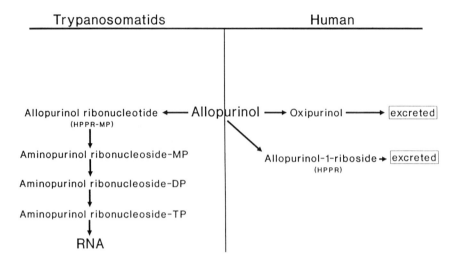

Fig. 2. Allopurinol metabolism in Trypanosomatids and humans. The metabolic avenues by which allopurinol is metabolized in trypanosomatids and humans are indicated. The pathway in trypanosomatids is conserved among *T. brucei*, *T. cruzi*, and *Leishmania*.

parasite that enables it to metabolize HPP selectively to the nucleotide level is the HGPRT enzyme, which also phosphoribosylates a second antiparasitic pyrazolopyrimidine, 4-thiopurinol. Therefore, to characterize this therapeutically germane enzyme further and to develop molecular and biochemical reagents for future studies directed toward a structure-based drug design strategy for the treatment of parasitic disease, this laboratory has embarked on a program to generate molecular and biochemical reagents to dissect the HGPRT enzymes from *Leishmania* and *Trypanosoma*.

Structure-Based Drug Design

The overall objective of this research program is to develop a structure-based drug design and discovery strategy for the treatment of parasitic diseases exploiting HGPRT as a paradigm. The vast majority of antiparasitic drugs or, for that matter, drugs employed in the treatment of any disease, have originated from indiscriminate screens. However, intimate knowledge of biological or biochemical mechanisms can facilitate otherwise empirical drug design. Recently, the ability to solve structures of important proteins or nucleic acids, either by nuclear magnetic resonance or x-ray crystallography, provides an exciting and promising new avenue for a structure-based approach to drug design. This structure-based strategy originates first and foremost with the solution of the tertiary structure of the macromolecule of interest, although if the structure has not been elucidated to an adequate resolution computer modeling of structures of families of related macromolecules can suffice for a solved structure.

For instance, a computational strategy involving a molecular docking computer program, DOCK 3.0, was successfully exploited to screen the Fine Chemicals Directory of >55,000 commercially available compounds to identify nonpeptide inhibitors of proteases involved in the establishment and maintenance of *Schistosoma mansoni* and *P. falciparum* infections (Ring et al., 1993). Although the structures of the parasite proteases have not been solved, their three-dimensional makeups were postulated from known structures of related proteases. Not only can these computer programs screen databases, but they can also make predictions for target inhibitors that require chemical synthesis. Recently, two potent inhibitors of influenza virus replication have been designed based on the crystal structure of the viral sialidase (von Itzstein et al., 1993). These compounds not only inhibit the enzyme but also obstruct the growth of the virus in cell culture and in animal models. This constitutes the first successful example of a rational-based computer-assisted drug design strategy that blocks the growth of an infectious agent in animals and offers promise for future developments in the treatment and eradication of all types of infectious organisms.

CLONING OF GENES ENCODING HGPRT

A major laboratory effort has been directed toward the isolation of the HGPRT genes (*hgprt*) from *L. donovani*, *T. cruzi*, and *T. brucei*. The justification for focusing on parasite HGPRTs is that the enzyme serves as a potential therapeutic target for the treatment of leishmaniasis, Chagas' disease, and African sleeping sickness. The basis for this is threefold. First, genetic and kinetic studies on promastigotes have indicated that HGPRT is probably indispensable for purine salvage in *Leishmania*, as it may very well be in *T. cruzi* and *T. brucei*. Second, hypoxanthine is a principal, if not the predominant, salvageable purine in the extracellular and intracellular host milieus in which these parasites reside. Third, as described above, HGPRT initiates the intracellular metabolism of the antiparasitic pyrazolopyrimidine analogs of hypoxanthine, one of which, HPP, has already proven efficacious against cutaneous leishmaniasis and Chagas' disease.

Initially, our efforts were directed toward the cloning of the *hgprt* gene from *L. donovani*, as the enzyme has been purified in small quantities to homogeneity and purine salvage has been most extensively examined in this species. Efforts to isolate the *L. donovani hgprt* by cross-hybridization to probes derived from other *hgprt* cDNAs, such as those from human (Jolly et al., 1983), *S. mansoni* (Craig et al., 1988), or *P. falciparum* (King and Melton, 1987), proved unsuccessful. Directional degenerate oligonucleotides derived from conserved stretches of amino acids among the human, *S. mansoni*, or *P. falciparum* also did not recognize *hgprt* sequences in genomic libraries, nor did they permit the amplification of specific *hgprt* sequences from *L. donovani* genomic DNA by the polymerase chain reaction (PCR). The failure of conventional cloning protocols to isolate the *L. donovani hgprt* gene necessitated the design of less straightforward gene cloning schemes. Therefore, this laboratory resorted to a "phylogenetic walking" strategy to isolate the *L. donovani hgprt* gene by undertaking the isolation of *hgprt* genes from related organisms, such as *T. brucei* and *T. cruzi*.

Initially, genomic libraries of *T. brucei* and *T. cruzi* DNA were hybridized with the cDNAs and degenerate oligonucleotides used in the screening of the *L. donovani* libraries without success. However, PCR-based strategies using oligonucleotides to conserved regions of HGPRT proteins amplified a 174 bp fragment of the *T. brucei* gene that was subsequently exploited as a homologous probe for the isolation of the entire *T. brucei hgprt* gene. After redesigning one of the PCR primers, due to an amino acid change in a region of the *T. brucei* HGPRT from which one of the primers was derived, a 174 bp fragment was amplified by PCR from *T. cruzi* DNA and the gene isolated from a genomic library. Unfortunately, however, neither the 174 bp probes nor the full-length *hgprt* genes from either *T. cruzi* or *T. brucei* enabled the detection of the *L. donovani* equivalent. Therefore, an NH_2-terminal amino acid sequence was obtained from the partially purified *L. donovani* HGPRT protein from which an appropriate degenerate oligonucleotide was designed. This oligonucleotide was designed in an antisense orientation, and its composition was biased according to the strong codon preference exhibited by *L. donovani* protein coding genes. Subsequently the 5′ fragment of the *L. donovani hgprt* mRNA was amplified from reverse transcribed RNA using PCR, the antisense primer to the NH_2 terminus and a sense primer derived from the sequence of the *L. donovani* miniexon. This anchored PCR strategy for amplifying probes from reversed transcribed cDNA for isolating genes has proven to be an effective cloning strategy for a number of genes for which NH_2-terminal amino acid sequence is available. The amplified fragment was then used to isolate the *L. donovani hgprt* gene from a cosmid library.

SEQUENCE ANALYSIS OF THE HGPRT GENES

The predicted amino acid sequences of the *T. brucei*, *T. cruzi*, and *L. donovani* HGPRT proteins are shown in Figure 3. The *T. brucei*, *T. cruzi*, and *L. donovani* HGPRTs are, respectively, 210, 221, and 211 amino acids in length, and their M_r's are 23.4, 25.5, and 23.6 kD, respectively. Alignment of the predicted amino acid sequences of the three trypanosomatid HGPRTs with the human, *S. mansoni*, and *P. falciparum* counterparts revealed three short regions of

```
T. brucei      1   MEPACK-----------------YDFA-----------TSVLFTEAEL  20
T. cruzi       1   MP--------------------REYEFA-----------EKILFTEEEI  18
L. donovani    1   MSNSAKSPSG-----PVGDEGRRNYPMS-----------AHTLVTQEQV  33
S. mansoni     1   MSSNMIKADC-----VVIEDSFRGFPTEYFCTSPRYDECLDYVLIPNGMI  45
P. falciparum  1   MPIPNNPGAGENAFDPVFVKDDDGYDLDSFMIPAHYKKYLTKVLVPNGVI  50
Human          1   MAT---RSPG-----VVISDDEPGYDLDLFCIPNHYAEDLERVFIPHGLI  42
                   *                 .                   .   .  .
```

```
T. brucei     21   HTRMRGVAQRIADDYSNCNLKPLENPLVIVSVLKGSFVFTADMVRILG--  68
T. cruzi      19   RTRIMEVAKRIADDYKGKGLRPYVNPLVLISVLKGSFMFTADLCRALS--  66
L. donovani   34   WAATAKCAKKIAEDYRSFKLTT-DNPLYLLCVLKGSFIFTADLARFLA--  80
S. mansoni    46   KDRLEKMSMDIVDYYEACN----ATSITLMCVLKGGFKFLADLVDGLERT  91
P. falciparum 51   KNRIEKLAYDIKKVY---N----NEEFHILCLLKGSRGFFTALLKHLSRI  93
Human         43   MDRTERLARDVMKEMGGHH-------IVALCVLKGGYKFFADLLDYIKAL  85
                    .                  . .***.  *  . .
```

```
T. brucei     69   ----DFGVPTRV---EFLRASSYGHDTKSCGRVDVKADGLCDIRGKHVLV  111
T. cruzi      67   ----DFNVPVRM---EFICVSSYGEGVTSSGQVRMLLDTRHSIEGHHVLI  109
L. donovani   81   ----DEGVPVKV---EFICASSYGTGVETSGQVRMLLDVRDSVENRHILI  123
S. mansoni    92   VRARGIVLPMSV---EFVRVKSYVNDVSIHEPILTGLGDPSEYKDKNVLV  138
P. falciparum 94   HNYSAVEMSKPLFGEHYVRVKSYCNDQSTGTLEIVS-EDLSCLKGKHVLI  142
Human         86   NRNSDRSIPMTV---DFIRLKSYCNDQSTGDIKVIGGDDLSTLTGKNVLI  132
                        . .  . ...  **     .              ..*.
```

```
T. brucei    112   LEDILDTALTLREVVDSLKKSEPASIKTLVAIDKPGGRKIPFTAEYVVAD  161
T. cruzi     110   VEDIVDTALTLNYLYHMYFTRRPASLKTVVLLDKREGRRVPFSADYVVAN  159
L. donovani  124   VEDIVDSAITLQYLMRFMLAKKPASLKTVVLLDKPSGRKVEVLVDYPVIT  173
S. mansoni   139   VEDIIDTGKTITKLISHLDSLSTKSVKVASLLVKRTSPRNDYRPDFVGFE  188
P. falciparum 143  VEDIIDTGKTLVKFCEYLKKFEIKTVAIACLFIKRTPLWNGFKADFVGFS  192
Human        133   VEDIIDTGKTMQTLLSLVRQYNPKMVKVASLLVKRTPRSVGYKPDFVGFE  182
                   .***.*.. *.                          *
```

```
T. brucei    162   VPNVFVVGYGLDYDQSYREVRDVVILKPSVYETWGKELERRK-------A  204
T. cruzi     160   IPNAFVIGYGLDYDDTYRELRDIVVLRPEVYAEREAARQKKQRAIGSADT  209
L. donovani  174   IPHAFVIGYGMDYPESYRELRDICVLSKKEYYEKYE-------------  208
S. mansoni   189   VPNRFVVGYALDYDNFRDLHHICVINEV--------GQKKFSVPCTSK  229
P. falciparum 193  IPDHFVVGYSLDYNEIFRDLDHCCLVNDE--------GKKKYK----AT  229
Human        183   IPDKFVVGYALDYNEYFRDLNHVCVISET--------GKAKYKA-----  218
                   .*. **.**..**  . .*.. .
```

```
T. brucei    205   AGEAKR------  210
T. cruzi     210   DRDAKREFHSKY  221
L. donovani  209   ---------SKV  211
S. mansoni   230   P----------V  231
P. falciparum 230  S----------L  231
Human        218   ------------  218
```

Fig. 3. Alignment of the amino acid sequences of the *T. brucei, T. cruzi, L. donovani, S. mansoni, P. falciparum,* and human HGPRTs. The predicted amino acid sequences of the trypanosomatid HGPRT genes were compared with those deduced from the nucleotide sequences of the human, *S. mansoni,* and *P. falciparum hgprt* cDNAs according to the CLUSTAL V program, a modification of that previously described by Higgins and Sharp (1988). Amino acids identities are indicated by asterisks below the aligned sequences, and nonidentical amino acids with similarity scores >10, as calculated by the log-odds amino acid similarity matix of Dayhoff (1978), are indicated with a dot. Amino acid positions are designated numerically on the right.

significant homology, each separated and flanked by much longer regions without substantial identity (Fig. 3). The stretches of homology correspond to the two putative substrate-binding domains and to a region proximal to the COOH terminus of HGPRT to which no function has been ascribed. In the 15 amino acid region encompassing the PRPP binding domain, corresponding to residues 108–122 of the *T. brucei* HGPRT, there are six completely conserved amino acids and eight other positions in which the substitutions are conservative in nature. A single change from Lys to a neutral amino acid found at position 120 of the *T. brucei* HGPRT is the only nonconservative change within the PRPP-binding domain. Similarly, the putative purine nucleobase binding domain, coinciding with residues 51–63 of the *T. brucei* HGPRT, is another region that is also fairly well preserved among the various HGPRTs. This purine binding motif contains four amino acid identities and four conservative differences among the mammalian and parasite HGPRTs.

Within this purine-binding domains lies a central Arg residue and a Thr-Ala dipeptide in the *P. falciparum* enzyme that distinguishes the malarial HGPRT purine-binding site from that of the others. A conserved aromatic amino acid and an Ala-Asp are found at these positions in the other HGPRTs. Elimination of the malarial protein from the alignment depicted in Figure 3 increases the number of identical amino acids within the purine nucleobase-binding regions of the other five HGPRTs to seven. As the malarial HGPRT protein has the capacity to recognize xanthine as a substrate, unlike the HGPRTs from mammals, *S. mansoni*, and trypanosomatids, it can be claimed that the ability to recognize xanthine can be attributed to the striking amino acid differences in this region of the malarial enzyme.

Finally, there is considerable sequence conservation at the region of unknown function located close to the COOH termini. Between residues 162 and 181 of the *T. brucei* HGPRT, there are eight amino acid identities and nine similarities. Although no known function has been imputed to this region of the protein, several naturally occurring missense mutations in this region confer HGPRT deficiency in humans and elevate apparent K_m values for both substrates dramatically, indicating the importance of this stretch of amino acids to both catalytic competence and substrate binding. Also, it is worth reiterating that the amino acid regions outside the three conserved areas are highly divergent among the HGPRTs with only an occasional single amino acid identical among the six aligned HGPRT sequences. Indeed, the longest stretch of amino acid identity outside the three conserved regions is two amino acids, a Ser-Tyr dipeptide corresponding to positions 83–84 of the *T. brucei* protein.

Alignments of the primary structures of the HGPRTs in a pairwise manner revealed that the *T. cruzi*, *T. brucei*, and *L. donovani* HGPRT proteins exhibited only a 21%–25% identity with the human, *S. mansoni*, and *P. falciparum* enzymes. The *T. cruzi* and *T. brucei* HGPRTs were identical in 49% of the amino acid positions, the *T. cruzi* and *L. donovani* HGPRT matched in 50% of the residues, and the *L. donovani* and *T. brucei* HGPRTs exhibited 34% identity. The extent of similitude among the various HGPRTs conformed to the phylogenetic divergence among the organisms expected from *rRNA* gene alignments (Sogin et al., 1986).

MOLECULAR CHARACTERIZATION OF THE *HGPRT* TRANSCRIPTS AND *HGPRT* CHROMOSOMAL LOCUS

Northern blot analyses confirmed *hgprt* transcripts of slightly less than 2 kb in all three pathogens. A single *hgprt* transcript was observed in both *T. cruzi* and *L. donovani*, whereas *T. brucei* contained two specific *hgprt* mRNAs of 1.4 and 1.9 kb. Amplification of the 5´ portion of the *T. brucei hgprt* transcripts by PCR generated only a single fragment, implying that the heterogeneity in the size of the two mRNAs could be attributed to differences in the length of the 3' terminus. Amplification of the 3' end of the mRNAs by PCR did produce two DNA fragments, differing in size by approximately the expected 500 bp. The spliced leader junction sites of the *T. brucei*, *T. cruzi*, and *L. donovani* transcripts were also determined by sequencing the DNA products amplified from cDNA by PCR. These experiments indicated that the *hgprt* mRNA began 30–180 bp upstream from the translation initiation site. Moreover, sequence analysis of the PCR product amplified from the 5´ portion of the *T. cruzi hgprt* transcript in four independent experiments suggested an apparently unusual nonconsensus 3´ splice site for the addition of the spliced leader RNA. However intriguing these results are, no conclusions should be drawn from them, as the atypical result could be ascribed to the transcript derived from the other *hgprt* allele that has not been sequenced or to a natural consequence of sequence differences in the upstream portions of the *hgprt* gene, since the gene was isolated from a library of *T. cruzi* CL strain DNA, whereas the PCR product amplified from the upstream region of the *hgprt* mRNA was obtained from *T. cruzi* Y strain RNA. Southern analyses of restriction digests of genomic DNA suggested that the *hgprt* gene was not tandemly repeated within any of the trypanosomatid genomes and appeared to be present in a single copy in *T. cruzi* and *L. donovani*, although *T. brucei* appeared to contain at least two nonidentical *hgprt* loci.

OVEREXPRESSION OF *HGPRT* GENES IN *ESCHERICHIA COLI* AND PURIFICATION OF HGPRTS

After appropriate PCR mutagenesis, the *T. brucei*, *T. cruzi*, and *L. donovani* *hgprt* genes were ligated into the pBAce bacterial expression plasmid, a vector that directs the high-level expression of soluble and enzymatically active foreign proteins in *E. coli* (Craig et al., 1991). The parasite *hgprt*-pBAce constructs were then transformed into the S_606 (*_gpt*, *hpt*) *E. coli* strain that is genetically deficient in the prokaryotic hypoxanthine and xanthine–guanine phosphoribosyltransferase activities (Jochimsen et al., 1975), and the genes were resequenced to confirm that the heterologously expressed products would be identical to the native protein.

The purine pathway of *E. coli* and the mutations in the S_606 strain are indicated in Figure 4. Under appropriate induction conditions, i.e., low phosphate medium, the transformants expressed 40–100 mg of enzymatically active recombinant HGPRT protein per liter of bacterial culture. Each of the parasite HGPRTs was then purified to homogeneity in a single step from a GTP-Agarose resin by elution in buffer containing 1.0 mM PRPP. The purified parasite HGPRTs were then analyzed with respect to substrate specificity and affinities for nucleobase substrates.

Each of the trypanosomatid HGPRTs phosphoribosylated hypoxanthine and guanine but did not recognize either adenine or xanthine for which biochemically distinct phosphoribosyltransferases exist in all three parasites. Lineweaver-Burk analyses revealed that the parasite HGPRTs exhibited a high affinity for their naturally occurring nucleobase substrates. K_m values of 2–5 µM and V_{max} values of 30-50 µmol/min/mg protein were calculated. HPP was a much less efficient substrate for all three parasite HGPRT proteins. Apparent K_m values between 200 and 800 µM and V_{max} values of 2–6 µmol/min/mg protein were determined. These data reveal that the antiparasitic pyrazolopyrimidine is a relatively inefficient HGPRT substrate and suggest that a

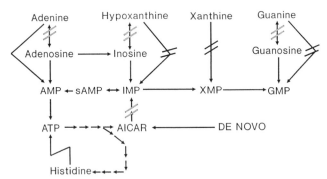

Fig. 4. Metabolism of purines in *E. coli*. The genetic lesions in S_606 (*_gpt*, *hpt*) and S_609 (*_gpt*, *hpt*, *pup*, *purHJ*) *E. coli* are indicated by double bars. Deficiencies found only in the S_609 strain are indicated by the hatched bars, whereas solid bars signify that the enzyme is lacking in both cell lines. The names of all of the enzymes are presented in Figure 1 of Jochimsen et al. (1975).

structure-based approach to the design of more efficient substrates of the trypanosomatid HGPRT enzymes might lead to the development of more valuable antiparasitic reagents that are better substrates for the parasite HGPRTs.

STRUCTURAL STUDIES ON *T. BRUCEI, T. CRUZI,* AND *L. DONOVANI* HGPRTS

Presently, little structural information is available on the pure HGPRT proteins. Preliminary estimates of the secondary structure content of the *T. brucei* and *T. cruzi* HGPRTs have been made by circular dichroism, and the data collected have confirmed many of the secondary structural predictions formulated using the Chou-Fasman (1974) algorithm. The computer-generated secondary structural analyses of the primary structures of the three HGPRT proteins revealed a highly conserved dinucleotide-binding motif in the NH_2 portions of the HGPRT proteins, which is also found in the mammalian, *S. mansoni*, and *P. falciparum* proteins despite the fact that the amino acid sequences within this region of the HGPRT protein are highly divergent. These higher order structure predictions indicate, therefore, that the catalytic sites of the HGPRT proteins are much more homologous than would be predicted from the divergent primary structures. Thus, the sequences of all the HGPRT proteins are far more divergent than their structures.

No information is currently available on the tertiary structures of any of the HGPRT proteins. As the structures of the HGPRTs are too large to solve by nuclear magnetic resonance, we will conduct crystallographic studies on the *T. brucei, T. cruzi,* and *L. donovani* enzymes in order to obtain a high-resolution structure of these HGPRTs. A high-resolution crystal structure of these HGPRTs in combination with the biochemical and molecular genetic studies described in the preceding paragraph should facilitate the complete elucidation of the catalytic mechanism of these proteins and may also provide some molecular insight into the interactions of these parasites with their hosts. Additionally, x-ray structures of these enzymes complexed with low-affinity substrates, e.g., HPP, will facilitate a knowledge-based approach to the design or discovery of novel HGPRT inhibitors or substrate analogs specific for the parasite HGPRT enzymes. Once a high-resolution structure of any HGPRT is determined, it will be possible to perform computer modeling on the HGPRTs from other organisms. Currently, crystals of all three trypanosomatid HGPRT proteins have been obtained in this laboratory by the hanging drop vapor diffusion method, but their diffractability has yet to be tested. It is clear, however, that the availability of large quantities of pure recombinant HGPRTs from *E. coli* provide an avenue for a structure-based strategy for the design and discovery of novel HGPRT substrate analogs or HGPRT inhibitors that can serve as effective agents in the treatment of trypanosomiasis, leishmaniasis, or any other parasitic disease for which the etiologic agent relies on HGPRT for purine salvage.

MOLECULAR DISSECTION OF FUNCTIONAL DETERMINANTS ON *T. BRUCEI, T. CRUZI,* AND *L. DONOVANI* HGPRTS

Future experiments on the *T. brucei, T. cruzi* and *L. donovani* HGPRTs will center on a molecular, as well as structural, characterization of the proteins. Alignments of the amino acid sequences from a variety of phylogenetically diverse phosphoribosyltransferases have afforded an opportunity to predict which amino acids in the protein might be responsible for the unique substrate specificity of the kinetoplastid HGPRTs. This laboratory is in the process of genetically altering several of these residues by site-directed mutagenesis. The mutated constructs, after sequencing, will be re-expressed in the S_606 *E. coli* and the proteins analyzed for substrate specificity and kinetic parameters before and after purification. The ability to express the parasite HGPRTs in *E. coli* should also facilitate a thorough molecular genetic dissection of the structural determinants within the proteins that mediate enzyme function. The *hgprt*–pBAce constructs will also be transformed into *E. coli* strain S_609 (_gpt, hpt⁻, pup, purHJ), a stock that is deficient in both phosphoribosyl-transferases and in purine nucleoside phosphorylase activity, and is also aux-otrophic for purines (Jochimsen et al., 1975) (Fig. 4). In this genetic background, we can easily select both for and against expression of HGPRT activity. Thus, we are capable of introducing by site-directed mutagenesis any and/or all conceivable mutations within any codon and select both for and against the expression of enzymatically active protein in *E. coli*. S_609 trans-formants that express enzymatically active HGPRT can be grown in low-phos-phate induction medium supplemented with hypoxanthine, while transformants that express inactive protein can be selected in a cytotoxic HGPRT substrate, such as 6-mercaptopurine or 6-thioguanine, as long as the medium is supple-mented with adenine and guanosine, two purines that circumvent the purine auxotrophy and the deficiencies in purine-metabolizing enzymes present in the S_609 strain. Once a crystal structure of an HGPRT protein is solved by x-ray crystallography, it will then be possible to construct knowledge-based mutations in specific amino acid residues within the active site of the pro-tein in order to further a dissection of the atomic determinants that con-tribute to substrate binding and catalytic function.

SUMMARY

The auxotrophy of parasitic protozoa for purines and the expression of their unique complement of purine salvage enzymes provide a rational avenue for the selective treatment and control of diseases of parasitic origin. Genetic, metabolic, biochemical, and clinical studies have suggested that the *L. donovani, T. brucei,* and *T. cruzi* HGPRT is a suitable target for rational drug development, since the enzyme plays an important, if not essential, nutritional function and initiates the selective antiparasitic effects of pyrazolopyrimidine nucleobases that are analogs of hypoxanthine. The breakthroughs in the isolation of the molecular clones encoding the HGPRT proteins from *T. brucei, T. cruzi,* and *L. donovani,* coupled with the production of large quantities of pure recombinant HGPRT protein from each of the parasites, provides a foundation for a structure-based strategy for drug design and discovery for African sleeping sickness, Chagas' disease, and leishmaniasis.

ACKNOWLEDGMENTS

This work was supported by grant AI-23682 from the National Institute of Allergy and Infectious Disease. T.A. was a recipient of an N.L. Tartar Trust Fellowship from the Medical Research Foundation of Oregon. B.U. is a Burroughs Wellcome Fund Scholar in Molecular Parasitology, and this work was supported in part by a grant from The Burroughs Wellcome Fund.

REFERENCES

Aronow B, Kaur K, McCartan K, Ullman B (1987): Two high affinity nucleoside transporters in *Leishmania donovani*. Mol Biochem Parasitol 22:29–37.

Baum KF, Berens RL, Marr JJ, Harrington JA, Spector T (1989): Purine deoxynucleoside salvage in *Giardia lamblia*. J Biol Chem 264:21087–21090.

Berens RL, Marr JJ, LaFon SW, Nelson DJ (1981): Purine metabolism in *Trypanosoma cruzi*. Mol Biochem Parasitol 3:187–196.

Boonlayangoor P, Albach RA, Booden T (1980): Purine nucleotide synthesis in *Entamoeba histolytica*: A preliminary study. Arch Invest Med (Mex) 11:83–88.

Chou PY, Fasman GD (1974): Prediction of protein conformation. Biochemistry 13:222–245.

Craig SP III, McKerrow JH, Newport GR, Wang CC (1988): Analysis of cDNA encoding the hypoxanthine–guanine phosphoribosyltransferase (HGPRTase) of *Schistosoma mansoni*: A putative target for chemotherapy. Nucleic Acids Res 16:7087–7101.

Craig SP III, Yuan L, Kuntz DA, McKerrow JH, Wang CC (1991): High level expression in *Escherichia coli* of soluble, enzymatically active schistosomal hypoxanthine/guanine phosphoribosyltransferase and trypanosomal ornithine decarboxylase. Proc Natl Acad Sci USA 88:2500–2504.

Dayhoff MO (1978): A model of evolutionary change in proteins. Matrices for detecting distant relationships. In Dayhoff MO (ed): Atlas of Protein Sequence and Structure, vol 5, suppl 3. Washington, DC: National Biomedical Research Foundation, pp 345–358.

Dwyer DM, Gottlieb M (1984): Surface membrane localization of 3′- and 5′-nucleotidase activities in *Leishmania donovani* promastigotes. Mol Biochem Parasitol 10:139–150.

Fairlamb AH (1989): Novel biochemical pathways in parasitic protozoa. Parasitology 99 (Suppl):S93–S112.

Fairlamb AH, Carter NS, Cunningham M, Smith K (1992): Characterization of melarsen-resistant *Trypanosoma brucei brucei* with respect to cross-resistance to other drugs and trypanothione metabolism. Mol Biochem Parasitol 53:213–222.

Fish WR, Marr JJ, Berens RL (1982): Purine metabolism in *Trypanosoma brucei gambiense*. Biochim Biophys Acta 714:422–428.

Gallerano RH, Sosa RR, Marr JJ (1990): Therapeutic efficacy of allopurinol in patients with chronic Chagas' disease. Am J Trop Med Hyg 43:159–166.

Garrett CE, Coderre JA, Meek TD, Garvey EP, Claman DM, Beverley SM, Santi DV (1984): Bifunctional thymidylate synthetase-dihydrofolate reductase in protozoa. Mol Biochem Parasitol 3:257–265.

Hammond DJ, Gutteridge WE (1984) Purine and pyrimidine metabolism in the Trypanosomatidae. Mol Biochem Parasitol 13:243–261.

Higgins DG, Sharp PM (1988): CLUSTAL: A package for performing multiple sequence alignment on a microcomputer. Gene 73:237–244.

Hill B, Kilsby J, Rogerson GW, McIntosh RT, Ginger DC (1981): The enzymes of pyrimidine biosynthesis in a range of parasitic protozoa and helminths. Mol Biochem Parasitol 2:123–134.

Iovannisci DM, Goebel D, Kaur K, Allen K, Ullman B (1984): Genetic analysis of adenine metabolism in *Leishmania donovani*: Evidence for diploidy at the adenine phosphoribosyltransferase locus. J Biol Chem 259:14617–14623.

Jochimsen B, Nygaard P, Vestergaard T (1975): Location on the chromosome of *Escherichia coli* of genes governing purine metabolism. Mol Gen Genet 143:85–91.

Jolly DJ, Okayama H, Berg P, Esty AC, Filpula D, Bohlen P, Johnson GG, Shively JE, Hunkapillar T, Friedman T (1983): Isolation and characterization of a full-length expressible cDNA for human hypoxanthine phosphoribosyltransferase. Proc Natl Acad Sci USA 80:477–481.

King A, Melton DW (1987): Characterization of cDNA clones for hypoxanthine-guanine phosphoribosyltransferase from the human malarial parasite, *Plasmodium falciparum*: Comparisons to the mammalian gene and protein. Nucleic Acids Res 15:10469–10481.

LaFon SW, Nelson DJ, Berens RL, Marr JJ (1982): Purine and pyrimidine salvage pathways in *Leishmania donovani*. Biochem Pharmacol 31:231–238.

Looker DL, Berens RL, Marr JJ (1983): Purine metabolism in *Leishmania donovani* amastigotes and promastigotes. Mol Biochem Parasitol 9:15–23.

Lindmark DG, Jarroll EL (1982): Pyrimidine metabolism in *Giardia lamblia* trophozoites. Mol Biochem Parasitol 5:291–296.

Lo HS, Wang CC (1985): Purine salvage in Entamoeba histolytica. J Parasitol 71:662–669.

Marr JJ, Berens RL (1983): Pyrazolopyrimidine metabolism in the pathogenic Trypanosomatidae. Mol Biochem Parasitol 7:339–356.

Marr JJ, Berens RL, Nelson DJ (1978): Purine metabolism in *Leishmania donovani* and *Leishmania braziliensis*. Biochim Biophys Acta 544:360–371.

Martinez S, Marr JJ (1992): Allopurinol in the treatment of American cutaneous leishmaniasis. N Engl J Med 326:741–744 (1992).

Miller RL, Linstead D (1983): Purine and pyrimidine metabolizing activities in *Trichomonas vaginalis* extracts. Mol Biochem Parasitol 7:41–51.

Ring CS, Sun E, McKerrow JH, Garson KL, Rosenthal PJ, Kuntz ID, Cohen FE (1993): Structure-based inhibitor design by using protein models for the development of antiparasitic agents. Proc Natl Acad Sci USA 90:3583–3587.

Schwartzman JD, Pfefferkorn ER (1982): *Toxoplasma gondii*: Purine synthesis and salvage in mutant host cells and parasites. Exp Parasitol 53:77–86.

Sogin ML, Elwood HJ, Gunderson JH (1986): Evolutionary diversity of eukaryotic small-subunit rRNA genes. Proc Natl Acad Sci USA 83:1383–1387.

Ullman B (1984): Pyrazolopyrimidine metabolism in parasitic protozoa. Pharmaceutical Res 1:194–203.

von Itzstein M, Wu W-Y, Kok GB, Pegg MS, Dyason JC, Jin B, Phan TV, Smythe ML, White HF, Oliver SW, Colman PM, Varghese JN, Ryan DM, Woods JM, Bethell RC, Hotham VJ, Cameron JM, Penn CR (1993): Rational design of potent sialidase-based inhibitors of influenza virus replication. Nature 363:418–423.

Walsh CJ, Sherman IW (1968): Purine and pyrimidine synthesis by the avian malaria parasite, *Plasmodium lophurae*. J Protozool 15:763–770.

Wang CC (1984): Parasite enzymes as potential targets for antiparasitic chemotherapy. J Med Chem 27:1–9.

Wang CC, Aldritt AL (1983): Purine salvage networks in *Giardia lamblia*. J Exp Med 158:1703–1712.

Wang CC, Cheng HW (1984): Salvage of pyrimidine nucleosides by *Trichomonas vaginalis*. J Exp Med 160: 987-1000.

Wang CC, Simashkevich PM (1981): Purine metabolism in the protozoan parasite *Eimeria tenella*. Proc Natl Acad Sci USA 78:6618–6622.

GENOMES

Preface

Like most eukaryotes, parasites often have more than just a simple nuclear genome. They can have organellar genomes, parasitic genomes (in the form of viral nucleic acid), and even nuclear genomes, which are far from "simple." In this section, some of the most striking examples of each are described.

The first chapter, by Paul Englund and colleagues, explores the current state of knowledge about replication of kinetoplast DNA. This network of mitochondrial DNA was the first major focus of studies on parasite nucleic acids in the 1970s, and, indeed, some claim it was the first extranuclear DNA discovered (at the turn of the century). Here Englund describes recent results on the mechanics of its replication and speculates on how the function of these molecules may relate to the mode of their replication.

The organellar DNA of *Plasmodium* is the next topic to be explored in this section in a chapter by Jean Feagin. Perhaps not surprisingly, given the remarkable results with trypanosomes, investigations into the unexplored organelles of this member of the Apicomplexa have revealed some unusual features and properties, including the discovery of an unsuspected organellar DNA that is still without a definite intracellular location.

The third chapter in this section, that by Alice and C.C. Wang, retells the discovery of an unusual double-stranded RNA in *Giardia* that, on further examination, proved to be the genome of a new virus in the Totiviridae family. The presence of this viral parasite in a protozoan parasite does more than just extend the famous poem of deMorgan.* Its presence may affect the biology of the *Giardia* "host," and it may also prove useful as a vector for transfection as has been the case for mammalian and bacterial viruses.

The final chapter in this section deals with the nuclear genome in nematodes. Fritz Muller describes the highly unusual phenomenon in ascarids known as *chromatin dimunition*. This is the process by which somatic cells systematically delete up to 80% of their DNA at an early embryo stage, leaving the essential "guts" of the genome to provide all the necessary functions. Clues are beginning to emerge as to the signals and machinery involved in this process and its possible role in development.

---

*Great fleas have little fleas upon their backs to bite 'em, And little fleas have lesser fleas and so *ad infinitum*. From "A Budget of Paradoxes" by Augustus deMorgan, 1872.

Molecular Approaches to Parasitology, pages 147–161
© 1995 Wiley-Liss, Inc.

The Replication of Kinetoplast DNA

Paul T. Englund, Martin Ferguson, D. Lys Guilbride,
Catharine E. Johnson, Congjun Li, David Pérez-Morga,
Laura J. Rocco, and Al F. Torri

*Department of Biological Chemistry, Johns Hopkins Medical School, Baltimore,
Maryland 21205 (P.T.E., D.L.G., C.E.J., C.L., D.P.M., L.J.R., A.F.T.);
Departments of Molecular Biophysics and Biochemistry and Genetics (M.F.),
Yale University, New Haven, Connecticut*

INTRODUCTION

Kinetoplast DNA (kDNA), the mitochondrial DNA of protozoan parasites related to the trypanosomes, consists of about 5,000 minicircles and a few dozen maxicircles (for reviews of kDNA, see Simpson, 1987; Ryan et al., 1988; Stuart and Feagin, 1992). An amazing property of kDNA, which is unique in nature, is that all of these circles are topologically linked, like chain mail, into a single giant network. Each parasite cell has only one network within its single mitochondrion. An electron micrograph (EM) showing part of a network isolated from the insect trypanosomatid *Crithidia fasciculata* is shown in Figure 1. The entire isolated network, an elliptical sheet of inter-locked rings, is about 10×15 µm in size. In this chapter, we discuss recent data on how this complex network is replicated in vivo and how this may relate to its biological function.

What is the function of kDNA? Although we still do not know why trypanosomatids are the only eukaryotes that organize their mitochondrial DNA in a network, there is considerable information about the genetic function of maxicircles and minicircles. The maxicircles resemble conventional mitochon-drial DNAs, in mammals or in yeast, in that they encode ribosomal RNAs and proteins involved in mitochondrial energy transduction (typical gene prod-ucts are subunits of cytochrome oxidase or NADH dehydrogenase; for re-view, see Simpson, 1987). However, the expression of maxicircle genes is highly complex. Most maxicircle transcripts undergo editing, a process in which uridine residues are added to or deleted from various positions in the tran-script to create open reading frames. The function of minicircles had been a mystery for many years, but recently it was discovered that they encode small guide RNAs which control editing specificity (for reviews on editing, see Benne, 1990; Simpson, 1990; Stuart and Feagin, 1992).

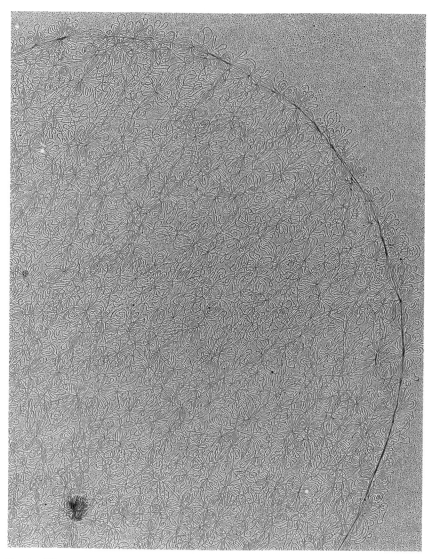

Fig. 1. Electron micrograph of a *C. fasciculata* kDNA network. Each small loop represents a 2.5 kb minicircle. The maxicircles (none shown) are 37 kb. The entire network is an elliptically shaped structure, about 10×15 μm. (Reproduced from Rauch et al., 1993, with permission of the publisher.)

REPLICATION OF A DNA NETWORK

Our laboratory began studying kDNA almost 20 years ago. Our initial objective, which still stimulates our research, was to understand how a DNA network could undergo replication. In every cell cycle the parasite starts with one network and must make two, one for each daughter cell. This process requires doubling the number of minicircles and the number of maxicircles. The two progeny networks must then segregate into the daughter cells during cell division. It is important to note that replication of kDNA, unlike that of other mitochondrial DNAs, occurs at about the same time as that of nuclear DNA, during a distinct S phase of the cell cycle (Cosgrove and Skeen, 1970).

Most of our work on kDNA has concerned the parasite *C. fasciculata.* This is a parasite of insects that does not infect humans. We chose this organism because it is an ideal experimental system for these studies. Among its many technical advantages, it grows rapidly in culture in an inexpensive medium to high cell density. We even grow 150 liter cultures in a fermentor for the purpose of enzyme purification. We would have made much less progress in this research if we had focused exclusively on one of the human pathogens such as *Trypanosoma* or *Leishmania,* especially as it is much more difficult to obtain sufficient material for biochemical studies. However, the basic information about kDNA that we have learned from *C. fasciculata* applies as well to the parasites of humans, and we have confirmed some of our findings in experiments with African trypanosomes.

THE ROLE OF FREE MINICIRCLES IN κDNA REPLICATION

An important finding, made nearly 15 years ago, was that minicircles do not replicate while attached to the network (Englund, 1979). Instead, they are first released from the central region of the network by the action of a topoisomerase II. The whole network does not suddenly dissociate into free minicircles, but instead there is a slow release of these molecules throughout the S phase. A few percent are free at any given time. Since the free minicircles are not linked to other circles in the network, there are no unusual topological problems associated with their replication. In fact they replicate as θ-structures, like other small DNA rings such as plasmid or viral molecules (extensive studies on the mechanism of replication of free minicircles have been published by our laboratory and Ray's laboratory) (reviewed in Ryan et al., 1988; Ray, 1987). One important characteristic of minicircles is that prior to replication they are covalently closed and after replication they contain nicks or gaps in their newly synthesized strand (Englund, 1978). It is thought that minicircle nicking plays a bookkeeping function, keeping track of which minicircles have undergone replication and ensuring that each minicircle replicates once and only once each generation.

After replication, the progeny minicircles are reattached to the network in another topoisomerase reaction. Since reattachment occurs exclusively at the network periphery, the replicating network develops two zones (Englund, 1978; Pérez-Morga and Englund, 1993b). The central zone contains covalently closed minicircles that have not yet replicated, and the peripheral zone contains nicked minicircles that have undergone replication. As replication proceeds the central zone shrinks and the peripheral zone enlarges. Since two minicircles are reattached for every one removed, the network grows in size. Figure 2 shows an EM autoradiograph of an isolated replicating network. This network had been radiolabeled by nick translation using [^{3}H]deoxynucleoside triphosphates, a treatment that labels only the nicked minicircles. The silver grains mark the peripheral location of the nicked minicircles; the clear central region contains covalently closed minicircles. Figure 3 shows a diagram of this model of network replication, emphasizing the role of free minicircles.

Finally, when all minicircles have replicated the network is double in size. Only then are all the nicks and gaps repaired (Pérez-Morga and Englund, 1993b). The final event is the splitting of the double-sized network in two. This scission, a mechanism not yet understood, probably involves unlinking of adjacent minicircles by a topoisomerase. Then the two progeny networks segregate into the daughter cells.

PACKING A κDNA NETWORK INSIDE THE CELL

The model described in the previous section was developed almost completely from studies of the structure of free minicircles and replicating networks that had been isolated from cells. Although this approach has proven valuable, it is limited as to what it can reveal about replication within the cell. The isolated kDNA network is a sheet of DNA rings that is actually larger in size than the parasite cell from which it was isolated. Yet inside the cell the network is condensed into a small disk that resides within the mitochondrial matrix. This condensed structure is the substrate for replication in vivo, and a complete description of this process must address the issue of how the network is compacted.

The first clue as to how the network is organized inside the cell came from EM study of thin sections. Almost 25 years ago, Delain and Riou (1969) noted that the thickness of a *Trypanosoma cruzi* kinetoplast disk in vivo is about half the circumference of a minicircle. They postulated that the network is packed as shown in the model in Figure 4A. This diagram shows a section through the kinetoplast disk. Each minicircle is elongated like a rubber band and linked to several neighbors. This model explains how a two-dimensional

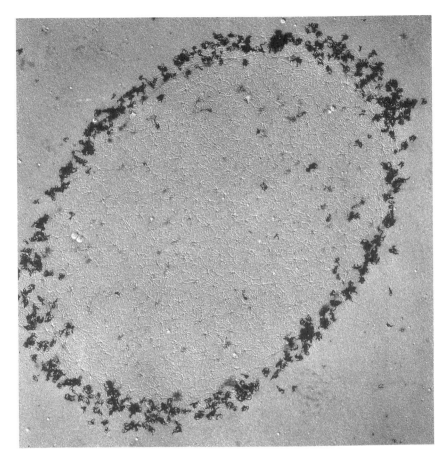

Fig. 2. Electron microscope autoradiograph of an early replicating kDNA network that had been labeled with [³H]deoxynucleoside triphosphates and DNA polymerase I. This nick translation reaction labels only those minicircles with endogenous nicks. The silver grains on the network periphery mark the location of the nicked circles. (Reproduced from Pérez-Morga and Englund, 1993b, with permission of the publisher.)

network, about 10 × 15 μm in size, can be condensed into a disk about 1 μm in diameter and 0.3 μm thick.

Support for this model came from fluorescence *in situ* hybridization of *C. fasciculata* cells using minicircle probes. These studies revealed that *replicating* kDNA looked not like a fluorescent disk as expected, but like a donut (Ferguson et al., 1992). The reason for the donut shape is that only nicked minicircles, and not covalently closed minicircles, can hybridize with the probe. As with the EM autoradiograph of the isolated network shown in Figure 2,

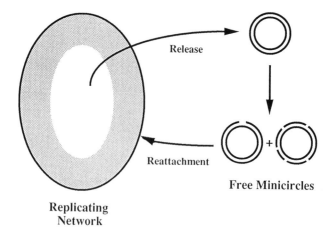

Fig. 3. Model of kDNA replication. The elliptical structure on the left represents a partly replicated isolated network. Covalently closed minicircles are released from the central region of the network. After replication of this free minicircle, the nicked or gapped progeny are reattached to the network periphery. The shaded region of the network represents the zone containing the nicked progeny minicircles. As replication proceeds, the peripheral zone grows and the central zone shrinks.

fluorescence microscopy revealed that the nicked minicircles are on the periphery of the kinetoplast disk. Covalently closed minicircles, which do not hybridize, form the donut hole in the central region of the disk. Figure 4B shows a diagram of a section through a partly replicated kinetoplast disk; the newly replicated nicked minicircles are drawn in bold.

What stabilizes the kinetoplast disk in this compact conformation? It is very likely that proteins are involved, but these remain to be isolated. Another important factor in stabilizing this structure could be the bent DNA helix found in minicircles from almost all trypanosomatid species (Marini et al., 1982; Ntambi et al., 1984). We can speculate that the bend is at the position indicated by the bold segment of each minicircle in Figure 4A, either at the top or bottom of the kinetoplast disk. Therefore, DNA bending could control the orientation of minicircles within the kinetoplast disk and could contribute to the stability of this structure in vivo.

COMPLEXES OF DNA REPLICATION PROTEINS

In 1988, Melendy, Sheline, and Ray showed by immunofluorescence that a *C. fasciculata* mitochondrial topoisomerase II localizes to two discrete sites on opposite sides of the kinetoplast disk in vivo. Subsequently, we found that

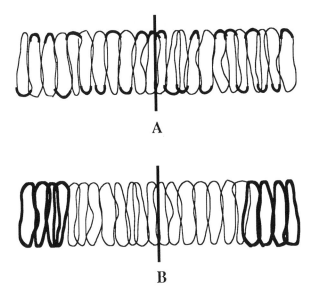

A

B

Fig. 4. **A:** Model for packing of the network in vivo (Delain and Riou, 1969). This diagram shows a section through the kinetoplast disk, and the axis of the disk is shown by the bold vertical line. Each stretched out minicircle is linked to several neighbors, both on the side and in front and behind. The bold segment of the minicircle is the postulated location of the bent helix, situated either at the top or bottom of the disk (see text for discussion). **B:** Section through a partly replicated kinetoplast disk in vivo. Bold minicircles on the periphery are nicked. Since only the nicked minicircles are available for hybridization, this model explains the donut structure observed by fluorescence *in situ* hybridization using a minicircle probe.

a mitochondrial DNA polymerase colocalizes with the topoisomerase (Ferguson et al., 1992). In addition we found with fluorescence *in situ* hybridization, using a minicircle probe, that minicircles are present in the same structures (Ferguson et al., 1992). Based on several criteria, these minicircles are very likely free minicircle replication intermediates. All of these data indicate that there are two complexes of replication enzymes, possibly containing all of the enzymes required for free minicircle replication, situated on opposite sides of the kinetoplast disk in vivo. We are currently purifying other enzymes that may be associated with these structures. Figure 5 shows a micrograph of a *C. fasciculata* cell. The kinetoplast (k), visualized from the edge of the disk, is stained with the fluorescent dye DAPI. On each side of the the kinetoplast (indicated by arrows) are the complexes of replication proteins. They are visualized with fluorescein-tagged antibodies against the DNA polymerase.

Based on these data, the diagram in Figure 6 shows the current view of

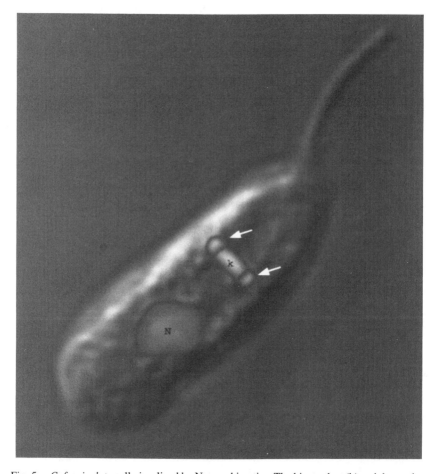

Fig. 5. *C. fasciculata* cell visualized by Nomarski optics. The kinetoplast (k) and the nucleus (N) are visualized by fluorescence after DAPI staining. The two complexes of replication proteins are visualized by fluorescence of fluorescein-labeled antibody to the mitochondrial DNA polymerase.

minicircle replication within a *C. fasciculata* cell. Minicircles are released from within the central region of the network, probably by a topoisomerase localized within the kinetoplast disk. A candidate topoisomerase II, distinct from the enzyme present in the two replication complexes and that could possibly serve to release minicircles, has been studied by Shlomai and coworkers (see Shlomai and Zadok, 1983). The free minicircles then migrate to one of the two peripheral complexes where they undergo replication. The minicircle progeny, containing nicks or gaps, then reattach to the network periphery.

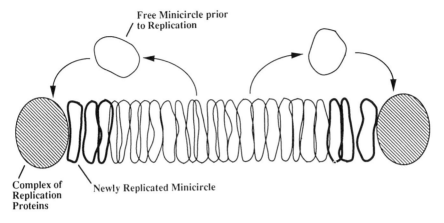

Fig. 6. Model for kDNA replication in vivo. Covalently closed minicircles are released from the central region of the network. They migrate to one of the two complexes of replication proteins where they undergo replication. The nicked progeny are then attached to the network periphery. Bold minicircles are nicked (see text for discussion).

This model explains an important early observation by Simpson and Simpson (1976). They used light microscopic autoradiography to study networks isolated from *C. fasciculata* that had been labeled in vivo for 1 minute with [³H]thymidine. Surprisingly, they found that the newly synthesized minicircles are located exclusively in two peripheral zones on opposite sides of the network. Now it seems clear that these minicircles had been attached to the network adjacent to the two complexes of replication proteins. Probably the topoisomerase II present in these complexes is responsible for attaching the newly replicated minicircles onto the network.

HOW ARE MINICIRCLES DISTRIBUTED UNIFORMLY AROUND THE KINETOPLAST PERIPHERY?

The model in Figure 6 predicts that newly synthesized minicircles should accumulate in the two zones on opposite sides of the network. However, the EM autoradiograph in Figure 2 demonstrates that nicked (recently replicated) minicircles are distributed *uniformly* around the network periphery. The same distribution, around the entire periphery, was also observed by Simpson and coworkers (1974) in light microscopic autoradiographs of networks labeled in vivo with [³H]thymidine for 10 minutes. How is this paradox explained?

To address this issue we used autoradiography of networks labeled in vivo with [³H]thymidine, exactly as done earlier by Simpson and coworkers. However, we used EM to study the labeled networks at higher resolution (Pérez-

Morga and Englund, 1993a). One example of an EM autoradiograph, a network labeled in vivo for 6 minutes, is shown in Figure 7. As expected, the silver grains are located on the periphery, and they are clearly in two zones. Surprisingly, the grains in each zone form a gradient in density; the gradient in the two zones is always in the same direction. This density gradient is due to the rising specific radioactivity of the DNA precursor during the course of the labeling. As the exogenous [^{3}H]thymidine mixes with the endogenous pool of DNA precursors, there is a gradual increase in specific radioactivity of the deoxynucleoside triphosphates. The presence of the two labeling zones is consistent with the minicircles being attached at two sites. However, the presence of the gradients of silver grains indicates that they are attached in an orderly and sequential manner around the network periphery. The fact that the silver grains on opposite sides of the network have approximately the same density indicates that the sites of reattachment are always on opposite sides of the disk.

The best explanation of these and related data is that there is a relative movement of the network and the two complexes (Pérez-Morga and Englund, 1993a). One possibility is that the two complexes are fixed and the kinetoplast disk actually rotates (see model in Figure 8). Another is that the disk is fixed and the complexes move around the circumference. Although based on incomplete data (Pérez-Morga and Englund, 1993a), we favor the first possibility. Since it takes about 6 minutes to radiolabel the entire network periphery, using two complexes of replication proteins, the kinetoplast disk must make about one turn in 12 minutes. Presumably after each turn it continues to rotate in the same direction, allowing minicircle reattachment to occur in a spiral pattern.

The concept of a rotating kinetoplast disk should still be considered speculative, and the idea must be tested rigorously. If true, then it will be very exciting to study the mechanisms which control this rotation.

MAXICIRCLE REPLICATION

Much less is known about the replication of maxicircles than of minicircles. In C. fasciculata, they appear to replicate while attached to the network, as rolling circles (Hajduk et al., 1984). When replication is complete, the rolling circle tail is cut off; the linearized molecule recircularizes and then reattaches to the network. These early studies had indicated that the maxicircle replication origin resides in the "variable region," a segment of the maxicircle that contains many repetitive sequences and therefore was difficult to clone. Recent sequencing of this region in T. brucei maxicircles revealed two copies of the GGGGTTGGTGT sequence, which is a crucial part of the minicircle replication origin in all species of trypanosomatids (Sloof et al., 1992; Myler et al., 1993). This finding suggests that the regulation of the initiation of minicircle and maxicircle replication may be similar.

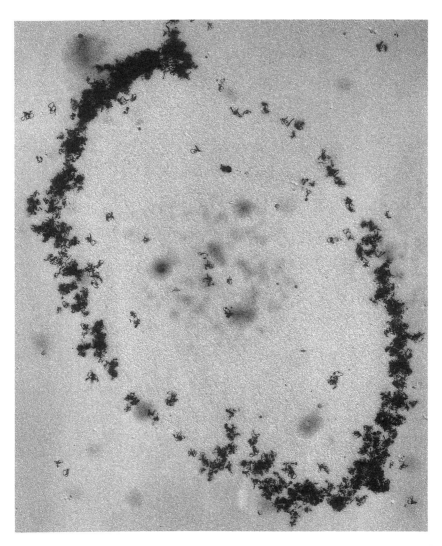

Fig. 7. EM autoradiograph of a network radiolabeled in vivo with a 6 minute pulse of [³H]thymidine. Silver grains represent newly synthesized minicircles attached to the network during the pulse. Note gradient of silver grain density in each of the labeling zones. (Reproduced from Pérez-Morga and Englund, 1993a, with permission of the publisher.)

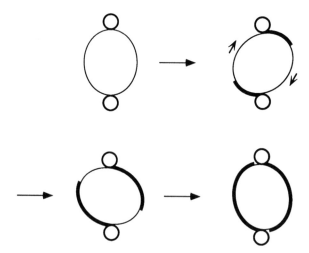

Fig. 8. Model for attachment of minicircles around the entire network periphery in vivo. The elliptical structure represents the kinetoplast disk, and the small circles represent the two complexes of replication proteins. The bold segments represent rows of newly attached minicircles. Small arrows indicate the direction of rotation of the kinetoplast disk. (Reprinted from Pérez-Morga and Englund, 1993a.)

There are several puzzling properties of maxicircles that must be addressed before their replication can be fully understood. For example, in isolated *T. brucei* double-sized networks, as observed by EM, all of the maxicircles appear clustered in the central region (Hoeijmakers and Weijers, 1980). In contrast, in *C. fasciculata* cells observed by fluorescence *in situ* hybridization using a maxicircle probe, the maxicircle signal is detected in 8–10 discrete foci embedded within the kinetoplast disk. The number of foci increases during replication, and they remain distributed throughout the disk (Ferguson, et al., 1994). From both of these observations it seems clear that maxicircles are not randomly distributed within the kDNA, but exactly how they are organized remains a mystery. Another unexpected finding with kDNA from *T. equiperdum* (a close relative of *T. brucei*) is that all of the network's maxicircles are topologically interlocked with each other, forming a "network within a network" (Shapiro, 1993). Maxicircle networks were detected in isolated kDNA after removing all of the minicircles by restriction enzyme cleavage. Their significance is not yet clear.

MINICIRCLE HETEROGENEITY AND SEQUENCE EVOLUTION

Study of kDNA replication has provided insight into some of the well-known characteristics of kDNA. For example, it has been known for many years that minicircles within a network are often highly heterogeneous. Now that we know the genetic function of minicircles, it is clear that a heterogeneous population is essential to encode multiple guide RNAs. *C. fasciculata,* in which editing is probably not extensive, has a small minicircle repertoire with one major class and a few minor ones (Sugisaki and Ray, 1987). In contrast, *T. brucei* apparently needs roughly 300 different types of minicircles in its network to support its very extensive editing (Steinert and Van Assel, 1980). Although minicircle heterogeneity is clearly selected by the needs of the editing machinery, it is not obvious why there are rapid changes in the minicircle repertoire. For example, several studies have revealed striking differences in minicircle restriction digests in different isolates of the same species (Borst et al., 1980; Morel et al., 1980). Even culturing trypanosomatid parasites for a year in the laboratory can result in detectable changes in minicircle restriction fragments (Hoeijmakers and Borst, 1982; Simpson et al., 1980).

What causes these rapid changes? One possibility is an error-prone DNA polymerase. We recently found that the *C. fasciculata* mitochondrial polymerase mentioned above has an error rate at least as high as any other DNA polymerase ever studied, including HIV reverse transcriptase and eukaryotic DNA polymerase-β. In an in vitro assay, it has an extraordinary error rate, about 1 mistake in roughly 1,200 nucleotides polymerized (Torri et al., 1994). Although it is possible that accessory proteins improve its fidelity in vivo, it is likely that this enzyme contributes to the rapid changes observed in minicircle sequences.

The replication model in Figure 6 suggests another mechanism for the rapid change in minicircle content of a network. According to this model, a free minicircle migrates to one of the two protein complexes, and, after replication, its two daughter minicircles attach to the network at neighboring sites. Then, when network division occurs during the G2 phase of the cell cycle, it would be likely that the two sister minicircles would segregate into the *same* daughter network. This might seem to be an unacceptable mechanism for inheritance of genetic information, as the guide RNAs encoded in that minicircle would be lost to one of the daughter cells. Nevertheless, it is possible that trypanosomatids could survive with this mechanism because each type of minicircle is present in multiple copies; there also could be related guide RNAs that could substitute for one that is lost. Since minicircle-encoded guide RNAs are assumed to be essential for parasite viability, there may be constant selection for maintenance of a critical repertoire of minicircles. If an essential minicircle is lost, then the parasite cell would die.

These thoughts on minicircle inheritance are highly speculative, and it is essential that they be tested experimentally. If it turns out that the idea is incorrect, then one would have to explain a precise mechanism for evenly distributing sister minicircles to daughter cells. To do this it would probably be necessary to refine the replication model in Figure 6. Whatever the case, it is certain that the most exciting work on kDNA replication lies in the future.

ACKNOWLEDGMENTS

We thank Viiu Klein and Kristen Gaines for invaluable support. Research in the authors' laboratory was supported by the NIH (GM27608) and the MacArthur Foundation.

REFERENCES

Benne R (1990): RNA editing in trypanosomes: Is there a message? Trends Genet 6; 177–181.

Borst P, Fase Fowler F, Hoeijmakers JH, Frasch AC (1980): Variations in maxi-circle and mini-circle sequences in kinetoplast DNAs from different *Trypanosoma brucei* strains. Biochim Biophys Acta 610:197–210.

Cosgrove WB, Skeen MJ (1970): The cell cycle in *Crithidia fasciculata*. Temporal relationships between synthesis of deoxyribonucleic acid in the nucleus and in the kinetoplast. J Protozool 17:172–177.

Delain E, Riou G (1969): DNA ultrastructure of the kinetoplast of *Trypanosoma cruzi* cultivated in vitro. CR Acad Sci [D] 268:1225–1227.

Englund PT (1978): The replication of kinetoplast DNA networks in *Crithidia fasciculata*. Cell 14:157–168.

Englund PT (1979): Free minicircles of kinetoplast DNA in *Crithidia fasciculata*. J Biol Chem 254:4895–4900.

Ferguson M, Torri AF, Ward DC, Englund PT (1992): In situ hybridization to the *Crithidia fasciculata* kinetoplast reveals two antipodal sites involved in kinetoplast DNA replication. Cell 70:621–629.

Ferguson ML, Torri AF, Pérez-Morga D, Ward DC, Englund PT (1994): Kinetoplast DNA replication: Mechanistic differences between *Trypanosoma brucei* and *Crithidia fasciculata*. J Cell Biol (in press).

Hajduk SL, Klein VA, Englund PT (1984): Replication of kinetoplast DNA maxicircles. Cell 36:483–492.

Hoeijmakers JH, Borst P (1982): Kinetoplast DNA in the insect trypanosomes *Crithidia luciliae* and *Crithidia fasciculata*. II. Sequence evolution of the minicircles. Plasmid 7:210–220.

Hoeijmakers JH, Weijers PJ (1980): The segregation of kinetoplast DNA networks in *Trypanosoma brucei*. Plasmid 4:97–116.

Marini JC, Levene SD, Crothers DM, Englund PT (1982): Bent helical structure in kinetoplast DNA. Proc Natl Acad Sci USA 79:7664–7668.

Melendy T, Sheline C, Ray DS (1988): Localization of a type II DNA topoisomerase to two sites at the periphery of the kinetoplast DNA of *Crithidia fasciculata*. Cell 55:1083–1088.

Morel C, Chiari E, Camargo EP, Mattei DM, Romanha AJ, Simpson L (1980): Strains and clones of *Trypanosoma cruzi* can be characterized by pattern of restriction endonuclease products of kinetoplast DNA minicircles. Proc Natl Acad Sci USA 77:6810–6814.

Myler PJ, Glick D, Feagin JE, Morales TH, Stuart KD (1993): Structural organization of the maxicircle variable region of *Trypanosoma brucei*: Identification of potential replication origins and topoisomerase II binding sites. Nucleic Acids Res 21:687–694.

Ntambi JM, Marini JC, Bangs JD, Hajduk SL, Jimenez HE, Kitchin PA, Klein VA, Ryan KA,

Englund PT (1984): Presence of a bent helix in fragments of kinetoplast DNA minicircles from several trypanosomatid species. Mol Biochem Parasitol 12:273–286.

Pérez-Morga D, Englund PT (1993a): The attachment of minicircles to kinetoplast DNA networks during replication. Cell 74:703–711.

Pérez-Morga D, Englund PT (1993b): The structure of replicating kinetoplast DNA networks. J Cell Biol 123:1069–1079.

Rauch CA, Pérez-Morga D, Cozzarelli NR, Englund PT (1993): The absence of supercoiling in kinetoplast DNA minicircles. EMBO J 12:403–411.

Ray DS (1987): Kinetoplast DNA minicircles: High-copy-number mitochondrial plasmids. Plasmid 17:177–190.

Ryan KA, Shapiro TA, Rauch CA, Englund, PT (1988): The replication of kinetoplast DNA in trypanosomes. Annu Rev Microbiol 42:339–358.

Shapiro TA (1993): Kinetoplast DNA maxicircles: Networks within networks. Proc Natl Acad Sci USA 90:7809–7813.

Shlomai J, Zadok A (1983): Reversible decatenation of kinetoplast DNA by a DNA topoisomerase from trypanosomatids. Nucleic Acids Res 11:4019–4034.

Simpson AM, Simpson L (1976): Pulse-labeling of kinetoplast DNA: Localization of 2 sites of synthesis within the networks and kinetics of labeling of closed minicircles. J Protozool 23:583–587.

Simpson L (1987): The mitochondrial genome of kinetoplastid protozoa: Genomic organization, transcription, replication, and evolution. Annu Rev Microbiol 41:363–382.

Simpson L (1990): RNA editing—A novel genetic phenomenon? Science 250:512–513.

Simpson L, Simpson, AM, Kidane G, Livingston L, Spithill TW (1980): The kinetoplast DNA of the hemoflagellate protozoa. Am J Trop Med Hyg 29:1053–1063.

Simpson L, Simpson AM, Wesley RD (1974): Replication of the kinetoplast DNA of *Leishmania tarentolae* and *Crithidia fasciculata*. Biochim Biophys Acta 349:161–172.

Sloof P, de Haan A, Eier W, van Iersel M, Boel E, Van Steeg H, Benne R (1992): The nucleotide sequence of the variable region in *Trypanosoma brucei* completes the sequence analysis of the maxicircle component of mitochondrial kinetoplast DNA. Mol Biochem Parasitol 56:289–299.

Steinert M., Van Assel S (1980): Sequence heterogeneity in kinetoplast DNA: reassociation kinetics. Plasmid 3:7–17.

Stuart K, Feagin JE (1992): Mitochondrial DNA of kinetoplastids. Int Rev Cytol 141:65–88.

Sugisaki H, Ray DS (1987): DNA sequence of *Crithidia fasciculata* kinetoplast minicircles. Mol Biochem Parasitol 23:253–263.

Torri AF, Kunkel TA, Englund PT (1994): A β-like DNA polymerase from the mitochondrion of the trypanosomatid *Crithidia fasciculata*. J Biol Chem 269:8165–8171.

Molecular Approaches to Parasitology, pages 163–177
© 1995 Wiley-Liss, Inc.

Exploring the Organelle Genomes of Malaria Parasites

Jean E. Feagin

*Seattle Biomedical Research Institute, Seattle, Washington 98109-1651;
Department of Pathobiology, School of Public Health and Community Medicine,
University of Washington, Seattle, Washington 98195*

INTRODUCTION

Malaria parasites have 14 chromosomes, as determined by pulsed field gel electrophoresis and counting of centromeres in serial sections. These chromosomes have been shown to have remarkable plasticity, with significant polymorphisms between different lines due to a variety of translocations, recombinations, and loss of telomeric sequences by breakage and telomere formation on the broken ends. In addition to these, there are two extrachromosomal DNAs that appear substantially less changeable. These are a 35 kb circular molecule and another DNA with varying numbers of a conserved tandemly repeated 6 kb sequence. Compared with the nuclear chromosomes, these DNAs make up a miniscule fraction of the cell's coding capacity. However, recent molecular analyses have imbued them with a fascination out of proportion with their size.

The role of the mitochondrion during the *Plasmodium falciparum* life cycle is not well understood. The parasite relies on glycolysis for energy production during the erythrocytic portions of the life cycle. There is, after all, little need to rely on more efficient methods when living in the vertebrate bloodstream where glucose is easily obtained. Several lines of evidence suggest that aerobic respiration is employed during insect stages of the life cycle, among them being more abundant mitochondrial cristae in insect stages and the detection, by cytochemical staining techniques, of some Krebs cycle enzymes in insect but not erythrocytic forms. While the basis and details of such a potential switch in energy metabolism remain to be determined, it adds another facet to the regulation of organelle genome expression, already potentially complex because of the need to coordinate nuclear and mitochondrial expression properly. In addition, despite the parasite's reliance on glycolysis in the erythrocytic cycle, inhibitors of organelle protein synthesis and the mitochondrial electron transport chain have antimalarial effects (Geary and Jensen, 1983; Divo et al., 1985; Ginsburg et al., 1986), arguing a crucial role for mitochondrial function in erythrocytic stages.

In 1975, a circular molecule was found in a partially purified mitochondrial fraction of *Plasmodium lophurae* (Kilejian, 1975). Since mitochondrial DNAs are often circular and the size was in the range normally seen for mitochondrial genomes of lower eukaryotes, it was cited as the mitochondrial DNA. Similar circular DNAs were subsequently detected in other *Plasmodium* species, and in 1988 a sequence for a small subunit rRNA was identified from this molecule (Gardner et al., 1988). It had the characteristics expected for an organelle rRNA, seemingly confirming a mitochondrial identity for this 35 kb circular DNA. Rapidly thereafter, however, two pieces of data appeared that muddied the waters. The first, in 1989, was sequence data from *P. gallinaceum* (Aldritt et al., 1989) and *P. yoelii* (Vaidya et al., 1989) that identified canonical mitochondrial protein coding genes on a tandemly repeated DNA element with a unit length of 6 kb. It was suggested that this DNA might be a mitochondrial episome or part of a bipartite mitochondrial genome. The second, in early 1991, was the identification of genes for RNA polymerase subunits on the circular molecule (Gardner et al., 1991b), a feature never before seen on mitochondrial genomes. This began to cast doubt on the identification of the circular molecule as mitochondrial DNA. Substantial data bearing on these extrachromosomal DNAs have been collected and, while it cannot yet be claimed that the identity and origins of either molecule are absolutely certain, the accumulated data now make the picture far clearer.

THE "6 KB ELEMENT"

The tandemly repeated DNA, now commonly called the 6 kb element, has been shown, by cross-hybridization, to be present in a variety of *Plasmodium* species (Vaidya and Arasu, 1987; Joseph et al., 1989). It has been estimated that there are as many as 150 copies of the 6 kb element in *P. yoelii* (Vaidya and Arasu, 1987) and 15 copies in *P. gallinaceum* (Joseph et al., 1989). The 6 kb element has been sequenced in three species of *Plasmodium: P. falciparum* (Feagin et al., 1992; Vaidya et al., 1993), *P. gallinaceum* (Aldritt et al., 1989; Joseph, 1990), and *P. yoelii* (Vaidya et al., 1989). The sequence is well conserved between these three species and encodes three open reading frames with homology to identified protein coding genes (Aldritt et al., 1989; Vaidya et al., 1989; Feagin, 1992). These are cytochrome *b*, cytochrome oxidase I, and, on the opposite strand of DNA, cytochrome oxidase III (Fig. 1). Cytochrome *b* and cytochrome oxidase I are the only two protein coding genes that have been invariably found in all mitochondrial genomes examined, and cytochrome oxidase III is nearly invariant, missing only from the *Chlamy-*

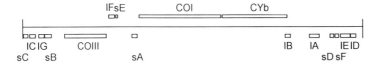

Fig. 1. Map of the *P. falciparum* 6 kb element. A schematic map of the 6 kb element is given, with genes shown by boxes above or below the line according to the direction of transcription (left to right above the line). CYb, cytochrome *b*; COI and COIII, cytochrome oxidase subunits I and III; lA-G and sA-F, regions homologous to large and small subunit rRNA sequences.

domonas mitochondrial genome. These three protein coding genes are therefore highly characteristic of mitochondrial genomes, and their presence has suggested that the 6 kb element, despite its small size, is the *Plasmodium* mitochondrial genome. This is an extremely abbreviated mitochondrial genome; those of vertebrates, which are among the smallest previously described, are generally about 16 kb in size and usually encode 13 proteins.

Further evidence in support of this interpretation comes from data about the subcellular location of the 6 kb element. Examination of materials generated during subcellular fractionation of *P. yoelii* showed that 6 kb element DNA tended to be most abundant in fractions containing mitochondrial enzyme activities (Wilson et al., 1992). Thus far, unfortunately, attempts to localize the 6 kb element more definitively by in situ hybridization have not been successful. As would be expected for a mitochondrial genome, the 6 kb element is uniparentally inherited (Creasey et al., 1993).

Unexpectedly, only the cytochrome *b* gene has an ATG at the expected 5′ location for translation initiation. The cytochrome oxidase I and III genes, when compared between the three sequenced *Plasmodium* species, are well conserved throughout the reading frame but diverge 5′ of the region where an ATG would be expected based on these genes in other species (Feagin, 1992). The 5′ end sequence of the cytochrome oxidase I transcript in all three species has been examined by RNA sequencing or sequencing of anchor polymerase chain reaction (PCR) products (Joseph, 1990; Suplick et al., 1990; Feagin, 1992). In each case, the transcripts match the DNA sequence exactly, and no evidence for alterations such as RNA editing was found. It seems likely that translation for these genes begins at alternate initiation codons, a feature seen in other mitochondrial genomes. In another somewhat unusual and thus far unexplained feature, database searches with the amino acid sequences for these three genes showed that their counterparts from the human mitochondrial genome, rather than those of other lower eukaryotes, were among the strongest matches (Feagin, 1992).

Transcripts for all three protein coding genes can be detected in RNA from the *P. falciparum* erythrocytic stages (Fig. 2A–C). This is not surprising, since

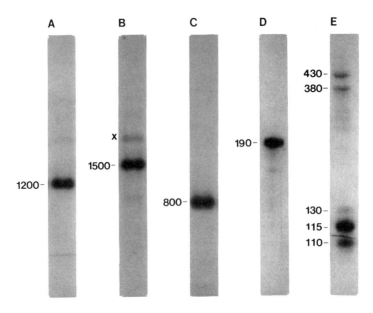

Fig. 2. Northern blot analysis of 6 kb element transcripts. Northern blots of *P. falciparum* erythrocytic stage RNA electrophoresed on agarose (**A–C**) or acrylamide (**D,E**) gels were probed with labeled oligonucleotides (A,B,D,E) or in vitro transcripts (C) complementary to 6 kb element genes. Sizes, given in nt, were determined based on RNA markers. The faint transcript in B marked x reflects spurious cross-hybridization with nuclear small subunit rRNA. Abbreviations as in Figure 1. A, CYb; B, COI; C, COIII; D, E, rRNA fragments.

the protein products of these genes are all components of the electron transport chain and inhibitors of its activity have antimalarial effects. The role that the electron transport chain plays in these stages, given the parasite's reliance on glycolysis, remains to be determined, however. The explanation for these apparently contradictory observations may lie in pyrimidine biosynthesis. *Plasmodium* species cannot salvage pyrimidines and instead have been shown to contain all the enzymes required for their de novo synthesis. One of these enzymes, dihydroorotate dehydrogenase, is mitochondrially located in mammals and passes electrons produced during the reduction of dihydroorotate to orotate to the electron transport chain via ubiquinone. It has been suggested that this may also be the case in *Plasmodium* (Gutteridge et al., 1979), unlike some other lower eukaryotes in which the enzyme is cytoplasmic. Both DNA and RNA synthesis during the erythrocytic cycle are greatest during the trophozoite and schizont stages; thus the need for pyrmidines is presumably highest at these times. Preliminary experiments have shown that transcripts of the electron transport chain components encoded by the 6 kb element are most abundant during the trophozoite and schizont stages (Feagin and Drew, unpublished results). While analyses of the protein products remain to be done, the timing of greatest transcript abundance for these genes is consistent with the proposed role for the electron transport chain in pyrimidine biosynthesis.

Besides the protein coding genes noted above, the only other genes invariably found in mitochondrial genomes are rRNAs. The 6 kb element does, indeed, contain regions that have homology to large and small subunit rRNA sequences (Aldritt et al., 1989; Vaidya et al., 1989; Joseph, 1990; Feagin et al., 1992). However, these are scattered in small blocks, interspersed between each other and the protein coding genes and on both strands of the DNA (Fig. 1). The scrambling of the rRNA fragments is such that it is impossible to construct a scenario in which a single transcript could be made and the unneeded intervening pieces removed to give either the large or small rRNA fragments in their proper order. While decidedly unconventional, this arrangement is not unheard of. Some other lower eukaryotes have fragmented rRNAs, and in a few cases the fragments are found out of order with respect to each other (Gray and Schnare, 1990). The *Chlamydomonas* mitochondrial rRNAs provide the best known example of these, having eight large subunit rRNA fragments and four small subunit rRNA fragments that are scrambled in order and found interspersed between each other and surrounding protein coding genes. However, the *Plasmodium* case differs from that of *Chlamydomonas* in one important feature, the aggregate size of the fragments. The *Chlamydomonas* rRNA fragments total approximately the size expected for bacterial rRNAs while the 6 kb element rRNA fragments are much smaller. The largest *P. falciparum* rRNA transcript detected thus far is only about 205 nt and the smallest is about 30 nt (Feagin and colleagues, unpublished results). Together, the *P. falciparum* large rRNA fragments identified by homology searches total 822 nt and the small subunit fragments total 429 nt (Feagin et al., 1992) compared with 2,904 and 1,542 nt, respectively, for *Escherichia coli* rRNAs.

In light of the highly unusual characteristics of the 6 kb element rRNA fragments, it is reasonable to ask if they can function in ribosomes. Although *Plasmodium* mitochondrial ribosomes have not yet been isolated to address this question directly, there are several lines of evidence that suggest that the 6 kb element-encoded rRNA fragments are functional. First, the regions with rRNA sequence homology are transcribed (Joseph, 1990; Suplick et al., 1990; Feagin et al., 1992). The transcripts detected are small, tending to correspond to approximately the size of the homology regions, and are relatively abundant (Fig. 2D,E). In a number of cases, oligonucleotide probes specific for single homology regions have detected only a single transcript, whereas in some cases multiple, often differentially abundant transcripts are seen. In the latter instance, it is not yet clear whether these data reflect processing of precursor molecules or simply spurious cross-hybridization to other small transcripts. It is possible that the larger low-abundance transcripts (up to 400–500 nt) that are occasionally seen represent ligation of the smaller fragments into larger molecules. However, the substantially greater abundance of the smaller transcripts suggests that these larger molecules, if not simply due to spurious cross-hybridization, are more likely to be precursor transcripts. The close spacing between many of the genes on the 6 kb element would lend itself to cotranscription and processing.

The sequences for the rRNA fragments are also extremely well conserved. Comparison of the homology between the *P. falciparum* and *P. yoelii* 6 kb element sequences shows that most of the rRNA regions are conserved at the 95%–100% level (Feagin et al., 1992). This is similar to the degree of conservation (about 98%) noted for the amino acid sequences of the three protein coding genes of the 6 kb element between these two species. In contrast, the overall nucleotide sequence homology rate for the 6 kb element between these two species is 89% and the homology at the nucleotide level for the protein coding genes is 86%. Thus the degree of sequence conservation noted for the rRNA fragments suggests they are under selective pressure to maintain specific nucleotide sequences.

The potential secondary structure of these rRNA fragments also suggests they are functional (Joseph, 1990; Feagin et al., 1992). rRNA sequence and secondary structure has been extensively studied in a wide variety of organisms, and certain areas have been found to be highly conserved. Unsurprisingly, many of the rRNA functions that have been mapped to specific sequences fall within these regions, called conserved core regions. When the rRNA fragments from the 6 kb element are aligned with the potential secondary structure of *E. coli* large and small subunit rRNAs, it can clearly be seen that the fragments correspond predominantly to the conserved core sequences (Fig. 3). In general, sequences corresponding to the more variable regions have not been found. This is in some senses a self-fulfilling prophecy, since these would be, by definition, more difficult to recognize. However, the coding capacity of the 6 kb element is highly limited, and the detection of sequences corresponding to much of the conserved core is telling. One might almost imagine that nature has performed a massive genetic deletion experiment, removing the more variable portions of the rRNA sequence and leaving behind only those absolutely required for function.

Fig. 3. Potential secondary structure of the fragmented small subunit rRNA of the *P. falciparum* 6 kb element. **A:** The potential secondary structure of the six fragments with homology to small subunit rRNA. Arrows indicate the junctions between fragments C and D, and E and F. **B:** The secondary structure of the *E. coli* small subunit rRNA with conserved core regions shown in thick lines and variable regions in dotted lines. Similar comparisons for the large subunit rRNA are presented by Feagin et al. (1992).

A

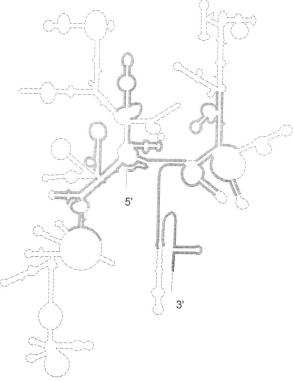

B

Figure 3.

Consideration of the predicted secondary structures for the large and small subunit rRNA fragments shows that almost all of them have the potential to interact with at least one other fragment by hydrogen bonding (Fig. 3) (Feagin et al., 1992). As noted above, there is little evidence from northern blots to support the idea that the fragments from each subunit become ligated into a single long molecule. Rather, the potential for intermolecular nucleic acid interactions suggests that these hydrogen bonds, possibly assisted by interactions with ribosomal proteins, may be sufficient to allow formation of functionally active ribosomes. At present there is no way to determine if the RNA fragments can self-assemble, followed by association with proteins, or if protein–RNA interactions are required earlier in the assembly process.

The 13 6 kb element rRNA fragments that were identified by homology searches do not include all of the expected conserved core sequences (Feagin et al., 1992). Regions such as the 790 loop and the 5′ end sequence of the small subunit rRNA are missing, as are some expected sequences from the large subunit rRNA. There are also short regions of the 6 kb element to which no genes have been mapped. We have employed these as probes on northern blots and have evidence for the existence of some additional small transcripts that are potential rRNA fragments (Feagin and colleagues, unpublished results). One step in verifying the identity of these as rRNAs is locating their potential positions in the secondary structure. Determining these has thus far proved difficult. In cases in which the highly conserved nucleotides for a region are few in number and interspersed with less conserved sites and in which one must consider the possibility that adjacent parts of a conserved sequence may be on two different RNA fragments, the complexity of the analyses rises astronomically. Also, mitochondrial rRNAs are sometimes significantly smaller than bacterial rRNAs, with correspondingly altered secondary structure. The mitochondrial rRNAs of *Trypanosoma brucei* provide an excellent example, being only 1,150 and 610 nt for the large and small subunit rRNAs, respectively, with quite unusual characteristics for portions of their proposed secondary structures. It is possible that the newly discovered small transcripts may provide necessary structures and interactive capabilities, even the specific nucleotides required for function, but will not conform to the structures expected based on bacterial rRNAs. The identity and role of these additional small RNAs are under study.

Thus the transcription, conservation, and correspondence to core sequences all suggest that these unusual rRNA fragments are functional. A further line of evidence supporting this contention comes from data about mitochondrial function. Cytochrome oxidase activity can be detected in the erythrocytic stages of *P. falciparum* (Scheibel and Sherman, 1988). Since two of the subunits crucial to this activity are encoded by the mitochondrial genome, it follows that the transcripts of the 6 kb element genes are translated. There are three possible ways in which this might occur. One possibility is that the rRNAs for the mitochondrial ribosomes are imported from the nucleus. However, while there is evidence supporting the import of small RNAs into the mitochondrion, large RNAs have not been shown to enter. In a second scenario, the mRNAs from the 6 kb element protein genes might exit the mitochondrion for translation on cytoplasmic ribosomes, and their protein products be reimported to the mitochondrion. However, there is no evidence that large RNAs can leave the mitochondrion. Furthermore, although it is by no means an absolute requirement, mitochondrial protein import usually relies on the presence of a cleavable protein presequence, and the protein genes encoded by the 6 kb element do not have such presequences. Finally, the fragmented rRNAs may be functional in the mitochondrial ribosomes of *Plasmodium* species, consistent with the evidence cited above. Experiments to examine the makeup of *Plasmodium* mitochondrial ribosomes are in progress. A greater understanding of these ribosomes may not only serve to indicate how mitochondrial proteins are made in malaria parasites but, because of the unusual and abbreviated structure of the rRNAs, may provide insight into structure–function correlations relevant to a more general understanding of ribosome function.

THE 35 KB CIRCULAR DNA

The second extrachromosomal DNA is the 35 kb circular DNA (Fig. 4). As noted above, this molecule was originally thought to be the mitochondrial DNA of *Plasmodium*. However, on closer examination, the characteristics and gene complement of this molecule suggest a more unexpected identification (Wilson et al., 1991; Palmer, 1992). The salient organizational feature of this molecule is a large inverted repeat that encompasses almost one-third of the molecule. Each half of the repeat encodes genes for large and small subunit rRNAs arranged in a head to head orientation. Unlike those of the 6 kb element, these rRNAs are intact and have lengths and potential secondary structures quite similar to those of the corresponding *E. coli* rRNAs (Gardner et al., 1991a, 1993). Between the rRNAs is a set of seven tRNAs, and additional single tRNAs flank the 3′ end of each of the rRNAs. Evidence gathered to date suggests that the duplication is perfect, with no nucleotide differences having yet been found to allow differentiation between the genes in one half versus the other half of the inverted repeat. An additional tRNA cluster is loctated to one side of the duplicated region, and some ribosomal protein genes are encoded in this area as well (R.J.M. Wilson, personal communication). The other protein coding genes that have been identified on this molecule are two subunits of a bacterial-type RNA polymerase, encoded by the *rpo*B and *rpo*C genes, respectively (Gardner et al., 1991b). Together, the known genes account for about two-thirds of the 35 kb DNA. The genetic complement of the remaining third of the molecule is as yet unknown.

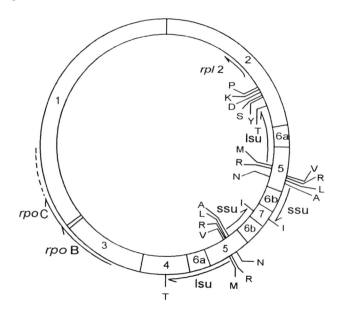

Fig. 4.   Map of the *P. falciparum* 35 kb DNA. A schematic map of the 35 kb circular DNA is shown with genes inside or outside the circle depending on direction of transcription (clockwise outside the circle). The dotted line indicates the expected extent of the *rpo*C gene. tRNAs are identified with the one letter code. *rpo*B and *rpo*C, RNA polymerase subunits; lsu and ssu, large and small subunit rRNAs; *rpl2*, ribosomal protein. Additional ribosomal proteins are also found in the *rpl2* region. *Hind*III sites are indicated.

The detailed studies of the 35 kb DNA undertaken in the last several years have undermined its originally assumed mitochondrial identification. Rather, the characteristics of the molecule appear more like those of a plastid DNA (Wilson et al., 1991; Palmer, 1992). For example, the presence of an inverted repeat containing rRNAs and tRNAs is rare in mitochondrial genomes but quite common in plastid genomes. It is the RNA polymerase genes, however, that are the most provocative. No mitochondrial genome has ever been found to encode its own RNA polymerase genes, whereas this is quite common in plastid genomes. Furthermore, the type of RNA polymerase genes normally found in chloroplast genomes are like those found in bacteria, while the only mitochondrial RNA polymerase (that of *Saccharomyces cerevisiae*) that has been sequenced is, in addition to being encoded in the nucleus, more similar to phage polymerases. In fact, phylogenetic analyses of the *rpo*B and *rpo*C genes of the 35 kb DNA suggest that they are even more related to their chloroplast DNA-encoded counterparts than to those in bacteria (Howe, 1992; R.J.M. Wilson, personal communication). Finally, examination of chloroplast genomes in nonphotosynthetic plants provides further evidence of the plastid genome similarities of the 35 kb DNA (Wolfe et al., 1992). The most studied plastid genome among the nonphotosynthetic plants is that of *Epifagus*. It is a circular molecule about 70 kb in size compared with the 120–180 kb size of chloroplast genomes in photosynthetic plants. The decrease in size has been accomplished by the loss of single copy sequences, leaving the inverted repeat with its rRNA sequences behind. In fact, all but four of the intact genes remaining are involved in either translation or transcription. The functions of the four remaining genes are unknown, and it has been argued that the reason for retention of the plastid genome in the absence of photosynthesis is that one or more of these genes may play a critical role in an as yet unidentified nonphotosynthetic process. One can easily imagine that, if the 35 kb DNA originated as a chloroplast DNA, the length of time since it last had to produce components for the photosynthetic apparatus is sufficiently long to have lost even more genes than *Epifagus*. Phylogenetic studies based on nuclear genes indicate that dinoflagellates are among the organisms most closely related to *Plasmodium* species (Gajadhar et al., 1991), providing additional support for the emerging picture of a photosynthetic algal-like ancestor for the malaria parasite. The reason for retention of 35 kb DNA, as with the plastid DNA of nonphotosynthetic plants, remains uncertain. It is ironic that all the genes identified to date are involved in either transcription or translation. Presumably, the reason for their retention is a gene (or genes) in the currently unknown region whose function is required for parasite survival.

The location of the 35 kb DNA within the cell is unknown. It does not colocalize with the 6 kb element in subcellular fractionation studies and thus is probably not in the mitochondrion (Wilson et al., 1992). However, given its organelle DNA-like characteristics, it is expected to be within a membrane-bound body. Electron micrography of *Plasmodium* species reveals the presence of a multiply membrane-bounded body with no known function, simply called the spherical body. It seems logical to suggest that the organelle DNA that lacks a home and the organelle that lacks a purpose may have a relationship (Kilejian, 1991). Indeed, the multiple membranes of the spherical body are reminiscent of what one might expect to see in a remnant chloroplast. However, hard evidence to document that the spherical body is the location of the 35 kb DNA has not yet been obtained.

As with the 6 kb element, transcriptional analysis of the 35 kb DNA indicates that it probably functions during the erythrocytic cycle. Transcription of both rRNAs (Fig. 5A,B) and some of the tRNAs has been verified in RNA from these stages. In fact, RNase protection analyses strongly suggest that the rRNAs are transcribed as precursor molecules containing at least some of their flanking tRNAs (Gardner et al., 1991a, 1993). The initial size of these precursors has not yet been determined, but processing appears to proceed slowly

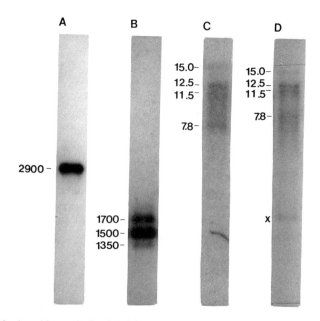

Fig. 5. Northern blot analysis of *P. falciparum* 35 kb DNA transcripts. Northern blots of *P. falciparum* erythrocytic stage RNA electrophoresed on agarose gels were probed with labeled oligonucleotides (**A,B**) or in vitro transcripts (**C,D**) complementary to 35 kb DNA genes. Sizes, given in nt (A,B) or kb (C,D), were determined based on RNA markers. Sizes >9 kb are approximations due to the lack of RNA markers in this range. The faint transcript in D marked x reflects spurious cross-hybridization with nuclear small subunit rRNA. Abbreviations as in Figure 4. A, Isu; B, ssu; C, *rpo*B; D, *rpo*C.

enough, at least in some steps, for a relatively abundant 1,700 nt potential precursor to the 1,500 nt small subunit rRNA to be detected on northern blots (Fig. 5B). The relationship of the faint 1,350 nt transcript detected with small subunit tRNA probes to the other transcripts is not known. No similar evidence of precursor molecules is seen in northern blot analysis of the large subunit rRNA (Fig. 5A), but RNase protection data suggest it is also processed from a larger molecule (Gardner et al., 1993), apparently more rapidly or completely than the small subunit rRNA. In contrast to the rRNAs, transcripts for the RNA polymerase subunits seem quite low in abundance and very large in size (Gardner et al., 1991b) (Fig. 5C,D), suggesting that they may be polycistronic. This would be entirely in keeping with the putative chloroplast DNA origin of the 35 kb DNA, since chloroplast genes are commonly polycistronic.

Rifampicin, an inhibitor of bacterial-type RNA polymerases, is known to have antimalarial effects at physiological concentrations (Geary and Jensen,

1983). The possibility that this action could be explained by inhibition of the RNA polymerase encoded by the 35 kb DNA has been very exciting. Unfortunately for that hypothesis, it has been recently shown that the kinetics of inhibition of parasite growth are different for rifampicin and another, more specific inhibitor of bacterial RNA polymerases, streptolydigin (Strath et al., 1993). Further, rifampicin-resistant lines of *P. falciparum* have been selected, and the RNA polymerase subunit genes of the 35 kb DNA show no nucleotide changes in the sites normally associated with changes from sensitive to resistant phenotypes in bacteria (Strath et al., 1993; N. Lang-Unnasch, personal communication). These data do not absolutely disprove the original hypothesis but suggest strongly that the principal effect of rifampicin may be on another molecule. Whether it also has some lesser effects on the RNA polymerase of the 35 kb DNA remains to be determined. The retention of the 35 kb DNA, requiring the allocation of cellular resources to replicate and segregate it properly, continues to suggest that something encoded by the molecule is important to cell survival.

Despite disappointment that rifampicin's antimalarial activity is probably not explained by inhibition of the 35 kb DNA RNA polymerase, the unusual evolutionary connotations of this extrachromosomal DNA make it eminently worthy of additional study. If, as suspected, there is a critical gene in the unknown region of the molecule, it might well provide an excellent target for development of new antimalarial chemotherapeutics. The likelihood is high that the product of a (presumably) remnant plastid gene would have significant differences from human gene products. For the 6 kb element, the evidence for the importance of its expression is unequivocal: Inhibitors of the electron transport chain, critical components of which are encoded by the 6 kb element, have antimalarial effects (Ginsburg et al., 1986). The antimalarial action of various inhibitors of organelle protein synthesis (Divo et al., 1985) could be explained by their action against ribosomes from either, or both, of the organelle genomes, since the rRNAs in both cases generally have the expected sites for antibiotic sensitivity.

CONCLUSION

Further study of both these extrachromosomal DNAs is expected to provide additional insights into novel genes and gene regulatory mechanisms, basic biochemical phenomena, and possible targets for new chemotherapeutics. The history of organelle genome studies in parasites has been full of surprises. The 6 kb element and the 35 kb DNA of *Plasmodium* species have certainly provided their share of these, and it is likely that they have yet more to offer.

ACKNOWLEDGMENTS

Dr. L.K. Read provided helpful comments on the manuscript. Work from the author's laboratory was supported by NIH grant AI25513 and NSF grant MCB-9205809. The author is also a Burroughs Wellcome Fund New Investigator in Molecular Parasitology.

REFERENCES

Aldritt SM, Joseph JT, Wirth DF (1989): Sequence identification of cytochrome *b* in *Plasmodium gallinaceum.* Mol Cell Biol 9:3614–3620.

Creasey AM, Ranford-Cartwright LC, Moore DJ, Williamson DH, Wilson RJM, Walliker D, Carter R (1993): Uniparental inheritance of the *mitochondrial* gene cytochrome b in *Plasmodium falciparum.* Curr Genet 23:360–364.

Divo AA, Geary TG, Jensen JB (1985): Oxygen- and time-dependent effects of antibiotics and selected mitochondrial inhibitors on *Plasmodium falciparum* in culture. Antimicrob Agents Chemother 27:21–27.

Feagin JE (1992): The 6 kb element of *Plasmodium falciparum* encodes mitochondrial cytochrome genes. Mol Biochem Parasitol 52:145–148.

Feagin JE, Werner E, Gardner MJ, Williamson DH, Wilson RJM (1992): Homologies between the contiguous and fragmented rRNAs of the two *Plasmodium falciparum* extrachromosomal DNAs are limited to core sequences. Nucleic Acids Res 20:879–887.

Gajadhar AA, Marquardt WC, Hall R, Gunderson J, Ariztia-Carmona EV, Sogin ML (1991): Ribosomal RNA sequences of *Sarcocystis muris, Theileria annulata* and *Crypthecodinium cohnii* reveal evolutionary relationships among apicomplexans, dinoflagellates, and ciliates. Mol Biochem Parasitol 45:147–154.

Gardner MJ, Bates PA, Ling IT, Moore DJ, McCready S, Gunasekera MBR, Wilson RJM, Williamson DH (1988): Mitochondrial DNA of the human malarial parasite *Plasmodium falciparum.* Mol Biochem Parasitol 31:11–17.

Gardner MJ, Feagin JE, Moore DJ, Rangachari K, Williamson DH, Wilson RJM (1993): Sequence and organization of large subunit rRNA genes from the extrachromosomal 35 kb circular DNA of the malaria parasite *Plasmodium falciparum.* Nucleic Acids Res 21:1067–1071.

Gardner MJ, Feagin JE, Moore DJ, Spencer DF, Gray MW, Williamson DH, Wilson RJM (1991a): Organization and expression of small subunit ribosomal RNA genes encoded by a 35-kb circular DNA in *Plasmodium falciparum.* Mol Biochem Parasitol 48:77–88.

Gardner MJ, Williamson DH, Wilson RJM (1991b): A circular DNA in malaria parasites encodes an RNA polymerase like that of prokaryotes and chloroplasts. Mol Biochem Parasitol 44:115–124.

Geary TG, Jensen JB (1983): Effects of antibiotics on *Plasmodium falciparum* in vitro. Am J Trop Med Hyg 32:221–225.

Ginsburg H, Divo AA, Geary TG, Boltand MT, Jensen JB (1986): Effects of mitochondrial inhibitors on intraerythrocytic *Plasmodium falciparum* in in vitro cultures. J Protozool 33:121–125.

Gray MW, Schnare MN (1990): Evolution of the modular structure of rRNA. In WE Hill, A Dahlberg, RA Garrett, PB Moore, D Schlessinger, JR Warner (eds): The Ribosome: Structure, Function, and Evolution. Washington, DC: American Society for Microbiology, pp. 589–597.

Gutteridge WE, Dave D, Richards WHG (1979): Conversion of dihydroorotate to orotate in parasitic protozoa. Biochim Biophys Acta 582:390–401.

Howe CJ (1992): Plastid origin of an extrachromosomal DNA molecule from *Plasmodium*, the causative agent of malaria. J Theor Biol 158:199–205.

Joseph JT (1990): The Mitochondrial Microgenome of Malaria Parasites. Ph.D. Thesis. Cambridge, MA: Harvard Medical School.

Joseph JT, Aldritt SM, Unnasch T, Puijalon O, Wirth DF (1989): Characterization of a conserved extrachromosomal element isolated from the avian malarial parasite *Plasmodium gallinaceum*. Mol Cell Biol 9:3621–3629.

Kilejian A (1975): Circular mitochondrial DNA from the avian malarial parasite *Plasmodium lophurae*. Biochim Biophys Acta 390:276–284.

Kilejian A (1991): Spherical bodies. Parasitol Today 7:309.

Palmer JD (1992): A degenerate plastid genome in malaria parasites? Curr Biol 2:318–320.

Scheibel LW, Sherman IW (1988): Plasmodial metabolism and related organellar function during various stages of the life cycle: Proteins, lipids, nucleic acids and vitamins. In WH Wernsdorfer, I McGregor (eds): Malaria: Principles and Practice of Malariology. Edinburgh: Churchill Livingstone, pp. 219–252.

Strath M, Scott-Finnigan T, Gardner M, Williamson D, Wilson I (1993): Antimalarial activity of rifampicin *in vitro* and in rodent models. Trans R Soc Trop Med Hyg 87:211–216.

Suplick K, Morrissey J, Vaidya AB (1990): Complex transcription from the extrachromosomal DNA encoding mitochondrial functions of *Plasmodium yoelii*. Mol Cell Biol 10:6381–6388.

Vaidya AB, Akella R, Suplick K (1989): Sequences similar to genes for two mitochondrial proteins and portions of ribosomal RNA in tandemly arrayed 6-kilobase-pair DNA of a malarial parasite. Mol Biochem Parasitol 35:97–108. Corrigendum (1990) Mol Biochem Parasitol 39:295–296.

Vaidya AB, Arasu P (1987): Tandemly arranged gene clusters of malarial parasites that are highly conserved and transcribed. Mol Biochem Parasitol 22:249–257.

Vaidya AB, Lashgari MS, Pologe LG, Morrisey J (1993): Structural features of *Plasmodium* cytochrome *b* that may underlie susceptibility to 8-aminoquinolines and hydroxy-naphthoquinones. Mol Biochem Parasitol 58:33–42.

Wilson RJM, Fry M, Gardner MJ, Feagin JE, Williamson DH (1992): Subcellular fractionation of the two organelle DNAs of malaria parasites. Curr Genet 21:405–408.

Wilson RJM, Gardner MJ, Williamson DH, Feagin JE (1991): Have malaria parasites three genomes? Parasitol Today 7:134–136.

Wolfe KH, Morden CW, Ems SC, Palmer JD (1992): Rapid evolution of the plastid translational apparatus in a nonphotosynthetic plant: Loss or accelerated sequence evolution of tRNA and ribosomal protein genes. J Mol Evol 35:304–317.

Molecular Approaches to Parasitology, pages 179–189
© 1995 Wiley-Liss, Inc.

The Double-Stranded RNA Genome of Giardiavirus

Alice L. Wang and C.C. Wang

Department of Pharmaceutical Chemistry, University of California, San Francisco, California 94143

INTRODUCTION

In 1986, while examining the nucleic acid extract of the binucleated flagellate *Giardia lamblia,* we noticed an unusual species of nucleic acid that turned out to be linear, double-stranded RNA (dsRNA) in the electrophoresed agarose gel. The detection of this new molecule in turn led to the discovery of its source, the giardiavirus (GLV), that readily infects many virus-free *Giardia* isolates (Wang and Wang, 1986). Here, we discuss the biology and genomic organization of GLV and how, in addition to its intrinsic interest, it may prove useful as a vector for transfection of *Giardia.*

GLV BIOLOGY

GLV infection occurs at rather high frequencies in nature, as approximately one-third of *Giardia* isolates we examined were found to harbour this virus, irrespective of the species or geographic distribution of its mammalian host (Miller et al., 1988a). The virus does not infect human intestinal cell lines or any other protozoa tested (Wang et al., 1988). The basis of this specificity cannot be simply attributed to the presence of GLV receptors on the cell of *G. lamblia.* We have observed that by introducing GLV RNA into *Tritrichomonas foetus* or *Trichomonas vaginalis* via electroporation there was no GLV replication in those cells thereafter. When the GLV RNA was electroporated into the *G. lamblia* isolates refractory to GLV infection, however, normal viral replication cycle could be completed to produce infectious GLV progeny (Sepp et al., 1994). Apparently, *G. lamblia* cells can provide a suitable environment for GLV replication, which is missing with *T. foetus* and *T. vaginalis.* The observation also suggests that the mechanism underlying GLV resistance among the refractory *G. lamblia* isolates are most likely due to the absence of cell surface receptors.

Giardiavirus is among the simplest of viruses. With electron microscopy the virion is seen as an icosahedron 36 nm in diameter with its electron-dense cores surrounded by a double shell (Miller et al., 1988b). Biochemically, the virus comprises a nonsegmented dsRNA genome of 6,277 nucleotides (nts), a major polypeptide of 100 kD (p100), and a much less abundant polypeptide of 190 kD (p190) (Miller et al., 1988b; Wang and Wang, 1991; Wu et al., manuscript in preparation). These characteristics place GLV taxonomically very close to the nonsegmented dsRNA viruses of fungi and yeast. In 1990, GLV was officially assigned the genus *Giardiavirus* in the family of Totiviridae by the International Committee on the Taxonomy of Viruses and became the first protozoan virus recognized by the Committee.

Attempts of direct peptide sequencing of the two viral proteins indicated that both p100 and p190 are blocked at the N termini. The identity of the blocking group is still to be determined. Further biochemical analysis indicated that these viral proteins contained no detectable sugar. Thus, p100 and p190 are apparently not glycosylated (Wang and Wang, unpublished data).

Similar to all dsRNA viruses, the replication cycle of GLV does not involve a DNA phase (Wang and Wang, 1988). In addition to the genomic dsRNA, a single-stranded full-length transcript (SS) of the GLV dsRNA was also detected in the nucleic acid extract of the virus-infected *Giardia* cells (Furfine et al., 1989). SS was fully infectious when electroporated into virus-free GLV-sensitive cells (Furfine and Wang, 1990). It is therefore most likely the viral messenger RNA as well as the replicative intermediate of the GLV genome. RNA-dependent RNA polymerase (RDRP) activity has been identified in the infected cell extract as well as purified GLV virion. Under the assay condition used, the polymerase product was exclusively the sense strand, therefore suggestive of a conservative replication model for the GLV dsRNA similar to that of yeast killer virus (ScV) (White and Wang, 1990).

To summarize, GLV is a small dsRNA virus that can be readily isolated from either the cellular extract or the culture medium supernatant of infected *G. lamblia*. The virus is being synthesized and shed to the culture medium at an astonishingly high level, yet imparts no obvious cytopathic effect on its protozoan host. Both the virus and its dsRNA can be prepared in reasonable quantities (virus in milligrams and dsRNA in micrograms), and are both stable upon storage. The ease of in vitro GLV infection and the feasibility of transfecting *Giardia* with SS distinguishes GLV from all the other known fungal and protozoan dsRNA viruses as the only one capable of permanent infection by either exposing sensitive cells to the free virions or electroporating with the viral messenger RNA.

ORGANIZATION OF THE GLV GENOME

General Features of the GLV dsRNA

Northern blot analysis indicated that the GLV genomic dsRNA and the SS are the only two identifiable GLV-derived RNAs in the infected *G. lamblia* cellular extract. Neither of these two molecules is polyadenylated (Wang et al., 1990). Similarly, no subgenomic transcript, spliced, or edited version of the viral RNA has been observed (Furfine et al., 1989). Using a combination of cDNA cloning strategies, we have synthesized a series of overlapping cDNA clones of GLV spanning the full length of the viral genome and determined its entire nucleotide sequence (GenBank accession No. L13218; Wang et al., 1993; Wu et al., manuscript in preparation). The contiguous 6,277 nt fragment revealed the presence of two major open reading frames (ORFs), both from the SS strand. ORF1 (nt 356–3025) encodes a polypeptide of 891 amino acid residues with predicted molecular mass of 99 kD and pI of 6.4. ORF2 (nt 2,806–5,976) overlaps ORF1 by 220 nt and is separated from the latter by a (–1) frameshift. ORF2 encodes a polypeptide of 1,057 amino acid residues with a predicted molecular mass of 120 kD and a pI of 9.65. All currently known RDRP consensus sequence motifs have been identified in the mid-third portion of this ORF (Poch et al., 1989) (Fig. 1).

Besides ORFs 1 and 2, no other ORF longer than 100 amino acid residues has been detected in all the six frames of this 6,100 nt cDNA. When these short ORFs were checked with the database from the GenBank, no significant homology to any known sequences or functional sequence motifs was found.

Identification of the ORFs With Viral Polypeptides and Evidences for a Frameshift Fusion Protein

Based on the amino acid sequence derived from the cDNA, four peptides from selected regions, their respective positions shown in Figure 1, were synthesized. These peptides were conjugated to keyhole limpet hemocyanin and used to immunize rabbits. Results from Western blots of purified GLV reacting to these antisera are shown in Figure 2. Peptide C and T are both located

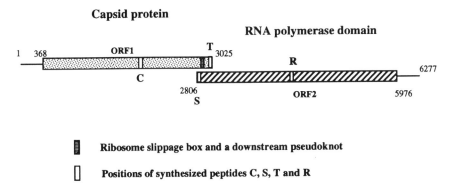

Fig. 1. Organization of the GLV dsRNA genome. Numerals refer to the positions of nucleotides in the 6,100 nt cDNA fragment. Synthesized peptides and their respective locations are as follows: C, NHITTTYAYEEEVTMAIK (nt 1,883–1,936); T, YSIRVSTLHHLMTTRAK (nt 2,952–3,002); R, MSYLEYIMADTIVDKAFTTT (nt 4,246–4,305); and S, LVLRHNLR (nt 2,809–2,832). Details of the ribosome slippage heptamer and pseudoknot are shown in Figure 3.

G   W

C   R   T   S

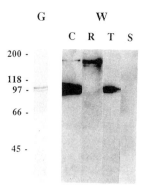

Fig. 2. Western blots of GLV proteins reacted to antisera against synthetic peptides. **G:** Coomassie blue–stained SDS-PAGE gel. p190 is not always visible in the stained gel. The lower band in the doublet is a cross-reacting protein that can be removed by an additional purification step of CsCl gradient centrifugation. **W:** Western blots of the same gel reacted with αC (lane C), αR (lane R), αT (lane T), and αS (lane S).

within ORF1. Antisera to peptide C and T (αC and αT) both recognize p100, indicating that ORF1 encodes p100. Similarly, αR, the antiserum to peptide R, which is located in ORF2, reacted to p190 only, assigning ORF2 to encode p190. However, in addition to p100, αC also reacted positively to p190, which was present at a level 2%–5% of p100. This result, together with the observation that αT and αR recognizes only the C terminus of the respective polypeptides, p100 and p190, suggests that these two viral proteins share a common domain at their N termini, but not the C termini (Wang et al., 1993).

Since ORF2 alone is too short to account for the observed molecular mass of p190, we suspected that the latter is in fact a fusion protein of both ORF1 and ORF2. The first indication that this may be true is that αC reacted with both p100 and p190. Further support of this possibility came from examining the cDNA sequence. Within the 220 nt region where the two ORFs overlap, we found a probable ribosomal slippage heptamer CCCUUUA (nt 2,836–2,842), which is followed 6 nt downstream by a pseudoknot (Fig. 3). These structural features agree with the frameshifting requirements found in many retroviruses (ten Dam et al., 1990) and ScV (Dinman, 1991). A third source of support for the formation of a frameshift fusion protein came from another immunostudy. A fourth peptide S was synthesized from the amino acid sequence at the N terminus of ORF2, upstream from the presumed ribosome slippage box. As expected from the frameshift model, which predicts that the portion of ORF2 before the slippage box should not have been expressed, αS did not react to either p100 or p190 (Fig. 2). The last and most direct support for the

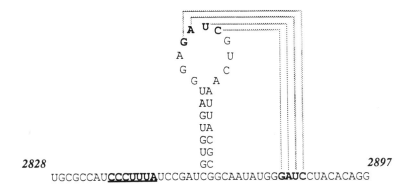

Fig. 3.   Ribosomal slippage heptamer and its downstream pseudoknot in GLV RNA. The sequence of the heptamer is underlined.

frameshifting in GLV derives from a yeast shuttle vector construct in which a 73 bp fragment from GLV cDNA (nt 2,826–2,888), which contains the presumed ribosomal slippage heptamer and the pseudoknot, was placed before an out-of-frame β-galactosidase (β-gal). A (–1) frameshift is required for the synthesis of β-gal fusion protein. It was observed that, from this construct, the β-gal fusion protein was synthesized at 10% level as compared with a separate in-frame construct (Tzeng, Bruenn, Wang, and Wang, unpublished data). We are therefore confident that GLV indeed uses the translational frameshift strategy to synthesize its larger polypeptide, the RDRP, in the form of a fusion protein.

Plausible Translational Start Site of GLV Proteins

ORF1 begins at nt 356 with Trp. The first Met in ORF1 is the fifth amino acid residue encoded by nt 368–370. Within 30 nt upstream from this Met there is a stop codon in each of the three reading frames, rendering this Met a probable start site for p100. The predicted molecular mass for a polypeptide commencing at this Met is 98.4 kD, a value reasonably agreeable to the estimated molecular mass of p100. In comparison, the next Met (nt 719–721) as translational start site would yield a much smaller polypeptide of 85 kD.

Assuming translational frameshifting for the synthesis of p190 takes place at the presumed CCCUUUA box, the resulting fusion protein starting from the same Met at nt 368 would have a predicted molecular mass of 210 kD, slightly larger than our estimate of the viral RDRP of 190 kD as determined from its mobility in SDS-PAGE. The discrepancy may simply be due to an anomalous mobility of this protein in gel electrophoresis at such high molecular weight range. However, other possibilities such as post-translational processing by proteases (Palmenberg, 1990) or initiation of translation at an alternate internal site (Pelletier and Sonenberg, 1988) cannot be ruled out.

5′ and 3′ Untranslated Regions and the Termini of GLV dsRNA

Within the 357 nt 5′ region upstream of ORF1, five ATGs and an ATGATG repeat are found on the sense strand. Each of these ATGs is followed by a small ORF comprising 3–46 amino acid residues, many of them overlapping one another. It is not known if any of these small ORFs is expressed. However, no peptide of such sizes has been detected in SDS-PAGE or immunoblot studies using polyclonal antibodies against the whole virus.

A computer-assisted search in the 357 nt 5′ region did not find any sequence motifs of known promotors or consensus translation initiation sequences used in vertebrates, *Drosophila,* or yeast (Cavener, 1987; Cigan and Donahue, 1987).

Following the termination codon of ORF2, there are 301 nt of untranslated regions at the 3′ terminus of the sense strand. Consistent with the observation that neither the GLV dsRNA nor the GLV SS is polyadenylated at the 3′ terminus, we did not find any consensus polyadenylation signal in this region either.

In contrast to the polymorphic termini noted in the *Leishmania* virus LRV (Widmer, 1993), the 3′ termini of GLV dsRNA appeared to be homogeneous, and both strands co-terminate (blunt-ended) at either terminus (Wu et al., manuscript in preparation).

COMPARISON OF GLV GENOMIC SEQUENCE WITH THOSE OF OTHER VIRUSES

The RDRP Domain

A computer-assisted search of GenBank using the program FASTA for sequences homologous to either ORF1 or ORF2 yielded nothing significantly above noise. After all the RDRP consensus motifs were uncovered from ORF2 by visual inspection, we decided to compare the GLV sequences surrounding these motifs with the genomic sequences from the other two viruses, ScV (Bruenn, 1980) and LRV (Tarr et al., 1988; Widmer et al.,1989), that have been considered taxonomically most closely related to GLV. The program LFASTA was used to align the three viral peptides pairwise until the RDRP motifs were correctly aligned. Subsequences taken from these paired fragments were then further aligned by PIMA. The results as shown in Figure 4 indicate that sequence homology among the three dsRNA viruses extends beyond the known RDRP consensus motifs. The percentages of identical amino acid residues within this region among the LRV:GLV, ScV:GLV, and LRV:ScV pairs are, respectively, 16.43, 16.71, and 27.11%, suggesting that GLV is equally distant from LRV and ScV, while the latter two are more closely related.

```
lrv LPQLVEMKCLLGRGVNEIDV ETEARRRLDV---GSLSMQR LDENELRAAVRLIYS-EELR RPVTYPLI--CDFWSSRWLW 347
scv --LFELAVLMNRGVGHVSW  QAEKDHRLN------PDVAV VDQARLYSCVRDMF--EGSK QTYKYFFMTWDDYTANRWEW 369
glv -TLLSDFETLLGKVSYKNPS IIEEQVVPWLTSDPIPRTPD FYSTYFKTAVQFMHRTFVPV TLRSAPPLTFHEYCGRPELW 415

lrv AANGS-HSRALE---HAHPE LATRKEGQAYRKAVMEQWQH NPMDRWDGTVYVTPSAKLEH GKTRLLLACDTLSYMWFEYA 423
scv VPGGSVHSQYEEDNYIYPG  QYTRNKFITVNK--MPKHKI SRMIASPPEVRAWTSTKYEW GKQRAIYGTDLRSTLITNFA 447
glv GTTGS--G------YIGYG  KRSFNKWSIYGA--YPAEEI YRLALYGDNPPLKPLEKPEL TKVRAVISASLQSYILMSYL 484

lrv LRPVERIWENSNVILDPGSM GNCGIATRINGWRNGM---P GQSFFAVDYDDFNSQHTLMS QKIVFEELFHHIGYN----- 495
scv M------FRCEDVLTHKFPV GDQAEAAKVHKRVNMML--D GASSFCFDYDDFNSQHSIAS MYTVLCAFRDTFSRNM---- 515
glv E------YIMADTYVDKAFT TTLMNDRQLENLERHMMTMT GGVRVPVDQSNFDRQPDLVQ IGIWQQLFHLASASAPYRA 558

lrv ---ASWVKTLVDSFDSM-E  LWIKGKCAGIMAGTLMSGHR ATSFINSVLNRAYIICAGGH ------VPTSMHVGDDILMS 564
scv SDEQAEAMNWVCESVRHMWV LDPDTKEWYRLQGTLLSGWR LTTFMNTVLNWAYMKLAGVF D--LDDVQDSVHNGDDVMIS 593
glv RDSVSLVISRLASTTTFPKV KVRMSDGDKRVLHGLFSGWK WTALLGALINVTQLLTMAEL SNTLASLRSTVVQGDDIALS 638

lrv C-TLGHADNLIANLNRKGVR LNASK-QVFSKTSGEFLRVA HREHTSHGYLAR 614
scv LNRVSTAVRIMDAMHRINAR AQPAKCNLFSIS--EFLRVE HGMSGGDGLGAQ 643
glv MTDREQATQLVDTYARQGFE VNPKK-FWISPDRDEFLRRV ATPGIVAGYPAR 689
```

Fig. 4. Alignment of computer-deduced amino acid sequences in the conserved RDRP domains from LRV, ScV, and GLV. Identical amino acids are shaded.

ORF1 and ORF2 Show Low Homology to the Viruses of the Pox, Flavi, and Picorna Families

Using the deduced amino acid sequences in ORFs 1 and 2 to search for homologies in the GenBank, program FASTA yielded a list of polypeptides with marginal homology scores. Not surprisingly, some of them seem to be a random assortment of unrelated proteins, such as chick spectrin α-chain or glucose transporter. However, when we expand the list and examine it more closely, we found that among the 80 sequences with the best scores, 68 of these were viral DNA-directed or RNA-directed RNA polymerases or other viral proteins. The identities of these proteins and their extent of homology to GLV are listed in Table 1. The list of best score includes many clusters of sequences from closely related strains that share identical sequences in regions involved in this match. Only one entry is represented in Table 1 in these instances.

Both ORFs 1 and 2 are homologous to a selected group of DNA- or RNA-directed RNA polymerases, especially from poxviruses. But the matched regions revealed by FASTA are either near the N terminus of ORF1 or in ORF2 but approximately 300–400 amino acid residues upstream from the consensus RDRP motifs. These polymerases may therefore share additional conserved domains in addition to the known polymerase sequence motifs.

The list of sequences with best homology score to GLV is dominated by viral proteins from three families, namely, the poxviruses, the insect-borne flaviviruses, and the picornaviruses. The poxvirus proteins identified are all RNA polymerases. The selection of flaviviruses and picornaviruses in this search cannot be based entirely on the presence of RNA-binding sequences expected of these viruses, since other families of RNA viruses are excluded by this comparison. It is not clear whether sequence homology at this level has any significant meaning. The hypothetical protein 3 from the *Leishmania* virus LRV (Stuart et al., 1992) was found among the 30 sequences of best scores in our most recent GenBank search using the same program. Except for the fact that a shorter region was selected by the computer, the alignment with GLV by this search was identical to that shown in Figure 4. It is interesting to note that none of the sequence derived from other dsRNA viruses besides LRV was included within the top 120 entries. Therefore, dsRNA viruses are a widely diverged group and might not have shared any common recent ancestor.

The sites of RNA binding and packaging on the dsRNA genome of ScV have been mapped (Shen and Bruenn, 1993; Wickner, 1993). However, no homology in sequence was found between corresponding regions in ScV and GLV. More thorough studies are needed to dissect the structural requirements for these functions in GLV.

GLV AS A GENETIC VECTOR?

Giardiavirus offers many features that make it a very attractive candidate as a transfecting vector: 1) it is small, stable, and easily purified; 2) GLV infec-

TABLE 1. Peptides Sharing Low Sequence Homology With GLV Proteins

GenBank code	Polypeptide	GLV region	Percent Identity	No. of AA overlap
ORF1				
POLH-POLIM or GNNY2P	Human poliovirus type 1[a]	60–295	16.0	237
CAPHIMS_1 or RNVZCA	Capripoxvirus ORF HM2 RNA polymerase	143–246	20.4	103
gp:M37415:VACRPO132_1	Vaccinia virus RNA polymerase subunit rpo132[b]	144–360	19.7	228
gp:M27157: TBECG_1	Tick-borne encephalitis (TBE) virus polyprotein[b]	186–296	14.5	110
S15010	Cryphonectria parasitica dsRNA hypothetical protein B	185–285	17.0	100
POLG_JAEV1	Japanese encephalitis virus genome polyprotein[b]	276–315	33.3	45
gp:M33668: TBEGNE_1	TBE virus nonstructural protein[b]	392–409	22.4	67
PWARPT_1	Powassan virus genomic RNA sequence	424–459	28.6	35
gp:M16572:CXA3G_1	Coxsackievirus A9 orB3[a]	452–527	26.7	75
gp:X01076: PIP03119_5	Human poliovirus type 3[a]	645–728	16.2	105
RCMMVBCRNA_1	Red clover mottle virus	649–733	21.4	84
gp:D11079:VACRHF_7	Vaccinia virus 29.9K protein or A37R protein	683–747	26.6	64
A42551 or S102321_1	Dengue virus polyprotein[b]	710–815	16.2	105
POLG_YEFV2	Yellow fever virus polyprotein[b]	780–819	17.9	39
ORF-2				
prp1-Send5 P27566	Sendai virus RNA polymerase β-subunit	236–318	21.6	88
CPVRPPO13A_1 P19798	Cowpox virus RNA polymerase 132 kD polypeptide	236–396	21.7	166
RPOL_EAV P19811	Equine arteritis virus RNA-directed RNA polymerase	250–307	14.0	57
P1; S26418	Rous sarcoma virus gene pol protein	262–328	25.8	66
Rrp1_Mease P12576	Measles virus RNA polymerase β-subunit	304–389	20.0	85
Vdmb_Bpt7 P03694	Phage T7 DNA maturase B	330–476	19.0	147
Fimd_Ecoli P30130	E. coli fimd protein precursor	390–470	20.2	89
Top2_Trycr P30190	Trypanosoma cruzi topoisomerase II	576–666	21.5	93
S27930	Leishmania RNA virus 1 hypothetical protein 3	609–692	26.5	83
DP3A_BACSU P13267	B. subtilis DNA polymerase III, α-chain	632–734	16.7	102
POLG_COXA2 P22055	Coxsackie virus genome polyprotein[a]	687–769	26.4	72
POLG_TBEVS P07720	TBE virus capsid protein C[b]	728–767	20.5	39
POLG HCVA P19712	Hog cholera virus genome polyprotein	984–1,043	25.4	59

[a]Members of the Picornavirus family.
[b]Members of the Flavisvirus family.

tion is efficient, specific, and permanent and does not cause any apparent pathological effect on the flagellate; 3) the GLV genome is small and can be manipulated through its cDNA; and GLV genes are replicated to a very high copy number and viral gene products are expressed in large amounts, suggesting the presence of a very strong viral promoter.

We have joined all our partial GLV cDNA clones into a contiguous 6,277 nt fragment and started to test the infectivity of its RNA transcript via electroporation. The sequence of this cDNA will be further substantiated and validated if successful transfection can be demonstrated by its transcript. It is also expected that the GLV promoter elements are present within the 367 nt 5´ untranslated region of the transcript of the cDNA. The GLV capsid gene is being replaced with the firefly luciferase or the neomycin phosphotransferase genes and will be tested in GLV-infected *Giardia* to examine if the chimeric transcripts can be packaged by GLV capsid protein in the form of dsRNA or expressed as functional proteins. We are only at the very beginning of this effort and need to learn much more about GLV. When this is all worked out, we will then hopefully have a viral vector in *Giardia*.

REFERENCES

Bruenn JA (1980): Virus-like particles of yeast. Annu Rev Microbiol 34:49–68.

Cavener DR (1987): Comparison of the consensus sequence flanking translational start sites in *Drosophila* and vertebrates. Nucleic Acids Res 15:1353–1361.

Cigan AM, Donahue TF (1987): Sequence and structural features associated with translational initiator regions in yeast—A view. Gene 59:1–18.

Furfine ES, Wang CC (1990): Transfection of the *Giardia lamblia* double-stranded RNA virus into *Giardia lamblia* by electroporation of a single-stranded RNA copy of the viral genome. Mol Cell Biol 10:3659–3663.

Furfine ES, White TC, Wang AL, Wang CC (1989): A single-stranded RNA copy of the *Giardia lamblia* virus double-stranded RNA genome is present in the infected *Giardia lamblia*. Nucleic Acids Res 17:7453–7467.

Miller RL, Wang AL, Wang CC (1988a): Identification of *Giardia lamblia* strains susceptible and resistant to infection by the double-stranded RNA virus. Exp Parasitol 66:118–123.

Miller RL, Wang AL, Wang CC (1988b): Purification and characterization of the *Giardia lamblia* double-stranded RNA virus. Mol Biochem Parasitol 28:189–196.

Palmenberg AC (1990): Proteolytic processing of picornaviral polyprotein. Annu Rev Microbiol 44:603–623.

Pelletier J, Sonenberg N (1988): Internal initiation of translation of eukaryotic mRNA directed by a sequence derived from poliovirus RNA. Nature 334:320–325.

Poch O, Sauvaget I, Delarue M, Tordo N (1989): Identification of four conserved motifs among the RNA-dependent polymerase encoding elements. EMBO J 8:3867–3874.

Sepp T, Wang AL, Wang CC (1994): Giardiavirus-resistant *Giardia lamblia* lacks a virus receptor on the cell membrane surface. J Virol 68:1426–1431.

Shen Y, Bruenn JA (1993): RNA structural requirements for RNA binding, replication, and packaging in the yeast double-stranded RNA virus. Virology 195:481–491.

Stuart KD, Weeks R, Guilbride L, Myles PJ (1992): Molecular organization of *Leishmania* RNA virus 1. Proc Natl Acad Sci USA 89:8596–8600.

Tarr PI, Aline RF Jr, Smiley BL, Scholler J, Keithly J, Stuart KD (1988): LR1: A candidate RNA virus of *Leishmania*. Proc Natl Acad Sci USA 85:9572–9575.

ten Dam EB, Pleij CWA, Bosch L (1990): RNA pseudoknots: Translational frameshifting and readthrough on viral RNAs. Virus Genes 4:121–136.

Wang AL, Furfine ES, Wang CC (1990) The double-stranded RNA virus of *Giardia lamblia*. In L.H.T. van der Ploeg, C. Cantor, and H.J. Vogel (eds): Immune Recognition and Evasion: Molecular Aspects of Host–Parasite Interaction. New York: Academic Press, pp. 261–268.

Wang AL, Miller RL, Wang CC (1988): Antibodies to the *Giardia lamblia* double-stranded RNA virus major protein can block the viral infection. Mol Biochem Parasitol 30:225–232.

Wang AL, Wang CC (1986): Discovery of a specific double-stranded RNA virus in *Giardia lamblia*. Mol Biochem Parasitol 21:269–276.

Wang AL, Wang CC (1988): Viruses of parasitic protozoa. In T.P. Singer, N. Castagnoli, C.C. Wang (eds): Molecular Basis of the Action of Drugs and Toxic Substances. New York: de Gruyter, pp. 126–137.

Wang AL, Wang CC (1991): Viruses of the protozoa. Annu Rev Microbiol 45:251–263.

Wang AL, Yang HM, Shen KA, Wang CC (1993): Giardiavirus double-stranded genome encodes a capsid polypeptide and a gag-pol-like fusion protein by a translational frameshift. Proc Natl Acad Sci USA 90:8595–8599.

White TC, Wang CC (1990): RNA-dependent RNA polymerase activity associated with the double-stranded RNA virus of *Giardia lamblia*. Nucleic Acids Res 18:553–559.

Wickner RB (1993): Double-stranded RNA virus replication and packaging. J Biol Chem 268:3797–3800.

Widmer G (1993): RNA circularization reveals terminal sequence heterogeneity in a double-stranded RNA virus. Virology 193:11–15.

Widmer G, Comeau AM, Furlong DB, Wirth DF, Patterson JL (1989): Characterization of an RNA virus from the parasite *Leishmania*. Proc Natl Acad Sci USA 86:5979–5982.

Molecular Approaches to Parasitology, pages 191–205
© 1995 Wiley-Liss, Inc.

Chromatin Diminution in Nematode Development: An Alternative Means of Gene Regulation?

Fritz Müller

Institute of Zoology, University of Fribourg, Pérolles, CH-1700 Fribourg, Switzerland

INTRODUCTION

It is generally believed that development and differentiation of multicellular organisms are based on regulation of a constant genome in the different cell types rather than on qualitative or quantitative changes in the genetic content. The early embryonic development of the intestinal parasites *Parascaris* and *Ascaris* represent the classic exception to this so-called DNA constancy rule. During germline–soma segregation in these two nematode species, the phenomenon of chromatin diminution takes place. It is defined as a process that involves fragmentation of the chromosomes and the concomitant elimination of chromatin from all presomatic cells during early cleavage stages (see Fig. 1). Consequently, chromatin diminution leads not only to a change in the chromosomal organization but also to different contents of DNA between the germline and the somatic cell lineages.

The phenomenon of chromatin diminution was discovered by T. Boveri in *Parascaris* more than 100 years ago. It provided the first direct proof for the early segregation and independent development of the germline and the somatic cell lines (Boveri, 1887), which was predicted by A. Weismann in his famous germline theory established in 1885. The aims of the present chapter are to recall briefly the classic and recent cytological observations on chromatin diminution in *Parascaris* and *Ascaris*, to summarize the molecular data, and to discuss the significance and possible functions of the chromatin diminution process.

CYTOLOGY

In the course of the first cleavage division of *Parascaris univalens*, the two large chromosomes are distributed in a regular fashion to the two daughter

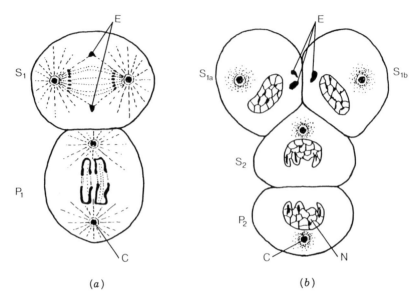

Fig. 1. Chromatin diminution in *P. univalens*. **a:** Anaphase of the second cleavage division in the two-cell stage. Chromatin diminution occurs in the top S_1 cell but not in the lower P_1 cell. **b:** Four-cell stage after completion of the second cell division. The cells S_{1a}, S_{1b} and S_2 give rise to somatic cells, whereas the P_2 cell represents the germline that later yields the germ cells. C, centrosome; E, eliminated chromatin; N, nucleus. (after Boveri, 1899, and Tobler et al., 1992.)

cells, designated S_1 and P_1 (see Fig. 1a). During the second cleavage division, the ventral P_1 cell again undergoes normal mitosis, giving rise to the cells S_2 and P_2 (Fig. 1a,b). In the dorsal S_1 cell, however, the central portions of the chromosomes break up into a large number of small chromosomes during metaphase (Fig. 1a). As anaphase progresses, only the diminished chromosomes migrate to the two daughter nuclei. The heterochromatic ends remain in the equatorial plate and are later expelled to the cytoplasm, where they eventually degenerate (Fig. 1b). As a result of the chromatin diminution process, the two postdiminution nuclei of the S_{1a} and S_{1b} cell now contain less chromatin than the nuclei of the cells S_2 and P_2. During the further embryonic development, chromatin diminution is repeated three more times in cells S_2, S_3, and S_4 (Fig. 2). Whereas elimination invariably takes place in these three blastomeres, chromatin diminution in the S_1 cell may be omitted. In this case, the diminution process is delayed to the third cleavage division, where it occurs simultaneously in the S_{1a} and S_{1b} cells (Boveri, 1910; Moritz, 1967). By careful analysis of the cell lineages, Boveri was able to show that all cells with a reduced amount of chromatin become somatic cells, whereas nuclei retaining the original integrity of chromosomes and full quantity of chromatin give rise to germline cells. The P_4 cell represents the primordial germ cell (see Fig. 2).

In *Ascaris suum,* an intestinal parasite of the pig, the process of chromatin diminution also occurs. In this nematode, however, the first elimination mitosis almost never takes place until the third cleavage division (see Fig. 2 and Table 1) (Meyer, 1895; Bonnevie, 1902). The fragmentation of the many small chromosomes ($2n = 38A + 10X$ in o and $38A + 5X$ in o) (Tobler, 1986) causes the elimination of terminal chromatin. It is not clear whether intercalarly located chromatin is also discarded, which could result in a change in the chromosome number, as is the case in *Parascaris.* Because of their small size it

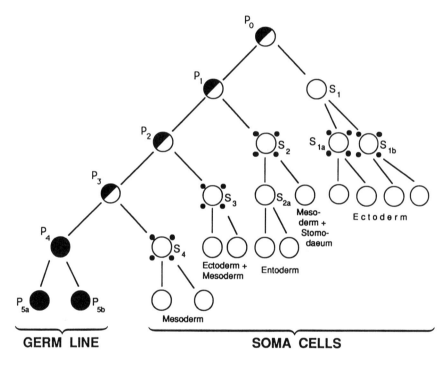

Fig. 2. Schematic representation of the cell lineage and segregation of germline and somatic cells in *A. suum.* The presumptive primordial germ cells (P_o–P_3) are indicated by half-filled circles and the primordial germ cells (P_4, P_{5a}, P_{5b}), giving rise to all germ cells, by large filled circles. The presomatic cells S_{1a}, S_{1b} and S_2–S_4 undergoing chromatin diminution are represented by small filled circles. These cells eventually form in a precisely determined manner the various parts of the embryo as designated. Early embryonic development of *P. univalens* is identical with the exception that the first chromatin diminution event usually occurs in the second cleavage division in the S_1 cell. (Modified from Boveri, 1910.)

TABLE 1. Occurrence of Chromatin Diminution in Nematodes

Species	Developmental stages at which chromatin diminution occurs	Reference
Parascaris univalens (= A. megalocephala var. univalens)	Second or third to fifth	Boveri (1887) Boveri (1899)
Ascaris suum (= A. lumbricoides)	Third to fifth	Meyer (1895) Bonnevie (1902)
Ophidascaris filaria (= A. rubicunda)	Second or third to fifth	Meyer (1895)
A. anguillae (= A. labiata)	—[a]	Meyer (1895)
Contracaecum incurvum (= A. incurva)	Third to fifth[a]	Goodrich (1916)
Toxocara canis (= A. canis)	Second to sixth	Walton (1917, 1924)
Toxocara cati (= Belascaris mystax)	Second or third to sixth	Walton (1924)
Toxocara vulpis (= Belascaris triquetra)	Third to sixth	Walton (1924)
Cosmocerca sp.	Third to eighth[a]	Yao and Pai (1942)

[a]The stages have either not been established or remain uncertain.

has not yet been possible to determine the exact number of chromosomes in any somatic tissue of *Ascaris*. Despite the very different genomic organization of *Parascaris* and *Ascaris*, the chromatin diminution process leads to the loss of all detectable heterochromatin in both species (Pimpinelli and Goday, 1989).

The chromosomes of *Parascaris univalens*, like those of all other nematode species studied thus far, are holocentric, that is, they have diffuse centromeres (Triantaphyllou, 1971). In gonial mitotic germ cells the continuous kinetochore plate extends over the whole chromatid surface (Goday et al., 1985), whereas in embryonic mitoses before and during chromatin diminution, it is confined only to the noneliminated euchromatic portion (Goday et al., 1992). Such a polycentric organization explains why during the elimination mitoses after chromosomal fragmentation the newly formed somatic chromosomes segregate independently to the poles and why the heterochromatic regions remain in the equatorial plate where they later degenerate. Thus, the centromeres located in the eliminated chromosomal regions must undergo developmentally regulated inactivation, which probably takes place soon after fertilization. This inactivation is an essential prerequisite for the diminution process and must depend on stage-specific factors.

No data about the centromeric organization of the *Ascaris* chromosomes are as yet available. However, the kinetic behavior of the chromosomes during the diminution process suggests that the eliminated chromatin, as in *Parascaris*, lacks centromeres and therefore remains in the equatorial plate.

OCCURRENCE

The process of chromatin diminution has thus far been reported to occur in nine different nematode species (Table 1). They all belong to the order of Ascaridida, a group of parasitic nematodes of vertebrates and occasionally invertebrates. However, not all nematodes undergo chromatin diminution, i.e., no chromatin diminution has been observed at the cytological level in at least 13 other nematode species (Walton, 1974). Particularly, biochemical and molecular techniques have revealed no evidence for chromatin diminution in the free-living nematode *Caenorhabditis elegans* (Sulston and Brenner, 1974; Emmons et al., 1979). Since this nematode contains no highly repetitive DNA, however, it is still possible that elimination of relatively small amounts of middle-repetitive and single-copy DNA sequences could remain undetected at both the cytological and biochemical levels. The genome of *Panagrellus redivivus*, a nematode related to *C. elegans*, contains two DNA satellite families, constituting together about 17% of the total genome, which are *not* eliminated from the presomatic cells during early development of this nematode (de Chastonay et al., 1990). Since in both *Ascaris* and *Parascaris* most of the highly repetitive satellite sequences are removed from the somatic genome, these findings indicate that chromatin diminution might not exist in *P. redivivus*. It still remains an enigma why some nematode species undergo chromatin diminution whereas others apparently do not.

ASCARIS SUUM AS AN EXPERIMENTAL SYSTEM

For the analysis of the process of chromatin diminution at the molecular level, we use *Ascaris suum* (*Ascaris lumbricoides* var. *suum*) rather than the horse parasite *Parascaris univalens,* which is almost extinct in central and northern Europe and in North America. *Ascaris*, like most ascarids, has a direct life cycle in a single host, which begins with the production of eggs by adult female worms in the distal small intestine of the host. The eggs are excreted in the feces. Under advantageous conditions (warm, moist, shaded soils) they become fully embryonated with an L2 stage larva that has molted once within the eggshell. The eggs are now infectious by ingestion and hatch, if swallowed, in the small intestine of the host. The larvae immediately penetrate the intestinal wall and are carried by the bloodstream, first to the liver and the capillaries of the portal circulation and then to the lungs. Here they pass into the alveoli, ascend the respiratory tract, and are swallowed to reach the intestine for a second time. Having terminated the migratory phase of their life cycle, the larvae remain in the intestine where they mature to become adult worms.

An interesting fact about *Ascaris* is the existence of two strains: human (*A. lumbricoides*) and porcine (*A.lumbricoides* var. *suum* or *A. suum*). Although the worms of both strains are almost identical in appearance, chemical composition, and details of the life cycle, they differ in the important respect that neither strain can easily infect the host of the other. Studies involving inoculation of pigs with ineffective eggs (L2 stages) from *A. suum* and *A. lumbricoides* revealed a number of physiological differences: The *Ascaris* of the pig completes its development in the lung and migrates to the intestine earlier, it requires less time to reach the egg lying stage, and, when taken to humans, develops to maturity less frequently and remains in the intestine for relatively short periods. A further important difference exists between the trypsin inhibitors of two *Ascaris* strains. Trypsin inhibitors of *A. suum* are unable to complex human trypsin effectively, which causes the death of *A. suum* worms in experiments where they were put in an environment containing human trypsin (Hawley and Peanasky, 1992). It is reasonable to speculate, that to resist digestion a parasitic nematode requires a complement of protease inhibitors that effectively inactivates digestive enzymes in the hostile environment of the host's intestine. Thus, trypsin inhibitors might be involved in the species specificity of the two *Ascaris* nematodes.

Ascaris lumbricoides is an important human parasite. The World Health Organization estimates that about 1 billion people are infected with this parasite (Warren, 1988). The disease occurs worldwide but is concentrated in warm, poorly sanitized areas, where it is maintained largely by the indiscriminate defecation and ingestion habits of children.

The related porcine strain *A. suum*, although not a human parasite, should not be neglected in public health planning, for larval migration occurs in abnormal hosts and may cause serious harm to humans. *A. suum*, however, can be readily obtained in large amounts from slaughterhouses. Its impressive size (females are about 8–16 inches long) has made it an ideal nematode for morphological, physiological, and biochemical studies. With regard to the chromatin diminution process, different germline and somatic tissues and stages from the adult animals can easily be dissected for the extraction of DNA, RNA, and proteins and for the preparation of in vitro extracts. Moreover, it is possible to isolate large amounts of fertilized eggs, which can be stored at 4°C for months. Upon incubation in vitro at 30°C they can be developed synchronously as far as the hatching L2 larvae. For further development, the infectious L2 larvae have to be ingested by the pig, where they undergo a migratory phase through various tissues and finally reach the adult stage in the intestine. Because of its parasitic life cycle, unfortunately, it is impossible to maintain *A. suum* in the laboratory and to use it for genetic analyses.

CHROMOSOME BREAKAGE

Using *A. suum* as an experimental organism, we have analyzed the chromatin diminution process at the molecular level. During this process, the heterochromatic termini of the many small *Ascaris* chromosomes break off, suggesting that new telomeres are added to the ends of the reduced somatic chromosomes. To gain further insight into this process, we have established a telomeric library from somatic DNA and randomly selected a few cloned somatic telomeres for further analysis (Müller et al., 1991, and unpublished data). Our data revealed that all of them were created during the process of chromatin diminution as a result of chromosomal fragmentation and subsequent addition of about 2–4 kb of telomeric TTAGGC repeats to the breakage sites (Fig. 3). No telomeric repeats were present at the equivalent position of the germline chromosomal regions, strongly arguing for a de novo generation of these sequences, probably by a telomerase-mediated process. Telomerases are specialized reverse transcriptases that carry their own RNA template for telomere synthesis. They appear to be widespread among eukaryotes as judged by the evolutionary conservation of telomeric DNA structures and by the identification of telomerase activity from diverse eukaryotes (for review, see Blackburn, 1991).

Telomere addition at a particular chromosomal breakage site, however, is not confined to a single spot, but rather occurs at many different positions that are scattered throughout a short chromosomal region of about 2–3 kb length, termed the chromosomal breakage region (CBR) (Müller et al., 1991). A complete nucleotide analysis of a cloned CBR revealed no evidence of repetitive

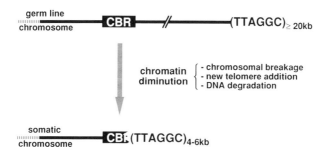

Fig. 3.   Schematic representation of germline and somatic DNA surrounding a chromosomal breakage region (CBR) in *A. suum*. The formation of a new somatic telomere during chromatin diminution involves chromosomal breakage, new telomere addition, and DNA degradation. Telomere addition occurs at many different sites within a CBR. Both the germline and the somatic telomeres consist of tandemly repeated TTAGGC sequences with an average length of ≥20kb for the germline telomeres and 4–6 kb for the somatic telomeres.

sequence motifs that might specify multiple chromosomal breakage and telomere addition sites. Rather, chromosomal breakage and telomere addition within this CBR seems to occur randomly, without any recognizable sequence specificity. Alternatively, an initial double-stranded DNA cleavage might occur at a single, yet unidentified specific DNA signal located at or near the 3´ end of the CBR. The resulting free chromosomal ends would then be randomly trimmed by a nonspecific exonuclease activity before being sealed by the addition of telomeric repeats (Fig. 3). At present, we cannot decide between the two alternatives.

The different chromosomal CBRs and/or their flanking regions are expected to contain target sites for specific elimination factors, including DNA binding proteins and other molecules involved in chromosomal breakage and telomere addition. However, on Southern blots, several cloned CBRs did not cross-hybridize to each other or to other sequences within the *Ascaris* genome. This rather unexpected finding indicates that the various genomic elimination sites do not share any conserved sequence motifs or, more likely, that such signal sequences are too short to be readily detected in Southern blot experiments. In a parallel approach we are currently analyzing and comparing the chromatin structures of a few selected CBRs and their flanking regions in developmental stages before and during the process of chromatin diminution. Putative recognition or regulation sequences important for the elimination process might be recognized as DNase hypersensitive sites. Once such sequences are identified, it should be interesting to establish their role in the elimination process and to look for specific binding factors.

Chromatin diminution must also depend on the presence or absence of regulatory factors that have to be distributed in a developmentally regulated manner in the different blastomeres. Thus far, no such factors have been isolated or characterized in *Ascaris*. However, classical experiments with *Parascaris* revealed that the eggs must contain a localized cytoplasmic substance, close to or at the vegetal pole, which becomes incorporated into the primordial germ cells, and whose function is to prevent chromatin diminution from taking place in all germ line cells (reviewed by Tobler, 1986).

TELOMERES

During the process of chromatin diminution some or all of the *A. suum* germline telomeres are removed and new somatic telomeres become attached directly to the chromosomal fragmentation sites. Developmentally regulated new telomere formation in all presomatic cells represents an interesting and unique feature among multicellular organisms. The telomeres of both cell lineages consist of tandemly repeated TTAGGC sequences, suggesting that the same telomerase activity might be responsible for the maintenance of telomeres in germ cells as well as for the de novo telomere addition onto the chromosomal breakage sites during the process of chromatin diminution (see Fig. 3). Neither germline nor somatic chromosomal ends seem to contain subtelomeric repetitive sequences such as, e.g., the X and Y′ DNA elements that are present at the ends of the *Saccharomyces cerevisiae* chromosomes (Biessmann and Mason, 1992). The *Ascaris* somatic telomeres differ from the germline telomeres not only in their different chromosomal location but also in that they are much shorter (≥20 kb vs. 4–6 kb length). Telomere shortening during development also occurs in human somatic cells, where it might be correlated with the number of DNA replications the cells have undergone and could lead to chromosomal instability and contribute to aging and senescence (reviewed by Biessmann and Mason, 1992).

Eukaryotic telomeres seem not to be randomly distributed within the nucleus. Rather, in a variety of different species two morphologically distinct kinds of telomeric associations have been observed to occur during the cell cycle: the clustering of telomeres to subnuclear sites and single end-to-end interactions resulting in a linear array of chromosomes. Both organizational forms may correspond to specific functions performed by the telomeres throughout an organism's life cycle (Gilson et al., 1993). Variations in the spatial distribution of telomeres in the nuclei of different cell types have been observed to take place in different mammalian species (Gilson et al., 1993). The formation of new somatic telomeres during the process of chromatin diminution is expected to interfere with the telomeric associations of the *Ascaris* chromosomes and might induce a change in the architecture of the interphase nuclei between the germ cells and the somatic cells. It is tempting to speculate that the developmentally regulated new telomere formation in *Ascaris* could be associated with important somatic differentiation events.

ELIMINATED CHROMATIN

The molecular data on the eliminated DNA in *P. univalens* are scarce; thus far two types of AT-rich DNA satellites have been reported in the germline genome (Moritz and Roth, 1976). These two satellites together represent about 85% of the germline DNA, a figure that approximately corresponds to the amount of eliminated DNA and indicates that the discarded sequences consist mainly of satellite DNA (Moritz and Roth, 1976).

In *A. suum*, about one-fourth of the total nuclear DNA, approximately 1.6×10^5 kb, is eliminated (Tobler, 1986; Tobler et al., 1972). A large portion of the germline DNA is composed of a single DNA satellite, which carries about 10^6 copies of an approximately 120 bp long, AT-rich repeating unit, whereas the somatic DNA contains at most 5,000 copies of this unit (Müller et al.,

1982). Thus, chromatin diminution removes more than 99.5% of the satellite DNA sequences from the presumptive somatic cells. As is the case for all eukaryotic DNA satellites analyzed thus far, nothing definitive is known about their function. However, the large difference in the amount of satellite DNA between germline and somatic cells in *Ascaris* is consistent with the hypothesis that satellite DNA exerts its biological function in processes that are inherent to the germline cells, for example, meiotic chromosome pairing or recombinational events (Bostock, 1980).

As well as large amounts of satellite DNA, the eliminated genomic fraction of *A. lumbricoides* var. *suum* also contains middle-repetitive and single-copy DNA sequences. Analysis of the genomic distribution of the middle-repetitive retrotransposon Tas in *Ascaris* revealed that some of these elements are discarded from the somatic cell lineages during chromatin diminution (Aeby et al., 1986). Tas elements are present in about 50 copies per haploid germline genome and exist in two structural variants (Tas-1 and Tas-2) in a ratio of about 2:1. Approximately 25% of the Tas-1 elements are expelled from the somatic cell lineages, as would be expected if they were randomly distributed in the *Ascaris* genome. The Tas-2 elements, however, are specifically localized within the eliminated portion of the genome, as demonstrated by their complete absence from all somatic cells (Aeby et al., 1986). They probably represent an inactive form of the Tas element, accidentally inserted into the heterochromatin and then amplified during evolution together with the surrounding DNA sequences. The eliminated copies of Tas do not excise independently, as is the case for the developmentally regulated elimination of some transposon-like elements during macronuclear formation in some ciliates (Cherry and Blackburn, 1985; Herrick et al., 1985; Baird et al., 1989), but are co-eliminated together with their flanking sequences (Aeby et al., 1986).

Thus far, three eliminated single copy genes have been identified (Etter et al., 1991, 1994; Spicher et al., 1994; Huang et al., manuscript in preparation), among them a gene for a protein homologous to the eukaryotic ribosomal protein S19 family. The genome of *Ascaris* encodes both a germline- and a soma-specific RpS19, which differ by 24 amino acid substitutions and which are both components of the small ribosomal subunits. In oocytes, the germline RpS19 homolog (RpS19G) predominates. During chromatin diminution, however, the gene is eliminated from all presomatic cells, and RpS19G is replaced by the product of the somatic gene (RpS19S). Chromatin diminution in *A. lumbricoides* causes a change in the protein composition of ribosomes during development. Experiments including two-dimensional gel electrophoresis of purified small ribosomal subunits from *Ascaris* oocytes and muscle tissue revealed a few other differences in the protein pattern between the two stages, suggesting that at least one additional small ribosomal protein gene could be eliminated during the process of chromatin diminution (Etter, personal communication).

The elimination of functional genes proves that the eliminated chromatin contains not just "useless" or "junk" DNA, but may be important for the germ line. Moreover, the three genes are also present in *P. univalens* where, as in *A. suum*, they are restricted to the germ cells (Etter et al., 1991, 1994; Spicher et al., 1994; Huang, et al., manuscript in preparation). Obviously, not only the sequences of these genes but also their behavior during the elimination process have been maintained during evolution of the two nematode species. In light of their completely different genomic organization, we suggest that the elimination of these genes could have an important function in the development and differentiation of the two parasites. It will be interesting to see whether the homologous genes are also expelled from the somatic genome of the other eliminating nematodes (Table 1).

CHROMATIN DIMINUTION: AN ALTERNATIVE MEANS TO GENE REGULATION?

Today, more than 100 years after its discovery by T. Boveri, the significance of the chromatin diminution process is still not known. The finding that the germline-specific DNA contains single-copy genes raises the question of whether chromatin diminution could represent an alternative means to gene regulation at the transcriptional level. This hypothesis is of particular interest in the context of the rather unexpected elimination of the ribosomal protein gene rpS19G. Eukaryotic ribosomal proteins are encoded by a group of coregulated "housekeeping" genes, which are thought to be constitutively expressed in all tissues and developmental stages of multicellular organisms. Somatic cells in *Ascaris* and *Parascaris* might therefore not be able to switch off their RpS19G genes by normal regulatory mechanisms, at least not independently from the other ribosomal protein genes. Thus, chromatin diminution could be used specifically to shut down the expression of the rpS19G, which is no longer needed during further development in the somatic lineages. Elimination of rpS19G results in a structural difference between ribosomes of the germ cells and of the somatic cells. Ribosome heterogeneity caused by changes in ribosomal proteins was found in cellular slime molds. Moreover, two putative genes coding for the mammalian rpS4 have recently been isolated from the sex chromosomes X and Y in humans. Their protein coding regions differ in 19 out of 263 amino acid residues, suggesting that ribosomes of human males and females might be structurally distinct (Fisher et al., 1990). The developmentally regulated ribosomal heterogeneity resulting from the elimination of rpS19G from the somatic cells of *Ascaris* and *Parascaris* could be related to a translational control mechanism, e.g., by selecting specific mRNAs to be translated or modulating the rate of translation in the different developmental stages. A potential role of structurally distinct ribosomes in the translational control of eukaryotic gene expression has been proposed but has not yet been proven (Ramagopal, 1992).

Apart from the elimination of single-copy genes, the chromosomal rearrangements during the process of chromatin diminution could influence *Ascaris* gene expression in additional ways. In a variety of eukaryotic organisms it has been well documented that pericentric heterochromatin can exert negative effects on the expression of adjacent genes, resulting, for example, in position-effect variegation in *Drosophila* (Tartof et al., 1989). Likewise, the large blocks of germline specific heterochromatin at the ends of the *Ascaris* germline chromosomes could repress the transcription of neighboring, noneliminated genes. Thus, in germ cells such genes would be silent. In somatic cells, however, upon removal of the telomeric heterochromatin, the inhibitory effect is abolished and the genes can be transcribed. In such a model, chromatin diminution would act as a mechanism specifically to activate *Ascaris* genes important for the development of the somatic cell lineages, which must not be expressed in germ cells.

A further possibility for the process of chromatin diminution to interfere with gene expression results from the process of new telomere formation. In general, telomeres exhibit heterochromatic characteristics such as condensed chromatin structure, late replication, and high amount of repetitive DNA sequences. In addition, *S. cerevisiae* telomeres have been shown to exert a position effect in that they repress the transcription of genes that were experimentally inserted close to chromosomal ends (Gottschling et al., 1990). The ability of telomeres to regulate gene expression, however, seems not to be restricted to transcriptional repression. In *Trypanosomes*, for example, the genes encoding various surface antigens are transcribed only when by DNA rearrangement events extra copies become located near telomeres (van der Ploeg et al., 1992). In the course of chromatin diminution in *Ascaris suum*, the reverse process takes place: De novo synthesized somatic telomeres are established in the vicinity of genes that are located close to the chromosomal breakage regions. Although there is no experimental evidence thus far, it is tempting to speculate that placement of somatic telomeres might have an influence on the transcription of nearby located genes and therefore could be used as a mechanism to control their transcriptional activity in a developmentally regulated manner.

CONCLUSION

Chromatin diminution in *Parascaris* and *Ascaris* undoubtedly represents *the* classic case of a developmentally programmed DNA rearrangement. It is a complex mechanism involving chromosomal breakage, new telomere addition, and DNA degradation (Müller et al., 1991). The process is highly specific with respect to its developmental timing as well as to its chromosomal localization. It will be interesting to learn more about the molecular mechanisms involved in chromatin diminution and to see how this phenomenon is regulated during development.

ACKNOWLEDGMENTS

I thank the members of the laboratory for their helpful comments on the manuscript and for the opportunity to discuss their unpublished results. This work was supported by the Swiss National Science Foundation and by the Sandoz-Stiftung zur Förderung der Medizinisch-Biologischen Wissenschaften.

REFERENCES

Aeby P, Spicher A, de Chastonay Y, Müller F, Tobler H (1986): Structure and genomic organization of proretrovirus-like elements partially eliminated from the somatic genome of *Ascaris lumbricoides*. EMBO J 5:3353–3360.

Baird SE, Fino GM, Tausta SL, Klobutcher A (1989): Micronuclear genome organization in *Euplotes crassus*: A transposonlike element is removed during macronuclear development. Mol Cell Biol 9:3793–3807.

Biessmann H, Mason JM (1992): Genetics and molecular biology of telomeres. Adv Genet 30:185–249.

Blackburn EH (1991): Structure and function of telomeres. Nature 350:569–573.

Bonnevie K (1902): Über Chromatindiminution bei Nematoden. Jena Z Naturwiss 36:275–288.

Bostock C (1980): A function for satellite DNA? Trends Biochem 5:117–119.

Boveri T (1887): Über Differenzierung der Zellkerne während der Furchung des Eies von *Ascaris megalocephala*. Anat Anz 2:688–693.

Boveri T (1899): Die Entwicklung von *Ascaris megalocephala* mit besonderer Rücksicht auf die Kernverhältnisse. In Festschr. für C. von Kupffer. Jena: Fischer, pp. 383–430.

Boveri T (1910): Die Potenzen der Ascaris-Blastomeren bei abgeänderter Furchung. Zugleich ein Beitrag zur Frage qualitativ-ungleicher Chromosomen-Teilung. In Festschr für R. Hertwig, vol. III. Jena: Fischer, pp. 131–214.

Cherry JM, Blackburn EH (1985): The internally located telomeric sequences in the germ-line chromosomes of *Tetrahymena* are at the ends of transposon-like elements. Cell 43:747–758.

de Chastonay Y, Müller F, Tobler H (1990): Two highly reiterated nucleotide sequences in the low C-value genome of *Panagrellus redivivus*. Gene 93:199–204.

Emmons SW, Klass MR, Hirsh D (1979): Analysis of the constancy of DNA sequences during development and evolution of the nematode *Caenorhabditis elegans*. Proc Natl Acad Sci USA 76:1333–1337.

Etter A, Aboutanos M, Tobler H, Müller F (1991): Eliminated chromatin of *Ascaris* contains a gene that encodes a putative ribosomal protein. Proc Natl Acad Sci USA 88:1593–1596.

Etter A, Bernard V, Kenzelmann N, Tobler H, Müller F (1994): Ribosomal heterogeneity from chromatin diminution in *Ascaris lumbricoides*. Science 265:954–956.

Fisher EMC, Beer-Romero P, Brown LG, Ridley A, McNeil JA, Lawrence JB, Willard HF, Bieber FR, Page DC (1990): Homologous ribosomal protein genes on the human X and Y chromosomes: Escape from X inactivation and possible implications for Turner syndrome. Cell 63:1205–1218.

Gilson E, Laroche T and Gasser SM (1993): Telomeres and the functional architecture of the nucleus. Trends Cell Biol 3:128–134.

Goday C, Ciofi-Luzzatto A, Pimpinelli S (1985): Centromere ultrastructure in germ-line chromosomes of *Parascaris*. Chromosoma 91:121–125.

Goday C, González-García JM, Esteban MR, Giovinazzo G, Pimpinelli S (1992): Kinetochores and chromatin diminution in early embryos of *Parascaris univalens*. J Cell Biol 118:23–32.

Goodrich HB (1916): The germ cells in *Ascaris incurva*. J Exp Zool 21:61–99.

Gottschling DE, Aparicio OM, Billington BL, Zakian VA (1990): Position effect at *S. cerevisiae* telomeres: Reversible repression of Pol II transcription. Cell 63:751–762.

Hawley JH, Peanasky RJ (1992): *Ascaris suum*: Are trypsin inhibitors involved in species specifity of *Ascarid* nematodes? Exp Parasitol 75:112–118.

Herrick G, Cartinhour S, Dawson D, Ang D, Sheets R, Lee A, Williams K (1985): Mobile elements bounded by C_4A_4 telomeric repeats in *Oxytricha fallax*. Cell 43:759–768.

Meyer O (1895): Celluläre Untersuchungen an Nematoden-Eiern. Jena Z Naturwiss 29:391–410.

Moritz KB (1967): Die Blastomerendifferenzierung für Soma und Keimbahn bei *Parascaris equorum*. II. Untersuchungen mittels Bestrahlung und Zentrifugierung. Wilhelm Roux Arch Entwickl Org 159:31–88.

Moritz KB, Roth GE (1976): Complexity of germline and somatic DNA in *Ascaris*. Nature 259:55–57.

Müller F, Walker P, Aeby P, Neuhaus H, Felder H, Back E, Tobler H (1982): Nucleotide sequence of satellite DNA contained in the eliminated genome of *Ascaris lumbricoides*. Nucleic Acids Res 10:7493–7510.

Müller F, Wicky C, Spicher A, Tobler H (1991): New telomere formation after developmentally regulated chromosomal breakage during the process of chromatin diminution in *Ascaris lumbricoides*. Cell 67:815–822.

Pimpinelli S, Goday C (1989): Unusual kinetochores and chromatin diminution in *Parascaris*. Trends Genet 5:310–315.

Ramagopal S (1992): Are eukaryotic ribosomes heterogeneous? Affirmation on the horizon. Biochem Cell Biol 70:269–272.

Spicher A, Etter A, Bernard V, Tobler H, Müller F (1994): Extremely stable transcripts may compensate for the elimination of the gene *fert-1* from all *Ascaris lumbricoides* somatic cells. Dev Biol 164:72–86.

Sulston JE, Brenner S (1974): The DNA of *Caenorhabditis elegans*. Genetics 77:95–104.

Tartof KD, Bishop C, Jones M, Hobbs CA, Locke J (1989): Towards an understanding of position effect variegation. Dev Genet 10:162–176.

Tobler H (1986): The differentiation of germ and somatic cell lines in nematodes. In W. Hennig (ed): Results and Problems in Cell Differentiation, vol 13, Germ line—soma differentiation. New York: Springer-Verlag, pp. 1–70.

Tobler H, Etter A, Müller F (1992): Chromatin diminution in nematode development. Trends Genet 12:427–432.

Tobler H, Smith KD, Ursprung H (1972): Molecular aspects of chromatin elimination in *Ascaris lumbricoides*. Dev Biol 27:190–203.

Triantaphyllou AC (1971): Genetics and cytology. In B.M. Zuckermann, W.F. Mai, R.A. Rohde (eds): Plant Parasitic Nematodes, vol. 2. New York: Academic Press, pp. 1–34.

van der Ploeg LHT, Gottesdiener K, Lee MGS (1992): Antigenic variation in African trypanosomes. Trends Genet 8:452–457.

Walton AC (1917): The oogenesis and early embryology of *Ascaris canis*. J Morphol 30:527–603.

Walton AC (1924): Studies on nematode gametogenesis. Z Zellen-Gewebel 1:167–239.

Walton AC (1974): Gametogenesis. In B.G. Chitwood, M.B. Chitwood (eds): Introduction to Nematology. Baltimore: University Park Press, pp. 191–201.

Warren K (1988): The Biology of Parasitism. New York: Alan R. Liss.

Weismann A (1885): Die Continuität des Keimplasmas als Grundlage einer Theorie der Vererbung. Jena: Fischer

Yao T, Pai S (1942): Heteropycnosis and chromatin diminution in *Cosmocerca* sp. Sci Rec Acad Sin 1:197–202.

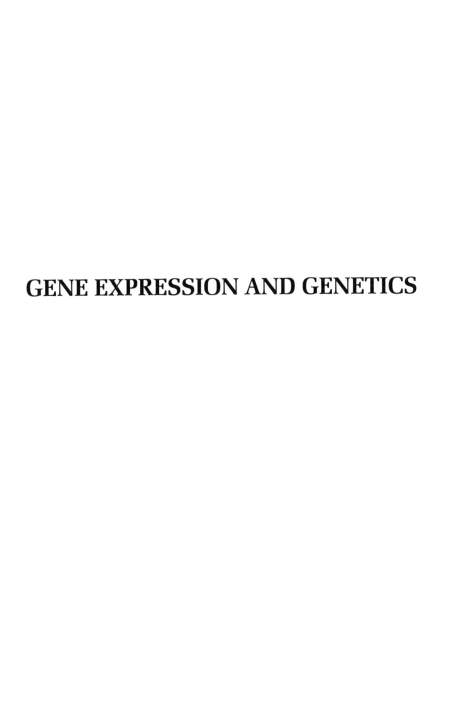

GENE EXPRESSION AND GENETICS

Preface

In the past 15 years, no subspecialty of parasitology has enjoyed more attention and generated more excitement than that dealing with gene expression in these organisms. In this, the longest of all the sections, eight chapters on this subject are presented. These range from relatively new systems in which genetics and detailed studies of gene expression have only recently begun to be applied, such as *Toxoplasma* and *Plasmodium*, to systems in which a remarkably detailed understanding is emerging (i.e., the trypanosomes).

The first chapter, from John Boothroyd's group, discusses the use of genetics and transfection to study gene expression and function in the Apicomplexan parasite *Toxoplasma*. The chapter is written with a view to showing how one can go about developing genetics as a tool for the study of relatively undeveloped systems, which, unfortunately, is the situation for all but a very few parasite systems today. Both classic "transmission" genetics and the more modern "reverse" genetics are discussed.

Dyann Wirth discusses how molecular biology and genetics have helped us understand the basis of one of the most serious problems in malaria: the emergence of multidrug-resistant lines of the parasite. She also describes the development of protocols for introducing DNA into this parasite for purposes of studying gene expression.

The next three chapters deal with gene expression in what is unquestionably the most studied of any group of parasites, at the molecular level, at least: the trypanosomes. Ken Stuart reflects on the most recent in a long list of unusual findings, RNA editing in the kinetoplast. He recounts the early discoveries and describes the evolution of current models. This chapter will undoubtedly be of special use to persons new to the field who may not appreciate the heresy that these findings initially represented to the general molecular biology community.

Chris Tschudi returns us to nuclear gene expression and reviews the state of knowledge about nuclear transcription and RNA processing in *T. brucei*, with an emphasis on the *trans*-splicing that is involved in the generation of apparently every mRNA in trypanosomes. John Swindle and coworkers take us into *T. cruzi* and discuss how polycistronic transcription may be involved in the regulation of many genes and how transfection and reverse genetics can be used to study gene function in this system.

The final three chapters in this section deal with gene expression in the nematodes. For many of us in parasitology, it is often hard to explain to "outsiders" that the helminths and protozoa are really totally unrelated and that as one moves deeper and deeper into molecular phenomena, the artifice of grouping these disparate organisms becomes more and more blatant. The exception is the finding that the nematodes and trematodes are similar to the kinetoplastida in their use of *trans*-splicing to process their mRNAs. Tom Blumenthal reviews the "state of affairs" in the nematodes and extends the parallels by arguing that polycistronic transcription is also occurring in these organisms, in a similar way to the trypanosomes. Dick Davis covers this subject in the trematodes and shows how *trans*-splicing can be exploited at the bench to help clone genes (anchored PCR has never been so simple!) and how the spliced leader genes may prove useful in deducing phylogenetic relationships. The final chapter in this section, by Gruidl and colleagues, shows how the model nematode *Caenorhabditis elegans* can be exploited to answer questions about gene expression that may be difficult to address in the less tractable parasites.

Molecular Approaches to Parasitology, pages 211–225
© 1995 Wiley-Liss, Inc.

Toxoplasma as a Paradigm for the Use of Genetics in the Study of Protozoan Parasites

John C. Boothroyd, Kami Kim, David Sibley, and Dominique Soldati

Department of Microbiology and Immunology, Stanford University School of Medicine, Stanford, California 94305

INTRODUCTION

Over the past century, genetics has been one of the most powerful tools available to the biologist. Yet, until recently, its impact on the study of parasites has been barely measurable. In this chapter, we discuss the ways that genetics *can* be used and how, in the past few years, it *has* been used to study the biology of the Apicomplexan parasite *Toxoplasma gondii*. It is hoped that the reader will take away the message that combining genetics with biochemistry, cell biology, molecular biology, and immunology can provide an extraordinarily powerful approach to answering many of the key questions that concern the modern parasitologist. It is also hoped that the lessons from this system will help others as they develop genetics as a tool for the study of different parasite systems.

GENETICS—THE APPROACH

In this section, the concepts that lie behind the theory and practice of genetics as it relates to any system are discussed.

What Is Genetics?

In the broadest sense, genetics is the study of genes and their function. However, the field is broken down into many discrete subspecialties dealing with such disparate subjects as population genetics, molecular genetics, and developmental genetics. For the purposes of this chapter, we consider genetics as the use of mutants to understand normal function. In practice, this means studying the way mutated genes disrupt the ability of an organism to do what it normally does.

Traditionally, genetics has proceeded from phenotype to genotype. That is, one first decides what property or phenomenon one is interested in, then devises and implements a strategy to select mutants that are defective in this, and, finally, maps and isolates the responsible gene. Later in this chapter, we discuss the reversal of this progression or "reverse genetics."

What Are the Advantages to Using Genetics?

Without doubt, the greatest advantage to using genetics is the fact that one need make no assumptions about what genes or what gene products are involved in a given function or attribute. Consider, for example, invasion. One could reasonably assume that microtubules and/or microfilaments of the parasite are involved, and one would probably be right. But what other components are involved? The beauty of genetics is that as long as there is a selection strategy for mutants, one need not guess; rather, genetics will do the work for you and lead you to the genes involved. In systems such as yeast, where genetics has a long history, this approach has revealed many surprises and more than justified its status as one of the most powerful tools available to the modern biologist.

The second major advantage of genetics is its ability to reveal interactions through the study of suppressor mutations. These are secondary mutations that restore a wild-type phenotype to a given mutant, i.e., in the presence of the suppressor mutation, the first mutation no longer results in a mutant phenotype. Suppressors can be intragenic (in the same gene as the first mutation) or extragenic (in a different gene).

Intragenic suppressors are useful for revealing interactions within a given gene's product. One simple example is that they may reveal salt bridges forming between two amino acids on the same polypeptide chain (i.e., a mutation that turns one amino acid from acidic to basic might be suppressed by a mutation that turns another from basic to acidic, thereby restoring the potential for ionic interactions between the two residues affected).

Extragenic suppressors are the more powerful variety, for they can reveal unsuspected interactions between different gene products. tRNA suppressors are the most well known, but these do not reveal much about new interactions because they are not gene specific (they suppress mutations in any gene harboring a particular type of coding error, for example, those harboring a nonsense mutation or stop codon).

Gene-specific suppressors are those that suppress mutations in one particular gene. Once the suppressor gene is identified, its identity can reveal clues as to how the first gene's product functions and how the two genes' products interact. For example, suppose one identified an invasion mutant with a mutation in a gene whose coding sequence revealed nothing about its identity. If one found that a mutation in one of the tubulin genes suppressed this first mutation, one might reasonably suppose that the first gene was specifically interacting with microtubules.

A third, more simple use of genetics is determining the number of genes that may contribute to a given phenomenon. This can be of academic interest (e.g., how many genes are involved in invasion) or great clinical importance (how many ways can drug resistance arise). For example, genetics has been used to argue that the multidrug resistance locus is not exclusively responsible for the resistance to certain drugs seen with some *Plasmodium* strains (see the chapter by Dyann Wirth for a detailed discussion of this).

How Does One Launch a Genetic Investigation?

The first requirement in launching a genetic investigation is to have a well-defined question. Although seemingly obvious, without a fair amount of thought into the question, the best genetic approach can sometimes be hard to pin down (i.e., it can be hard to determine an effective selection strategy, and thus crude screening may be necessary).

Next, one should have at least one clonal wild-type population. Use of a cloned line gives confidence that any mutant obtained is a true mutant rather than a natural variant selected out of a mixed population. Comparisons can then be made between a defined parent and the mutant progeny to determine the exact basis of the genetic difference. Multiple cloned lines are needed for easy genetic mapping using natural polymorphisms (e.g., restriction fragment length polymorphisms). Ideally such lines should have the most genetic differences while showing the least biological or phenotypic differences. For genetic analysis, they must obviously be readily mated with no bias for self-mating over a true cross.

Some means for generating (as opposed to selecting) mutants is needed. The most common forms of mutagenesis are chemical to generate point mutations, radiation to produce chromosomal breaks and deletions and transposon mutagenesis to insert a defined sequence element into the genome at random. Using the latter method, genes that are disrupted are also "tagged" with the transposon sequence used.

Undoubtedly the most intellectually challenging (and thus fun) part of any genetic project is devising selection strategies that allow the work to be done by the *experiment* rather than by the researcher! A good selection strategy results in only the desired mutants emerging, eliminating the need for laborious screening. For mutations that are expected to be lethal under normal growth conditions, alternative conditions must be found where this is not the case. Examples of such conditional lethal mutations include not only the common temperature sensitivity (cold or heat sensitive) but might also include host-range mutants, cell-type mutants (for intracellular parasites), auxotrophic mutants that can grow only in the presence of some metabolite, or developmental mutants that might show altered development or have an abbreviated life cycle.

Once a mutant is in hand, it must be cloned to ensure that all subsequent analyses are on a uniform line, thus avoiding selection of different subpopulations under different conditions.

The next task is to identify the gene harboring the responsible mutation. The two most common means to do this are by mapping the gene through analysis of genetic crosses or by attempting to complement the mutation through introduction of a gene library harboring, for example, the wild-type gene that can then be selected. If using crosses to map the mutation, a large number of progeny is a great advantage in allowing precise mapping.

In this way, it is possible to move from interesting phenotype to responsible gene and that is the often referred to "power" of genetics.

Reverse Genetics as a Tool to Refining Structure–Function Relationships

As the name implies, *reverse genetics* is a conceptual inversion of transmission genetics (which is now sometimes irreverantly but usefully referred to as *forward genetics*); that is, instead of going from a mutant organism or phenotype to finding the mutated gene, one starts by mutating a particular gene and then creating a mutant organism and assessing its phenotype. In practice, forward genetics is very useful for *identifying* genes involved in a given phenomenon, but reverse genetics allows precise *structure–function* determinations to be made. Of course, reverse genetics suffers from requiring many assumptions and guesses in deciding what mutations to make that contrasts dramatically with the assumptionless nature of forward genetics.

But, reverse genetics makes fewer demands of a system than does transmission genetics: It requires only that one be able to introduce genetic material back into an organism and obtain expression. For this to be accomplished, one must have a reporter gene (whose expression will be measured) and, ideally, some sort of selectable marker to allow stable progeny to be selected out for analysis.

Mutation of a cloned gene in preparation for reverse genetics can be by any of a wide variety of techniques, although many now lean on polymerase chain reaction (PCR) to generate precise constructs. Similarly, reintroduction of the resulting plasmids can be by many means but electroporation has come to be the almost exclusive means for introducing DNA into protozoan parasites because of its simplicity and efficiency.

Once introduced, the DNA may be retained only transiently, or, if appropriate selection techniques are available, stable transformants may be obtained.

Transient transfection is quick and easy for screening large numbers of constructs. However, it suffers from the fact that not all members of a population are alike, and thus any result obtained might simply be an average of a wide range of values (varying, for example, with the number of copies of a given plasmid taken up by each parasite). Consequently when one wishes to examine subtle aspects of biology, stable transformants are needed.

TOXOPLASMA AS A PARADIGM

The remainder of this chapter focuses on *Toxoplasma gondii* as a paradigm for genetic analyses, both forward and reverse. For excellent reviews on the biology of *Toxoplasma gondii*, see Dubey (1977); for immunology, Kasper and Boothroyd (1992); for molecular biology, Kasper and Boothroyd (1992) and McLeod et al. (1991); for cell biology, Joiner and Dubremetz (1993) and Pfefferkorn (1991); and for clinical aspects, see Luft and Remington (1992) and Frenkel (1988).

Biology of Toxoplasma

T. gondii has an extremely complex life cycle that includes three major, distinct stages: the sporozoite, the tachyzoite, and the bradyzoite. Sporozoites are the ultimate product of the sexual cycle that occurs exclusively in felines. Oocysts that are shed in the feces of infected cats contain eight sporozoites.

Oocysts are infectious and, if ingested by another feline, can initiate a new sexual cycle. Alternatively, if ingested by a grazing animal, they can initiate an asexual cycle in almost any warm-blooded land vertebrate (i.e., mammals and birds). Within such hosts, the parasite initially replicates as the fast-growing (hence its name) tachyzoite. Although the parasite can reproduce only within a host cell, it is nonfastidious in its choice and can be found in many different tissues.

Once the initial, acute phase of the infection is past, the parasite is found as the differentiated bradyzoite ("slow" grower). The bradyzoites are antigenically distinct from the tachyzoite and reside within a "tissue cyst." These tissue cysts are relatively long lived and infectious if ingested.

If a tissue cyst is ingested by a cat (e.g., feeding on an infected rodent), then the sexual cycle ensues with the generation of oocysts. If the prey was infected with two strains or if two prey are consumed each of which harbors a different strain, then the resulting mixed infection in the cat can result in a genetic cross.

If the tissue cysts are ingested by a scavenger or carnivore other than a feline, then another asexual cycle ensues with, presumably, no genetic recombination. Hence, in nature, it is at least theoretically possible for a strain to reproduce asexually indefinitely.

Genome and Gene Expression

The genome of *T. gondii* is haploid and has an estimated mass of 8×10^7 bp per nucleus. Using a combination of physical and genetic means, it is believed that there are 11 chromosomes in the nuclear genome (Sibley and Boothroyd, 1992).

Beyond these 11 nuclear chromosomes, there are probably two other genomes, one mitochondrial (Joseph et al., 1989) and the other derived from an uncharacterized organelle but possibly the spherical body, a multimembrane limited organelle. These are largely undescribed in *T. gondii*, and most of what is thought stems from analogy to the situation in *Plasmodium* (see the chapter in this volume by Jean Feagin). Interestingly and importantly, the nuclear genome is "contaminated" with sequences that are clearly mitochondrial in origin (Ossorio et al., 1991). The function of these sequences is unknown; they are presumed to be examples of "selfish" DNA.

All known protein-coding genes thus far studied in *Toxoplasma* are present in a single copy per nucleus. The only possible exception, the B1 gene cloned several years ago and the template for many PCR-based diagnoses, is present in 35 copies, but its protein-coding function has not yet been firmly established.

The 5′-end of the mRNA for *Toxoplasma* genes has been mapped in only a few cases and, in all, apparently shows no evidence of *trans*-splicing (e.g., the same result is obtained using primer extension and RNase protection). Based on recent results using transfection, it is clear that in the four cases examined, a promoter lies in or around the transcription start site (Soldati and Boothroyd, 1993). No detailed analysis of a *Toxoplasma* promoter has yet been published (but see below).

Genetics

Toxoplasma meets all of the prerequisites stated above for development of a genetic system, and for most properties it does so to a superb degree:

1. "A well-defined question": as an obligate intracellular parasite from a class of organisms that are relatively little studied, there is no shortage of questions for the biologist, whatever his or her particular bent. These can range from issues of cell biology to pathogenesis to molecular biology, and so forth.

2. "At least one clonal wild-type population": Toxoplasma can be grown indefinitely in an asexual, vegetative form in culture or in intermediate hosts such as mice. Clones are readily obtained, since a single organism can give rise to a plaque in tissue culture that is readily seen and picked.

3. "Multiple cloned lines with reasonable polymorphism and no bias for self-mating": Using molecular biology, markers are not a problem for any organism as long as there is a reasonable degree of polymorphism between

members of the species. Although the degree of polymorphism is not high in *Toxoplasma,* it is sufficient to enable sequence differences to be found in almost any gene. In collaboration with Elmer Pfefferkorn, we have crossed two strains and generated a genetic map on which 64 markers have been positioned (Sibley et al., 1992). This was done through identification of restriction fragment length polymorphisms (RFLPs) for each probe followed by analysis of how these RFLPs segregate in a cross. The resulting map appears to encompass the entire nuclear genome, as the number of genetic linkage groups was the same as the number of chromosomes physically resolved.

4. "Easy to handle in the laboratory": *Toxoplasma* can be readily passed in tissue culture, although, because it is a human pathogen, some care must be exercised to avoid infection. Selection strategies are relatively easy to devise for any organism that one can culture or otherwise maintain in the laboratory (e.g., in animals).

In addition to these properties, *Toxoplasma* has several other attributes that make it particularly well suited to genetic analyses. Among these are

5. Its haploid genome means one does not generally have to worry about mutations being recessive to a wild-type allele. Hence, generating mutants is relatively easy.

6. As already mentioned, all known protein-coding genes are single copy (as compared with the situation with the kinetoplastida, where many genes are tandemly reiterated). This again means that there is a far higher chance that a given mutation will be revealed in the phenotype of the organism.

7. Its gene expression is apparently conventional in that there is no evidence of *trans*-splicing or polycistronic transcription. Promoters for protein-coding genes have been defined and appear thematically similar in organization (but different in sequence motifs) to those found in higher eukaryotes.

8. The sexual cycle shows all the hallmarks of a classic mating, including meiosis, and it results in the generation of many, highly stable progeny (~10^7 oocysts are obtained per cross). Hence, the progeny from a single cross can be sufficient to do genetic mapping to very high resolution.

9. The oocysts are believed to contain all of the progeny of meiosis, making "tetrad analyses" possible. This allows evidence of unequal crossovers, gene conversions, and other nonreciprocal events to be obtained. It also permits synthetic lethality to be easily established (*synthetic lethality* is the inverse of suppression and means that two mutations that are individually not lethal, in combination are; crosses between two such mutants will result in oocysts that have one-fourth nonviable progeny. (Note that realization of this potential will depend on development of efficient means to dissect out and expand the eight sporozoites within the oocyst).

10. The crosses are relatively easy to perform in that no insect is involved (insect vectors are anathema to many regulatory agencies). As yet, however, cats are still required, which poses both ethical and financial concerns.

11. The disease it causes is of growing importance internationally and thus while a horrible price to pay (most would gladly give up their grants to see it disappear as a problem), there is great motivation on the part of many funding agencies to find new solutions to dealing with it. In an era of shrinking funding in all areas of science, launching a major effort on a new system of little health or economic importance can be a major struggle.

12. They can be efficiently cryopreserved, making the maintenance and storage of strains relatively simple.

13. There is a substantial background of information on their biology and much work going on in other aspects of their study (e.g., immunology, cell biology, population biology, and pathology).

What Are the Disadvantages of Using *Toxoplasma?*

Although the advantages are many, no system is without its drawbacks, least of all one that is a pathogen. For *Toxoplasma,* most of the major disadvantages are inherent to the very aspects of its biology that make it so interesting and important: pathogenicity and intracellular parasitism. In discussing the limitations of this system, we also include ways in which they may be circumvented.

1. Toxoplasma is a human pathogen, albeit one that is relatively mild in the vast majority of cases (in one published study, ~85% of women of child-bearing age in Paris were found to be seropositive and thus infected [Desmonts and Couvreur, 1974]). Women must be especially careful in handling the parasite, and anyone who is pregnant and seronegative should obviously not handle infectious material. Indeed, in the opinion of most workers (male and female), anyone actively trying to get pregnant should not handle the parasite. Similarly, HIV-positive individuals should probably not handle infectious parasites. As with any pathogen, serum antibody titers should be checked before beginning work with the parasite to serve as a baseline in the event of a suspected infection.

To circumvent this, it should be possible to engineer the parasite, using the gene replacement technology discussed below, so that it is less pathogenic. Such an attenuated strain may well emerge from efforts to design a human or animal vaccine, but the requirements are less stringent if the goal is only to develop a safe laboratory strain (since protective immunity would not be the goal, only lack of virulence if infected). One particularly attractive possibility would be to engineer the parasite such that it cannot survive as a bradyzoite through, for example, deleting several bradyzoite-specific genes. Assuming growth of tachyzoites was unaltered, if an infection did occur, one could be confident that once the acute stage had been dealt with no chronic infection would ensue (and thus should the person subsequently become immunosuppressed, he or she would not suffer from reactivated disease as is thought to be the case for most AIDS patients).

2. The second limitation is that *Toxoplasma* is an obligate intracellular parasite, which means one must allow for the influence of the host cell in every experiment, be it metabolic labeling, drug resistance, or response to environmental changes (e.g., temperature or other stresses). The reason why the host cell is indispensable is unknown, and thus it may eventually prove possible to grow the parasites extracellularly. Unlike the situation with the very fragile *Plasmodium* merozoites, extracellular *Toxoplasma* actively metabolize for up to 12 hours; once the essential contributions of the host cell are identified, it should be possible to provide these to the parasite via the medium.

3. Genetic crosses must be done in cats. There are obvious economic and ethical issues involved in the use of any animals, and, for many, this is especially so for cats. Fortunately, the large numbers of progeny obtained and the fact that the infection causes only relatively minor illness in the cat mitigate against this potential shortcoming. Even so, the ability to do crosses in vitro would obviously be a great advantage, and the existence of strains bearing drug-resistance markers (i.e., one can select for recombinants based on their possessing resistance markers from both parents) may facilitate this. Use of feline cell lines will likely be important, as, in nature, it is thought that only the cat can serve as a host for the sexual cycle (although what felines specifically provide over mice or other mammals is not known).

4. There is no stable diploid stage. In yeast, the existence of a stable diploid allows lethal mutations to be analyzed (because of the presence of a second, complementing wild-type allele). This need may be partially replaced by the development of stable episomal vectors that allow a second copy of a given gene to be maintained. Generating diploids may be possible through fusion techniques that have been developed for mammalian cells in combination with selection strategies that require two alleles of a particular locus to be present or even simple selection for resistance to two or more drugs as outlined for the in vitro crosses discussed above.

Where Are We Now?

Genetic mapping. We have generated a genetic map that includes markers on all 11 of the known nuclear linkage groups or chromosomes (Fig. 1). While this map may appear relatively low resolution, in fact this limited number of markers is sufficient to map any mutation relative to one or more of them (i.e., no matter where a mutation lies in the nuclear genome, at least one of the markers will show linkage). Since it is possible to analyze thousands of progeny, this limited set of markers allows relatively precise mapping.

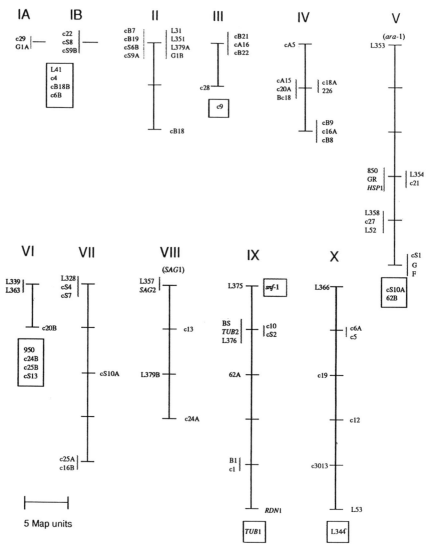

Fig. 1. Linkage maps for the 11 nuclear chromosomes. A cross was done between the PLK and CEP strains, and 19 recombinant progeny were analyzed for the segregation patterns of over 60 RFLP probes. The CEP parent was resistant to sinefungin (the *snf-1* allele) and adenosine arabinoside (*ara-1*); the PLK parent was sensitive to both drugs, and recombinant progeny were identified based on resistance to one but not the other drug. The probes have been ordered based on the minimum number of recombination events that explain the inheritance in all 19 progeny. Probes that have been mapped solely by hybridization to gel-separated chromosomes are indicated in a solid line box below the genetic map of their respective chromosomes. The two markers that were mapped with a statistical accuracy of only $P < 0.05$ are indicated in brackets. All other linkages are supported by a statistical significance of $P < 0.01$. (Reproduced from Sibley et al., 1992, with permission of the publisher.)

Generation of mutants.   As already stated, mutants for a wide variety of phenotypes have been reported. These include lines that are temperature sensitive for growth (Pfefferkorn and Pfefferkorn, 1976), deficient in one or other surface antigen (Kasper, 1987; Kasper et al., 1982), and resistant to one or more drugs (Pfefferkorn et al., 1992a,b).

In addition, we have generated mutants that are cold sensitive for attachment/invasion. These were obtained by repeated cycles of selecting for parasites that would not attach/invade at 32°C but would function as wild type at 38°C. Selection was by placing a mutagenized population of parasites in a flask of host cells, allowing invasion to occur at the cold, restrictive temperature, and then removing those that had not invaded: Because the host cells are attached to the plastic, only parasites that do not invade at this temperature will be recovered. The resulting population could then be expanded at the warmer, permissive temperature. Following three cycles, the mutants shown in Figure 2 were obtained. The molecular basis of this phenotype has not yet been established.

Transient transfection (structure/function analysis).   Transfection is an essential tool for reverse genetics and for forward genetics when using complementation to identify the responsible gene. We have developed protocols for efficient transfection that rely on electroporation in the appropriate medium (Soldati and Boothroyd, 1993). These protocols have been used to determine the sequences involved in the expression and regulation of *SAG1*.

Our initial studies focused on the elements necessary for transcription in tachyzoites. When the gene was originally cloned and analyzed (Burg et al.,

Cold sensitive mutants

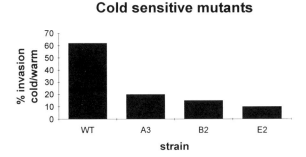

Fig. 2.   Invasion efficiency of three cold-sensitive mutants. Duplicate cultures of human foreskin fibroblasts were infected with each of four strains of parasites and placed at either 32°C or 38°C. The efficiency of invasion was measured at each temperature and plotted as the percentage seen at 32°C vs. 38°C. WT, the wild-type RH strain parent; A3, B2, and E2, three cloned mutants resulting from mutagenesis of RH and selection for cold-sensitivity, as described in the text.

1988), we observed at least two discrete transcription start sites ~35 basepairs apart. The start codon for translation (see above) lies ~150 bp downstream of the second initiation site. Beginning ~35 bp upstream of the first initiation site are six nearly identical, tandem, 27 bp repeats. These were obvious candidates for binding of a transcription factor. Constructs were generated in which these repeats have been moved downstream, upstream, inverted, and reduced in number (Soldati, Tomavo, and Boothroyd, manuscript submitted). Figure 3 shows an example of the sort of results obtained; in this case, when the number of repeats was increased from 5 to 10, the expression of the reporter gene chloramphenicol acetyl transferase (CAT) went up proportionately, indicating that the usual number of repeats (6) is apparently not saturating and presumably has been selected over time for appropriate expression of the *SAG1* gene.

Taken together, the results show that these repeats are best described as promoter elements because they are absolutely necessary for transcription of the *SAG1* locus and their position determines the start site for transcription. They can function in either orientation, which is highly unusual for a promoter and, when placed upstream of a heterologous promoter (a truncated promoter of TUB1) they can result in substantially more activity (data not shown).

Stable transformation. We have taken two tacks to achieving stable transformation in *Toxoplasma*: 1) complementation of a mutant of *Toxoplasma* and 2) introduction of heterologous drug resistance genes. In the first approach (Kim and Boothroyd, 1994), we have complemented the Sag1⁻ mutant (PTgB) of Kasper (1987), which is unable to express *SAG1*

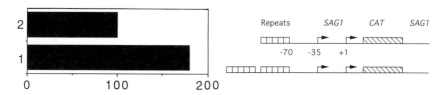

Fig. 3.   More upstream repeats from the *SAG1* promoter give increased *CAT* expression. Two plasmids were constructed. In the first, the natural arrangement of 5.5 27-bp repeats from the *SAG1* gene are positioned about 35 bp upstream of the first of two transcription start sites. This is the promoter driving expression of chloramphenicol acetyl transferase (*CAT*). Downstream *SAG1* sequences are also located 3′ of *CAT* to provide the polyadenylation and termination functions. The second construct is identical to the first except that an additional five repeats have been inserted with a small spacer between the two clusters (the spacer derives from the HindIII site used in the engineering). The CAT activity resulting from transfection of equal amounts of the two plasmids into RH strain tachyzoites is shown, with the first construct being used to define 100% activity. The second construct gives about 180% of the level of the first, indicating that the additional repeats increase the level of expression. The transcription start sites in the second construct are presumed to be the same as in the first, but this has not been confirmed.

due to the presence of a nonsense mutation near the middle of the gene (Kasper et al., 1992).

The second selection strategy utilizes drug selection. We have exploited the previously unrecognized susceptibility of *Toxoplasma* tachyzoites to chloramphenicol and the often ignored fact that the common reporter gene *CAT* is in fact a chloramphenicol resistance gene. Thus chloramphenicol can be used to select for stable integration into the genome of *CAT*-expressing constructs (Kim et al., 1993).

As an example of use of stable transformation, we have been interested in the function of *ROP1*, a rhoptry gene product that has been implicated in invasion (Ossorio et al., 1992). One of the quickest (and bluntest) ways to examine the function of a gene is to delete it entirely and examine the phenotype of the resulting mutants. To do this, we transfected in *CAT* flanked by upstream and downstream *ROP1* sequences and selected with chloramphenicol so that stable transformants expressing *CAT* would be obtained. The expectation was that a subset of these would be the result of a double crossover event involving the replacement of the *ROP1* coding sequences with *CAT*. We used a linearized plasmid to increase the probability of gene replacement since a single crossover with a circular plasmid would not generate a deletion.

This proved successful with 2 of 18 CAT-expressing stable transformants lacking *ROP1* by Western blot analysis. Southern blotting established that the desired homologous replacement had occurred (Fig. 4 of Kim et al., 1993). The phenotype of these mutants is currently being examined for changes in ultrastructure and growth in vitro and in vivo.

WHERE DO WE GO FROM HERE?

In terms of developing this system for genetic analysis, most of the major tools are now in hand. Some of the things that would improve the situation further were discussed above. There are a few other tools that should be developed to enhance this system. Fortunately, efforts are underway in various laboratories to develop these additional tools, and it should not be long before many are available. Some of the major needs are

1. A mini "genome-project" to produce defined genomic clones that span the entire genome (nuclear and non-nuclear). These will be cataloged and/or arrayed so as to give contiguous representation, allowing one to walk from one gene to another.

2. "Sequence tag sites," which have become a key tool in the development of any genetic mapping project. These allow for investigators easily to define and use specific sequences as their genetic markers. In combina-

tion with PCR, they make the need for central repositories of probes or strains relatively unnecessary.

3. A physical map to mesh with the genetic map. That is, we do not know with any accuracy what a single map unit corresponds to in basepairs and thus what physical distance separates the various markers.

4. Ability to microdissect viable sporozoites out of oocysts.

CONCLUSION

Genetics, be it forward or reverse, is inevitably going to be used more and more in modern parasitology. Although still in its infancy, the study of *Toxoplasma gondii* through such means presents a superb case study for how a relatively unstudied organism can quickly come to benefit from the application of such tools. It is likely that the learning curve will be as steep as the results curve, but equally sure is that there are many experiments waiting to be done and now only the number of investigators is limiting.

ACKNOWLEDGMENTS

We are grateful to our colleagues who provided unpublished information and to members of this laboratory who provided useful insight into the work described here. This work was supported by grants from the NIH, the MacArthur Foundation, and the Burroughs Wellcome Fund.

REFERENCES

Burg JL, Perelman D, Kasper LH, Ware PL, Boothroyd JC (1988): Molecular analysis of the gene encoding the major surface antigen of *Toxoplasma gondii*. J Immunol 141:3584–3591.
Desmonts G, Couvreur J (1974): Congenital toxoplasmosis. A prospective study on 378 pregnancies. N Engl J Med 290:1110–1116.
Dubey JP (1977): Toxoplasma, Hammondia, Besnoita, Sarcosystis, and other tissue cyst-forming coccidia of man and animals. In J.P. Kreier (ed) Parasitic Protozoa. New York: Academic Press, pp. 101–237.
Frenkel JK (1988): Pathophysiology of toxoplasmosis. Parasitol Today 4:273–278.
Joiner KA, Dubremetz J-F (1993): *Toxoplasma gondii*: A protozoan for the nineties. Infect Immun 61:1169–1172.
Joseph JT, Aldritt SM, Unnasch T, Puijalon O, Wirth DF (1989): Characterization of a conserved extrachromosomal element isolated from the avian malarial parasite *Plasmodium gallinaceum*. Mol Cell Biol 9:3621–3629.
Kasper LH (1987): Isolation and characterization of a monoclonal anti-P30 resistant mutant of *Toxoplasma gondii*. Parasitol Immunol 9:433–445.
Kasper LH, Boothroyd JC (1992): *Toxoplasma gondii*: Immunology and molecular biology. In K. Warren (ed): Immunology and Molecular Biology of Parasites. Oxford: Blackwell, pp. 269–301.
Kasper LH, Crabb JH, Pfefferkorn ER (1982): Isolation and characterization of a monoclonal antibody-resistant antigenic mutant of *Toxoplasma gondii*. J Immunol 129:1694–1699.

Kasper LH, Khan IA, Ely KH, Buelow R, Boothroyd JC (1992): Antigen specific (P30) mouse CD8⁺ T cells are cytotoxic against *Toxoplasma gondii* infected peritoneal macrophages. J Immunol 148:1493–1498.

Kim K, Boothroyd JC (1994): *Toxoplasma gondii*: Stable complementation of *sag1* mutants using *SAG1* transfection and fluorescence activated cell sorting. Exp Parasitol (in press).

Kim K, Soldati D, Boothroyd JC (1993): Gene replacement in *Toxoplasma gondii* with chloramphenicol acetyltransferase as selectable marker. Science 262:911–914.

Luft BJ, Remington JS (1992): Toxoplaxmic encephalitis in AIDS. Clin Infect Dis 15:211–222.

McLeod R, Mack D, Brown C (1991): *Toxoplasma gondii*—New advances in cellular and molecular biology. Exp Parasitol 72:109–121.

Ossorio PN, Schwartzman JD, Boothroyd JC (1992): A toxoplasma rhoptry protein associated with host cell penetration has unusual charge assymetry. Mol Biochem Parasitol 50:1–16.

Pfefferkorn ER (1991): Cell biology of *Toxoplasma gondii*. In D.J. Wyler, M.E.A. Pereira, D. Wirth (eds): Cell Biology, Molecular Biology and Immunology of Parasites. New York: Freeman Press, pp. 26–50.

Pfefferkorn ER, Borotz SE, Nothnagel RF (1992a): *Toxoplasma gondii*: Characterization of a mutant resistant to sulfonamides. Exp Parasitol 74:261–270.

Pfefferkorn ER, Nothnagel RF, Borotz SE (1992b): Parasiticidal effect of clindamycin on Toxoplasma gondii grown in cultured cells and selection of a drug-resistant mutant. Antimicrob Agents Chemother 36:1091–1096.

Pfefferkorn ER, Pfefferkorn LC (1976): *Toxoplasma gondii*: Isolation and preliminary characterization of temperature-sensitive mutants. Exp Parasitol 39:365–376.

Sibley LD, Boothroyd JC (1992): Construction of a molecular karyotype for *Toxoplasma gondii*. Mol Biochem Parasitol 51:291–300.

Sibley LD, LeBlanc A, Pfefferkorn ER, Boothroyd JC (1992): Generation of a restriction fragment length polymorphism linkage map for *Toxoplasma gondii*. Genetics 132:1003–1015.

Soldati D, Boothroyd JC (1993): Transient transfection of the obligate intracellular parasite, *Toxoplasma gondii*. Science 260:349–352.

Molecular Approaches to Parasitology, pages 227–241
© 1995 Wiley-Liss, Inc.

Drug Resistance and Transfection in *Plasmodium*

Dyann F. Wirth

Department of Tropical Public Health, Harvard School of Public Health, Boston, Massachusetts 02115

INTRODUCTION

Malaria remains a major threat to world health. Efforts to control the disease have focused on chemotherapy, mosquito control, and, most recently, vaccine development. These efforts have been hampered by the emergence and spread of drug-resistant parasites, the breakdown of malaria control programs due both to insecticide resistant mosquitoes and upheavals in spraying programs, and the complicated problems of vaccine development and testing. The world is facing an increasing threat of malaria in the 1990s with few new tools to combat the parasite and disease (Targett, 1991).

One of the underlying problems in developing newer methods of control is that the basic biology of the parasite has not been fully investigated, primarily due to the lack of a method for functional analysis of genes and their products. The goal of the work presented here is to develop such methods using DNA transfection. This type of methodology is required for a detailed examination of the control of expression of parasite genes. Such methods also have been critical in dissecting the mechanisms of bacterial pathogenesis and in the development of vaccines for several important bacterial pathogens.

THE CHALLENGE OF MALARIA IN THE 1990s

Malaria continues to plague the world as a health threat to both indigenous populations and travelers alike. The parasite is a complex microorganism with multiple life cycle stages and a highly evolved system for evading the immune response (Coppel, 1986; Cryz, 1991; Good et al., 1988; Gordon, 1990; Kaslow, 1990; Nussenzweig and Nussenzweig, 1989). During the majority of its life cycle in the mammalian host, the parasite is intracellular and thus protected both from the immune system and potentially from several chemotherapeutic agents because of the barrier of the host cell membranes. The parasite has also evolved a mechanism for the rapid development of drug resistance and today resistance has been reported to all commonly used antimalarial drugs (White and Pukrittayakamee, 1993; Peters, 1989; Looareesuwan et al., 1992). One of the themes in malaria research today is to identify the Achilles heel of the parasite, whether it be for immune intervention, for the development of new drugs, or for interventions in the vector phase of the parasite's life cycle.

The challenges facing the scientific community with regard to malaria also represent opportunities to understand the biology of this fascinating microorganism. The malaria parasite has evolved to survive and thrive in the invertebrate vector and the mammalian host. In the invertebrate vector, the parasite is extracellular and in direct contact with molecules in the mosquito gut, hemolymph, and salivary glands. It undergoes a complex set of programmed developmental changes in its transit from ingested bloodmeal to infective sporozoite stage parasites. Relatively little is known regarding the signals and responses that lead to this progression. Similarly, once in the mammalian host, the parasite first invades hepatic cells where it undergo both developmental changes and a large expansion in numbers of parasites and subsequently infects erythrocytes where the majority of the organisms undergo cyclical development and reinvasion of the red cells. A small subset of the organisms follows a different developmental pathway, namely, the development of male and female gametocytes. The gametocytes remain relatively dormant in the infected erythrocytes but once taken up in a mosquitoes blood meal, the gametes are released from the erythrocytes and begin their developmental cycle in the mosquito. Again, at each stage in the parasite's life cycle, there are a programmed series of developmental changes, and little is known of the signals or events that trigger these changes. Not only is the parasite a complex microorganism, but it has the added feature of adaptation for interaction with its host. Clearly the parasite has evolved mechanisms for the evasion of the mammalian host's immune response, but in addition the parasite has developed a dependence on the host for certain nutrients and other cellular functions.

ACHILLES HEEL: LESSONS FROM THE PARASITE'S UNIQUE BIOLOGY

Genetic analysis has demonstrated that the parasite's genome is haploid throughout the entire exoerythrocytic and erythrocytic stages of the life cycle. The genome is divided into 14 chromosomes and two extrachromosomal elements that are organellar in their localization (see the chapter by Feagin in this volume and Walker et al., 1992). After fertilization of the female gametes, the parasite is diploid for a brief interval. Sexual exchange of genetic material occurs during this stage of the parasite's life cycle (Vaidya et al., 1993). Thus, at each mosquito bloodmeal there is an opportunity for exchange of genetic information between parasites. This must contribute to both the genetic diversity and polymorphism found in the parasite and may play an important role in the spread of certain genetic characteristics such as drug resistance.

Studies are now beginning on the cell biology of the malaria parasite (see, for example, the chapter in this volume by Haldar and colleagues). Important insights have been gained regarding the molecules critical to the invasion of the malaria parasite into erythrocytes, with both putative ligands and receptors being identified on the parasite and red blood cell surface. In addition, the rhoptry organelle, unique to this family of parasites, has been implicated in the invasion process. From a cell biological perspective, perhaps one of the most fascinating aspects of the malaria parasite is its ability to invade mature erythrocytes that have no existing mechanism for phagocytosis. This distinguishes the malaria parasite from many other intracellular parasites that invade cells capable of phagocytosis. The careful and stepwise analysis currently in progress will hopefully serve to dissect this process into its component parts and may serve as an ideal target for intervention, based on either immunological or chemotherapeutic approaches to interfere with receptor–ligand interactions or with the unique membrane-forming processes associated with rhoptry-mediated invasion of the parasite into the red blood cell.

The malarial food vacuole is a specialized organelle primarily for the digestion of hemoglobin and other red cell cytoplasmic components, and there is a significant amount of evidence indicating that many of the currently used antimalarial drugs such as chloroquine, quinine, their derivatives, and artemisinin compounds interfere with the activity of the food vacuole, and the food vacuole may indeed be the primary target of these drugs. In addition, the recent discovery of another food vacuole enzyme activity, one that polymerizes the heme molecules and converts them from a toxic to nontoxic form, indicates that several distinct and unique activities may exist in the food vacuole (Slater and Cerami, 1992).

One approach to thinking about weaknesses in the parasite's life cycle may be to focus on the stages when the parasite is present in relatively small numbers. Both for immunological intervention and for chemotherapeutic intervention, the smaller the number of organisms, the easier it may be to eliminate the infection effectively. The parasite presents two opportunities in this regard, namely, the early stages in liver infection and the mosquito midgut. These are the targets of intensive vaccine development efforts, and intervention at these points may indeed prove successful (Nardin and Nussenzweig, 1993; Kaslow, 1993).

Vaccine development in malaria has focused on vaccines directed at specific polypeptides of the malaria parasite, including surface proteins in the sporozoite, merozoite, and gamete stages. While promising results have been obtained in animal models, human trials have been limited in both scope and success. Establishing immunity to malaria may in fact be more difficult than originally hypothesized. There may be multiple components in any immune response and immunity, at least to the blood stages, is not sterile immunity but instead a type of antidisease immunity. That is, individuals are still infected with the parasite but do not have the morbidity and mortality associated with the disease in nonimmune states. Recent work has been directed at developing antidisease or antipathology approaches to intervention, the most notable of which is the current trial of antibody to tumor necrosis factor (TNF) as a treatment for cerebral malaria.

DRUG RESISTANCE IN MALARIA: CHALLENGE OF THE LATE 20TH CENTURY

Malaria continues as a major health threat throughout the tropical world, and the potential demand for antimalarial drugs is higher than for any other medication yet the world faces a crisis; drug resistance is emerging and spreading faster than drugs are being developed, and the flow in the pipeline of new drugs has all but stopped. In a short time there may be parts of the world where no effective antimalarial drug is available. The recent emergence of multidrug resistant malaria parasites has intensified this problem (Oduola et al., 1992; Peters, 1989; Bray and Ward, 1993; Nosten et al., 1991). Recognizing this emerging crisis, it is necessary to identify new strategies for the identification and development of new antimalarial drugs.

Current drugs are based on a small number of target molecules or lead compounds, and in most cases the target of drug action is yet to be identified (Ginsburg and Krugliak, 1992). Resistance is emerging rapidly, and the mechanisms of resistance are poorly understood (Fontanet et al., 1993; Milhous et al., 1989). The identification of new targets or new candidate drugs based on an understanding of the parasite biology are key elements in this new strategy. The goal of our work is to use a molecular genetic approach both in the investigation of mechanisms of drug resistance and in the identification of new drug targets.

Drug resistance has emerged as a major problem in the treatment of all microbial agents and in many cancer chemotherapies. This has necessitated continuous development of new chemotherapeutic agents both for treatment of infectious agents and for cancer chemotherapy. Often resistance develops through selection of a mutation in the target enzyme of the drug or in the overexpression of that enzyme. For example, resistance to antifolate drugs is frequently associated with mutations in the dihydrofolate reductase enzyme or in its overexpression (Foote, et al., 1990a; Peterson, et al., 1990). An alternative type of resistance, namely, multidrug resistance, has emerged as a major problem in the treatment of many cancers and remains a major obstacle to the successful control of certain neoplasias with chemotherapy. This type of resistance is characterized by several unique features and the molecular basis for this resistance is under extensive investigation (Gros et al., 1986; Raymond, et al., 1990; Roninson, et al., 1986). In the case of multidrug resistance, resistance is observed to a number of structurally distinct drugs each with a different target. Selection of cells resistant to one drug results in the cross-resistance to several structurally and functionally unique drugs. The genes associated with this resistance are the multidrug resistance *mdr* genes. The *mdr* gene encodes a membrane glycoprotein, the P-glycoprotein, which mediates the efflux of drugs from the cell. Amplification of the *mdr1* gene in resistant cells results in increased expression of the P-glycoprotein and thus increased efflux of drugs. Thus, the cells are resistant because drug is rapidly removed from the cell before significant toxicity occurs. Use of transfection of the *mdr1* cDNA has demonstrated that overexpression of this gene is sufficient to confer the multidrug resistance phenotype. Drug resistance can be modulated by the use of several compounds, including verapamil, that appear to inhibit drug efflux. The current hypothesis is that verapamil and related compounds directly bind the P-glycoprotein molecule and block efflux, and evidence for direct binding of radiolabeled verapamil to the P-glycoprotein molecule supports this hypothesis.

In the case of malaria, the similarity in the pharmacological features of the chloroquine resistance in *P. falciparum*, namely, the proposed efflux mechanism and the reversal of resistance by verapamil, desipramine, and related compounds led to the proposal that a similar mechanism for drug resistance was operating in *P. falciparum* (Martin et al., 1987; Krogstad et al., 1992; Kyle et al., 1990). Both our group and David Kemp's group identified genes that had sequence and predicted structural similarity to the *mdr* genes and analyzed the expressed mRNA and protein (Foote et al., 1989; Foote et al., 1990b; Wilson et al., 1989; Wilson et al., 1993; Volkman et al., 1993). These genes and their encoded proteins are indeed related to genes in the ATP-binding cassette family and have the highest homology with the *mdr* genes from mouse and human. Thus, the hypothesis was proposed that these genes are involved in drug resistance in *P. falciparum*. Further evidence for this proposal was presented in identifying several polymorphisms within the pfmdr1 gene that appeared to be associated with chloroquine resistance in field isolates (Foote et al., 1990b). This evidence was in contrast to the analysis by Wellems et al. (1990, 1991) in performing a genetic cross between cloned chloroquine resistant and chloroquine sensitive parasite (Wellems et al., 1990; Wellems et al., 1991). In the genetic analysis, both the *pfmdr1* gene and its assorted polymorphism could be dissociated from chloroquine resistance. This was confirmed by a collaboration between our group and the NIH group in which we sequenced the relevant regions of the polymorphism from the resulting progeny. Further evidence to refute the association of polymorphism in the *pfmdr1* gene associated with chloroquine resistance was obtained by sequencing recent isolates of drug-resistant *P. falciparum*. We have completed this and have demonstrated in 12 new isolates of chloroquine-resistant parasites that the *pfmdr1* gene sequence is identical to that predicted for the chloroquine-sensitive phenotype, thus refuting the original claim (1990b) of Foote et al. (Wilson et al., 1993). Further RFLP analysis of the genetic cross by the Wellems group has determined linkage of the resistant phenotype to a small region of chromosome 7, a location distinct from the known location of either *pfmdr1* or *pfmdr2*. Thus, the conclusion from this work is that neither the *pfmdr1* nor the *pfmdr2* gene is linked to chloroquine resistance.

The mechanism of chloroquine resistance remains unknown, but progress has recently been reported on a putative target for chloroquine drug action. Slater and Cerami (1992) have reported an enzyme activity, heme synthetase, that is hypothesized to be involved in the formation of hemozoan pigment and is a method for detoxification of the heme. This enzyme activity in cell extracts is inhibited by chloroquine and related quinones. Interestingly, the enzyme activity is equally sensitive to chloroquine whether derived from chloroquine sensitive or chloroquine resistant parasites. These results indicate progress toward identifying the primary target of chloroquine action and are consistent with the hypothesized importance of efflux of the chloroquine in drug resistance. The increased efflux phenotype remains associated with chloroquine resistance both in the genetic cross experiments and in new chloroquine-resistant field isolates. In addition, reversal of chloroquine-resistance with verapamil is observed in all chloroquine resistant strains tested. Thus, the pharmacology of this system remains consistent and has many similarities to the efflux-mediated multidrug resistance in mammalian cells. However, the genetic evidence argues strongly that the identified *pfmdr1* and *pfmdr2* genes are not linked to the chloroquine resistance phenotype.

The role of *pfmdr* genes in other drug resistance mechanisms remains an open and important question. This is particularly the case for mefloquine resistance in Southeast Asia. In our original work, we demonstrated that in a laboratory selected mefloquine-resistant cloned parasite, W2mef, the *pfmdr1* gene was amplified when compared with the cloned parent parasite W2 (Wilson et al., 1989). In subsequent work, Peel and coworkers have demonstrated that under increased mefloquine selection pressure the *pfmdr1* gene is further amplified approximately 8–10-fold. We also demonstrated an increased expression of *pfmdr1* mRNA in W2mef compared with W2. This work has now been expanded to include several field-isolated mefloquine-resistant parasites, and our data suggest that in mefloquine-resistant parasites in Southeast Asia an amplification of the *pfmdr1* gene and an increased expression of mRNA is associated with this resistance. Furthermore, analysis of the mefloquine-resistant strains from Southeast Asia demonstrates that they are cross-resistant, in vitro, to other unrelated drugs, similar to the cross-resistance observed in multidrug-resistant mammalian cells (Shanks, et al., 1991; Wilson et al., 1993). Similar results have recently been reported for additional laboratory isolates (Cowman et al., 1994). Resistance to all drugs can be reversed by penfluoridol and other reversal compounds (Kyle et al., 1993). Thus, it appears that mefloquine-resistant *P. falciparum* has many of the characteristics in common with multidrug-resistant mammalian cells; however, definitive proof of this relationship awaits functional analysis.

DEVELOPMENT OF A MOLECULAR GENETICS SYSTEM FOR THE MALARIA PARASITE

Functional analysis of malaria genes using the method of DNA transfection should allow us to investigate the biology of the parasite at a mechanistic level and to engineer the parasite genetically both to identify new targets for chemotherapeutic intervention and to develop new approaches to vaccines for malaria. Among the most successful vaccines for microorganisms, both bacterial and viruses, are attenuated whole organism vaccines. In fact, in malaria, the most effective vaccine has been irradiated sporozoites. Thus, one future goal of this work is the development of genetically engineered, attenuated *P. falciparum* for use as a vaccine candidate. The advantage to using attenuated vaccines for complex organisms like malaria is that multiple antigens are presented in a native context, and this may lead to a better and longer lasting immunity.

Choice of the Sexual Stage Parasites for the Initial Transient Transfection System

At the outset of this work it was clear that there were numerous barriers to the development of a transfection system in the malaria parasite. We divided the problem into its component parts and set about developing methods and approaches at solving each. One problem that made the malaria parasite unique was that the form of the parasite available in long-term in vitro culture was intracellular, with the extracellular merozoite form viable for only a brief time. Thus, to introduce DNA into the parasite, it would be necessary to cross three membranes, the erythrocyte membrane, the parasitophorous vacuolar membrane, and the parasite plasma membrane. In addition, for expression from DNA the introduced plasmid would most likely need to enter the nucleus. This problem is analogous to that posed by the transfection of intracellular organelles such as mitochondria and chloroplasts. Recent progress in these areas included the use of the microprojectile method of DNA delivery; however, the efficiency of this method remains quite low for intracellular organelles.

Based on this analysis, we decided to explore other potential life cycle stages as targets for transfection. After an examination of the literature and a careful look at parasite biology, a decision was made to use the sexual stages of the model malaria system *Plasmodium gallinaceum*, an avian malaria (see Goonewardene et al., 1993). There are several advantages to this system. First, the sexual stages of the parasite are extracellular, thus eliminating the problem of the introduced DNA crossing multiple membrane barriers. Second, methods had previously been developed and standardized for the purification of the extracellular gamete and fertilized zygote stages of the parasite in relatively large numbers, and recent work has demonstrated that these parasites may be carried in vitro for up 96 hours and still retain viability and infectivity for mosquitoes. The feasibility of in vitro development to the sporozoite stage using this system had been demonstrated, and thus the potential for future experiments using selectable markers is theoretically possible even if technically difficult at the moment. The clear disadvantage to this parasite stage is that studies will be limited to transient expression unless significant technical advances are forthcoming in either in vitro systems or in vivo selection. However, at a minimum, this system should allow the feasibility testing of a transfection system and allow identification of promoter and other controlling elements necessary for gene expression in the sexual stage of the parasite. Clearly, the information learned by these experiments must be transferred to the asexual stages for studies on drug resistance and other biologic properties of the parasite related to pathology and disease development.

A second problem that we faced in the development of this system was the identification of sequences that control and direct gene expression in the parasite. Some work has been published on transcriptional mapping for two of the asexual stage parasite genes, pf195 and pf130, but no similar information regarding those genes expressed at the sexual stages was available (Lanzer et al., 1993). No in vitro system for protein coding gene transcription in the malaria parasite is reliably available. Several genes of *P. gallinaceum* have been identified that are expressed at high level in the gamete–zygote stages of the parasite, and one of these, pgs28, had been cloned with adequate flanking DNA to ensure that necessary 5′ and 3′ controlling elements for the expression of this gene were present (Duffy et al., 1993). In choosing the pgs28 gene as our initial gene for this work, several different considerations were made. First, previous work had demonstrated that this gene was expressed at high levels in the sexual stage parasites shortly after fertilization and continued throughout ookinete development. Second, the work of Duffy et al. (1993) had demonstrated that the pgs28 mRNA was approximately 1.4 kb in length with a coding region of 800 bp. A cloned 3.0 kb HindIII fragment of *P. gallinaceum* DNA contained the coding region of the pgs28 gene in the central portion of the fragment. Thus, based on the size of mRNA, we concluded that both the 5′ and 3′ flanking regions of the mature mRNA were contained within this cloned fragment.

Choice of Transient Transfection Assay and Luciferase as Reporter Gene

As mentioned above, by choosing the sexual stages as the target stage for these initial experiments, a transient assay was the only feasible choice for the initial experiments. The zygotes can only survive for a few days in vitro, and selection of transfectants in the mosquito and subsequently in the avian host are technically difficult with current methodologies. In addition, as we demonstrated in the development of a transfection system for *Leishmania spp.*, the initial development of a transient system allows relatively rapid testing and only requires expression of the reporter gene for a short period. In contrast, long-term selectable transfection vectors are the eventual goal of this work, but they require continuous maintenance of the introduced DNA and expression of the selectable marker. Thus, the transient assay was the appropriate choice for this system.

The next decision was the choice of reporter genes. Two considerations were made. One, the sensitivity of the assay for the reporter gene; and, two, the knowledge from other fields regarding the expression of the reporter gene in widely diverse biological systems. Two genes fit this criteria, the firefly luciferase gene and the bacterial ß-galactosidase gene. The ß-galactosidase gene is a large gene with a coding region approximately 3 kb, and the potential problem of malaria codon usage was a concern. In contrast, the firefly luciferase gene is small with a coding region of less than 800 bp. The luciferase assay is also quite sensitive, but this gene has not been used as extensively as the ß-galactosidase gene in diverse systems.

Development of the Transient Expression Vector

The firefly luciferase gene was inserted in frame into the coding region of the pgs28 gene, creating a chimeric gene. These represent first-generation vectors in which a minimum manipulation of gene is needed to retain potential important controlling elements in their native position. The development of a second generation of transfection vectors in which the coding region of pgs28 has been exactly replaced by the reporter genes is underway. The advantage of these vectors is that the reporter gene will be synthesized as a native protein rather than a fusion protein, and potential problems associated with efficient expression of fusion proteins and stability or transport of these proteins will be reduced. This will also allow us to develop a cassette vector in which different reporter genes or selectable markers can be inserted and used for transfection.

Choice of Electroporation as a Method for the Introduction of DNA Into the Parasite

There are several potential methods available for the introduction of exogenous DNA into organisms. These include calcium phosphate, DEAE, lipofection, electroporation, and microprojectiles. Each of these has worked in some biological systems and with varying efficiency. The plan of this work was to use each of these methods systematically for the attempted transfection of the malaria parasite. We chose to begin our transfection experiments using the method of electroporation. This method is appealing in that it is a general method for the introduction of DNA into cells, and we had previous extensive experience with the use of this methodology in transfecting *Leishmania sp.*

Our approach to determining appropriate electroporation conditions was to use a measure of ookinete development after electroporation. Purified gametes–zygotes were resuspended in Cytomix and subjected to electroporation conditions ranging from 0.5 to 5 kV/cm with 25 µF. Parasites were incubated in ice, washed, resuspended in ookinete maturation media, and analyzed for ookinete development after 48 hours.

At voltages greater than 3 kV/cm, no ookinetes were recovered. At voltages of less than 1.5 kV/cm, ookinete development was similar to that in the mock treated controls. In the range of 1.5 to 3 kV/cm, ookinete development was retarded and several retort forms were observed. In addition, overall recovery of mature ookinetes was reduced 30–70% depending on the experiment. Based on these observations, we chose 2.5 kV/cm and 25 µF as the initial electroporation conditions. We also noted during these experiments that ookinete development was dependent on the cell concentration during ookinete maturation. At cell concentrations less than 2×10^7/ml, there was a significant reduction in mature parasite forms.

Characterization of a Transient Transfection System

The initial step in the development of a transfection system for malaria has been achieved, namely, the transient expression of a reporter gene in the malaria parasite. The data indicate that the gene expression is under the control of malaria sequences, as plasmids containing the reporter gene in the absence of malaria sequences or in the opposite orientation as the malaria sequences do not express reporter activity.

The next goal is a clear delineation of the sequences necessary for the expression of the reporter gene. The work focuses on the luciferase-containing plasmid as that plasmid is currently available. Based on work in other eukaryotic systems and on the initial transcriptional mapping work in *P. falciparum,* we concentrate our analysis of controlling elements on the 5´ flanking sequences. The sequence of the region 5′ to the protein coding region is sequenced using standard methodology. A systematic series of nested deletions is made in the 5′ flanking regions of the pgs28.1LUC plasmid, and each of these is tested for expression of luciferase. Our hypothesis is that if a sequence necessary for expression is deleted, expression of luciferase will be prevented or reduced. In these experiments, a second reporter gene with a fully intact 5' flanking region is used as an internal control for transfection efficiency. For most systems, this approach has proven highly useful.

Once a region is identified as critical in luciferase expression, we examine it in detail. First, the DNA sequence is analyzed and compared with known promoter and other controlling elements in other eukaryotic systems and the putative promoters described for asexual genes. The putative promoter and other controlling sequences are cloned adjacent to the luciferase reporter gene and analyzed using linker scanning mutagenesis to identify key sequences for luciferase expression.

TESTING OF THE PGS28.1LUC PLASMID AND ITS DERIVATIVES IN OTHER PARASITE STAGES

The pgs28 gene is expressed in the gamete–zygote and ookinete stages of the *P. gallinaceum* life cycle, and therefore, we anticipate that the controlling elements necessary for this stage-specific expression will be associated with the gene. We however do not know if this stage-specific expression element is within the cloned sequence. Some information regarding sequence-controlling elements will be obtained from the deletion analysis above. A likely outcome, based on analogies with other eukaryotic systems, is that there will be a core promoter region and then sequences that direct the stage-specific expression, similar to tissue-specific expression for many mammalian genes. Thus, one of our approaches to developing a transfection system for the asexual stages will be to test in asexual stage parasites the pgs28.1LUC plasmid and its derivatives, which contain only a putative core promoter adjacent to the luciferase gene.

DEVELOPMENT OF OTHER TRANSIENT TRANSFECTION VECTORS FOR USE WITH ASEXUAL STAGE PARASITES

A second parallel approach is to develop another transient transfection vector based on a gene that is expressed throughout the parasite life cycle and thus is likely to be expressed upon transfection in both sexual and asexual parasites. This would allow us to develop and test the vector in the sexual stage system that we have already characterized and then, with this vector, move to an attempt at transfection in the asexual stage. We could then test different types of DNA delivery (microprojectiles, lipofection, or electroporation) to the asexual parasite. There are relatively few genes cloned in *P. gallinaceum,* and, therefore, based on the *P. falciparum* literature, either the tubulin genes or calmodulin genes appear to be candidates for this type of vector. These genes should be relatively easy to clone as they are highly conserved in sequence. Both of these genes have proven extremely useful in the development of transfection vectors for *Leishmania* and *Trypanosome spp.*

DEVELOPMENT OF TRANSIENT TRANSFECTION VECTORS FOR *P. FALCIPARUM*

One of the eventual goals of this work is the development of vectors for the human malaria parasite *P. falciparum.* We do not yet know whether the vectors developed for the avian *P. gallinaceum* will be functional in *P. falciparum.* Our experience in the case of *Leishmania spp* is that vectors developed for one species worked extremely efficiently in other species, and thus a single set of vectors could be developed and used in all the parasites. Clearly, we will test the *P. gallinaceum* vectors in *P. falciparum.* We will initiate these experiments with the Honduras strain of *P. falciparum,* which produces high levels of gametes.

DEVELOPMENT OF STABLE TRANSFECTION VECTORS

The development of a stable transfection vector will proceed along two parallel lines. First, should one of our transient vectors prove active in *P. falciparum* asexual stages, we will attempt to develop a stable vector based on our successful transient transfection vector. The luciferase gene will be replaced by a selectable marker, the *neo^r* gene, transfected into parasites and the parasites placed under selection with G418. We have already determined that *P. falciparum* is killed at a concentration of 25 µg/ml of G418. This approach has worked successfully in numerous other systems, and the *neo^r* gene is expressed in wide variety of cell types.

An alternate approach that is technically more difficult and cumbersome is to select resistant parasites at the ookinete stage and then pass them through mosquitoes and hosts. This part of the project will be attempted if we fail to identify a vector that will work in the asexual stages. The luciferase gene will be replaced by a selectable marker, transfected into the zygotes–gametes and the resulting transfectants incubated under selection. The zygotes can be incubated for up to 100 hours in vitro and still retain infectivity for mosquitoes. Based on our experience in the *Leishmania enriettii* system, this would be an adequate amount of time for the killing of the nontransfected parasites. Parasites would then be fed to mosquitoes using the membrane feeding method and the infected mosquitoes allowed to develop sporozoites and then used to infect chickens. In such a manner, transfected parasites could be isolated from the infected chickens. For certain applications, this approach may be practical, but clearly is not the optimal choice.

One problem that must be addressed in the development of a stable transfection system is how the introduced DNA will be maintained in the cells. In the case of Leishmania, the introduced DNA remained as an extrachromosomal plasmid, whereas in the case of trypanosomes the introduced DNA was incorporated into the chromosome at a homologous site. In the case of mammalian cells, the introduced DNA is generally incorporated at a nonhomologous site. There is no way to predict what will happen in the case of malaria, and therefore we would try different approaches. In the case of homologous integration, it is particularly important to design the vector so as not to destroy an essential gene. This is a haploid parasite, and thus integration and knockout of an essential gene would kill the parasite.

CONCLUSIONS

Malaria remains the major parasitic disease in the world today, causing morbidity and mortality in individuals and negative economic and social impacts on society. Efforts to control the disease have been hampered by the emergence and spread of drug-resistant parasites, the breakdown of malaria control programs due to both insecticide-resistant mosquitoes and upheavals in spraying programs, and the complicated problems of vaccine development and testing. The world is facing an increasing threat of malaria in the 1990s with few new tools to combat the parasite and disease. Recognizing this emerging crisis, it is necessary to design new strategies for the identification and development of interventions. One approach, namely, a focus on identifying key targets in the parasite and using those to develop new interventions, vaccines, or drugs, is emphasized in this chapter. This reports the first successful step in this strategy, namely, the genetic engineering of the malaria parasite.

REFERENCES

Bray PG, Ward SA (1993): Malaria chemotherapy: Resistance to quinoline containing drugs in *Plasmodium falciparum*. Fems Microbiol Lett, 113:1–7.
Coppel RL (1986): Prospects for a malaria vaccine. Microbiol Sci, 3:292–295.
Cowman AF, Galatis D, Thompson JK (1994): Selection for mefloquine resistance in Plasmodium falciparum is linked to amplification of the pfmdr1 gene and cross-resistance to halofantrine and quinine. Proc Natl Acad Sci USA, 91:1143–1147.
Cryz S, Jr J (1991): Molecular parasitology: Progress towards the development of vaccines for malaria, filariasis, and schistosomiasis. Experientia, 47:146–151.
Duffy PE, Pimenta P, Kaslow DC (1993): Pgs28 belongs to a family of epidermal growth

factor-like antigens that are targets of malaria transmission-blocking antibodies. J Exp Med, 177:505–510.

Fontanet AL, Johnston DB, Walker AM, Rooney W, Thimasarn K, Sturchler D, Macdonald M, Hours M, Wirth DF (1993): High prevalence of mefloquine-resistant falciparum malaria in eastern Thailand. Bull WHO, 71: 77–83.

Foote SJ, Galatis D, Cowman AF (1990a): Amino acids in the dihydrofolate reductase-thymidylate synthase gene of Plasmodium falciparum involved in cycloguanil resistance differ from those involved in pyrimethamine resistance. Proc Natl Acad Sci USA 87:3014–3017.

Foote SJ, Kyle DE, Martin RK, Oduola AM, Forsyth K, Kemp DJ, Cowman AF (1990b): Several alleles of the multidrug-resistance gene are closely linked to chloroquine resistance in *Plasmodium falciparum* [see comments]. Nature, 345:255–258.

Foote SJ, Thompson JK, Cowman AF, Kemp DJ (1989): Amplification of the multidrug resistance gene in some chloroquine-resistant isolates of *P. falciparum*. Cell, 57:921–930.

Ginsburg H, Krugliak M (1992): Quinoline-containing antimalarials—Mode of action, drug resistance and its reversal. An update with unresolved puzzles. Biochem Pharmacol 43:63–70.

Good MF, Kumar S, Miller LH (1988): The real difficulties for malaria sporozoite vaccine development: nonresponsiveness and antigenic variation. Immunol Today 9:351–355.

Goonewardene R, Daily J, Kaslow D, Sullivan TJ, Duffy P, Carter R, Mendis K, Wirth D (1993): Transfection of the malaria parasite and expression of firefly luciferase. Proc Natl Acad Sci USA, 90:5234–5236.

Gordon DM (1990): Malaria vaccines. Infect Dis Clin North Am 4:299–313.

Gros P, Ben NYB, Croop JM, Housman DE (1986): Isolation and expression of a complementary DNA that confers multidrug resistance. Nature 323:728–731.

Kaslow DC (1990): Immunogenicity of *Plasmodium falciparum* sexual stage antigens: Implications for the design of a transmission blocking vaccine. Immunol Lett 25:83–86.

Kaslow DC (1993): Transmission-blocking immunity against malaria and other vector-borne diseases. Curr Opin Immunol 5:557–565.

Krogstad DJ, Gluzman IY, Herwaldt BL, Schlesinger PH, Wellems TE (1992). Energy dependence of chloroquine accumulation and chloroquine efflux in *Plasmodium falciparum*. Biochem Pharmacol 43(1):57–62.

Kyle DE, Milhous WK, Rossan RN (1993): Reversal of *Plasmodium falciparum* resistance to chloroquine in Panamanian aotus monkeys. Am J Trop Med Hyg 48:126–133.

Kyle D. E., Oduola AM, Martin SK, Milhous WK (1990): *Plasmodium falciparum:* Modulation by calcium antagonists of resistance to chloroquine, desethylchloroquine, quinine, and quinidine in vitro. Trans R Soc Trop Med Hyg. 84(4): 474-478.

Lanzer M, et al. (1993): *Plasmodium:* Control of gene expression in malaria parasites. Exp Parasitol 1993. 77:121–128.

Looareesuwan S, Harinasuta T, Chongsuphajaisiddhi T (1992): Drug resistant malaria, with special reference to Thailand. Southeast Asian J Trop Med Public Health 23:621–634.

Martin SK, Oduola AM, Milhous WK (1987): Reversal of chloroquine resistance in *Plasmodium falciparum* by verapamil. Science 235(4791):899–901.

Milhous WK, Gerena L, Kyle DE, Oduola AM (1989): In vitro strategies for circumventing antimalarial drug resistance. Prog Clin Biol Res 313:61–72.

Nardin EH, Nussenzweig RS (1993): T cell responses to pre-erythrocytic stages of malaria: Role in protection and vaccine development against pre-erythrocytic stages. Annu Rev Immunol 11:687–727.

Nosten F, ter Kuile F, Chongsuphajaisiddhi T, Luxemburger C, Webster HK, Edstein M, Phaipun L, Thew KL, White NJ (1991): Mefloquine-resistant falciparum malaria on the Thai-Burmese border [see comments]. Lancet 337(8750):1140–1143.

Nussenzweig RS, Nussenzweig V (1989): Antisporozoite vaccine for malaria: Experimental basis and current status. Rev Infect Dis 3:s579–s585.

Oduola AM, Sowunmi A, Milhous WK, Kyle DE, Martin RK, Walker O, Salako LA (1992): Innate resistance to new antimalarial drugs in *Plasmodium falciparum* from Nigeria. Trans R Soc Trop Med Hyg 86:123–126.

Peters W (1989): Changing pattern of antimalarial drug resistance. J R Soc Med 17:14–17.

Peterson DS, Milhous WK, Wellems TE (1990): Molecular basis of differential resistance to cycloguanil and pyrimethamine in *Plasmodium falciparum* malaria. Proc Natl Acad Sci USA 87:3018–3022.

Raymond M., Rose E, Housman DE, Gros P (1990): Physical mapping, amplification, and overexpression of the mouse mdr gene family in multidrug-resistant cells. Mol Cell Biol 10(4):1642–1651.

Roninson IB, Chin JE, Choi KG, Gros P, Housman DE, Fojo A, Shen DW, Gottesman MM, Pastan I (1986): Isolation of human mdr DNA sequences amplified in multidrug-resistant KB carcinoma cells. Proc Natl Acad Sci USA 83(12):4538–4542.

Shanks GD, Watt G, Edstein MD, Webster HK, Suriyamongkol V, Watanasook C, Panpunnung S, Kowinwiphat W (1991): Halofantrine for the treatment of mefloquine chemoprophylaxis failures in *Plasmodium falciparum* infections. Am J Trop Med Hyg 45(4):488–491.

Slater AF, Cerami A (1992): Inhibition by chloroquine of a novel haem polymerase enzyme activity in malaria trophozoites [see comments]. Nature 355:167–169.

Vaidya AB, Morrisey J, Plowe CV, Kaslow DC, Wellems TE (1993): Unidirectional dominance of cytoplasmic inheritance in two genetic crosses of Plasmodium falciparum. Mol Cell Biol 13:7349–7357.

Volkman SK, Wilson CM, Wirth DF (1993): Stage-specific transcripts of the Plasmodium falciparum pfmdr 1 gene. Mol Biochem Parasitol 57:203–211.

Walker JA, Dolan SA, Gwadz RW, Panton LJ, Wellems TE (1992): An RFLP map of the *Plasmodium falciparum* genome, recombination rates and favored linkage groups in a genetic cross. Mol Biochem Parasitol 51:313–320.

Wellems TE, Panton LJ, Gluzman IY, do Rosario VE, Gwadz RW, Walker JA, Krogstad DJ (1990): Chloroquine resistance not linked to mdr-like genes in a *Plasmodium falciparum* cross [see comments]. Nature 345:253–255.

Wellems TE, Walker JA, Panton LJ (1991): Genetic mapping of the chloroquine-resistance locus on *Plasmodium falciparum* chromosome 7. Proc Natl Acad Sci USA 88:3382–3386.

White NJ, Pukrittayakamee S (1993): Clinical malaria in the tropics. Med J Aust 159:197–203.

Wilson CM, Serrano AE, Wasley A, Bogenschutz MP, Shankar AH, Wirth DF (1989): Amplification of a gene related to mammalian mdr genes in drug-resistant *Plasmodium falciparum*. Science 244:1184–1186.

Wilson CM, Volkman SK, Thaithong S, Martin RK, Kyle DE, Milhous WK, Wirth DF (1993): Amplification of pfmdr 1 associated with mefloquine and halofantrine resistance in *Plasmodium falciparum* from Thailand. Mol Biochem Parasitol 57:151–160.

Molecular Approaches to Parasitology, pages 243–254
© 1995 Wiley-Liss, Inc.

RNA Editing: An Overview, Status Report, and Personal Perspective

Kenneth Stuart

Seattle Biomedical Research Institute, Seattle, Washington 98109-1651

BACKGROUND

It may be that selection of a research field and certainly a research problem may be as important as the decision to embark on a research career. My studies on RNA editing stem from the beginning of my graduate training, when as an M.A. student I began to explore the role of an unusual mitchondrial (mt) DNA called *kinetoplast DNA* (kDNA) in a Leptomonad parasite, using acridine mutagenesis and (unsuccessful) DNA transformation. During this time I learned of the global health importance of parasites and recognized their value as study systems for fundamental biological questions. The protozoan parasites were particularly intriguing to me since they were simultaneously single cells and organisms and I was interested in phenomena at the cellular and molecular levels. The switch between glycolysis and cytochrome-mediated mt oxidative phosphorylation for energy production during the life cycle of African trypanosomes fascinated me. I thought that the regulation of these fundamental processes must involve important control mechanisms. I focused on the mt respiratory system, since some of its components are encoded in the mt genome, which is much less complex than the nuclear genome, and essentially nothing was known about organellar gene regulation. African trypanosomes, unlike other kinetoplastids and most organisms, also seemed able to survive kDNA loss and hence substantial mutation. I thus turned to *Trypanosoma brucei* for my doctoral studies, received infected mice (shipped to me in a tobacco tin), and isolated the dyskinetoplastic (Dk) mutants, which are devoid of kDNA and which have been useful in many later experiments.

The path to RNA editing began with the characterization of kDNA, initially with the determination of kDNA complexity, restriction mapping of the maxicircle, and cloning of the maxicircle and minicircles. The substantial work that has elucidated many aspects of RNA editing can be traced from several recent reviews (Benne, 1993a,b; Stuart, 1991, 1993a,b; Simpson et al., 1993; Coleman and Stuart, 1993;). The first direct step toward the discovery of RNA editing came from sequencing maxicircle DNA. We found that a sequence in *T. brucei* predicted a protein with homology to cytochrome oxidase subunit II (COII) genes, but the homology was encoded in two different reading frames. We sequenced about 100 independent clones to convince ourselves (and skeptical reviewers of the paper) of the result. The same result was obtained at about the same time in the laboratories of Rob Benne and Larry Simpson. These studies naturally included preliminary characterization of maxicircle transcripts, and unusual features were noticed, especially in *T. brucei*. Rob Benne an coworkers sequenced the COII transcript of *Crithidia* and found four noncoded uridines (Us) in the RNA that eliminated the encoded frameshift (Benne et al., 1986) and went on to assess the possibility of an alternate gene. In my laboratory the apocytochrome *b* (CYb) transcript was being studied since we had found substantial variation in its abundance in different life cycle stages of *T. brucei* and multiple transcript sizes. Although this was also true for the COII transcripts, we focused on CYb transcripts because of Benne's efforts on COII. Although reviewers of our papers strongly suggested we do nuclease protection mapping studies, we chose to sequence the RNA since our primer extension studies suggested CYb transcripts with different 5′ ends. The autoradiograms of the initial sequencing gels were confusing until we realized that it contained two superimposed related sequences, one of which matched the gene sequence and the other which had additional Us. The RNA sequence determined by Jean Feagin revealed 34 Us added at 12 sites, which was confirmed by cDNA cloning and sequencing by Doug Jasmer. These results concerned us since both relied on reverse transcriptase, but Northern blot analyses with oligonucleotides specific for edited and unedited RNA showed the presence of both sequences in cellular RNA, each with a characteristic size, and also revealed that the edited RNA was essentially restricted to the procyclic forms. (Feagin et al., 1987) This study also showed that editing can create an initiation codon and revealed partially edited RNA.

Subsequent studies revealed that editing creates initiation codons in 10 mRNAs, suggesting that editing may regulate translation of the mRNAs since editing occurs in the 3′ to 5′ direction, as discussed below. Editing also creates termination codons in eight mRNAs and open reading frames that predict proteins with homology to other mt proteins. Hence, the edited mRNAs appear to be competent for translation. Interestingly, some RNAs, such as CYb and COII in *T. brucei*, appear competent for translation both before and after editing, although translation of the unedited mRNA would result in a truncated protein. Thus, it is conceivable that proteins with different domain contents are produced depending on RNA editing, and this may have physiological significance.

Were these findings not sufficiently dramatic, we also found that several mRNAs are extensively edited. For example, the cytochrome oxidase subunit

III (COIII) gene of *T. brucei* was not recognizable from the gene sequence. However, a COIII probe from *Leishmania* detected the edited mRNA in normal but not Dk mutants, and determination of the edited COIII sequence showed that editing adds hundreds of Us and removes tens of encoded Us from COIII mRNA. (Feagin et al., 1988) The COIII mRNA sequence is thus more the result of editing than transcription of the maxicircle. This finding led to reviewers comments such as "the results reported in this manuscript are so shocking that I searched for a fatal flaw but could find none" and "I personally find these results difficult to accept; thus, they are potentially fascinating." We noted that the COIII gene sequence has a pronounced G versus C strand bias as we had noticed for several other maxicircle regions. We have now shown that all of these regions in *T. brucei* encode RNAs that are extensively edited as summarized in Table 1. The extensive editing highlighted the question of how the edited sequence was specified, as is discussed in some detail later.

The study of RNA editing stimulated new experimental directions that include mechanisms of RNA editing, the characterization of the editing machinery, and the interesting developmental control of editing, as discussed below. In addition, the mechanisms that regulate mt mRNA abundance, the processing of polycistronic primary RNA, mt mRNA polyadenylation, and

TABLE 1.   Edited and Unedited mt mRNAs in *Trypansoma brucei*

Gene[a]	Us added	Us deleted	mRNA
COI	—	—	1,680
COII	4	0	659
COIII	547	41	969
ND1	—	—	1,046
ND4	—	—	1,358
ND5	—	—	1,810
ND7	553	89	1,238
ND8	259	46	562
ND9	345	20	649
CR3	148	13	299
CR4	325	40	567
CR5 (ND3)	710	13	452
RPS12 (CR6)	132	28	325
A6 (MURF4)	447	28	811
MURF1	—	—	1,352
MURF2	26	4	1,111
CYb	34	0	1,151

CYb, apocytochrome b; COI, COII, COIII, cytochrome oxidase subunits I, II, and III; MURF1 and 2, maxicircle unidentified reading frames 1 and 2; ND1, 4, 5, 7, 8, 9, NADH dehydrogenase subunits 1, 4, 5, 7, 8, and 9; A6, ATPase subunit 6 (alias MURF4); CR3, 4, 5, 6 (alias G3, 4, 5, and 6), C-rich template sequences 3, 4, 5, and 6; RPS12, CR6 may encode ribosomal protein S12.

the consequence of editing at the levels of protein synthesis and mt respiratory physiology wait to be explored.

WHAT IS RNA EDITING?

RNA editing is a type of post-transcriptional RNA processing with the hallmark that it adds and removes Us. It has only been found to affect the mt RNAs of kinetoplastid flagellates. It is distinct from RNA splicing, since additional sequence is created after transcription. It is also distinct from other types of RNA processing currently termed *RNA editing* that either modify nucleotides, such as the C to U and U to C modifications in plant organelle and mammalian apolipoprotein b mRNAs and the A to I modifications of several dsRNAs in several species, or add or replace various nucleotides as in *Acanthamoeba* tRNA and *Physarum* mt RNAs. These forms of processing have been recently reviewed (Benne, 1993; Gesteland and Atkins, 1993). The mechanism of editing is uncertain, as discussed below, but appears to entail small complementary RNAs called *guide RNAs* (gRNAs), gRNA/mRNA chimeras, and macromolecular complexes.

The genes for all of the RNAs known to be involved in editing are encoded in kDNA. The maxicircle encodes 18 mRNAs, 12 of which are edited. The 9S and 12S rRNAs and a stable transcript from an unidentified sequence (US) that does not appear to encode a protein are not edited. The variable region of the maxicircle, which is composed of A+T-rich repeated sequences and which probably does not encode protein, encodes a heterogeneous set of transcripts that have not been thoroughly studied. The maxicircle also encodes a small number of gRNAs, at least in *Leishmania* and *Crithidia,* but most of the gRNAs are encoded in the minicircle of *T. brucei*, with each minicircle encoding three or four gRNAs. It is conceivable that other RNAs are important for RNA editing, perhaps analogous to the U RNAs of the spliceosome, and multiple proteins are probably required to catalyze the editing process. The molecules must be encoded in the nucleus since kDNA has insufficient unaccounted coding capacity.

WHICH RNAS ARE EDITED?

The COII, CYb, and MURF2 mRNAs are edited to limited extents as summarized in Table 1. Four Us are added to COII mRNA (as described above), 34 are added to CYb (creating the initiation codon and extending the open reading frame [ORF], and 26 are added and 4 deleted in the 5′ end of MURF2 mRNA, (again creating an initiation codon and extending the ORF). ND7, ND8, ND9, COIII, A6, RPS12, and CR3, CR4, and CR5 mRNAs are extensively edited by the addition of hundreds of Us and deletion of tens of encoded Us. The editing in both ND7 and CR5 mRNAs occurs in two separate domains. The A6 and RPS12 homologies are low, and CR5 may have homology to ND3; these restricted homologies require additional study to confirm gene identities. The five mRNAs that encode ND1, ND4, ND5, MURF1, and COI are not edited. Thus, there is no correlation between which mRNAs are edited and the respiratory complexes of which they are a part. Noncoded Us also occur in poly(A) tails, and the 3′ ends of rRNAs and gRNAs but are probably not added by the editing process. They may be added by the direct action of the mitochondrial 3′ terminal uridylyl transferase (TUTase). Despite the extensive editing that adds a total of about 3,600 Us and removes over 300, the edited mRNAs predict proteins with homology to those encoded mRNAs of other organisms that do not edit these mRNAs. Thus, the edited RNAs appear to be the functional mRNAs.

WHAT SPECIFIES THE EDITED SEQUENCE?

Several lines of evidence suggest that gRNAs, initially found and characterized by B. Blum in Larry Simpson's laboratory, specify the edited sequence. This includes their coding by mt DNA, existence in the mt, complementarity to edited mRNA, existence in chimeras that are described below, and absence of normal edited mRNA in mutants devoid of most gRNA genes. Each minicircle in T. brucei can encode three of four gRNA and these gRNAs are encoded in cassettes defined by pairs of 18 bp sequences that flank the gRNA coding region in an inverted orientation. gRNAs can be radiolabeled using guanylyltransferase, indicating that they have di- or triphosphate 5′ termini, thus implying that they are primary transcripts. However, the possibility that minicircles are transcribed into polycistronic transcripts that are processed cannot be excluded. The minicircle complexity is ample to encode sufficient gRNA for all the editing. Its over 400 minicircle classes can encode 1,200 different gRNAs, but only about 240 are needed for all the editing that appears to occur in T. brucei. Multiple gRNAs have been found in T. brucei that can guide the same final sequence, indicating considerable guiding redundancy consistent with the excess gRNA coding capacity. While some RNAs appear to be encoded in the maxicircle, most are encoded in minicircles. In T. brucei, the vast majority of the gRNAs are encoded in minicircles. Leishmania tarentolae encodes a single gRNA per minicircle, and it is on the opposite strand relative to T. brucei. The kDNA complexity of T. brucei is greater than that of L. tarentolae. This reflects more extensive editing in the former species as well as the absence of wild-type editing in laboratory strains of the latter species, apparently due to loss on minicircles and their gRNA genes. The differences in editing between species may reflect their relative evolutionary position and/or physiological difference.

THE EDITING PROCESS

The genetic information for each edited mRNAs is dispersed among multiple genes: the gene that encodes the encrypted pre-edited mRNA and one or more genes for the gRNA that specify the edited sequence. How, then, is the edited sequence specified? This question must be considered at three levels: that of the whole mRNA molecule, that of the sequence specified by a single gRNA, and that of a single site where one or more Us are added or deleted.

Editing of the whole mRNA molecule proceeds in the 3′ to 5′ direction, as suggested by the characteristics of partially edited molecules and gRNAs. The numerous partially edited molecules are edited in the 3′ portions of the editing domains and are unedited in the 5′ portions of the editing domains. All gRNAs have characteristic features that are probably important to their function. They are just under 60 nts in size and have 3′ oligo-U tails that are not encoded by the genome but are probably added by the mt TUTase. The gRNAs are complementary to the edited sequence and can thus form a stable gRNA–mRNA duplex with this RNA. However, the gRNAs for the 3′ limit of the editing domain can form a duplex with the unedited RNA. This duplex is between the 5′ end of the gRNA and the approximately 6–12 nt sequence 3′ to the editing domain. A subset of gRNAs can form a partial duplex with unedited mRNA, and the other gRNAs can form a duplex between the 5′ end of gRNA and edited but not unedited mRNA. This partial duplex between the 5′ end of gRNA and mRNA is called the *anchor duplex* since it may anchor the gRNA with its mRNA. In addition, many examples have been found in which one gRNA can specify the edited mRNA sequence that is able to form an anchor duplex with the next gRNA. Thus, the editing in the 3′ to 5′ direction appears to result from the order of gRNA utilization, based on anchor duplex formation with one gRNA specifying the sequence that allows selection of a subsequent gRNA. *L. tarentolae* has limited gRNA diversity, especially in laboratory strains, and thus can have little variation in the order of gRNA utilization. *T. brucei,* however, has substantial gRNA diversity that includes multiple gRNAs for the same sequence, which is possible because of the use of G/U and Watson-Crick basepairing, and gRNAs for substantially overlapping sequences and thus probably has a more complex pattern of gRNA utilization. The use of G/U and Watson-Crick basepairing also allows the generation of slightly different edited sequences. This has been observed but appears to result in conservative replacements at the protein level and thus is of no physiological consequence. Furthermore, some misediting appears to occur where gRNA for one mRNA appears to be used to edit another pre-mRNA. This is presumably due to fortuitous formation of a gRNA–mRNA duplex and may be observed more frequently in species or strains in which gRNA complexity is low.

The junctions between the edited and unedited sequences in partially edited RNA probably correspond to regions where editing was occurring at the time of RNA isolation. The sequence transits from fully edited directly to unedited RNA in only a very small fraction of partially edited RNAs. Most junctions have a region with added and/or removed Us, but its sequence does not match mature mRNAs. The sizes of these junctions are such that their editing could be specified by a single gRNA. In addition, chimeric mRNA–gRNA molecules have been isolated from cellular RNA using polymerase chain reactions (PCR). The gRNAs are attached by oligo-U to internal sequences in the editing domains. This has the important implication that the Us that are added and removed in editing are derived from and possibly transferred to the gRNA U tails, respectively. The gRNA portions of the chimeras vary in size, which is of unknown significance. The mRNA sequence in a minor fraction of the chimeras is partially edited, supporting the notion that junctions are regions of editing by single gRNAs. The junctions and incompletely edited sequences in chimeras have incompletely edited sites interspersed among fully edited sites which suggests that editing by each gRNA does not necessarily proceed precisely in the 3′ to 5′ direction. The initial model for editing suggested that the most 3′ mismatch between gRNA and mRNA was selected for editing, and thus editing proceeded precisely 3′ to 5′. This appears inconsistent with the interspersion of edited and unedited sites, and thus a second model proposed that sites were edited in a random order until protected by gRNA–mRNA duplex formation. However, neither model explained the deletion of Us 3′ to Cs since there would be no mismatch according to the first model and a protected site that is edited according to the second. Thus, a third model proposed preferential selection of the least stable (more frequently single-stranded) regions of RNA duplex. This model suggested that thermodynamic parameters drives editing toward completion. This model fits all current data, including occasional mismatch between gRNA and mRNA.

Elucidation of the process of editing at each site would be advanced by identification of the molecules that catalyze editing. Several candidate catalytic activities have been detected in the mt. These include endoribonuclease, TUTase, and RNA ligase, but the molecules responsible for these activities and their functions in editing have not been characterized. Detection of these activities led to the "cleavage/ligation" hypothesis (Fig. 1) that editing is catalyzed by a series of enzymatic steps whereby the pre-mRNA is cleaved, Us are added or removed, and the RNA is then religated. The gRNA would specify the editing by selecting the sites in the gRNA–mRNA duplex for cleavage. However, detection of chimeric molecules suggested that editing might be catalyzed by transesterification. The transesterification reaction has the same result as "cleavage/ligation" but accomplishes this in a single concerted step. In addition, transesterification has the attractive features that it is energeti-

Models for RNA Editing

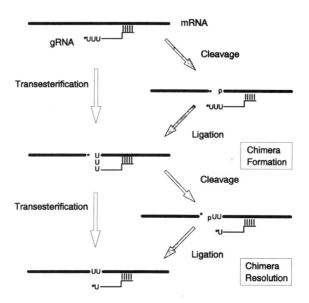

Fig. 1. The transesterification (left column) and cleavage/ligation (right column) models of editing. Both models assume that Us are added (and deleted) by the 3′ U tail of gRNA and that chimeras are editing intermediates. Transesterification forms and resolves chimeras directly, while cleavage/ligation entails separate steps. The asterisk indicates a 3′ OH, and p indicates a 5′ phosphate.

cally conservative and is used in RNA splicing. Transesterification also implies that the reactions may be catalyzed by RNA enzymes.

Experiments to date do not allow determination of which mechanism is used in RNA editing. Submitochondrial fractionation studies reported by the Hajduk and Simpson laboratories at the 1993 Cold Springs Harbor RNA processing meeting show that the endoribonuclease does not cofractionate with macromolecular complexes that contain gRNA. Fractions containing these gRNA complexes are able to form chimeras in vitro and can incorporate Us into added pre-edited RNA. These experiments imply transesterification but are not definitive. For example, endoribonuclease may not retain a stable association with the editosome or retain activity after fractionation, and the in vitro activities have not been shown to be true editing activities. There is limited evidence that editing does occur in vitro, since studies by Donna Koslowsky in my laboratory reported at the RNA processing meeting showed that several cDNA clones derived from added A6 pre-edited mRNA have deletion of two

Us, which is what normally occurs at the most 3´ editing site. While encouraging, these experiments are also not definitive.

THE EDITOSOME

Editing is very likely to be catalyzed by a macromolecular complex, perhaps by analogy to the catalysis of RNA splicing by the spliceosome and protein synthesis by the ribosome. The absence of a definitive assay for RNA editing led to the analysis of complexes that occur in vivo and complexes that form in vitro. The gRNAs, pre-edited mRNAs, TUTase and RNA ligase activities cosediment as two broad peaks of about 20S and 35–40S. (Pollard et al., 1992). In addition, Uli Göringer showed that incubation of isolated or synthetic gRNA with mt extracts led to the formation of four specific complexes designated G1, G2, G3 and G4 based on their mobility in native polyacrylamide gels (Göringer et al., 1993). G1 has the greatest mobility and is often resolved into three distinct bands. Several experiments showed that these complexes were specific to gRNAs, and mt extract and required protein as well as the gRNA. Laurie Read in my laboratory has found that addition of mRNA enhanced the formation of the complexes, and the added mRNA appeared to be incorporated into the same complexes as gRNA. However, the complexes formed with gRNA alone using micrococcal nuclease-treated extract, suggesting that mRNA can be incorporated into the complexes but is not required for the formation of the complexes that are visualized on the gels. Competition with oligo-U blocks the formation of the complexes, and subcomponents of the G1 band do not form with gRNAs that lack the U tail or the anchor sequence. These experiments suggest the existence of a multiprotein complex that forms specifically with gRNA. Studies in which the gRNA or mRNA probes are cross-linked to the proteins reveal two distinct proteins that have clear specificity for gRNA. These are a 25 kD protein that is primarily localized in the G1 complex and a 90 kD protein that is primarily cross-linked with the probe in the G3 complex. The 90 kD protein appears to have specificity for the U tail of gRNA.

The abundance of edited RNA is developmentally regulated. For example, edited CYb and COII transcripts are much more abundant in procyclic than in bloodstream form *T. brucei;* they are also at very low abundance in the slender bloodstream forms compared with the stumpy bloodstream forms. Conversely, edited ND7 and CR4 transcripts are more abundant in the bloodstream forms. Edited MURF2 RNA is similar in abundance in both life cycle stages. The basis for this regulation is unclear, but it may occur at the level of the editing process. CYb gRNAs are encoded in the maxicircles in *L. tarentolae* and *C. fasciculata* but not in *T. brucei*. George Riley in my laboratory found that there are three related minicircles that encode CYb gRNAs. These gRNAs have sequences that differ by as much as 30%, but they specify the same edited sequence, which is possible because of G/U basepairing. All three gRNAs appear functional, since they occur in chimeras. Interestingly, some chimeras have gRNAs with 3´ sequence that is about 20 nts longer than in all other gRNAs examined. These "extra" sequences may have a role in developmental regulation of editing, for example, as recognition sequences for regulatory factors. The gRNAs are also encoded outside the 18 bp repeats, unlike all of the numerous other minicircle encoded gRNAs found in *T. brucei*.

Quantitative PCR analysis revealed that there are tens of molecules per cell of CYb pre-edited mRNA and CYb gRNAs. Surprisingly, CYb chimeras are very low in abundance, with only one molecule or less per several thousand cells. This suggests that chimeras are short lived, assuming they are editing intermediates. Pre-edited CYb mRNA is similar in abundance in bloodstream and procyclic forms, and there is approximately 10 times more edited CYb mRNA in the procyclic forms than in the bloodstream forms. The CYb gRNAs appear slightly less abundant in procyclic forms than in bloodstream forms, and there is about 10 times more CYb chimeras in procyclic than in bloodstream forms. The higher level of CYb chimeras and lower level of CYb gRNA in procyclic forms suggest that regulation of editing occurs at the level of gRNA utilization. It implies that gRNAs may be consumed by the editing process; this may be the basis for the different gRNA sizes in chimeras.

Other processes affecting mt transcripts also appear to be developmentally regulated in *T. brucei*. Many of the mt transcripts occur in two size classes one of which has about 20 nt poly(A) tails and the other about 150 residue tails. Edited transcripts that preferentially accumulate in different life cycle stages tend to have longer poly(A) tails. This implies transcript-specific developmental regulation of poly(A) tail size. This may affect RNA stability and/or translation. In addition, there may be regulation of the processing of polycistronic transcripts. Several maxicircle genes overlap in the sense that the same sequence encodes portions of different mRNAs in these cases. For example, the same 37 bp sequence encodes the 3´ UTR of RPS12 mRNA and the 5´ UTR of ND5 mRNA; the former, but not the latter, sequence is edited in the mature mRNAs. Northern blot analysis reveals potential processing precursor transcripts that are large enough to encode both RPS12 and ND5. PCR analysis shows the presence of both sequences on the same molecule, and, interestingly, the RPS12 3´ UTR sequence is edited in some precursors, indicating that editing can precede the processing of the precursor molecules. Thus, the same precursor molecule cannot be processed to produce both mature RPS12 and ND5 mRNAs unless some mechanism exists to add 5´- or 3´-terminal sequences. Editing of the precursor may result in cleavage of the precursor at the RPS12 poly(A) addition site to produce functional RPS12 mRNA and perhaps nonfunctional ND5 mRNA. Cleavage at the 5´ terminus of ND5 mRNA prior to editing may do the reverse. This suggests the possible existence of a system that regulates gene expression at the level of transcript processing.

CONCLUSION

RNA editing is a form of RNA processing that regulates the expression of mt genes, since it results in the formation of mature translatable mRNA. Since edited mRNAs encode components of the mt respiratory system, editing probably functions to regulate this metabolic process. The production of edited mRNA is developmentally regulated, and this is especially evident in *T. brucei*, in which production of the mt respiratory system is regulated during the life cycle. Thus, editing among other regulatory process appears to adjust the composition and function of terminal respiration at least during the life cycle of *T. brucei*. The origins of RNA editing are unknown. Its occurrence in the mt and the early divergence of trypanosomes in the eukaryotic lineage suggest an early origin. However, its accuracy, regulation, apparent coordination with processes that regulate mRNA abundance, polyadenylation, and processing suggest a high level of integration into cellular regulatory processes. Editing probably provides a selective advantage to trypanosomes and thus was retained. RNA editing is probably catalyzed by a macromolecular complex. The editing process and the editing machinery may have some distant relationships to RNA splicing or other cellular processes that may shed light on its origins.

ACKNOWLEDGMENTS

I thank my laboratory colleagues for numerous stimulating discussions and G. Riley for assistance in preparation of Figure 1. This work received support from NIH grants AI14102 and GM42118 to K.S., who is a Burroughs Wellcome Scholar in Molecular Parasitology.

REFERENCES

Benne R (1993a): RNA editing, an overview. In R. Benne (ed): RNA Editing: The Alteration of Protein Coding Sequences of RNA. Chichester, West Sussex. England: Ellis Horwood, Ltd., pp. 13–24.

Benne R (1993b): RNA editing in mitochondria of *Leishmania tarentolae* and *Crithidia fasciculata*. Semin Cell Biol 4:241–249.

Benne R. (ed) (1993c): RNA Editing: The Alteration of Protein Coding Sequences of RNA. Chichester, West Sussex, England: Ellis Horwood, Ltd.

Benne R, van den Burg J, Brakenhoff JP, Sloof P, Van Boom JH, Tromp MC (1986): Major transcript of the frameshifted *coxII* gene from trypanosome mitochondria contains four nucleotides that are not encoded in the DNA. Cell 46:819–826.

Colman A, Stuart K (eds) (1993): Seminars in Cell Biology: RNA Editing. London: Academic Press.

Feagin JE, Abraham JM, Stuart K (1988): Extensive editing of the cytochrome *c* oxidase III transcript in *Trypanosoma brucei*. Cell 53:413–422.

Feagin JE, Jasmer DP, Stuart K (1987): Developmentally regulated addition of nucleotides within apocytochrome *b* transcripts in *Trypanosoma brucei*. Cell 49:337–345.

Gesteland RF, Atkins JF (eds) (1993): RNA World. Cold Spring Harbor, NY: Cold Spring Harbor Laboratory.

Göringer HU, Koslowsky DJ, Morales TH, Stuart KD (1994): The formation of mitochondrial ribonucleoprotein complexes involving gRNA molecules in *Trypanosoma brucei*. Proc Natl Acad Sci USA 91:1776–1780.

Pollard VW, Harris ME, Hajduk SL (1993): Native mRNA editing complexes from *Trypanosoma brucei* mitochondria. EMBO J 11:4429–4438.

Simpson L, Maslov DA, Blum B (1993): RNA editing in *Leishmania* mitochondria. In R. Benne (ed): RNA Editing: The Alteration of Protein Coding Sequences of RNA. Chichester, West Sussex, England: Ellis Horwood Ltd., pp. 53–85.

Stuart K (1991): RNA editing in trypanosomatid mitochondria. Annu Rev Microbiol 45:327–344.

Stuart K (1993a): RNA editing in mitochondria of African trypanosomes. In R. Benne (ed): RNA Editing: The Alteration of Protein Coding Sequences of RNA. Chichester, West Sussex, England: Ellis Horwood Ltd., pp. 25–52.

Stuart K (1993b): The RNA editing process in *Trypanosoma brucei*. Semin Cell Biol 4:251–260.

Molecular Approaches to Parasitology, pages 255–268
© 1995 Wiley-Liss, Inc.

Transcription and RNA Processing in *Trypanosoma brucei*

Christian Tschudi

*Department of Internal Medicine, Yale University School of Medicine,
New Haven, Connecticut 06520*

INTRODUCTION

The study of transcriptional events has revealed a complex and diverse set of biochemical interactions between sequence-specific DNA-binding proteins, promoter and enhancer elements, and the basal transcriptional apparatus consisting of RNA polymerase and a variety of accessory factors. In addition, remarkable progress has been made in identifying components of RNA processing reactions and deciphering the mechanism of the reactions. Compared with what we know about these machineries in a number of organisms, including yeast and higher eukaryotes, our understanding of these processes in trypanosomes is extremely limited. Although DNA transfection has become recently available, a detailed and exhaustive biochemical analysis of the enzymes and protein factors involved in transcription and RNA processing will only be possible with the development of *in vitro* systems. Nevertheless, despite this limitation, the study of transcription and RNA processing in trypanosomes has provided the scientific community with a number of unexpected and exciting discoveries, some of which I would like to discuss in this chapter.

PROTEIN CODING GENES ARE ORGANIZED AS POLYCISTRONIC TRANSCRIPTION UNITS

In trypanosomes, an unusual number of genes coding for housekeeping as well as developmentally regulated proteins are organized in tandemly repeated gene families. Examples include the genes for tubulin, calmodulin, heat shock proteins, procyclic acidic repetitive proteins (PARP), and a number of genes coding for glycolytic enzymes. The spacing between protein coding regions is quite small, ranging in size from less than one hundred to a few hundred nucleotides. This is the case between repeating units within a gene cluster as well as between different genes. This degree of packaging of genetic information is higher than in other eukaryotic organisms, where genes are generally separated from each other by several kilobases.

In most eukaryotic organisms, each gene has its own promoter, that is transcription is monocistronic. Soon after transcription is initiated, the 5′ end of the pre-mRNA is capped. Processing of the pre-mRNA then occurs by the addition of a poly(A) tail at the 3′ end and in some cases by the removal of intervening sequences. This is in contrast to what we have learned in trypanosomes, where transcription appears to encompass more than one gene unit, thus generating a polycistronic pre-mRNA that contains information for more than one protein. For most transcription units we do not know where transcription begins, and it appears that these pre-mRNAs do not contain the cap structure present on mature mRNA. Two RNA processing reactions then generate mature mRNAs coding for individual proteins. The cap at the 5′ end is provided by *trans*-splicing, and the 3′ end is formed by polyadenylation.

What is the experimental evidence for polycistronic transcription units in trypanosomes? When we analyzed the RNA transcripts derived from the calmodulin locus, we found mature mRNAs from all four tandemly repeated copies of the calmodulin genes. In addition, the upstream region of the calmodulin genes gives rise to two stable RNA molecules of 2 and 4 kb, which in steady-state RNA are 100-fold less abundant than the mature calmodulin mRNAs. However, when we analyzed the transcription rates of the various genes, they appeared approximately constant across the entire locus. More importantly, by this technique we did not detect any discontinuity in the RNA polymerase density between the individual calmodulin genes and between the calmodulin genes and the 3' end of the upstream 4 kb RNA coding region, which would have been indicative of a putative promoter region. In addition, we were able to identify in steady-state RNA polygenic transcripts spanning adjacent calmodulin coding regions as well as polycistronic transcripts in which calmodulin sequences were continuous with sequences coding for the 4kb RNA. Since these polygenic and polycistronic transcripts are the most abundant transcripts detected after a brief pulse with radioactive nucleotides, we reasoned that they are the precursors to mature mRNA (Tschudi and Ullu, 1988). These results are corroborated by the observation that treatment of trypanosome cells with cycloleucine, which in other systems has been shown to inhibit RNA processing reactions, induced an accumulation of these polygenic and polycistronic transcripts. Similarly, maturation of pre-mRNA can be disrupted by heat shock which causes an increase in abundance of multimeric precursors (Muhich and Boothroyd, 1989). With other model systems, inactivation of transcription by UV irradiation provided additional evidence for polycistronic transcription units (Johnson et al.,1987). Since RNA polymerases cannot traverse pyrimidine dimers induced in the DNA by UV irradiation, synthesis of long RNA molecules is more sensitive to UV inactivation than that of shorter ones. Using this technique, it was shown that the gene for the variant specific glycoprotein (VSG) 221 is in a transcription unit of about 60 kb. This unit comprises several other stable mRNAs, thus providing evidence for a polycistronic transcription unit. Finally, by DNA transfection it was demonstrated that sequences separating protein coding regions in tandemly repeated gene families do not possess detectable promoter activity to drive expression of a reporter gene.

In conclusion, it is now generally accepted that trypanosome protein coding genes are organized as polycistronic transcription units. Trypanosomes and nematodes represent the only examples of eukaryotic organisms that transcribe their genes in this peculiar way. However, polycistronic transcription units are typical of prokaryotic organisms and of some viruses. At present there is no conclusive evidence that the various genes encoded in polycistronic transcription units in trypanosomes are related in functional terms as is the case in operons in bacteria. Likewise, for most transcription units we do not know the transcription start site; thus, the average size of a transcription unit in trypanosomes is yet unknown.

RNA POLYMERASES, PROMOTER STRUCTURES, AND TRANSCRIPTION FACTORS OF PROTEIN CODING GENES

Eukaryotic gene transcription involves the complex interaction of *trans*-acting factors with different *cis*-regulatory elements of the gene. Nuclear RNA polymerases recognize their respective transcription units by binding to specific initiation complexes assembled on short promoter elements. In all eukaryotic cells studied, including trypanosomes, transcription is carried out by three different classes of RNA polymerases, each responsible for the synthesis of a unique set of RNAs. RNA polymerase I (pol I) is responsible for the synthesis of the large ribosomal RNAs. RNA polymerase II (pol II) transcribes all of the genes coding for proteins and most of the genes encoding the uridine-rich small nuclear RNAs (U-snRNAs), which are involved in various RNA processing reactions. RNA polymerase III (pol III) transcribes tRNA and 5S RNA genes and a number of small cytoplasmic and nuclear RNAs. The three RNA polymerases can be distinguished from each other by their different sensitivity to two transcription inhibitors, namely α-amanitin and tagetitoxin. Pol I is insensitive to α-amanitin, pol II is very sensitive to this inhibitor, whereas pol III is moderately sensitive to α-amanitin. Tagetitoxin, on the other hand, is a specific inhibitor for pol III and has no effect on pol I or pol II. Until recently, the particular division of labor described above was characteristic of all eukaryotic organisms. However, there are now a few examples that question the generality of this concept. In trypanosomes, the U2 and U4 snRNA genes and in plants, the U3 snRNA genes are transcribed by pol III. This is in contrast to what is known in all other organisms studied to date, where these genes are transcribed by pol II. These genes represent the only known examples that are transcribed by different RNA polymerases in different organisms. Even more surprising was the finding that in trypanosomes the gene families coding for VSG of bloodstream forms and PARP are transcribed by pol I and not by a typical α-amanitin–sensitive pol II (Kooter and Borst, 1984; Rudenko et al., 1989; Clayton et al., 1990). Although initially pol I transcription of protein coding genes was challenged by many investigators in the field, these findings can be rationalized by considering the pathway of 5´ end formation in trypanosomes. Pre-mRNAs are polycistronic, and the mature 5´ end, including the cap structure, is generated post-transcriptionally by an RNA processing reaction and not by transcription initiation. Thus, in trypanosomes maturation of the 5´ end is independent of the RNA polymerase that synthesizes the pre-mRNA, and therefore theoretically any of the three RNA polymerases could mediate transcription of protein coding genes. Thus far, the VSG and PARP genes are the only known examples of pol I–mediated expression of eukaryotic protein coding genes. It would be interesting to determine whether there are additional α-amanitin–resistant transcription units in trypanosomes and whether any of the polycistronic transcription units in nematodes are transcribed by pol I.

The initial report of the α-amanitin–resistant transcription of the VSG and PARP genes was followed by a detailed functional analysis of the PARP promoter, which revealed an organization reminiscent of a typical promoter for pol I (Sherman et al., 1991; Brown et al., 1992). Further experiments demonstrated that the PARP and pol I promoters are indeed functionally equivalent, since different regulatory elements of the *T. brucei* ribosomal RNA gene promoter can replace the corresponding sequences in the PARP promoter. The next challenge will be to identify *trans*-acting factors interacting with the VSG and PARP promoter elements and to establish a structural and functional relationship with transcription factors involved in rRNA gene expression in other eukaryotic organisms.

In the past years, the analysis of promoter structures in trypanosomes has concentrated primarily on the VSG and PARP genes. However, we should not forget that the majority (over 95%) of protein coding genes are transcribed by an RNA polymerase with the typical α-amanitin sensitivity of eukaryotic pol II. Thus far, experiments aimed at localizing promoter elements for these genes have failed and major questions that remain to be answered are the localization and number of transcription start sites for pol II–mediated gene transcription. It is possible that the mechanism of transcription initiation by pol II in trypanosomes is different from that in other eukaryotic organisms as suggested by the structure of the large subunit of pol II (Evers et al., 1989). The C-terminal domain (CTD) is a highly conserved feature of the large subunit of pol II, composed of a heptapeptide repeat that varies between 26 and 52 copies in yeast and mouse, respectively. Recently, it was shown that the CTD directly interacts with the transcription initiation complex through contacts with the TATA-binding protein (Koleske et al., 1992; Usheva et al., 1992). Although the large subunit of the trypanosome pol II contains a C-terminal extension, this region lacks the characteristic repeated heptapeptide structure. The CTD of trypanosomes has a high proportion of serine and tyrosine residues, which are potential phosphorylation sites. Most likely, phosphorylation of the CTD is involved in the transition from transcription initiation to elongation, as it is becoming apparent in other systems. It remains to be seen whether the unusual structure of the trypanosome CTD changes the way pol II recognizes an initiation complex, and whether this interaction occurs through a homolog of the TATA-binding protein.

MECHANISM OF U-sn RNA GENE EXPRESSION

One of the essential steps of gene expression in trypanosomes, the processing of pre-mRNAs by *trans*-splicing, requires the participation of U-snRNAs. Evolutionary considerations suggest that snRNAs may have a catalytic role and that they are descendants of the oldest enzymes, the ribozymes of the RNA world. Unlike nuclear mRNA splicing, splicing of nuclear pre-rRNA of the ciliated protozoan *Tetrahymena* occurs *in vitro* in the absence of proteins (Cech, 1986). Originally, it was not clear whether this self-splicing RNA (group I intron) was an example of a general mechanism or a molecular fossil. The subsequent discovery of a new class of self-splicing introns (group II introns) in fungal mitochondria suggested an answer. These group II introns combine self-splicing and lariat formation (the hallmark of nuclear mRNA splicing), therefore providing the missing link between group I introns and nuclear mRNA introns. The implication of this finding is that nuclear mRNA splicing has evolved from self-splicing group I or group II introns. In the course of evolution, nuclear mRNA introns could have lost the original autocatalytic function and transferred it to the snRNA components of snRNPs. Thus, U-snRNAs may originate from one of the oldest enzymes of the RNA world, the ribozyme. Consequently, the transcription units themselves might represent descendants of some of the oldest genes.

We are using DNA transfection of procyclic trypanosome cells to dissect the regulatory elements involved in transcription of U-snRNA genes in trypanosomes (Fantoni et al., 1994). These experiments showed that the U2 snRNA gene promoter consists of three distinct elements necessary for expression: one element located in the coding region close to the transcription start site and two elements upstream of the coding region. Interestingly, inspection of the upstream sequences revealed that they closely resemble the intragenic promoter elements of tRNA genes. Expression of eukaryotic tRNA genes depends predominantly on a bipartite intragenic promoter including an A box and a B box (Geiduschek and Tocchini-Valentini, 1988). The A box is found 8–25 bp downstream of the transcription start site, and the B box is located 30–90 bp downstream of the A box. The tRNA-like A and B boxes of the U2 snRNA gene are positioned and oriented in a way normally found in tRNA coding regions. However, in this case they do not appear to be part of a *bona fide* tRNA gene, since the surrounding sequences cannot be folded into a convincing cloverleaf structure. The finding that a B box was required for expression of the U2 snRNA gene is most intriguing. In tRNA genes, the B box is the primary binding site for transcription factor (TF)IIIC, which then recruits TFIIIB to the transcription initiation complex. Thus, both transcription factors are implicated in trypanosome U2 snRNA gene expression.

The unprecedented structure of the trypanosome U2 snRNA gene promoter raised the question whether similar sequence elements are located upstream of other U-snRNA and small RNA genes. We therefore inspected the corresponding regions of small RNA genes for which upstream sequences are available, namely, the genes coding for U6 snRNA, U-snRNA B, and 7SL RNA, a small cytoplasmic RNA that is part of the signal recognition particle. In all three cases we found an A and a B box in approximately the same positions and in the same orientation as in the U2 5′ flanking region. Most surprising, however, was the discovery that in all three cases the A and B boxes are part of a previously identified tRNA gene. The 5' end of a threonine tRNA gene is located 97 bp upstream of the U6 snRNA gene, an arginine tRNA gene is found 95 bp upstream of the U-snRNA B gene, and a lysine tRNA gene is located 95 bp upstream of the 7SL RNA gene. Remarkable in these arrangements is the strict conservation of the distance between the tRNA gene and the respective small RNA gene. In addition, all three tRNA genes are transcribed in the opposite direction relative to the small RNA gene. Site-directed mutagenesis determined that the A and B boxes of these tRNA genes are required for expression of the associated small RNA genes, and at least the tRNA gene upstream of the U6 snRNA gene is expressed and functional in vivo. Thus, our experiments identified promoter elements shared by two different transcription units. This novel promoter strategy adds yet another layer of complexity to the pol III transcription machinery, since it suggests that the tRNA control regions serve as bifunctional regulatory elements.

Is there an evolutionary or functional significance for the promoter structure of snRNA genes in trypanosomes? Until recently, it was assumed that each of the three RNA polymerases in eukaryotic cells had its own set of associated factors. This general belief has been challenged by the recent discovery that the TATA-binding protein is a ubiquitous transcription factor for all three RNA polymerases (Hernandez, 1993). This finding together with the notion that the large subunit of the three eukaryotic RNA polymerases derive from a common progenitor underscore the possibility that modern promoter structures were built from modular elements and that the variety of modern promoters is a result of different combinations of these modular structures. In this light, the discovery that elements corresponding to the internal control regions of a tRNA gene serve as promoter elements for transcription of the U6 snRNA gene in trypanosomes is quite puzzling. Because trypanosomes are ancient eukaryotes, one would be tempted to speculate that this genetic arrangement represents a molecular fossil in the evolution of snRNA gene promoters. If this were true, one should consider the possibility that the RNA polymerase III intragenic promoter of tRNA genes provided the first modular elements for assembly of extragenic promoters as we observe in the trypanosome U6 snRNA gene. How does the promoter structure of the trypanosome U2 snRNA gene fit into this picture? We have inspected the region surrounding the B box element of the U2 snRNA promoter for remnants of a tRNA. We have found that, indeed, it is very likely that the B box consensus sequence was originally part of a tRNA gene. Thus, the U2 snRNA gene promoter would represent yet another intermediate in the evolution of the modern U-snRNA promoter structure.

We should also consider whether or not there is a functional significance for the close linkage of tRNA and small RNA genes in trypanosomes. Clustering of functionally related genes is most common in bacteria, where enzymes needed for a particular pathway are coded for by adjacent genes organized in operons. This arrangement allows all the genes in the unit to be coordinately regulated. In yeast, the genes encoding the enzymes responsible for galactose utilization are clustered, and two of these genes, GAL1 and GAL10, are divergently transcribed from a common promoter. However, genetic linkage is not a prerequisite for coordinate expression of a set of genes. Interestingly, when *Escherichia coli* are deprived of one or more amino acids, the synthesis of rRNA and tRNA is reduced 10–20 fold by a phenomenon called *stringent response*. The signal for the stringent response is an accumulation of uncharged tRNA, and this signal is transduced into the second messenger ppGpp (magic spot). A similar control mechanism has recently been identified in *S. cerevisiae*, where amino acid starvation leads to increased expression of more than 30 biosynthetic enzymes. The genes we have characterized in our studies encode small stable RNAs that are required by the cell for essential functions, namely, RNA processing (U6 snRNA), translation (tRNAs), and targeting of membrane proteins to the endoplasmic reticulum (7SL RNA). It is tempting to speculate that trypanosomes have a mechanism to express these genes coordinately and that the elaborate and unusual promoter structure suggests regulatory strategies.

POST-TRANSCRIPTIONAL PROCESSES FORM BOTH THE 5′ AND 3′ ENDS OF MATURE mRNAS

We now need to turn to the mechanisms that generate mature mRNA from polycistronic pre-mRNAs. In trypanosomes, the structure of every mature mRNA is characterized by the same identical sequence of 39 nt. at the very 5′ end. This sequence is called the mini-exon or spliced leader (SL) sequence. Initially, the SL sequence constitutes the 5′ end of a small RNA, the SL RNA, which in *T. brucei* is about 140 nt long. There are approximately 200 SL RNA genes clustered at one or two sites in the genome. These SL RNA genes are not found nearby mRNA genes, and for a number of protein coding genes it has been shown that the SL RNA genes are actually located on a different chromosome. Joining of the SL sequence to the mRNA body occurs by a splicing mechanism referred to as "*trans*-splicing" (Murphy et al., 1986; Sutton and Boothroyd, 1986; Laird et al., 1987). *Trans*-splicing is an intermolecular reaction involving two separate RNA precursors, unlike *cis*-splicing, which is an intramolecular event and removes intervening sequences in eukaryotic pre-mRNAs (Green, 1991). Both reactions are best described by a two step model (Figure 1). First, the 5′ splice site is cleaved and the newly generated 5′ end of the intron is ligated via a 2′–5′ phosphodiester bond to the branch site located upstream from the 3′ splice site. This generates the intron-exon lariat in *cis*-splicing and in *trans*-splicing the so called Y-structure. In the second step, the SL exon is covalently joined to the mRNA body to form the mature 5′ end of the mRNA, whereas the Y-structure is released and resolved by a specific debranching enzyme. There is as yet no direct evidence that *trans*-splicing in trypanosomes proceeds through the pathway outlined in Figure 1. Although all the predicted intermediates and products have been identified in trypanosome cells, the lack of an *in vitro* system precludes the confirmation of this pathway. Nevertheless, *trans*-splicing is mechanistically very similar to *cis*-splicing, since it was demonstrated that small ribonucleoprotein particles containing U-snRNAs are essential for this process (Tschudi and Ullu, 1990). *Cis*-splicing requires a number of small ribonucleoprotein particles containing U1, U2, U5, and U4/U6 snRNAs. Trypanosomes contain homologs of the U2, U4 and U6 snRNAs, and it was shown that destruction of these small ribonucleoprotein particles blocks *trans*-splicing. One major difference between *cis*- and *trans*-splicing is that in trypanosomes no U1 and U5 snRNAs have been identified thus far. These two RNAs have been shown to be required for identification of the 5′ splice site of the intron during *cis*-splicing. How 5′ splice site identification is achieved in trypanosome *trans*-splicing is not known. It has been hypothesized that the SL RNA itself can substitute for U1 and U5 snRNA function, but this model needs to be tested.

The 3′ end of trypanosome mRNAs, as in most eukaryotic mRNAs, is de-

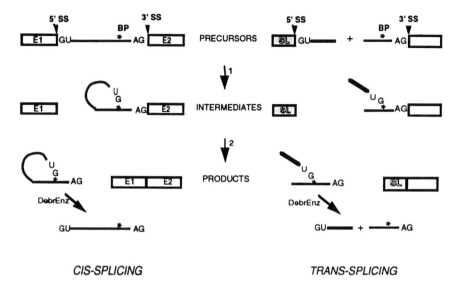

Fig. 1.   Pre–mRNA splicing pathways. Exons are shown as boxes and the introns as a solid line.

fined by a tail of adenylate residues, the poly(A) tail. Although there is no experimental evidence, the formation of the trypanosome mRNA 3´ end is thought to occur as in higher eukaryotes and yeast, namely, through an RNA processing reaction that involves cleavage at the polyadenylation site with the concomitant addition of the poly(A) tail to the newly formed mRNA 3´ end. However, no consensus sequence similar to the AAUAAA polyadenylation signal has been identified in trypanosome mRNAs.

The main lesson is that in trypanosomes the 5´ end of the mRNA is formed by an RNA processing reaction rather than by transcription initiation as is the case in most eukaryotes. In this context the function of *trans*-splicing can be viewed as an alternate and unusual pathway of mRNA 5´ end formation. How such a mechanism evolved is a matter of speculation. Because trypanosomes are ancient eukaryotes that separated very early from the main branch of the eukaryotic lineage, it is possible that *trans*-splicing is a molecular fossil that operated in eukaryotic cells at the time when promoter sequences were still evolving.

METHYLATION OF THE UNIQUE CAP 4 STRUCTURE OF THE SL RNA IS REQUIRED FOR *TRANS*-SPLICING

It has long been argued that studies on the biosynthesis of mRNA in trypanosomes could potentially provide means of chemotherapeutic intervention, because the 5´ end of each mRNA is generated by the unusual process of *trans*-splicing. Most interestingly, work in several laboratories has shown that the very 5′ end of the SL sequence bears a highly unusual mRNA cap structure (Perry et al., 1987; Freistadt et al., 1988; Bangs et al., 1992). Whereas eukaryotic cap structures contain no more than two modified nucleotides, the *T. brucei* cap structure has four modified nucleotides (referred to as cap 4 structure). Furthermore, detailed structural analysis of this cap structure revealed the presence of two nucleosides, $N^6,N^6,2′$-O-trimethyladenosine and 3,2′-O-dimethyluridine, which were previously unknown in nature (Bangs et al., 1992). Since the same cap structure is found on mRNA from *Leptomonas collosoma* and since the first six nucleotides of the SL sequence are highly conserved among trypanosomatids, these data suggest that this unusual cap structure is present in all trypanosomatids.

We have been able to address the function of this unique cap structure in *T. brucei*. In permeable cells we have clearly established that inhibition of "de novo" methylation with *S*-adenosylhomocysteine, a competitive inhibitor of *S*-adenosyl-methionine–mediated methylation reactions, abolishes the utilization of the SL RNA in *trans*-splicing (Ullu and Tschudi, 1991). This essential role of the 5′ end of the SL RNA was confirmed by two other approaches: removing the first 10 nucleotides of the SL RNA by cleavage with a complementary oligonucleotide and ribonuclease H, and masking the first 17 nucleotides with complementary 2′-*O*-methyl RNA oligonucleotides blocked *trans*-splicing of the SL RNA. In view of the cap structure of the SL RNA which is so drastically different from its mammalian counterparts, and in light of the demonstration that methylation of this structure is absolutely required for mRNA formation in *T. brucei*, this seems an attractive field of research to explore as a potential target for chemotherapeutic intervention. In addition, since the cap structure appears to be conserved among trypanosomatids, the mechanism of cap methylation might be similar in different organisms, such as *T. brucei, T. cruzi,* and *Leishmania*, to allow the identification of a common chemotherapy target.

Why is it that utilization of the SL RNA in *trans*-splicing requires methylation of the cap 4 structure? There are several possible explanations. First, the modified nucleosides could be required for assembly of the SL RNA into a ribonucleoprotein particle (RNP). We have examined this possibility by analyzing the electrophoretic mobility of the SL RNP assembled in cells in which methylation has been inhibited. The results showed that the core SL RNPs isolated by DEAE chromatography have indistinguishable electrophoretic mobilities. Thus, if a protein interacts with the cap 4 structure, this association is probably salt labile or perhaps only transient. The second possibility is that the cap 4 structure is part of an extended nuclear location signal required for nuclear import of the SL RNP. This hypothesis is based on the idea that, similar to the maturation of U-snRNPs in higher eukaryotes, the SL RNA, after synthesis in the nucleus, would exit into the cytoplasm to acquire the cap 4 structure and the proper complement of proteins. After assembly, the SL RNP would move back to the nucleus and enter the *trans*-splicing pathway. However, an analysis of the time course of SL RNA synthesis does not favor this possibility, because the SL RNA is modified within less than 30 seconds from its synthesis and is *trans*-spliced within 2 minutes. Finally, we should consider that the modified nucleosides are recognized by a protein component of the *trans*-splicing machinery or that the addition of methyl groups forces the 5' end of the SL RNA into a particular structural conformation. Clearly, identifying the methyltransferases involved in maturation of the cap 4 and determining the function of the cap 4 structure are important areas of investigation that deserve more attention.

SEQUENCES IN THE PRE-ᴍRNA REQUIRED FOR *TRANS*-SPLICING AND 3´ END FORMATION?

Sequences in the trypanosome pre-mRNA, where the SL sequence is joined, resemble the consensus sequence established for the 3´ splice acceptor site of mammalian introns: Upstream of the invariant AG dinucleotide there is a polypyrimidine tract of variable length. However, no branch site consensus sequence has been identified thus far. The sequence requirements at trypanosome 3´ splice sites have been studied at the PARP and α-tubulin genes. The efficiency of *trans*-splicing of the PARP pre-mRNA has been shown to be extremely sensitive to minor sequence changes in the polypyrimidine tract at the 3´ splice site. On the other hand, when we analyzed the region at the 3´ splice site of the α-tubulin gene, we found that the extent of the polypyrimidine tract can be substantially manipulated without causing severe effects. From these experiments we are led to conclude that the definition of a 3´ splice site is quite relaxed. The AG dinucleotide at the 3´ splice site appears to be essential, but the sequence context around it seems to be variable. This is different from *cis*-splicing in mammalian systems, where the polypyrimidine tract is an essential component of the 3´ splice site. Why would *trans*-splicing signals in the pre-mRNA be so loose? Perhaps *trans*-splicing does not need to be very precise because the consequences of *trans*-splicing are very different from *cis*-splicing of intervening sequences. In particular, *trans*-splicing of the SL sequence does not modify the open reading frame of the messenger RNA, and therefore the site of addition of the SL sequence need not be exquisitely precise.

Processing of polycistronic pre-mRNAs by polyadenylation of the upstream mRNA and *trans*-splicing of the downstream mRNA occurs within a relatively short distance. To ensure successful production of mature mRNAs there

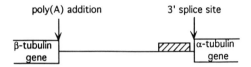

Fig. 2. RNA processing sites. The hatched box denotes the polypyrimidine stretch involved in 3´ end formation and *trans*-splicing.

must exist some level of coordination between these two RNA processing reactions. Evidence for this model is provided by the observation that inhibition of *trans*-splicing in *T. brucei* cells blocks the formation of the 3´ end of mature mRNA molecules. This finding also suggests that in trypanosomes there is a hierarchical order in the pathway of pre-mRNA processing reactions. In this model, *trans*-splicing, or perhaps assembly of a *trans*-splicing complex on the pre-mRNA, is a prerequisite for subsequent recognition of the mRNA 3´ end formation and polyadenylation signals. An alternative and intriguing possibility is that in the pre-mRNA the signals required for *trans*-splicing partially or perhaps completely overlap with those determining the choice of the polyadenylation sites.

To gain further insight into the potential mechanistic relationship between *trans*-splicing and 3´ end formation, we have mutagenized by block substitutions the region between the *T. brucei* β- and α-tubulin genes (Fig. 2). All mutations were introduced in the context of a synthetic dicistronic construct consisting of two reporter genes, namely, the bacterial chloramphenicol acetyltransferase gene placed upstream and the firefly luciferase gene placed downstream. The results of this analysis demonstrated that the integrity of two blocks of pyrimidine residues upstream of the α-tubulin 3´ splice site is required to specify accurate 3´ end formation of the upstream β-tubulin mRNA. Since the same sequences are also essential for *trans*-splicing, our results are consistent with the interpretation that the polypyrimidine tracts upstream of the α-tubulin 3´ splice site have a dual role in RNA processing. They are required for the identification of the β-tubulin poly(A) site upstream and of the α-tubulin 3´ splice site downstream (Fig. 2). In this scenario, the polypyrimidine-rich sequences could be recognized by different component(s) of the *trans*-splicing and 3´ end formation machineries. Alternatively, the primary role of the pyrimidine-rich sequences could be to bind a factor common to 3´ end formation and *trans*-splicing. This shared factor could be a protein or a protein complex, or even an snRNP since a role for the U1 snRNP in the coupling of *cis*-splicing and polyadenylation at terminal exons is suggested by recent in vitro cross-linking experiments.

CONCLUDING REMARKS

Although we still have much to learn, considerable progress has been made in laying a foundation for understanding the mechanisms of transcription and RNA processing in *T. brucei*. In this highly selective progress report, I have presented some of the unique and fascinating aspects that have been discovered by studying these processes in trypanosomes. Because trypanosomes are ancient eukaryotic organisms, that separated very early from the main branch of the eukaryotic lineage, their peculiar mechanisms of gene expression might reflect ancient eukaryotic functions that have been preserved to the present. By studying the process of gene expression in trypanosomes not only do we hope to identify parasite specific functions that might be exploited against the parasites themselves, but we will also learn about the evolution and functioning of the modern eukaryotic cell.

REFERENCES

Bangs JD, Crain PF, Hashizume T, McCloskey JA, Boothroyd JC(1992): Mass spectrometry of mRNA cap 4 from trypanosomatids reveals two novel nucleosides. J Biol Chem 267:9805–9815.

Brown SD, Huang J,Van der Ploeg LHT (1992): The promoter for the procyclic acidic repetitive protein (PARP) genes of *Trypanosoma brucei* share features with RNA polymerase I promoters. Mol Cell Biol 12:2644–2652.

Cech TR (1986): The generality of self-splicing RNA: Relationship to nuclear mRNA splicing. Cell 44:207–210.

Clayton CE, Fueri JP, Itzhaki JE, Bellofatto V, Sherman DR, Wisdom GS, Vijayasarathy S, Mowatt MR (1990): Transcription of the procyclic acidic repetitive protein genes of *Trypanosoma brucei*. Mol Cell Biol 10:3036–3047.

Evers R, Hammer A, Kock J, Jess W, Borst P, Memet S, Cornelissen AWCA (1989): *Trypanosoma brucei* contains two RNA polymerase II largest subunit genes with an altered C-terminal domain. Cell 56:585–597.

Fantoni A, Dare AO, Tschudi C (1994): RNA polymerase III-mediated transcription of the trypanosome U2 small nuclear RNA gene is controlled by both intragenic and extragenic regulatory elements. Mol Cell Biol 14:2021–2028.

Freistadt MS, Cross GAM, Robertson HD (1988): Discontinuously synthesized mRNA from *Trypanosoma brucei* contains the highly methylated 5′ cap structure, m7 GpppA*A*C(2′-O)mU*A. J Biol Chem 263:15071–15075.

Geiduschek EP, Tocchini-Valentini GP (1988): Transcription by RNA polymerase III. Annu Rev Biochem 57:873–914.

Green MR (1991): Biochemical mechanisms of constitutive and regulated pre-mRNA splicing. Annu Rev Cell Biol 7:559–599.

Hernandez N (1993): TBP, a universal eukaryotic transcription factor? Genes Dev. 7:1291–1308.

Johnson PJ, Kooter JM, Borst P (1987): Inactivation of transcription by UV irradiation of *Trypanosoma brucei* provides evidence for a multicistronic transcription unit including a VSG gene. Cell 51:273–281.

Koleske AJ, Buratowski S, Nonet M, Young RA (1992): A novel transcription factor reveals a functional link between the RNA polymerase II CTD and TFIID. Cell 69:883–894.

Kooter JM, Borst P (1984): Alpha-amanitin-insensitive transcription of variant surface glyco-protein genes provides further evidence for discontinuous transcription in trypanosomes. Nucleic Acids Res 12:9457–9472.

Laird PW, Zomerdijk JCBM, de Korte D, Borst P (1987): In vivo labelling of intermediates in the discontinuous synthesis of mRNAs in *Trypanosoma brucei*. EMBO J 6:1055–1062.

Muhich ML, Boothroyd JC (1989): Polycistronic transcripts in trypanosomes and their accu-mulation during heat shock: Evidence for a precursor role in mRNA synthesis. Mol Cell Biol 8:3837–3846.

Murphy WJ, Watkins KP, Agabian N (1986): Identification of a novel Y branch structure as an intermediate in trypanosome mRNA processing: Evidence for *trans*-splicing. Cell 47:517–525.

Perry K, Watkins KP, Agabian N (1987): Trypanosome mRNAs have unusual "cap 4" structure acquired by addition of a spliced leader. Proc Natl Acad Sci USA 84:8190–8194.

Rudenko G, Bishop D, Gottesdiener K, Van der Ploeg LHT (1989): Alpha-amanitin resistant transcription of protein coding genes in insect and bloodstream form *Trypanosoma brucei*. EMBO J 8:4259–4263.

Sherman D, Janz L, Hug M, Clayton C (1991): Anatomy of the *parp* gene promoter of *Trypanosoma brucei*. EMBO J 10:3379–3386.

Sutton RE, Boothroyd JC (1986): Evidence for trans splicing in trypanosomes. Cell 47:527–535.

Tschudi C, Ullu, E (1988): Polygene transcripts are precursors to calmodulin mRNAs in try-panosomes. EMBO J 7:455–463.

Tschudi C, Ullu E (1990): Destruction of U2, U4, or U6 small nuclear RNAs blocks *trans* splicing in trypanosome cells. Cell 61:459–466.

Ullu E, Tschudi C (1991): *Trans* splicing in trypanosomes requires methylation of the 5′ end of the spliced leader RNA. Proc Natl Acad Sci USA 88:10074–10078.

Usheva A, Maldonado E, Goldring A, Lu H, Houbavi C, Reinberg D, Aloni Y (1992): Specific interaction between the nonphosphorylated form of RNA polymerase II and the TATA-binding protein. Cell 69:871–881.

Molecular Approaches to Parasitology, pages 269–280
© 1995 Wiley-Liss, Inc.

Gene Replacements and Genetics in *Trypanosoma cruzi*

John Swindle, R. Dean Gillespie, Sobha Hariharan, Sul-Hee Chung, and Janet Ajioka

Department of Microbiology and Immunology, University of Tennessee, Memphis, Tennessee 38163

INTRODUCTION

Historically, scientific interest in the trypanosomatidae has been driven by the global impact on human populations of diseases caused by these organisms. The trypanosomatidae constitute a diverse family of parasitic protozoa, including three important species of insect-borne mammalian pathogens: *Trypanosoma cruzi*, which causes Chagas' disease in humans, is found throughout South and Central America. African sleeping sickness, caused by the *Trypanosoma brucei* complex, is endemic throughout much of sub-Saharan Africa. *Leishmania* species also cause devastating disease in human populations throughout much of China, Southeast Asia, India, Africa, and South and Central America. As a group, this family of parasites inflicts suffering on over 200 million people directly and millions more indirectly through economic hardships due to decreased productivity.

Over the last 15 years members of the family trypanosomatidae have evolved into productive alternative model systems for the study of eukaryotic gene expression. This evolution, to a large extent, has been driven by four observations. Molecular biologists were first attracted to African trypanosomes because of the gene rearrangements responsible for antigenic variation (Cross, 1978; Vickerman, 1978). Interest was further heightened by the discovery of *trans*-splicing, through which each messenger RNA is capped by a 5´ terminal miniexon, or spliced leader (Boothroyd and Cross, 1982; van der Ploeg et al., 1982). Although initially thought to be unique to the trypanosomatids, *trans*-splicing has since been described in a number of higher eukaroytes, further broadening the interest in the molecular biology of the trypanosomatidae (Agabian, 1990). The discovery of *trans*-splicing was followed closely by experiments indicating that transcription of most nuclear genes in trypanosomatids may be polycistronic, once again suggesting that gene expression in the trypanosomatidae is unusual among eukaryotes. This subject is discussed in detail by Tschudi in this volume. Last, and undoubtedly the most bizarre, was the discovery of extensive post-transcriptional editing of mitochondrial RNAs in *T. brucei* (see the chapter by Stuart in this volume; see also Benne et al., 1986; Feagin et al., 1987).

During the last 4 years the evolution of the trypanosomatids as viable model systems has accelerated more rapidly as efficient DNA-mediated transformation systems have been developed for many species, including *T. brucei*, *Leishmania*, and *T. cruzi* (see Gillespie et al., 1993, for a list of published transformation systems). With the advent of these technologies the ability to manipulate a parasite's genome at will has become a practical reality, thus opening doors to investigations that in the recent past would have been difficult and in some cases impossible to undertake. Examples of the use of gene replacements to study the expression of the ubiquitin-calmodulin gene complex of *T. cruzi* are discussed below.

GENE REPLACEMENTS AND THE ANALYSIS OF MULTICOPY GENE FAMILIES

In trypanosomes many highly expressed proteins, such as calmodulin (Tschudi et al., 1985; Chung and Swindle, 1990), tubulin (Thomashow et al., 1983), and ubiquitin (Swindle et al., 1988), are frequently encoded by multicopy, tandemly repeated gene families. Although transcriptions of such gene families have been extensively studied, it has been difficult to analyze the expression of individual genes. Therefore, much of our understanding of how the genes are transcribed, and their mRNAs processed, is based on analysis of mixed RNA populations potentially including the transcripts of each member of the gene family. One approach to overcoming this drawback is to replace a specific member of a gene family with a unique reporter gene whose expression can be used as an indirect measure of the expression of the replaced gene. In this manner, a multicopy gene family can be operationally reduced to a single copy gene whose transcription and mRNA processing can be accurately analyzed.

The ubiquitin genes of T. *cruzi* provide good examples of multicopy gene families. We have previously shown that the *T. cruzi* genome contains at least two types of ubiquitin genes, polyubiquitin (*PUB*) and ubiquitin-fusion (*FUS*) genes (Swindle et al., 1988). There are in fact five *PUB* and five *FUS* genes distributed between two chromosomal loci (Fig. 1). The *2.65* locus contains a single *FUS* gene (*FUS1*) followed by the *PUB12.5* polyubiquitin gene. The *2.8* locus contains *FUS2* followed in order by *PUB2.65*, *PUB2.0*, *PUB5.2*, and *PUB1.7*, and then by *FUS3*, *FUS4*, and *FUS5*. The *PUB* genes appear to be constitutively expressed at a low level in all stages of the parasite's life

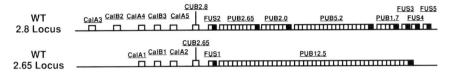

Fig. 1.   Genomic map of the *2.65* and *2.8* ubiquitin–calmodulin loci: ubiquitin-fusion (*FUS*) and polyubiquitin (*PUB*) genes. The open boxes represent the 228 bp ubiquitin coding sequence, and the closed boxes represent the coding sequence for the 52 amino acid nonubiquitin domain. Calmodulin–ubiquitin-associated genes are denoted *CUB2.65* and *CUB2.8*. The positions of the calmodulin genes (*CalA* and *CalB*) are also indicated.

cycle as well as during periods of stress such as heat shock or starvation (Swindle et al., 1988; J. Swindle, unpublished observations]. Furthermore, since each *PUB* gene generates a different length mRNA, it is clear that all five genes are expressed at similar levels in each developmental stage (Swindle et al., 1988). The *FUS* genes present a different picture. Although the *FUS* gene transcripts represent a major mRNA species in rapidly dividing epimastigotes, the transcripts are not detectable in either starved epimastigotes (Swindle et al., 1988) or metacyclic trypomastigotes (J. Swindle, unpublished observations). Based on these observations, it is clear that the *PUB* and *FUS* genes are differentially expressed, although the underlying mechanisms responsible in the regulation are unknown.

Analysis of ubiquitin gene expression is complicated by several factors that may also be encountered during the analysis of other multicopy gene families. For instance, the *FUS* genes and their flanking 5' and 3' intergenic regions are nearly identical. Consequently, neither Northern blot analysis nor nuclease S1 protection analysis can be used to identify actively expressed *FUS* genes. Without knowing how many *FUS* genes are expressed, the differences in *FUS* and *PUB* gene expression are difficult to quantitate accurately. The different levels of *PUB* and *FUS* gene expression may also suggest that the genes represent separate transcription units. However, nuclear run-on analysis, which measures transcription by pre-engaged RNA polymerases in isolated nuclei and has evolved into the "gold standard" for defining transcription units in trypanosomes, cannot be used in this case. This is because a complete copy of the *FUS* gene sequence is contained within each *PUB* gene, making it virtually impossible to distinguish between transcription of the two types of ubiquitin genes in nuclear run-on experiments.

Although the factors described above hinder biochemical analyses of *PUB* and *FUS* gene expression, they can, to a large extent, be circumvented by using site-specific gene replacements. Gene replacements can be used to identify an actively expressed gene within a multicopy gene family and to quantitate the level of expression of the replaced gene. When using gene replacements to study expression of a targeted gene indirectly it is important that there is no overt selection for expression of the reporter gene. If selective pressure such as that for antibiotic resistance were exerted, the pattern of expression of the targeted gene could be altered, thus invalidating the analysis. This pitfall can be avoided by replacing the gene of interest with a nonselected reporter gene. Expression of the reporter gene can then be analyzed in stable transformants isolated based on expression of a gene conferring antibiotic resistance from a different locus (Gillespie et al., 1993). Two variations of this strategy have been used successfully to demonstrate that, within the *FUS* gene family, *FUS1* and at least one other *FUS* gene are expressed in epimastigotes (Gillespie et al., 1993; Chung et al., 1993). In one case, stable G418-resistant transformants were isolated by simultaneously replacing the tandemly arrayed *CUB2.65* and FUS1 genes with the neomycin phosphotransferase (*neo^r*) and chloramphenicol acetyl transferase (*CAT*) gene, respectively (Gillespie et al., 1993). Since *CUB2.65* was known to be expressed (Ajioka and Swindle, 1993), a cryptic transcription unit was unlikely to have been activated. Consequently, the fact that all tandem transformants also expressed CAT activity indicated that *FUS1* was expressed in nontransformed parasites. Furthermore, since the tandem transformants continued to express *FUS* mRNAs, at least one other member of the *FUS* gene family must be expressed.

As described above, the *FUS* mRNAs constituted a major RNA species while each polyubiquitin gene was expressed at a much reduced level. At face value this observation suggested that *FUS* genes were more highly expressed than were *PUB* genes. However, since the five *FUS* genes may generate identical mRNAs while unique transcripts are produced for each *PUB* gene, the observed abundance of *FUS* over *PUB* transcripts may simply reflect the different numbers of genes contributing the the various ubiquitin mRNA populations. Therefore, whether or not specific *FUS* and *PUB* genes were expressed at significantly different levels remains an open question. Once again, gene replacements provide the ideal experimental tool with which to resolve this issue. CnFc7, one of the transformed *T. cruzi* lines in which *FUS1* was replaced by the *CAT* gene, was used to measure *FUS1* expression indirectly (Fig. 2). Polyubiquitin gene expression was quantitated using a second tandem transformant, Cl-CAT12.5, in which *FUS1* was replaced with the *neo^r* gene and the first ubiquitin coding sequence in *PUB12.5* was replaced with the *CAT* gene (Fig. 2). As shown in figure 2, CnFc7 produced over 16 times the CAT activity of Cl-CAT12.5 in mid-log epimastigotes, suggesting that in nontransformed parasites FUS1 is expressed at a significantly higher level than PUB12.5. Although the mechanism responsible for the different levels of expression has not been identified, these results establish that the tandemly arrayed FUS1 and *PUB12.5* genes are expressed at dramatically different lev-

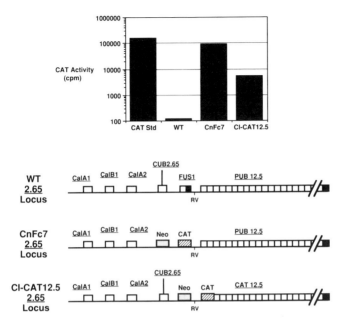

Fig. 2.   Analysis of *PUB12.5* and *FUS1* expression. The bar graph represents the results of CAT assays performed on stable transformants in which either *FUS1* (CnFc7) or the first ubiquitin coding sequence of *PUB12.5* (Cl-CAT12.5) had been replaced by the *CAT* gene. Electroporation and isolation of stable transformants were carried out precisely as described by Gillespie et al. (1993). All CAT assays were carried out within the linear range of the assay, also as described by Gillespie et al. (1993). CAT Std, chloramphenicol acetyltransferase standard assay (0.1 units of purified enzyme, 5′, 3′ INC.); WT, wild-type extract. Genomic maps of the *2.65* calmodulin–ubiquitin loci of wild-type (WT), CnFc7, and Cl-CAT12.5 *T. cruzi* are shown below the bar graph. CAT and Neo represent the *CAT* and *Neo* genes, respectively.

els. Furthermore, CnFc7 and Cl-CAT12.5 are now being subjected to nuclear run-on analysis to measure transcription of *FUS1* and *PUB12.5* indirectly. If the *CAT* genes are transcribed at the same rate in the two transformed *T. cruzi* lines the different levels of expression must be due to post-transcription events such as RNA processing or mRNA stability. If the genes are, however, shown to be transcribed at different rates, FUS1 and *PUB12.5* are likely to be expressed from separate transcription units.

GENETIC ANALYSIS OF *TRANS*-SPLICING

Trans-splicing has been one of the most intensively studied aspects of trypanosome gene expression. *Trans*-splicing results in the transfer of a 39 nucleotide miniexon (or spliced leader) sequence from the 5′ terminus of the miniexon primary transcript to the 5´ end of each *T. cruzi* mRNA (Boothroyd and Cross, 1982; van der Ploeg et al., 1982). Mechanistically, *trans*-splicing has much in common with *cis*-splicing as carried out in higher eukaryotes. Although initially thought to be unique to trypanosomes, *trans*-splicing has since been observed in other eukaryotes (Agabian, 1990). Both *trans*- and *cis*-splicing proceed through branched intermediates and utilize 5– GpU dinucleotide splice donor and ApG dinucleotide 3´ splice acceptor sites. To maintain the correct reading frame during *cis*-splicing the selection of 5´ donor and 3´ splice acceptor sites must be tightly regulated. In contrast, during *trans*-splicing the 3´ splice acceptor site invariably resides within the 5´ untranslated region of the target mRNA. Therefore, since *trans*-splicing plays no role in establishing the reading frame of the encoded protein, it has been believed that 3´ splice acceptor site selection could be more imprecise. Generally, nuclease S1 protection and cDNA nucleotide sequence analyses have been the methods used to identify the site of miniexon addition. Much of the data have, however, been obtained from the analysis of the expression of multicopy gene families. Consequently, distinguishing between the transcript of one gene using multiple miniexon addition sites and different members of the gene family each using unique but different sites is difficult unless the nucleotide sequence of the intergenic region preceding each gene within the gene family has been determined. Sequencing all intergenic regions within a gene family can be a formidable task especially in cases such as the tubulin genes of T. *brucei* (15 a- and b-tubulin gene repeats) (Thomashow et al., 1983) and the calmodulin genes of *T. cruzi* (5 *CalA* and 3 *CalB* genes) (Chung and Swindle, 1990).

When studying processing of the calmodulin transcripts of *T. cruzi* by cDNA sequence and nuclease S1 protection analyses, a major miniexon addition site was identified 94 bp upstream of the protein coding sequence (Fig. 3, position –94), (Chung et al., 1993). In addition, a second, minor miniexon addition site was identified 24 bp upstream of the protein coding sequence (position –24). This result raised the possibility that multiple miniexon addition sites were used during processing of the *CalA2* transcript. However, it was also possible that the minor site represented the miniexon addition site of one of the other seven calmodulin genes. To test this possibility, a *T. cruzi* line, Cl-A2, was generated in which *CalA2* was replaced with the *neo*[r] gene and the miniexon addition site for the *neo*[r] transcript was identified. This analysis indicated that only the miniexon addition site at position –94 was used during processing of the *neo*[r] mRNA (Fig. 3). Miniexon addition at position –24 was never observed either by nuclease S1 or cDNA sequence analyses. This result suggested that, in all likelihood, the miniexon addition site at position –24 was used during *trans*-splicing of one of the other calmodulin transcripts. This result further suggested that *trans*-splicing of the *CalA2* transcript was very precise, using only one of seven potential ApG 3' splice acceptor sites (the

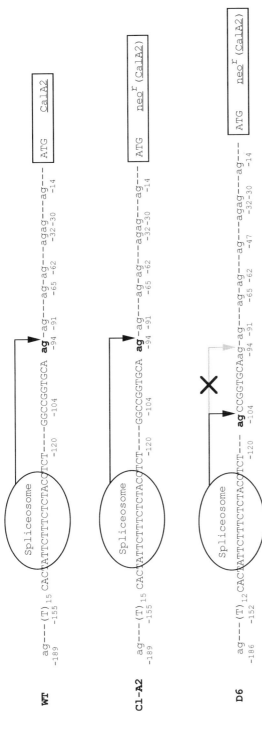

Fig. 3. Scanning model for 3′ splice acceptor site selection. WT, wild-type trypanosomes. *T. cruzi* lines Cl-A2 and D6 are as described in the text. The arrow indicates the position of miniexon addition. The 3′ splice acceptor sites used in each trypanosome line are indicated by the **ag** dinucleotide written in bold. All other potential 3′ splice acceptor sites are indicated as ag (not bold) dinucleotides. The positions of the possible 3′ acceptor sites are numbered relative to the ATG translation initiation codon (the A nucleotide of the ATG translation initiation codon is nucleotide +1). The large **X** indicates that the native splice acceptor site at position −94 is not used in this line. The spliceosome is drawn as a circle and has been arbitrarily positioned upstream of the 3′ splice acceptor site.

other potential sites are at positions −14, −30, −32, −62, −65, and −91). The contention that 3´ splice acceptor site selection is a precise event was further supported by the identification of a mutation that quantitatively shifted miniexon addition to position −104 of the *CalA2* intergenic region in the *T. cruzi* line *D6* (Fig. 3) (Chung et al., 1993). Although the native 3´ splice acceptor site at position −94 was unaltered, it was not used at a detectable level. Although all *cis*-acting elements involved in 3´ splice acceptor site selection have not been identified, the data are most consistent with a scanning model in which the spliceosome recognizes a sequence (possibly a polypyrimidine tract or branch point) and scans downstream, splicing at the nearest ApG dinucleotide (Fig. 3). It would have been difficult to reach these conclusions without the use of gene replacements, which permitted the analysis to focus on RNA processing within a specific intergenic region.

CUB GENE EXPRESSION IS REQUIRED FOR *T. CRUZI* VIABILITY

Although both the calmodulin and ubiquitin proteins have been extensively studied in trypanosomes and other eukaryotes, nothing is known about the role of the potential *CUB* gene product. We have previously shown that the genome of *T. cruzi* contains two *CUB* genes, *CUB2.65* and *CUB2.8,* which are both expressed as *trans*-spliced, polyadenylated mRNAs and encode potential proteins of 208 amino acids (Ajioka and Swindle, 1993). Although a *T. brucei* homolog of the *CUB* protein has been shown to bind calcium when expressed in *E. coli* (Wong et al., 1992), the protein has not been identified in either parasite. One puzzling feature of the *CUB* genes is their nucleotide sequence composition, which has more similarity to *T. cruzi* intergenic regions than to protein coding sequences. Although the average G plus C content of *T. cruzi* protein coding sequences is greater than 60%, the *CUB* coding sequences are less than 38% G plus C. The aberrant G plus C composition raises obvious questions, such as are the *CUB* genes functional protein coding genes or, alternatively, do they represent inactive pseudogenes? The facts that the 624 bp open reading frame of both *CUB* genes is conserved and that a *CUB* gene analog is found in all kinetoplastids analyzed, suggest that there is positive selection for maintenance of the possible protein coding sequence (Ajioka and Swindle, 1993; Wong et al., 1992; J. Swindle, unpublished observations).

As a first step towards studying the *CUB* gene and identifying possible functions of the encoded protein, a series of *T. cruzi* lines carrying various *CUB* gene deletions was generated (Fig. 4). In wild-type *T. cruzi*, *CUB2.65* and *CUB2.8* are fully contained within two BglII restriction fragments of 2.65 and 2.8 kb, respectively. In *T. cruzi* line Cl-neo2.65, *CUB2.65* has been replaced by the *neo^r* gene, and, in line Cl-hyg2.8, *CUB2.8* has been replaced by

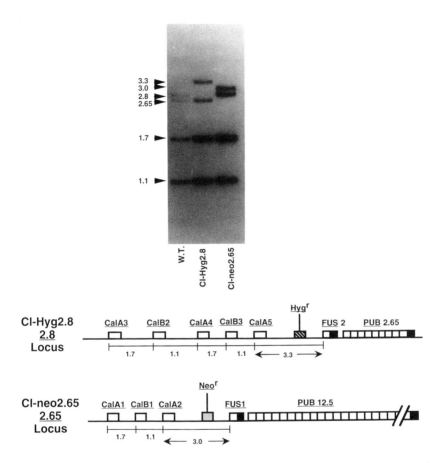

Fig. 4. *CUB* gene replacements. For each lane in the Southern blot 2.0 μg of *T. cruzi* genomic DNA was digested with *Bgl*II. After transfer the blot was probed with the calmodulin coding sequence. Lane designations: WT, wild-type *T. cruzi*; Cl-Hyg2.8, *CUB2.8* gene replaced with *hyg^r* (notice that the 2.8 kb *Bgl*II restriction fragment has been enlarged to 3.3 kb); Cl-Neo2.65, *CUB2.65* replaced with *neo^r* (notice that the 2.65 kb *Bgl*II restriction fragment has been enlarged to 3.0 kb). The genomic maps of the Cl-Hyg2.8 *2.8* locus and the Cl-Neo2.65 *2.65* locus are shown below the Southern blot. The lengths of the hybridizing restriction fragments are shown on the left. The position and size of the *Bgl*II restriction fragments that will hybridize to the calmodulin coding sequence probe are shown below each genomic map.

the *hyg^r* gene. It has not, however, been possible to delete the remaining *CUB* gene from Cl-neo2.65. These data suggest that, although *T. cruzi* tolerates deletion of either *CUB2.65* or *CUB2.8*, deletion of both genes is a lethal event, indicating that at least one active *CUB* gene is required for parasite viability. Therefore, although a gene product has yet to be identified, *CUB* gene expression has been shown to play an important role in the parasite based on genetic analysis.

DISCUSSION

The pitfalls inherent in investigating the expression of multicopy gene families are encountered when analyzing expression of the ubiquitin–calmodulin gene complex of *T. cruzi*. Three examples in which site-specific gene replacements were used to facilitate analysis of the complex genetic locus were described. Gene replacements were used to establish that *FUS1* was expressed and to demonstrate that its expression exceeded that of *PUB12.5* by approximately 16-fold. Although the mechanisms responsible for the differential regulation are unknown, likely possibilities include either differential transcription or mRNA stability or a combination of both. Gene replacements will undoubtedly continue to play a significant role in discerning the mode of regulation.

In the second example, gene replacements were used to study *trans*-splicing of the calmodulin transcripts indirectly. By focusing on the processing of the *neo*^{r} mRNA, it was found that although multiple potential miniexon addition sites existed within the 5′ untranslated region of the *neo*^{r} mRNA, only the site at position –94 bp was used. These data suggested that 3′ splice acceptor site selection was tightly controlled and led to the proposal that a scanning model was used in the selection process. This conclusion conflicts with past assumptions that 3′ splice acceptor site selection is promiscuous, with any ApG dinucleotide within the 5′ untranslated region of a transcript serving as a potential splice acceptor site. In contrast to past in vitro analyses, tandem gene replacements are currently being used to introduce specific mutations designed to alter the expression of a reporter gene, thus permitting critical testing of the scanning model for 3′ splice acceptor selection in vivo (Gillespie et al., 1993).

The final example described a series of preliminary genetic experiments that indicated that, although it was possible to delete either *CUB* gene individually, it was not possible to delete both genes. These results suggested that at least one expressed *CUB* gene was essential for parasite viability. By first carrying out a genetic analysis it was possible to pinpoint quickly the *CUB* genes as playing a central role in the parasite's survival and therefore meriting further study.

THE PAST REVISITED

Historically, the study of genetics has proven to be one of the most powerful tools available to investigators studying the regulation of gene expression in a wide variety of organisms from *E. coli* and their viruses to humans. With few exceptions, however, the parasitic protozoa have not been amenable to classic genetic analysis. Although this imposed a serious impediment to the removal of the mysteries surrounding gene expression in parasites, significant progress was made. *Trans*-splicing, polycistronic transcription, and RNA editing were all discovered. However, when investigations turned to the mechanisms underlying these processes the analyses were severely hindered by the inability to carry out a careful genetic analysis. With the advent of efficient DNA-mediated transformation systems, however, genetic analysis is being rapidly brought to the forefront and certain conclusions drawn from past *in vitro* analyses may have to be re-evaluated and some possibly thrown out.

CONCLUSION

The mechanisms of transcription and *trans*-splicing are ideal candidates for genetic analysis. Although the idea that most transcription in trypanosomes is polycistronic has become nearly dogmatic, much of the evidence was derived from *in vitro* analyses that are open to alternative interpretations. This is clearly an example of a conclusion that should be revisited using genetic criteria either to support or to refute the model. The mechanism of *trans*-splicing provides another example in which genetic criteria could be used to support or deny proposed models. Using genetics, it should be possible to identify all the *cis*-acting elements in the primary transcript involved in *trans*-splicing and to define potential interactions between them. Also as described above, genetics is an invaluable tool when studying newly characterized genes and defining possible functions of the encoded proteins.

Although models for various cellular processes in trypanosomes could be generated, until very recently it was nearly impossible to test them in a meaningful way in vivo. To a large extent this is no longer true. Within the framework of transformation based genetic analysis, most models can be tested in vivo, and investigators are limited only by their imagination and determination.

ACKNOWLEDGMENTS

This work was supported by grants from the USPHS (AI26587) and World Health Organization (TDR:920169) awarded to J.S. and by Biomedical Research Support Grant RR05423 awarded to the University of Tennessee, Memphis.

REFERENCES

Agabian N (1990): *Trans*-splicing of nuclear pre-mRNAs. Cell 61:1157–1160.
Ajioka J, Swindle J (1993): The calmodulin-ubiquitin associated genes of *Trypanosoma cruzi:* Their identification and transcription. Mol Biochem Parasitol 57:127–136.

Benne R, Van der Burg J, Brakenhoff JPJ, Sloof P, Van Boom JM, Tromp MC (1986): Major transcripts of the frameshifted *coxII* gene from trypanosome mitochondria contains four nucleotides that are not encoded in the DNA. Cell 46:819–826.

Boothroyd JC, Cross GAM (1982): Transcripts coding for surface glycoproteins in *Trypanosoma brucei* have a short identical exon at their 5′ end. Gene 20:281–289.

Chung S-H, Gillespie RD, Swindle J (1993): Analyzing expression of the calmodulin and ubiquitin-fusion genes of *Trypanosoma cruzi* using simultaneous independent gene replacements. Mol Biochem Parasitol Manuscript in submission.

Chung SH, Swindle J (1990): Linkage of the calmodulin and ubiquitin loci in *Trypanosoma cruzi*. Nucleic Acids Res 18:4561–4569.

Cross GAM (1978): Antigenic vatiation in trypanosomes. Proc R Soc Lond Ser Biol 202:55–72.

Feagin JE, Jasmer DJ, Stuart K (1987): Developmentally regulated addition of nucleotides within apocytochrome *b* transcripts in *Trypanosoma brucei*. Cell 49:337–345.

Gillespie RD, Ajioka J, Swindle J (1993): Using simultaneous tandem gene replacements to study expression of the multicopy ubiquitin-fusion (*FUS*) gene family of *Trypanosoma cruzi*. Mol Biochem Parasitol 60:281–292.

Swindle J, Ajioka J, Eisen H, Sanwal B, Jacquemot C, Browder Z, Buck G (1988): The genomic organization and transcription of the ubiquitin genes of *Trypanosoma cruzi*. EMBO J 7:1121–1127.

Thomashow LS, Milhausen M, Rutter WJ, Agabian N (1983): Tubulin genes are tandemly linked and clustered in the genome of *Trypanosoma cruzi*. Cell 32:35–43.

Tschudi C, Young AS, Ruben L, Patton CL, Richards FF (1985): Calmodulin genes in trypanosomes are tandemly repeated and produce multiple RNAs with a common 5′ leader sequence. Proc Natl Acad Sci USA 82:3998–4002.

van der Ploeg LHT, Liu AYC, Michels PAM, Delange T, Majumder HK, Weber H, Veenemen GH, Van Boom J (1982): RNA splicing is required to make the messenger RNA for the variant surface antigen in trypanosomes. Nucleic Acids Res 10:3591–3604.

Vickerman K (1978): Antigenic variation in trypanosomes. Nature 273:613–617.

Wong S, Kretsinger RH, Campbell DA (1992): Identification of a new EF-hand superfamily member from *Trypanosoma brucei*. Mol Gen Genet 233:225–230.

Molecular Approaches to Parasitology, pages 281–298
© 1995 Wiley-Liss, Inc.

Trans-Splicing Specificity and Polycistronic Transcription Units in *Caenorhabditis elegans*

Tom Blumenthal and John Spieth

Department of Biology, Indiana University, Bloomington, Indiana 47405

INTRODUCTION

In all nematodes thus far examined some mRNAs receive a 22 nucleotide 5´ leader by a process known as *trans*-splicing. The function or functions of this leader, called the *spliced leader* (or SL), remain a mystery. Whereas the pre-mRNA products of some genes receive this leader, other pre-mRNAs do not, yet they function apparently normally. Furthermore, it has proven possible to convert *trans*-spliced genes into conventional genes and vice versa without obviously affecting mRNA function. Thus it appears that the SL is not required for any mRNA-specific functions, although it may well enhance one or more functions, such as translatability, stability, or subcellular localization. Our laboratory has been studying, not the function of *trans*-splicing, but the mechanism. Specifically, we became interested in the question of what marks a pre-mRNA for *trans*-splicing. That is, why do some pre-mRNAs receive the SL while others do not? With the discovery of a second SL (SL2) in the Hirsh laboratory, the question was extended to what signals the pre-mRNA products of some genes to receive SL1 and others to receive SL2. This latter question led us to the discovery of operons in *Caenorhabditis elegans*. This paper recounts the scientific events leading up to that discovery.

TRANS-SPLICING

The process of trans-splicing has recently been reviewed by Huang and Hirsh (1992) and by Nilsen (1993). The chapter by Davis in this book discusses *trans*-splicing in flatworms, while those by Tschudi and Swindle cover the subject in the trypanosomes. As discussed in detail by these authors, *trans*-splicing was discovered first in trypanosomes, where genes are transcribed as polycistronic precursors without introns. *Trans*-splicing of a 39 nt SL serves to separate the individual mRNAs from the polycistronic precursor and provide them with a capped 5′ end. In trypanosomes all splicing is *trans*-splicing and all mRNAs receive SL, so no splicing-specific decisions need be made. In contrast, nematodes are relatively advanced metazoan animals, so virtually all of their pre-mRNAs do contain introns. Since *trans*-splicing and *cis*-splicing (intron removal) are fundamentally similar processes, except for the location of the 5′ splice site, the problem in nematodes would appear to be how to keep the inappropriate event from occurring at each 3′ splice site. To understand how that is successfully accomplished, it is necessary to consider the basic rules that govern splice site choice in nematodes. While these rules are not yet fully understood in even the intensively studied yeast or mammalian cells, we have learned enough about splicing in *C. elegans* to formulate testable hypotheses about how *trans*- and *cis*-splicing are specified and kept separate and what signals *trans*-splicing on those pre-mRNAs that receive them. As is elaborated below, we even have some tentative answers.

Trans-splicing in nematodes was first discovered by Krause and Hirsh (1987) in *C. elegans*, and subsequently in numerous other nematode species, both free-living and animal and plant parasitic. It was originally estimated that about 15% of *C. elegans* genes encode products destined for *trans*-splicing (Bektesh et al., 1988). The percentage now appears to be substantially higher, perhaps 70% or more, based on the fraction of cloned genes that are *trans*-spliced (our unpublished observations). It has been estimated that as many as 90% of *Ascaris lumbricoides* genes encode *trans*-spliced products (Nilsen, 1993). While it has generally been found that either all or none of a given pre-mRNA is *trans*-spliced, the mechanism of *trans*-splicing does not require that to be so, as we shall see. Indeed, in a handful of cases a single gene has been shown to produce both *trans*-spliced and non-*trans*-spliced mRNAs.

Trans-splicing is very similar to *cis*-splicing. It is catalyzed by at least some of the same small nuclear ribonucleoprotein particles (snRNPs), U2, U4, U5, and U6; it proceeds through an equivalent branched intermediate, although it is a lariat in *cis*-splicing and a Y-branch in *trans*-splicing; and the 5′ and 3′ consensus splice sites are the same for *trans*- and *cis*-splicing. The SL is donated by a small RNA, about 100 nt long, SL RNA, which contains the SL at its 5′ end, followed by a canonical 5′ splice site. Thus SL RNA can be visualized as half of a substrate for a conventional splicing event, an exon (the SL) followed by the 5′ end of an intron. Bruzik et al. (1988) proposed that this RNA could be folded to resemble one of the spliceosomal snRNAs, with the 5′ splice site basepaired to sequences within SL. They also noted that the SL RNA contains an Sm-protein binding site, characteristic of U1-U5 snRNPs. They hypothesized that SL RNA is itself found in the form of an snRNP. This prediction turned out to be correct (Thomas et al., 1988; Van Doren and Hirsh,

1988): SL RNA is indeed bound to Sm proteins and also contains the unusual trimethylguanosine cap at its 5´ end, as do U1–U5. This cap is transferred to the mRNAs by *trans*-splicing, and the mRNAs are translated with this unusual cap structure (Liou and Blumenthal, 1990). Production of mRNAs with trimethylguanosine caps may be a major role of *trans*-splicing in worms, although the functional consequences for an mRNA of having such a cap are unknown.

Because the SL RNA contains the 5´ splice site, exists in the form of an snRNP, and contains sequence basepaired to the 5´ splice site, which is the function performed by U1 snRNP in cis-splicing, Bruzik et al. (1988) hypothesized that the SL snRNP replaces U1 snRNP in *trans*-splicing. Although some evidence in support of this idea has been adduced, it remains controversial. If U1 does not function in *trans*-splicing, it is not clear how formation of a spliceosome is initiated, since in both yeast and mammals interaction between U1 and the 5´ splice site on the pre-mRNA is the obligatory first step in splicing (reviewed by Green, 1991). In any case, it is worth noting that the SL snRNP is the only snRNP thus far identified that serves as a substrate in pre-mRNA splicing. It may represent an evolutionary link between the self-splicing group 2 introns, which are also spliced through a branched intermediate, and nuclear pre-mRNA processing.

WHAT IS THE SIGNAL ON THE PRE-ᴍRNA FOR *TRANS*-SPLICING?

Several ideas have been proposed (outlined in Fig. 1). Since most RNAs involved in splicing seem to get together by basepairing (U1–5´ splice site, U4–U6, U2-branch site, U2–U6, U5–5´ exon, U5–3´ exon, U1–3´ splice site), the most obvious idea is a direct basepairing interaction between SL RNA and the 5´ region of pre-mRNA destined for *trans*-splicing. However, as more such pre-mRNAs were identified and sequenced, it became clear that they did not share any obvious sequences in common, much less sequences that could basepair with SL RNA. This observation also argues against a second proposal (Sharp, 1987) that *trans*-spliced pre-mRNAs contain a binding site for a specialized U2 snRNP that in turn has an SL snRNP binding site. Although *C. elegans* does have genes for variant U2 RNAs (Thomas et al., 1990), the variation is relatively small and does not seem likely to specify interactions with both *trans*-spliced pre-mRNAs and the SL RNA.

To resolve these difficulties, we proposed a third model, a default model (Conrad et al., 1991). Since the SL RNA is composed of an exon followed by the 5´ half of an intron, we proposed that the sole signal for *trans*-splicing is the presence of the missing part of SL RNA's splicing substrate: the 3´ half of an intron followed by the 3´ exon. Specifically, we posited that the presence of intron-like RNA followed by a 3´ splice site, but without a 5´ splice site

Cis-splicing

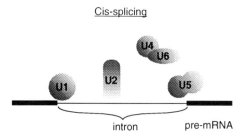

Trans-splicing Models

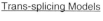

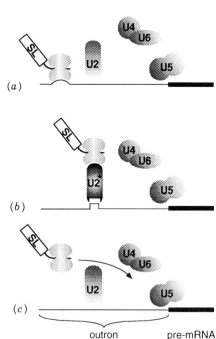

Fig 1. Three models for what signals the pre-mRNA for *trans*-splicing. Cis-splicing is shown for comparison. **a:** SL snRNP interacts with the pre-mRNA by a direct, basepairing interaction. **b:** The pre-mRNA contains a binding site for a specialized U2 snRNP, which in turn has an SL snRNP binding site. **c:** The presence of intron-like RNA followed by a 3′ splice site, but without an upstream 5′ splice site, is sufficient information to specify *trans*-splicing.

upstream, is sufficient information to specify *trans*-splicing. We tested this idea by creating modified genes, injecting them into *C. elegans*, isolating transgenic worms, and asking what sort of splicing events their RNA products underwent in vivo.

To do this we needed to know something about how introns are recognized in *C. elegans*. Our survey of sequenced *C. elegans* introns showed two rather interesting properties (Blumenthal and Thomas, 1988). *C. elegans* introns tend to be quite short; while some were found to be upwards of 15 kb in length, most (more than 75%) were around 50 bp. Thus there appears to be selective pressure for unusually short introns. Second, whereas the 5´ splice site consensus is the same as in other metazoans, the 3´ splice site consensus is a highly conserved six base sequence, UUUCAG. Furthermore, no consensus branch point sequence can be discerned, even though *C. elegans* U2 does contain the precise sequence known to basepair with the branch point in other metazoans. Finally, *C. elegans* introns can be easily identified by their base composition: extreme A+U-richness (>70%) compared with surrounding exons (about 50%). Based on these observations we modified our hypothesis as follows: any A+U-rich sequence, followed by a good match to UUUCAG but without a 5´ splice site should, if properly positioned, be able to convert a conventional gene into a *trans*-spliced gene. A corollary hypothesis was that it might be possible to do the symmetrical conversion by careful introduction of a 5´ splice site into the region serving as the 3´ half of the "intron" in *trans*-splicing.

As an initial test, we attempted to convert a vitellogenin fusion gene we had been studying in the laboratory for other reasons into a *trans*-spliced gene by transplanting an authentic intron, minus its 5´ splice site, into its 5´ untranslated region (Fig. 2). The *vit-2/6* gene, which is not normally *trans*-spliced, begins with an 11 bp 5´ untranslated region, into which we inserted an entire intron except the 5´-most G from a different *vit* gene. This modified gene was injected into the nuclei of oocytes, and stable transgenic strains were isolated. When RNA isolated from these strains was analyzed by RT-PCR and by primer extension with sequencing, over 80% of the products were found to be *trans*-spliced at the site that normally serves as the intron 3´ splice site (Conrad et al., 1991). This result demonstrated that *cis*- and *trans*- splice sites were functionally interconvertible. It also suggested that there is no specific sequence required to specify *trans*-splicing, although it left open the unlikely possibility that the transplanted intron fortuitously contained such a sequence. Finally, the experiment provided strong experimental support for the model that *trans*-splicing occurs at splice sites preceded by intron-like sequences without a 5´ splice site. We named the sequence between the 5´ end of the pre-mRNA and the *trans*-splice site an *outron*, to indicate an intron that is not intervening, but outside all exons.

Conventional ⟶ Trans-spliced

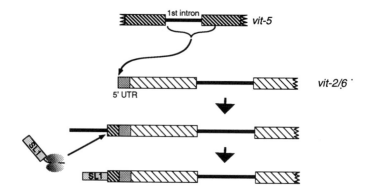

Trans-spliced ⟶ Cis-spliced

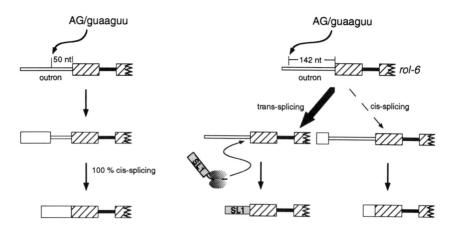

Fig. 2.   Interconversion of *trans*-spliced and conventional genes. A conventional gene, *vit 2/ 6*, was converted into a *trans*-spliced gene by transplanting an intron (from *vit-5*) lacking its 5´ splice site into the 5´ untranslated region. A *trans*-spliced gene was converted into a *cis*-spliced gene by inserting a perfect match to the consensus 5´ splice site into the outron. When this insertion site was 50 nt upstream of the *trans*-splice site, *trans*-splicing was completely suppressed and replaced by *cis*-splicing. When the insertion site was 142 nt upstream of the *trans*-splice site, the 5´ splice site was used less efficiently.

To control for the possibility that the intron we used happened to contain a *trans*-splicing signal, we designed additional experiments in which synthetic sequences of varying lengths and base compositions were inserted into the *vit-2/6* 5′ untranslated region just upstream of a synthetic 3′ splice site (Conrad and Blumenthal, manuscript in preparation). This experiment should indicate whether we are in command of all parameters involved in encoding *trans*-splicing. In this series of experiments, the DNA was injected into the gonadal syncytium, and unstable transgenic lines containing the DNA on large extrachromosomal arrays were selected. The results were unequivocal: *Trans*-splicing occurred at the introduced 3′ splice site, and its efficiency was dependent on both the length and the base composition of the synthetic outron. When the sequence was about 50% A+T, no *trans*-splicing was observed. In contrast, A+T contents of greater than 75% led to efficient *trans*-splicing. Furthermore, a strict, outron length dependence was observed. Outrons of 41 nt were spliced inefficiently (8–15%), while outrons of 50 nt were spliced relatively well (38–69%). When the synthetic outron was greater than about 180 nt, all of the transgene products were found to be *trans*-spliced. These experiments demonstrate that *trans*-splicing occurs whenever a 3′ splice site near the 5′ end of a pre-mRNA is preceded by A+U-rich RNA. Furthermore they demonstrate that there is no specific sequence required for interaction of the SL snRNP with the remainder of the splicing machinery, although the possibility remains that there are sequences within the outron that influence the efficiency of *trans*-splicing.

How important is it that there be no 5′ splice site upstream? To answer this question we asked whether it would be possible to convert a natural *trans*-spliced gene into a conventional one by introduction of a 5′ splice site into its outron (Conrad et al., 1993a). We used the *rol-6* gene, which encodes a cuticle collagen and begins with a 173 nt outron. A dominant allele of *rol-6* results in an easily observable rolling phenotype. We inserted a perfect match to the consensus 5′ splice site at two different positions within the outron, either 142 nt or 50 nt upstream of the *trans*-splice site (Fig. 2). When the site was introduced 50 nt upstream of the *trans*-splice site we found that *trans*-splicing was completely suppressed and was replaced by *cis*-splicing between the introduced site and the *trans*-splice site. This result demonstrates that lack of a site recognized as a 5′ splice site is part of the signal for *trans*-splicing. It also confirms the earlier conclusion that *cis*- and *trans*-splice sites are functionally interchangable.

When the 5′ splice site was introduced 142 nt upstream, it was recognized much less efficiently. Although some product was *cis*-spliced, the majority was still *trans*-spliced (Fig. 2). In this artificial situation the two processes competed for use of the same 3′ splice site. For whatever reason, the introduced 5′ splice site functioned less efficiently when it was present at this location than when it was closer to the 3′ splice site. Since most *C. elegans* introns are about 50 nt long, we thought that intron length might be the key difference between the two locations. However, we found that when we introduced 200 extra bp of DNA into the small intron, it was still *cis*-spliced efficiently. That result suggests that the key variable could be the sequence context surrounding the introduced splice site that controls how efficiently it is used. In this light it is evident that the competition between *cis*- and *trans*-splicing is strongly affected by how well any matches to the 5′ splice site consensus present in the outron are recognized by the splicing machinery. It seems likely that natural cases of alternative *cis*- and *trans*-splicing will be uncovered as more *C. elegans* genes are characterized at the molecular level. Indeed, several good candidates have recently been reported (e.g., Nonet and Meyer, 1991) but in no case has it been unequivocally demonstrated that a single pre-mRNA species can give rise to both *cis*- and *trans*-spliced products.

We have also analyzed the *rol-6 trans*-splice site in some detail in order to determine which parameters are important in *trans*-splice site definition (Conrad et al., 1993b). When the *trans*-splice site is mutated from AG to AA, *trans*-splicing nevertheless occurs, but at a site that is normally completely cryptic, 20 bp upstream of the normal site (Fig. 3). We used this observation to analyze the importance of individual bases in the *trans*-splice site. By mutating individual bases in the UUCC immediately preceding the AG, we showed that these highly conserved pyrimidines are necessary components of *trans*-splice site recognition. We also demonstrated that the upstream site is normally cryptic because it does not lie at a boundary between A+U-rich and non-A+U-rich RNA. When several As and Us between the two sites were changed to Gs and Cs, splicing occurred at the upstream site even though the downstream *trans*-splice site was unchanged. Although no *C. elegans cis*-splice site has been analyzed in such detail, we expect the same principles to apply: a 3' splice site must be a good match to the UUUCAG consensus and must be near a boundary between A+U-rich and non-A+U-rich RNA.

Our view of how *trans*-splicing occurs is still somewhat primitive. We suggest that after a spliceosome begins to assemble on a 3′ splice site, it searches for a 5′ splice site with which to interact. When none is found upstream on the same pre-mRNA, the mobile 5′ splice site on SL RNA serves the same role and donates the SL as the 5′ exon. A possible mechanism by which the SL snRNP interacts with the remainder of the spliceosome is suggested by a recent finding from the Nilson laboratory. Hannon et al. (1992) demonstrated that SL RNA and U6 RNA can interact by basepairing. They proposed that this interaction, combined with the basepairing of U6 to U2, and the basepairing of U2 to the branch site on the pre-mRNA provide a mechanism for bringing the two splicing substrates (SL RNA and pre-mRNA) together. If this idea is correct, then U6 must play a role quite early in *trans*-spliceosome formation.

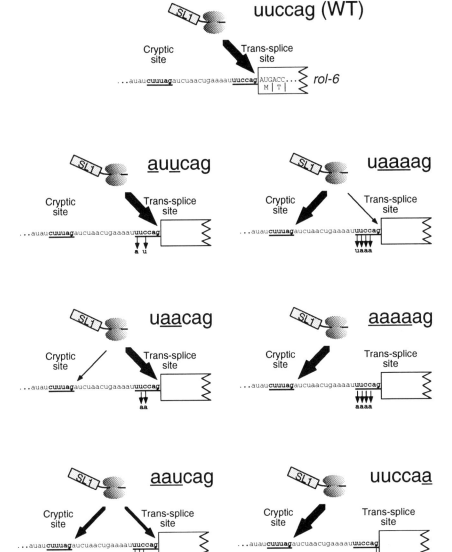

Fig. 3. Analysis of a *trans*-splice site. The *trans*-splice site of *rol-6* was analyzed in detail by mutating the wild-type site (UUCCAG) and assaying for the frequency with which splicing switched from the normal site to a cryptic site 20 nt upstream. The relative frequency of splicing to each site is indicated by the thickness of the arrow. The cryptic site is not used when the normal site is intact.

SL2 *TRANS*-SPLICING

In the preceding discussion we ignored the second SL in *C. elegans*, SL2. That is because SL2 did not turn out to be relevant, as is discussed below. SL2 was originally found by Huang and Hirsh (1989) at the 5' end of one of the four GAPDH-encoding genes, *gpd-3* (the other three were all reported to receive SL1). It was found that SL2 was delivered by a different snRNP, very similar in size and predicted secondary structure to the SL1 snRNP. Since its original discovery, SL2 has been found on only a handful of additional gene products, while SL1 has been reported on over 100 *C. elegans* gene products. Furthermore, while SL1 has been found unchanged in all nematodes examined, SL2 has been found thus far only in *C. elegans* and a close relative, *C. briggsae*. Even within *C. elegans*, several SL2 variants have been found (Kuwabara et al., 1992; C. Rubin, personal communication). In addition, while there are 110 SL1 RNA genes, all contained as a tandem cluster with the 5S rRNA genes (Krause and Hirsh, 1987), only a few SL2 RNA genes have been found, and these are scattered throughout the genome (Huang and Hirsh, 1989).

What determines which SL is spliced onto the 5' end of a given mRNA? For the purposes of this discussion, we assume that, for any particular gene, all of its pre-mRNA receives either SL1 or SL2, never both. Later, however, we discuss recent discoveries that show that both SL1 and SL2 can be accepted by products of a single gene. From the relative distribution of SL1 and SL2 on *C. elegans* mRNAs and from the wide phylogenetic distribution of SL1, one might expect SL1 *trans*-splicing to be a default process, while SL2 *trans*-splicing might require some additional information. Indeed, the results we obtained in the experiments described above support that idea strongly. All of the synthetic outrons and the outron created by the transplanted intron were *trans*-spliced exclusively to SL1, never to SL2 (Conrad et al., 1991; Conrad and Blumenthal, manuscript in preparation). This observation demonstrates that SL1 *trans*-splicing requires no sequence-specific information; just the presence of an A+U-rich sequence followed by a 3' splice site is enough. So where is the information to encode SL2-specific *trans*-splicing? A first guess might be the presence of some specific sequence in the outron. However, a comparison of the *gpd-3* outrons of *C. briggsae* and *C. elegans*, both of which receive SL2, did not reveal much in common upstream of the 3' 20 bases (Lee et al., 1992). When these 20 bases were moved to an identical position in the *rol-6* gene, they resulted in *trans*-splicing, but only of SL1. In a similar experiment, when Church and Wickens (personal communication) fused the last 70 bases of the *tra-2* outron, which normally receives SL2, to the 5' end of the *unc-54* gene, which is normally not *trans*-spliced, the gene product was *trans*-spliced, but to SL1. These experiments suggested that the sequences just upstream of SL2 *trans*-splice sites do not contain SL2 specificity information.

One unusual aspect of the SL2-accepting *gpd-3* gene is its chromosomal location. This gene is just downstream of another gene, *gpd-2*, which is oriented in the same direction (Huang et al., 1989). The distance between the 3' end of *gpd-2* and the *trans*-splice site of *gpd-3* is only about 100 basepairs. With the discovery of a gene a similar distance upstream of *tra-2* (the second SL2-accepting gene to be reported), again with the same orientation (Kuwabara and Kimble, personal communication), we began to entertain the possibility that this unusual chromosomal arrangement had something to do with specifying SL2 *trans*-splicing. We hypothesized that, unlike all other metazoan genes, SL2-accepting genes do not have their own promoters. Instead they are transcribed by readthrough transcription from the promoter of the upstream gene. That is, we proposed that SL2-accepting genes are part of polycistronic transcription units, not unlike bacterial operons (Spieth et al., 1993). In this model, the purpose of SL2 is to separate the polycistronic precursor into individual mRNAs, much like *trans*-splicing in trypanosomes.

When a third gene pair, the *lin-15* genes, with spacing almost identical to the first two was discovered by Linda Huang in Paul Sternberg's laboratory (personal communication) and by Scott Clark in Bob Horvitz's lab (personal communication), we predicted that the downstream member of this pair, *lin-15A*, would turn out to be *trans*-spliced to SL2. The first indication that the model was correct was provided by the verification of this prediction. When Charles Rubin reported two more SL2-accepting genes, the gene for protein kinase C, *kin-13*, and the gene for casein kinase II, *kin-10*, we decided to investigate whether there were genes just upstream. We discovered a gene in the same orientation just upstream of each, with spacing of 100 bp for the first pair and about 300 bp for the second (Spieth et al., 1993). Thus the model was found to predict correctly both that a gene would be an SL2 gene if it was found just downstream of another gene in the same orientation and that a closely spaced gene would be found just upstream of any gene that is *trans*-spliced to SL2.

The gene just upstream of *gpd-3*, *gpd-2*, was originally reported to be an SL1-accepting gene (Huang et al., 1989). However, when we investigated the 5′ end of *gpd-2* mRNAs we found that a substantial portion began with SL2. That suggested there would be a gene just upstream of *gpd-2*. About the same time, Ralph Hecht's laboratory discovered the presence of a short open reading frame (which they named *ORF88*) upstream of *gpd-2* in both *C. elegans* and *C. briggsae* (Lee et al., 1992). We determined that this was indeed a real gene by selecting cDNA clones for ORF88. Once again the spacing was about 100 bp: The 3′ end of the ORF88 gene was just about 100 bp upstream of the *gpd-2 trans*-splice site (Spieth et al., 1993). This gene encodes the worm homolog of the mitochondrial ATPase inhibitor, which is a subunit of the ATP synthetase. It prevents the enzyme from running in reverse and breaking down

ATP. We named the gene *mai-1*, and we discuss later the possible regulatory implications of this interesting juxtaposition of genes involved in ATP biogenesis. Its presence in this location and the fact that *gpd-2* receives SL2 suggests that we may have uncovered a three-gene operon, 5′–*mai-1*–*gpd-2*–*gpd-3*–3′, but the fact that *gpd-2* receives both SLs suggests an additional complication (see below).

The idea that *mai-1* and *gpd-2* are cotranscribed was confirmed by our isolation of two unusual classes of cDNA clones (Fig. 4). The first class comes from polycistronic RNA. These clones are presumably copies of incompletely spliced precursors to mature mRNAs. The introns of both genes have been spliced out, but the *trans*-splicing of *gpd-2* has not occurred. Thus the sequences of both mature mRNAs are connected by the intercistronic region in these clones. In the second class, only *mai-1* sequences are present, but the clones are from mRNAs that were polyadenylated at the 3′ end of the intercistronic space instead of the normal site following the AAUAAA 100 bases upstream. These clones may have arisen by polyadenylation at the free 3′ end of *mai-1* created by *trans*-splicing of *gpd-2* from the polycistronic precursor. This would require that *trans*-splicing occurs at a site in the middle of a long, intronless RNA, which might be possible if the *trans*-splice site follows an A+U-rich region without a 5′ splice site upstream. It would also require that the *mai-1* RNA be de-branched before cDNA synthesis.

mai-1 cDNA Clones

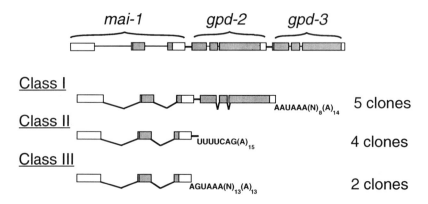

Fig. 4. Three classes of *mai-1* cDNA clones. Class I clones come from polycistronic RNA in which all the introns have been spliced out but *trans*-splicing to *gpd-2* has not occurred. Class II clones contain only *mai-1* sequences and are from mRNAs polyadenylated 100 nt downstream of the normal site. Class III clones are from *mai-1* mRNAs polyadenylated at the normal site.

It is worth noting that although *mai-1/gpd-2* polycistronic cDNA clones provide unequivocal evidence for the operon idea, polycistronic precursors are not typical of the other proposed operons. In no other case have we been able to detect the presence of a polycistronic precursor, even with RT-PCR. We believe that in most cases cleavage and polyadenylation of the upstream mRNA precedes temporally the transcription of the downstream gene. Thus, although the genes are polycistronic in the sense that they are transcribed from a single promoter, no polycistronic precursor ever exists because the 3′ end processing is cotranscriptional. We suggest that we were able to isolate polycistronic precursors in the case of *mai-1/gpd-2* because for some reason the *mai-1* polyadenylation signal is suboptimal.

We have also performed several experiments that support the idea of the *mai-1/gpd-2/gpd-3* operon and suggest that being a downstream gene in a polycistronic transcription unit is sufficient to specify SL2 *trans*-splicing (Spieth et al., 1993) In the first, we simply asked what sequences were required for expression of *gpd-3* in vivo. We found that sequences upstream of *mai-1* were necessary for high-level expression of *gpd-3* and that sequences upstream of *gpd-2* were required for any detectable expression of *gpd-3*. While the needed upstream sequences could be enhancers, these results are certainly consistent with the idea of an upstream promoter. Our results suggest that there are two promoters: an upstream one that serves all three genes and another one just upstream of *gpd-2*. *gpd-3* is a downstream gene with both, so it always receives SL2. However, *gpd-2* is the first gene when transcription begins downstream of *mai-1*, so in that case it would be expected to receive SL1. This hypothesis explains why both SL1 and SL2 are found on *gpd-2*.

When we inserted the *gpd-2/gpd-3* gene pair downstream of a heat-inducible promoter, we obtained strictly heat-inducible expression of *gpd-3* and *trans*-splicing exclusively to SL2. This experiment showed that *gpd-3* lacks its own promoter, that when transcription is known to begin upstream of an upstream gene proper SL2 specificity occurs and that transcription intitiated upstream of *gpd-2* does not terminate between *gpd-2* and *gpd-3*. When the heat shock promoter was moved closer to the 5′ end of *gpd-3, trans*-splicing specificity was lost, suggesting that full SL2 specificity requires a gene to be in a downstream position. In contrast, changing the spacing between the two genes to 200 bp in this context did not interfere with full SL2 specificity.

To determine whether being a downstream gene was a sufficient condition to specify SL2 *trans*-splicing, we inserted the SL1-accepting gene, *rol-6*, into the position normally occupied by *gpd-3*, but with *rol-6* outron sequences serving as the intercistronic region (Fig. 5). This construction was placed under the control of the heat shock promoter upstream of *gpd-2*. *rol-6* inserted directly downstream of the heat shock promoter, without the intervening *gpd-2* gene, served as the control. When the latter was induced, the *rol-6* mRNA

Conversion of an SL1- to an SL2-accepting gene

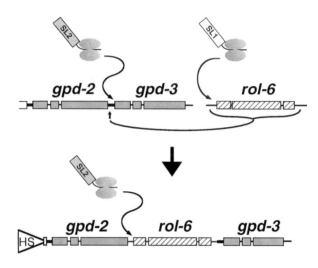

Fig. 5. Transplantation of an SL1-accepting gene into a site normally occupied by an SL2-accepting gene. An SL1-accepting gene, *rol-6*, was placed into the position normally occupied by *gpd-3*, an SL2- accepting gene. This construction was placed under the control of the heat shock promoter upstream of *gpd-2*.

was found to be *trans*-spliced primarily to SL1, as expected. However, when the *rol-6* gene was inserted downstream of *gpd-2*, its product was *trans*-spliced primarily to SL2, although some SL1 splicing was observed. Clearly, *rol-6* can be transcribed when it is placed (promoterless) downstream of *gpd-2*. The finding that most of its product is *trans*-spliced to SL2 when it is in this un-natural position suggests strongly that this chromosomal arrangement leads to SL2 *trans*-splicing.

What might the mechanism be? Since almost all of the gene pairs are spaced very close to 100 bp apart, we hypothesized that somehow the process of 3´ end formation of the upstream gene was interacting with the process of *trans*-splicing of the downstream gene. To test this idea we deleted the AAUAAA cleavage and polyadenylation signal of *gpd-2* in the heat shock promoter context. This resulted in accumulation of a polycistronic precursor RNA (*gpd-2* + *gpd-3*). Unfortunately, however, it only made cleavage inefficient; it did not eliminate it. Correctly *trans*-spliced *gpd-3* mRNA was still formed because a cryptic cleavage signal 13 bp upstream was utilized. The experiment nevertheless did demonstrate the key role played by the AAUAAA in maturation of what would otherwise be a polycistronic mRNA. The role, if any, played by the cleavage and polyadenylation signal of the upstream gene in determining SL2 specificity remains to be determined.

Since the initial publication of the discovery of operons in *C. elegans*, three more have been clearly demonstrated, and evidence for several more is accumulating. For those operons in which the spacing is known, two different spacings have been found. In general, when the genes are separated by about 100 bp (six instances), the downstream gene is found to receive exclusively SL2. However in the three cases where spacing is about 300 bp, the product of the downstream gene receives both spliced leaders. Again, this correlation points to the importance of spacing in the mechanism of SL2 specificity, but exactly how the proximity of the upstream gene influences *trans*-splicing specificity remains to be discovered. The simplest possibility is that a protein involved in the polyadenylation of the upstream gene has affinity for a protein that forms a part of the SL2 snRNP. In this idea, when the *trans*-splice site is close it has a greater chance of receiving the SL2 snRNP bound to the polyadenylation complex.

Another reason why spacing may be important concerns the connection between cleavage at the poly(A) site and transcription termination. While not all signals required for termination in eukaryotes have been identified, it is clear that cleavage at the poly(A) site is required for termination to occur (reviewed by Wahle and Keller, 1992). In general it has been found that termination occurs well downstream of the cleavage site. But in an operon there might be a special problem: Termination following upstream genes must be prevented. Since some of the cleavage and polyadenylation machinery is known to bind downstream of the cleavage site, it would remain attached to the downstream pre-mRNA following cleavage. If this is the machinery involved in termination, it might be necessary to separate it from the transcription complex in order to prevent termination from occurring before the end of the downstream gene or genes is transcribed. *Trans*-splicing would accomplish this separation. It may be necessary for the *trans*-splice site to be close to the cleavage site so that separation occurs before transcription termination.

How likely is it that operons and a specialized SL will be found in other nematodes or in even more distantly related organisms? Thus far SL2 has been found only in *Caenorhabditis* species. Failure to find it by cross-hybridization even in the relatively closely related, *Dolichorhabditis* (Winter and Blumenthal, unpublished observations), may be due to sequence divergence. It is clear that SL2 has diverged far more rapidly than SL1, based on the active variants found in *C. elegans*. Thus it may be more fruitful to search by other methods. For example, attempts to clone homologous gene pairs from other nematodes might provide evidence that these gene arrangements are ancient. Additionally, sequencing the 5′ ends of cDNA clones from other nematodes corresponding to genes that have been found to accept SL2 in *C. elegans* could reveal the sequence of alternative SLs from these species. Eventually the presence of alternative SLs, as well as operons, will turn up as more and more genes from other nematodes are characterized, if the phenomenon is not restricted to *Caenorhabditis*. While it seems improbable that such a basic aspect of gene expression would have arisen since the divergence of *C. elegans* and other nematodes, it does seem possible that it could have developed independently from operons in bacteria and the polycistronic transcription units of trypanosomes. It seems unlikely that operons are a primitive trait that has been retained in bacteria, the most primitive eukaryotes, and nematodes, but lost in all the well-characterized forms of life in between (e.g., yeast, plants, protists). On the contrary, it seems reasonable to suggest that the presence of *trans*-splicing in nematodes allowed the development of polycistronic transcription units because it provided a mechanism for processing individual mRNA species from precursor RNAs. However, it is very difficult to rationalize the existence of a specialized SL snRNP to do this.

However they may have evolved, it is interesting to consider whether the operons in *C. elegans* serve the purpose of coordinate regulation of genes of related function, as they do in bacteria. In most of the cases identified thus far, the function of only one member of the pair of genes is known, so it is not yet clear whether the genes are coregulated so as to coordinate their functions. However, there are a few intriguing observations that suggest that the operons do serve this purpose. The clearest case is the pair of *lin-15* genes. These two genes are not related to each other by sequence, but they clearly are by function: They collaborate in the process of vulva determination (reviewed by Horvitz and Sternberg, 1991). A second example that is easy to rationalize is the three-gene operon composed of *mai-1* and the *gpd* genes. The latter are involved in glycolysis, a relatively expensive pathway of ATP biogenesis, while *mai-1* serves to prevent the mitochondrial ATP synthetase from breaking down ATP. It makes sense to coexpress them under conditions where the worm requires maximum production of ATP. Third, the gene upstream of *kin-13*, the PKC gene, encodes a protein of unknown function, but contains a clear tyrosine kinase recognition site adjacent to an ATP binding site, suggesting it might in some way be related to kinase function. Finally, there are two recently discovered cases in which the downstream genes encode members of a family of RNA binding proteins. Many members of this family are known to regulate splice-site choice. Hence their cotranscription with other genes could be needed to regulate splicing of the mRNA of the upstream gene (or genes).

CONCLUSIONS

As a consequence of studying how decisions about which pre-mRNAs are *trans*-spliced and to which SL, we discovered a surprising and novel aspect of the basic mechanism of gene expression in *C. elegans*. Most pre-mRNAs that are *trans*-spliced receive SL1. They do so simply because they begin with an outron (an intron-like sequence at the 5′ end followed by a 3′ splice site, but with no exon upstream). No specific sequences on the pre-mRNA are required for SL1-specific splicing. Similarly, there are no specific sequences required for SL2-specific splicing. Instead, SL2 is reserved for splicing onto downstream gene products in polycistronic transcription units equivalent to bacterial operons. Preliminary evidence suggests that these operons have regulatory significance. In at least some cases they appear to effect the coordinate regulation of genes that function together. How widespread this phenomenon will turn out to be in the eukaryotes is still a matter for conjecture.

REFERENCES

Bektesh S, Doren KV, and Hirsh D (1988): Presence of the *Caenorhabditis elegans* spliced leader on different mRNAs and in different genera of nematodes. Genes Dev 2:1277–1283.

Blumenthal T, Thomas J (1988): *Cis* and *trans* mRNA splicing in *C. elegans*. Trends Genetics 4:305–308.

Bruzik JP, Van Doren K, Hirsh D, Steitz JA (1988): *Trans* splicing involves a novel form of small nuclear ribonucleoprotein particles. Nature 335:559–562.

Conrad R, Liou RF, Blumenthal T (1993a): Conversion of a *trans*-spliced *C. elegans* gene into a conventional gene by introduction of a splice donor site. EMBO J 12:1249–1255.

Conrad R, Liou RF, Blumenthal T (1993b): Functional analysis of a *C. elegans trans*-site acceptor. Nucleic Acids Res 21:913–919.

Conrad R, Thomas J, Spieth J, Blumenthal T (1991): Insertion of part of an intron into the 5′ untranslated region of a *Caenorhabditis elegans* gene converts it into a *trans*-spliced gene. Mol Cell Biol 11:1921–1926.

Green MR (1991): Biochemical mechanisms of constitutive and regulated pre-mRNA splicing. Annu Rev of Cell Biol. 7:559–599.

Hannon GJ, Maroney PA, Yu Y-T, Hannon GE, Nilsen TW (1992): Interaction of U6 snRNA with a sequence required for function of the nematode SL RNA in *trans*-splicing. Science 258:1775–1780.

Horvitz HR, Sternberg PW (1991): Multiple intercellular signalling systems control the development of the *Caenorhabditis elegans* vulva. Nature 351:535–541.

Huang X-Y, Barrios LAM, Vonkhorporn P, Honda S, Albertson DG Hecht RM (1989): Genomic organization of the glyceraldehyde-3-phosphate dehydrogenase gene family of *Caenorhabditis elegans*. J Mol Biol 206:411–424.

Huang X-Y, Hirsh D (1989): A second *trans*-spliced RNA leader sequence in the nematode *Caenorhabditis elegans*. Proc Nat Acad Sci USA 86:8640–8644.

Huang X-Y, Hirsh D (1992): RNA *trans*-splicing. *Genetic Engineering*. New York: Plenum, pp. 211–229.

Krause M, Hirsh D (1987): A *trans*-spliced leader sequence on actin mRNA in *C. elegans*. Cell 49:753–761.

Kuwabara PE, Okkema PG, Kimble J (1992): *tra-2* encodes a membrane protein and may mediate cell communication in the *Caenorhabditis elegans* sex determination pathway. Mol Biol Cell 3:461–473.

Lee YH, Huang X-Y, Hirsh D, Fox GE, Hecht RM (1992): Conservation of gene organization and *trans*-splicing in the glyceraldehyde-3-phosphate dehydrogenase-encoding genes of *Caenorhabditis briggsae*. Gene 121:227–235.

Liou R-F, Blumenthal T (1990): *Trans*-spliced *Caenorhabditis elegans* mRNAs retain trimethylguanosine caps. Mol Cell Bio 10:1764–1768.

Nilsen TW (1993): *Trans*-splicing of nematode pre-messenger RNA. Ann Rev Cell Biol 47:413–440.

Nonet ML, Meyer BJ (1991): Early aspects of *Caenorhabditis elegans* sex determination and dosage compensation are regulated by a zinc-finger protein. Nature 351:65–68.

Sharp PA (1987): *Trans* splicing: Variation on a familiar theme. Cell 50:147–148.

Spieth J, Brooke G, Kuerston S, Lea K, Blumenthal T (1993): Operons in *C. elegans:* Polycistronic mRNA precursors are processed by *trans*-splicing of SL2 to to downstream coding regions. Cell 73:521–532.

Thomas JD, Conrad RC, Blumenthal T (1988): The C. elegans *trans*-spliced leader RNA is bound to Sm and has a trimethylguanosine cap. Cell 54:533–539.

Thomas J, Lea K, Zucker-Aprison E, Blumenthal T (1990): The spliceosomal snRNAs of *Caenorhabditis elegans*. Nucleic Acids Res 18:2633–2642.

Van Doren K, Hirsh D (1988): *Trans*-spliced leader RNA exists as small nuclear ribonucleoprotein particles in *Caenorhabditis elegans*. Nature 335:556–559.

Wahle E, Keller W (1992): The biochemistry of 3´-end cleavage and polyadenylation of messenger RNA precursors. Ann Rev Biochem 61:419–440.

Molecular Approaches to Parasitology, pages 299–320
© 1995 Wiley-Liss, Inc.

Trans-Splicing in Flatworms

Richard E. Davis

*Department of Biology, San Francisco State University, San Francisco,
California 94132*

INTRODUCTION

Trans-splicing is an RNA processing event that accurately joins exons
derived from distinctly transcribed RNAs. In one form of *trans*-splicing, a
leader sequence (the spliced leader [SL]) is donated from the 5´ end of a
small, nonpolyadenylated RNA (the spliced leader RNA [SL RNA]) to
pre-mRNAs to form the 5´ terminal exon of the mature mRNAs. This form
of RNA maturation was first described in trypanosomes (see the chapters
by Tschudi and Swindle) and has subsequently been demonstrated in other
kinetoplastida and flagellated protozoa *(Euglena)*, nematodes, and flatworms (see the chapter by Blumenthal for detailed discussion of *trans*-
splicing in nematodes). Although once considered an anomaly of the
kinetoplastida, the subsequent identification of *trans*-splicing in multiple
members of two distinct invertebrate phyla, first in nematodes and then in
flatworms, suggests that this particular form of RNA processing may be
common among invertebrates and likely represents an evolutionarily important form of gene expression.

The recent developments of permeabilized cell and transformation systems in the kinetoplastida and, particularly, of in vitro transcription, *trans*-
splicing, and transformation systems in nematodes have significantly
increased our understanding of aspects of the regulation, mechanism, and
function of *trans*-splicing. However, the primary function(s) of most *trans*-
splicing in metazoa remain somewhat of an enigma. Excellent reviews and
perspectives on these studies can be found elsewhere and, as already mentioned in preceding chapters in this volume (Blumenthal, 1993; Boothroyd,
1985; Donelson, 1990; Huang, 1992; Laird, 1989; Nilsen, 1989, 1992, 1993;
Agabian, 1990; Blumenthal and Thomas,1988). Current research and interest in *trans*-splicing are focused on several interrelated areas: 1) characterization of the specificity and regulation of *trans*-splicing with reference

to its role in post-transcriptional gene regulation and its temporal relationship with other concurrent RNA processing events; 2) the distribution and functional signficance of *trans*-splicing as a mechanism of gene expression, particularly in metazoa; 3) elucidation of aspects of the mechanism and determinants of *trans*-splicing and their potential evolutionary relationship or similarities with self-splicing and snRNA mediated *cis*-splicing; and 4) *trans*-splicing as a potential common drug target in several different groups of human, veterinary, and agriculturally important parasites.

The focus of this chapter is limited to a summary of current knowledge regarding *trans*-splicing in flatworms from a phylogenetic perspective and a brief discussion of the perplexing question of the functional signficance of *trans*-splicing in metazoa. It is not meant to be comprehensive and, due to its limited scope, omits reference to many interesting studies conducted in trypanosomes and nematodes. The current lack of flatworm cell lines, in vitro systems, and transformation systems precludes direct analysis of the mechanism and regulation of *trans*-splicing in these organisms. However, characterization of several aspects of *trans*-splicing in schistosomes and other flatworms has contributed to our understanding of the prevalence, importance, and properties of *trans*-splicing in early metazoa. Studies on flatworms and other simple metazoa may provide additional information regarding the distribution, signficance, and perhaps function of *trans*-splicing among early metazoans. In addition, phylogenetic characterization of metazoan SL RNAs and *trans*-splicing might provide information regarding the evolutionary origins of *trans*-splicing, the relationships among lower metazoa, and perhaps contribute to our understanding of the signficance (or lack thereof) of conserved elements or secondary structures associated with *trans*-splicing in these groups.

At the outset, it is essential to recognize that although both nematodes and flatworms are often lumped together in discussions of parasites as worms or helminths, these two unique phyla (Nematoda and Platyhelminthes) represent quite evolutionarily divergent organisms, and observations on one group may not always be valid on the other, as illustrated by some differences described below. Flatworms are a more diverse and disparate assemblage of organisms than the nematodes. A simplistic classification (Fig. 1A) of the majority of Platyhelminthes or flatworms for this chapter can be subdivided into at least four major classes: Turbellaria (predominantly free-living, aquatic, planaria-like organisms), Trematoda (endoparasites of vertebrates with complex, indirect life cycles–flukes), Monogenea (ectoparasites of fishes and amphibians with simple, direct life cycles), and Cestoidea (endoparasites of the intestines of vertebrates and elasmobranchs with complex, indirect life cycles–tapeworms).

PHYLUM PLATYHELMINTHES

Class Turbellaria
Order Tricladida
Dugesia spp
Bdelloura candida
Order Polycladida
Stylochus zebra

Class Trematoda
Order Strigeata
Schistosoma spp.
Order Echinostomata
Superfamily Echinostomatoidea
Family Echinostomatidae
Echinostoma caproni
Family Fasciolidae
Fasciola hepatica
Order Plagiorchiodea
Superfamily Plagiorchioidea
Family Haematolechus
Haematolechus spp.
Superfamily Allocreadioidea
Family Acanthocolpidae
Stephanostomum spp.

Class Monogenea
Order Monoopisthocotylea
Order Polyopisthocotylea

Class Cestoidea
Order Cyclophyllidea
Hymenolepis diminuta
Order Pseudophyllidea
Species unidentified
Order Tetraphyllidea
Calliobothrium spp.
Order Trypanorhynchida
Lacistorynchus tenuis

(A)

Fig. 1. Classification of flatworms and an evolutionary scheme for the metazoa. **A:** General classification of flatworms used in this chapter including organisms mentioned in the text. The parasitic flatworms including the Trematoda, Monogenea, and Cestoidea are generally considered to be a monophyletic group having arisen from progenitor(s) within the Turbellaria. One phylogeny of parasitic groups based on molecular and morphological data currently suggests an evolutionary progression from Trematoda to Monogenea to Cestoidea.

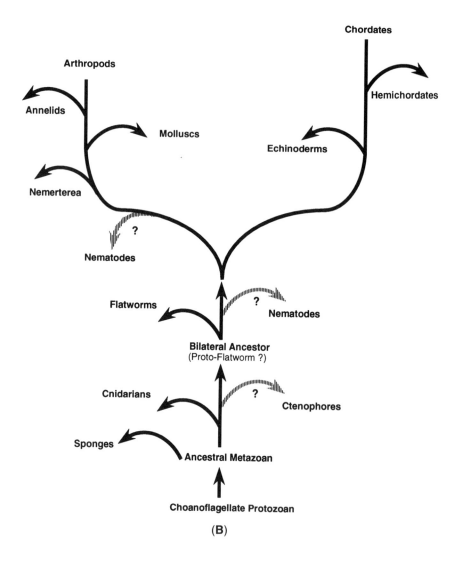

Fig. 1 (cont'd). **B:** One possible monophyletic evolutionary scheme for the metazoa illustrating relationships among the early metazoa. This representation illustrates a potential role for a flagellate ancestor of metazoa, a protoflatworm as an ancestor of bilateral metazoa, and the questionable origins of the nematodes and ctenophores. It should be noted that this scheme represents one possible view and that the evolutionary origin and relationships among the early metazoa remain controversial and not well resolved. Furthermore, it is unlikely that a kinetoplastid flagellate was the flagellate protozoan ancestor of the metazoa.

TRANS-SPLICING IN SCHISTOSOMES

Evidence for *Trans*-splicing

Trans-splicing in flatworms was first observed in schistosomes (Trematoda) (Rajkovic et al., 1990). Discovery of *trans*-splicing in *Schistosoma mansoni* was fortuitous, as it was in flagellated protozoa and nematodes, following from the characterization and comparison of the 5′ terminal sequences of an mRNA with the genomic organization of its corresponding gene. In *S. mansoni*, the 5′ terminal 36 nucleotides of the HMG CoA-reductase mRNA are not encoded within the genomic locus for HMG-CoA reductase, but are derived from a 90 nucleotide, nonpolyadenylated RNA transcribed from small RNA (SL RNA) genes organized as tandemly repeated arrays located elsewhere in the schistosome genome. The 5′ terminal 36 nucleotides of the HMG CoA-reductase mRNA originate from the 5′ terminus of the 90 nucleotide SL RNA. In the SL RNA, the 5′ terminal 36 nucleotides are immediately followed by a splice donor site. Characterization of the genomic organization of HMG CoA-reductase gene indicated that a splice acceptor site is located at the position within the gene where the mRNA acquires the terminal 36 nucleotides (the SL). Significantly, the identical 5′ terminal 36 nucleotides acquired by the HMG CoA-reductase mRNA are also found at the termini of other mRNAs in *S. mansoni*. These observations indirectly suggest that the 5′ terminal sequences of some *S. mansoni* mRNAs are derived from *trans*-splicing.

Examination of the Specificity and Function

We were interested in studying *trans*-splicing in schistosomes not only to expand the general knowledge of the process but also to provide an evolutionary perspective. All mRNAs in *S. mansoni* do not undergo *trans*-splicing and thus only a subset of mRNAs acquire the SL sequence (Rajkovic et al., 1990). Our estimate of the percentage of mRNAs in schistosomes that undergo *trans*-splicing is extremely rough: 10%–20% based on mRNAs described in the literature and on several different approaches we used to identify and characterize *trans*-spliced mRNAs. Potential errors in estimates have recently been discussed (Nilsen, 1993 #14). In comparison, all mRNAs in trypanosomes are thought to be *trans*-spliced whereas a large percentage of nematode mRNAs are *trans*-spliced (*Caenorhabditis. elegans* ca. 70%+ and *Ascaris* ca. 80%–90%) (Nilsen, 1993) (Blumenthal, personal communication). The high percentage of mRNAs that are *trans*-spliced in nematodes suggests that rather than conferring selective properties on nematode mRNAs that *trans*-splicing more likely is related to some general process of gene expression in these organisms.

Since only a relatively small subset of mRNAs appear to acquire the spliced leader in schistosomes, we identified, characterized, and compared *trans*-spliced and non-*trans*-spliced mRNAs and their genes in schistosomes as one approach to determine if the type or organization of genes that are *trans*-spliced could provide information on the potential function(s) and regulation of *trans*-splicing in flatworms. We used several approaches to construct cDNA libraries enriched for mRNAs that contain spliced leaders and isolated and characterized over 30 *trans*-spliced mRNAs. These were used to determine if there are any discernible patterns in the type of computer-predicted proteins encoded, general sequence or secondary structure characteristics of these mRNAs, any unusual temporal or spatial expression, or if there is a potential relationship between spliced leader addition and the translation of these mRNAs. Our analyses suggest that there are no obvious patterns in *trans*-spliced schistosome mRNAs (Davis et al., 1994b). Furthermore, although the schistosome spliced leader contributes a potential initiator methionine to the 5′ end of the mRNA (see Figs. 2, 3), we have found no computer-predicted evidence that it consistently contributes an essential initiator methionine for open reading frames, improves the translation initiation context, or confers a conserved 5′ length or secondary structure on *trans*-spliced mRNAs. A 3′ terminal ATG is conserved in all other known flatworm SLs (see below and Fig. 2), yet in all cases lacks what is generally considered a good translation initiation context. Although computer predictions indicate that *trans*-splicing may be required to provide an initiator AUG for open reading frames in a few cDNAs we have characterized, it appears unlikely that the primary function of SL addition is associated with translation initiation. Analyses of *C. elegans* (Bektesh et al., 1988; Blumenthal, personal communication) and *Ascaris trans*-spliced mRNAs (Nilsen, 1992, 1993) also indicate that there appear to be no discernible patterns or specific properties attributable to *trans*-spliced mRNAs in nematodes either.

One of the *trans*-spliced schistosome mRNAs we have characterized in detail putatively encodes the glycolytic enzyme enolase based on high amino acid similarity with known enolase proteins. We used the glycolytic pathway as a paradigm to determine if proteins in a common pathway (i.e., glycolysis) might be derived from *trans*-spliced mRNAs. We characterized the 5′ terminal sequences of four other schistosome glycolytic enzymes (G3PDH, TPI, aldolase, and PFK) using 5′ RACE and direct sequencing to determine if these mRNAs were *trans*-spliced. None of these other glycolytic enzymes are *trans*-spliced (nor do they have any 5′ terminal sequences in common) indicating that glycolytic enzyme mRNAs do not appear to be *trans*-spliced as a group in schistosomes (Davis, et al., 1994b; dos Reis et al., 1993). Furthermore, there is no general conservation of particular genes that are *trans*-spliced in metazoa, since, for example, G3PDH is *trans*-spliced in *Caenorhabditis* spp., but not in schistosomes, and the homolog of the mitochondrial ATPase inhibitor in *Caenorhabditis* spp. is not *trans*-spliced while the analogous mRNA in schistosomes acquires an SL (Spieth et al., 1993).

Secondary structure and basepairing interactions have been implicated as phylogenetically conserved elements associated with self-splicing and snRNA-mediated *cis*- and *trans*-splicing. We have isolated and examined four single copy *trans*-spliced schistosome genes (enolase and an unknown gene in their entirety, portions of HMG CoA reductase, and synaptobrevin) in the region of their *trans*-splice acceptor sites for homologous sequences or potential secondary structures that might be involved in facilitating the interaction of the two RNA substrates, the *trans*-splicing reaction, and/or the specificity of the *trans*-splicing reaction. We identified a conserved octamer 40–50 nucleotides upstream of the *trans*-splice acceptor site in several genes whose sequence has the potential to basepair with the 5´ splice site of the SL RNA to form an eight-nucleotide intermolecular duplex (Davis et al., 1994b). If this interaction occurred in vivo, it might enhance the efficiency and specificity of the *trans*-splicing reaction. However, this element does not appear to be essential, since it is not found in all the *trans*-spliced genes we have examined. There are currently no systems in schistosomes to determine if such potential interactions occur and if they are of functional importance.

All four schistosome *trans*-spliced genes examined also undergo *cis*-splicing raising questions regarding the regulation of *trans*- versus *cis*-splicing within the same gene. We compiled and compared the sequences of 5 *trans*-splice acceptor sites and over 50 *cis*-splice acceptor site sequences (including 10 *cis*- splice acceptor sites from *trans*-spliced genes) from characterized schistosome genes to determine if there are any differences in consensus sequences for *trans*- versus *cis*-splice acceptor sites. Comparison of the small set of *trans*-splice acceptor sites with *cis*-splice acceptors did not demonstrate any discrete differences between these two types of acceptor sites with the exception that the *trans*-splice acceptor site appears to be more G/C rich within the first 10 nucleotides of intron (or outron) (Davis et al., 1994b). Thus, factors that might facilitate regulation of discrimination of *cis*- versus *trans*-splice acceptor sites within a gene undergoing both types of splicing in schistosomes remain to be determined. Interestingly, in HMG CoA reductase the SL can be joined to two separate exons generating two different mRNAs (Rajkovic et al., 1990). The downstream exon thus undergoes both *cis*- and *trans*-splicing. This has also been observed recently in several nematode genes. It remains to be determined whether this is alternative *trans*-splicing within the same primary transcript, if distinct transcription initiation sites exist for the different mRNAs, or if inefficient *cis*-splicing is responsible for the generation of these different mRNAs.

To explore the regulation and differentiation of *cis*- versus *trans*-splicing, Blumenthal and coworkers analyzed splice acceptor site context in transgenic *C. elegans* strains and demonstrated that if the primary transcript of a *C. elegans* gene begins with an intron-like sequence, which lacks an upstream splice donor site and is followed by a 3′ splice site, that these elements may be sufficient to identify a transcript as an appropriate *trans*-splice acceptor substrate (Conrad et al., 1991, 1993). Our attempts to identify transcription initiation sites of *trans*-spliced genes in schistosomes have not been successful, and consequently the primary transcription units for schistosome *trans*-spliced genes are not known. Clearly, information on the location of transcription initiation sites, the organization of primary transcription units, and attributes of promotors for *trans*-spliced genes will be essential to facilitate our understanding of the functional significance of *trans*-splicing and the factors that regulate the specificity of *trans*-splicing in either schistosomes or nematodes.

Comparison of the exon–intron organization of the schistosome enolase gene (composed of seven exons spanning 5000 bp) with other enolase genes (plant, yeast, *Drosophila*, amphibians, birds, and mammals) indicates that specific features in gene organization that might be related to or correlated with *trans*-splicing are not clearly evident. However, preliminary polymerase chain reaction (PCR) and RNAase mapping analyses to detect enolase pre-mRNA intermediates suggest that *cis*-splicing of the 5′ most exons and polyadenylation precede *trans*-splicing. In this *trans*-spliced gene, the fidelity of SL addition to the *trans*-splice acceptor site is extremely high, since using PCR analyses we have not been able to detect SL addition to internal *cis*-splice acceptor sites. In contrast, similar PCR analyses of several well-characterized non*trans*-spliced genes indicates that internal *cis*-spliced sites can inappropriately acquire the SL (Davis et al., 1994b). Such data might suggest that attributes or processing of *trans*-spliced genes may contribute to the fidelity of the *trans*-splicing reaction.

One other possible function of *trans*-splicing could be associated with restricted expression of SL RNAs and *trans*-spliced genes to particular cells or tissues. Analysis of the expression of the spliced leader in adult schistosomes by in situ hybridization indicates that both males and females express the SL RNA and that the SL RNA is expressed in virtually all tissues and cells (Davis et al., 1994b). Interestingly, the SL RNA accumulates to high levels in the nuclei of cells, and there is assymmetry in the abundance of the SL RNA in various cell nuclei. This variation in levels of SL RNA in nuclei might be related to expression of the SL RNA during the cell cycle, but this remains to be investigated. No identifiable patterns of expression of *trans*-spliced mRNAs were observed. Genes that are *trans*-spliced in *C.elegans* have been found to be expressed in many different tissues and cell types, suggesting that *trans*-splicing is also not associated with specific tissues or cells in nematodes either.

In summary, the results described above suggest that schistosome genes and their mRNAs that undergo *trans*-splicing do not fall into any obvious patterns or categories, nor do the proteins they encode. From sequence analysis of several *trans*-spliced genes, consensus sequences or secondary structures that appear essential for facilitating the interaction of the two RNA substrates, the *trans*-splicing reaction, or the discrimination of splice acceptor sites are not readily apparent. However, basepairing between the SL RNA and the pre-mRNA substrate might potentially occur in some *trans*-spliced genes that may enhance the efficiency and/or specificity of the *trans*-splicing reaction. Finally, in situ hybridization studies suggest that there is no tissue- or cell-specific expression of *trans*-splicing in schistosomes. These data further suggest that identifying potential functions of *trans*-splicing in flatworms and factors that regulate *trans*-splicing specificity await the development of functional systems to address these questions.

TRANS-SPLICING IN OTHER TREMATODES AND FLATWORMS

Although some recent molecular phylogenetic analyses support a monophyletic origin of the metazoa (Wainright et al., 1993), there are a number of conflicting studies and views. Furthermore, many questions remain unanswered regarding the origin, evolution, and relationships among early metazoa. In one view, flatworms may represent the earliest bilateral animals, and one possible evolutionary tree places a flatworm ancestor as a putative progenitor of a number of other invertebrates groups (see Fig. 1B). Current molecular and morphological studies on flatworms support the contention that the parasitic Platyhelminthes represent a monophyletic group (Blair, 1993; Rhode, 1990) most likely derived from other free-living flatworms. However, the possible identity of the parasitic flatworm progenitor(s) is still not certain. An understanding of the characteristics and distribution of *trans*-splicing within flatworms and early metazoan phyla might provide additional insight into the importance of this form of RNA processing in the evolution of early metazoa, flatworms, and parasitic groups of flatworms. Such studies might also provide information addressing the evolutionary or convergent origins of *trans*-splicing in early metazoa and could add to our knowledge of the importance and conservation of secondary structure, SL sequences, and other elements in *trans*-splicing metazoans.

The sequence of the *S. mansoni* spliced leader is absolutely conserved in two other human schistosomes, *S. haematobium* and *S. japonicum* (Simonsen et al., unpublished data). However, we noted from a lack of hybridization in low-stringency Northern blots that the schistosome spliced leader did not appear highly conserved in other trematodes or other members of the flatworm phylum (Rajkovic et al., 1990). Considering that all nematodes have been shown to have an absolutely conserved spliced leader and that spliced leaders within the kinetoplastida are homologous (typically > 75%–80%), the Northern blot data were somewhat unexpected. Although schistosomes exhibit many of the general characteristics of trematodes, they are unusual in several respects, including the presence of separate sexes, a relatively rare occurrence in trematodes. Considering the unusual lack of SL conservation in flatworms, we were interested in determining 1) if *trans*-splicing was absent in other trematodes and restricted only to schistosomes, 2) if *trans*-splicing was present in other nontrematode flatworms, and 3) if *trans*-splicing was present in other flatworms, then would the SLs and SL RNAs exhibit any conserved sequence elements, secondary structures, or other properties.

Trans-Splicing in the Trematode *Fasciola hepatica*

Our initial hybridization experiments suggesting a lack of sequence similarity of the schistosome spliced leader with small RNAs in other flatworms precluded the use of hybridization as a general detection method for new SL RNAs. Consequently, the development of novel methods for the identification, cloning, and characterization of SL RNAs and their genes was required to determine if *trans*-splicing is present in other members of the flatworm phylum or early metazoa. One approach we have explored involves the use of 5′ RACE to identify the terminal sequences of flatworm enolase mRNAs. These terminal sequences are then characterized and assayed to determine if they represent spliced leaders. To test the applicability of this approach, we initially examined enolase mRNAs in another trematode, *Fasciola hepatica*. We hypothesized that if the related trematode *Fasciola* lacked a spliced leader homologous to the schistosome SL, mechanisms of gene expression including *trans*-splicing might remain conserved within homologous genes of evolutionarily related organisms. If true, characterization of the 5′ terminal nucleotides of the homologous mRNA, in this case the mRNA for enolase, might then lead to the identification and characterization of an SL in *Fasciola hepatica*.

To obtain *Fasciola* enolase-specific sequences, we screened a *Fasciola hepatica* cDNA library using the schistosome enolase cDNA as a probe and isolated a cDNA corresponding to the 3′ terminal portion of the *Fasciola* enolase mRNA. Using sequences derived from the enolase cDNA, we designed *Fasciola* enolase-specific oligonucleotide primers and used them successfully in 5′ RACE to clone and determine the 5′ terminal nucleotide sequence of the *Fasciola* enolase mRNA. Complementary oligonucleotides corresponding to the enolase 5′ terminal sequence were found to hybridize to a small trimethylguanosine (TMG) precipitable RNA, a smear on poly (A)+ Northern blots, and high copy number sequences in the *Fasciola* genome. These results are typically observed when sequences corresponding to SLs are used in hybridization analyses in *trans*-splicing organisms and thus suggested that the terminal sequences of enolase might be an SL. Subsequent analyses demonstrated that the 5′ terminal sequences of the enolase mRNA are likely to be derived from a 108- nucleotide nonpolyadenylated, TMG precipitable RNA.

This RNA is transcribed from genes independently located within approximately 100 tandem repeats of ca. 1.1 kb. RNAase mapping and sequence analysis of the small RNA gene and its transcribed RNA demonstrated that the 5´ terminal 37 nucleotides of the enolase mRNA were located at the 5´ terminus of the small RNA and were immediately followed by a 5´ splice site (Davis et al., 1994a). As predicted by our original hybridization analysis, the *Fasciola* SL exhibits only 65% sequence similarity with the schistosome SL, and sequence similarity between the SL RNA intron regions is extremely low.

If the 5´ terminal 37 nucleotides on the enolase mRNA and the small RNA represent an SL exon, we predicted that the sequence should be present at the termini of other *Fasciola* mRNAs. We subsequently identified approximately 20 SL-containing cDNAs in several different cDNA libraries and demonstrated that their corresponding mRNAs contained the identical 37 nucleotide exon at their 5´ termini. It thus seems likely that the SL RNA in *Fasciola hepatica* serves as a donor substrate for the addition of the SL exon to mRNAs (Davis et al., 1994a). This reaction, by analogy with trypanosomes and nematodes, is likely to occur by *trans*-splicing. mRNAs that acquire the SL in *Fasciola*, however, represent a subset of mRNAs since other mRNAs have been characterized in *Fasciola* that are not *trans*-spliced (A. Rice-Ficht, personal communication). Based on the frequency of SL-containing cDNAs in two cDNA libraries constructed in parallel for *Fasciola* and *Schistosoma*, the percentage of *Fasciola* mRNAs with the SL is several times greater than that in schistosomes.

Conserved, Degenerate Enolase Oligonucleotides and 5´ RACE as an Assay for Spliced Leaders in Flatworms

The studies on *Fasciola hepatica* indicated that *trans*-splicing in flatworms was not restricted to schistosomes. This observation prompted us to determine further if other flatworms exhibited *trans*-splicing and if a common feature was a general lack of spliced leader sequence conservation. The presence of spliced leaders on enolase mRNAs in both trematodes and the high degree of sequence similarity among eukaryotic enolase proteins led us to explore the possiblity of designing degenerate, oligonucleotide primers corresponding to conserved regions in these proteins that could be used directly in a 5´ RACE strategy to identify the terminal sequences of other trematode or flatworm enolase mRNAs. These terminal sequences could then be compared with known flatworm spliced leaders and tested by Northern blot hybridization to determine if sequences homologous to the enolase termini were associated with a small RNA, i.e., a potential SL RNA, using methods described above.

The direct 5´ RACE strategy with conserved, degenerate oligonucleotides successfully amplified the terminal portions of three new trematode enolase mRNAs representing several orders of trematodes (Fig. 1A). Northern blot hybridizations and cloning of putative spliced leader RNA genes (cloning of spliced leader RNA genes was facilitated by using a PCR amplification strategy exploiting opposing SL primers and the organization of SL RNA genes in tandem repeats to amplify the SL RNA containing genomic repeat) from several of these trematodes indicates that the respective terminal enolase sequences appear to be derived from the 5′ ends of small RNAs and thus are likely to be spliced leaders involved in *trans*-splicing (Davis et al., 1994c).

Comparison of the *Fasciola* SL sequence with the three new trematode SL sequences demonstrated very high conservation of the spliced leaders among these four trematodes (86%–100%). These data suggest that there is typically a high degree of conservation among most trematode spliced leaders. The lack of conservation of the schistosome SL compared with other trematode SLs might be attributed to an early and/or rapid divergence of schistosomes in trematode evolution, convergent evolution within the phylum, or perhaps is in part a consequence of an increased potential for recombination and variation related to the unusual presence of separate sexes in schistosomes.

The successful use of degenerate, enolase 5′ RACE within trematodes led us to analyze several other groups of flatworms including turbellaria (free living and symbiotic) and tapeworms (representing four orders) considered to represent early and later clades within the phylum, respectively (Fig. 1A). In all flatworms examined, the degenerate, enolase 5′ RACE cloning strategy was successful in specifically amplifying enolase mRNAs. Preliminary data suggest that four tapeworms and several triclad turbellarians do not appear to *trans*-splice their enolase mRNAs. Significantly, however, data from Northern blot hybridization and sequence analyses on a polyclad turbellarian, *Stylochus zebra,* suggest that a 51 nucleotide spliced leader on the enolase mRNA is likely to be derived from an SL RNA by *trans*-splicing (Davis et al., 1994c). Interestingly, *Stylochus zebra* (the zebra flatworm is found in snail shells occupied by large hermit crabs) is one representative of early and distantly related flatworm clades that could include the ancestor of parasitic flatworms.

PHYLOGENETIC COMPARISON OF FEATURES OF SL AND SL RNA

Alignment of all the flatworm SLs and SL RNAs we have identified suggests that although they exhibit limited sequence similarity there are two extended regions of absolute sequence conservation within the 34–51 nucleotide sequences of the spliced leaders. These are shown in Figure 2.

The alignments suggest that the flatworm spliced leaders can be placed into three groups based on sequence similarity: turbellarian (*Stylochus*), schistosome, and general trematode (*Fasciola hepatica, Echinostoma caproni, Haematolechus* spp., *Stephanostonum* spp.). Pairwise comparisons of the general trematode SLs indicates that sequence similarities are 86%–100%, with

```
TGCCG                    AAAA                 GCAATA
  WACYKWNACGGTYYY     MTBYBSTGTWTMTT        RKTGCATG
```

Fig. 2.   General consensus sequence of flatworm spliced leaders. The consensus represents
the schistosome SL, four other trematode SLs, and the *Stylochus* SL. Spliced leader lengths
vary from 34 to 51 nucleotides. Bold and underlined letters represent sequences absolutely
conserved in all flatworm spliced leaders. Normal text represents the consensus nucleotides at
the respective positions. Elevated and italicized nucleotides represent sequences that are insertions or deletions of nucleotides and thus are not present in all spliced leaders.

the *Fasciola* and *Echinostoma* SLs exhibiting a 100% match. Interestingly,
the degree of sequence similarity among the trematode spliced leaders correlates well with their traditional systematic classification (Fig. 1). Optimal alignment of the turbellarian spliced leader (*Stylochus zebra*) with either the
schistosome or *Fasciola* SL (general trematode) indicates sequence identities
of only about 50%, with several large insertions and deletions required for
alignment. Sequence conservation in the 5′ splice site and several nucleotides
3′ is very high. However, sequence conservation further 3′ of the splice donor
site in flatworm SL RNAs is extremely low, analogous to that observed within
nematode or kinetoplastid SL RNAs. Overall, although flatworm SLs and SL
RNAs exhibit limited sequence and length identity, high nucleotide conservation in several short regions within the SL and SL RNA suggest that flatworm
SL RNAs are likely to be derived from a common ancestor. Notably, aside
from the 5′ splice site, the conserved residues within the flatworm SL are not
present in flagellate or nematode SL RNAs.

Bruzik et al. (1988) first noted that, although kinetoplastid and nematode
SL RNAs exhibited no sequence homology, a comparison of energy minimi-
zation derived secondary structures predicted that SL RNAs from both groups
exhibited a similar, conserved secondary structure. This structure consisted of
three stem loops with the Sm analogous region located between stems II and
III. The SL and spliced donor site are located within stem I with a loop preceding the splice donor site and the close of a loop formed by two basepaired
G residues (Fig. 3). The phylogenetic conservation of this structure suggests
that the secondary structure of the SL RNA may be important in the *trans*-
splicing process. The three stem structure is also predominantly conserved in
Euglena SL RNAs. Recent biophysical and secondary analyses of the spliced
leader RNA from *Leptomonas collosum* confirmed the general features of the
two stem loops in the 3′ half of the kinetoplastid SL RNA but suggest that the
first stem loop can exist as two alternate structures that may switch between
the two forms (LeCuyer and Crothers, 1993). The more stable form exhibits a
paired helix derived from the 5′ end sequences of the SL and the splice donor
site. Some support for the alternate 5′ paired helix structure may be derived

from studies in permeabilized cells of *T. brucei* that indicate that the 5´ splice site must be accessible for *trans*-splicing (Ullu and Tschudi, 1993).

Computer generated secondary structures for four flatworm SL RNAs indicate that the Sm-analogous region is located between two stem loops and that with the exception of the schistosome SL RNA, three stem loops are present as observed in nematode and kinetoplastid SL RNAs (Fig. 3) (Rajkovic et al., 1990; Davis et al., 1994a,c). A long stem comprised of the first 48–64 nucleotides (varying as function of the length of the SL: 34–51 bases), including the SL and splice donor site, is a universally conserved secondary structure feature in all flatworm SL RNAs, as seen for *S. mansoni* in Figure 3. This stem is contributed to by both very high sequence conservation within particular regions of the SL and the 5´ splice site of the SL RNA and other nonconserved regions which exhibit compensatory nucleotide changes to facilitate the maintenance of the stem. Although LeCuyer and Crother [LeCuyer and Crothers, 1993) suggested that potential base pairing within the *S. mansoni* SL RNA could form the alternate paired 5´ helix in their revised structure of stem I of the kinetoplastida, we have not seen conservation of such base pairing in other flatworm SL RNAs.

Bruzik et al. (1988) suggested that intramolecular basepairing of the 5´ splice site within stem I might autonomously activate the SL RNA splice donor site in *trans*-splicing, thus obviating the need for U1 snRNA required for 5´ splice site recognition in *cis*-splicing. Notably, however, the ability of the SL RNA to *trans*-splice in vitro is not affected by disruptions of basepairing in stem I of the *Ascaris* SL RNA. Furthermore, sequences in the snRNA-like domain apparently confer the determinants for *trans*-splicing on the SL RNA, and there are few sequence or length requirements on the exon sequences upstream from 5´ splice site for *trans*-splicing in vitro (Maroney et al., 1991). Thus, specific sequences within the SL and the apparent conservation of basepairing in stem loop I of the SL RNA are not absolutely necessary for *Ascaris trans*-splicing in vitro. The limited sequence conservation and variable length of the flatworm SL is perhaps a good biological illustration of the *Ascaris* in vitro experiments, implying that neither high sequence conservation nor exon size appear to be essential for *trans*-splicing in flatworms. If the general mechanism and determinants of *trans*-splicing are phylogenetically conserved in metazoa as one might expect, the conservation of the stem I structure in flatworms is not likely to be essential for *trans*-splicing. It seems unlikely, how-

Fig. 3. Comparison of possible computer-generated secondary structure predictions for representative spliced leader RNAs from flatworms, nematodes, and the kinetoplastida. All structures are generated under the constraint that the Sm-analogous region (underlined) remains single stranded. Secondary structures for *C. elegans* and *T. cruzi* were taken from Bruzik et al. (1988), the *S. mansoni* from Rajkovic et al. (1990), and *Fasciola hepatica* from Davis et al. (1994a). Arrows indicate the 5´ splice sites.

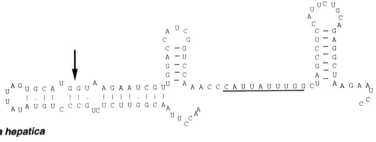

Schistosoma mansoni

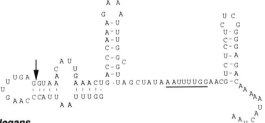

Fasciola hepatica

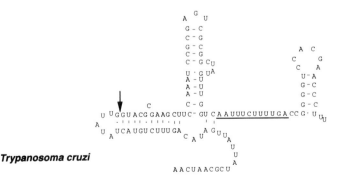

Caenorhabditis elegans

Trypanosoma cruzi

Figure 3.

ever, that the phylogenetic conservation of a 5′ stem involving the SL in all SL RNAs is fortuitous, but must contribute some essential attribute or functional importance to SL RNAs that has yet to be determined. Maroney et al. (1990) suggested that the observed absolute conservation of the nematode spliced leader sequence is not related to the *trans*-splicing reaction, but can be explained by their SL RNA transcription data, indicating that the SL sequence acts as a promoter element and is associated with the binding of transcription factors in *Ascaris*. Notably, flatworm SLs exhibit the greatest diversity in sequence and length. The limited sequence conservation in flatworm spliced leaders might be sufficient to facilitate transcription of the SL RNA, impart specific properties on recipient mRNAs, or contribute some essential attribute to the SL RNA. Although less likely, it cannot be ruled out that *trans*-splicing in flatworms may not be entirely analogous to *Ascaris* and that the secondary structure and/or limited sequence conservation observed in flatworms could be essential requirements for the *trans*-splicing reaction.

Sequences apparently analogous to the Sm antigen binding region observed in other SL RNAs appear to be present in all the flatworm SL RNAs, although they are heterogeneous in length and sequence and deviate signficantly from the $RAU_{n>3}GR$ consensus. Antisera to the human Sm antigen recognize and immunoprecipitate both U1 and U2 snRNPs in schistosome extracts, but do not precipitate the SL RNA RNP (El-Meanawy et al., 1994). In contrast, the Sm-binding region is highly conserved in nematode SL RNAs and the SL RNA RNP is effectively immunoprecipitated from nematode extracts by anti-Sm antisera (Nilsen, 1993).

Elegant experiments in the *Ascaris* in vitro system have recently demonstrated that extended basepairing (18 bases) between sequences in the U6 snRNA and the SL RNA may play an important role along with a phylogenetically conserved U2–U6 interaction in bringing the pre-mRNA and SL RNA substrates efficiently together for *trans*-splicing (Hannon et al., 1992). Cloning of the schistosome U2 and U6 snRNAs to examine for potential phylogenetic conservation of this interaction suggests that, based on visual inspection, basepairing between the schistosome U6 snRNA and the SL RNA could also occur, although the extent of basepairing is significantly less (seven bases) than that observed in *Ascaris* (El-Meanawy et al., 1994).

Several, although not all, nematodes (*Ascaris, Brugia malayi, C. elegans, Onchocerca volvulus*, and *Dirofilaria immitis*) and flagellates (*Trypanosoma vivax, Trypanosoma rangelis, Herpetomonas*, and *Euglena*) have spliced leader genes located within the same genomic tandem repeat as the 5S gene. The phylogenetic conservation of this linkage has been suggested to imply some functional significance. Interestingly, none of the flatworm SL RNAs characterized to date appear to be linked with 5S RNA genes. Whether this observation has phylogenetic implications remains to determined.

Phylogenetic Overview

The presence of a spliced leader on all trematode enolase mRNAs could be due to conservation of *trans*-splicing of the enolase locus in these organisms or merely a random consequence of the high frequency of *trans*-spliced mRNAs in trematodes. The latter seems less likely based on our estimates of the relatively low percentage of mRNAs that are *trans*-spliced in schistosomes and the absence of *trans*-splicing of enolase in several flatworm groups examined. Whether the conservation of enolase *trans*-splicing has functional implications with respect to either the enolase mRNA or *trans*-splicing in general would be interesting to know. The presence of *trans*-splicing in a clade of flatworms generally considered to be primitive suggests that *trans*-splicing may have been an ancestral feature within the phylum and present in a flatworm progenitor. The apparent absence of spliced leaders at the termini of several other flatworm enolase mRNAs we have examined (and other lower metazoan enolase mRNAs; Davis et al., unpublished observations) clearly does not imply that these metazoa lack *trans*-splicing, but only that there is a lack of conservation of *trans*-splicing of enolase in these organisms. We are currently exploring the use of oligonucleotides, corresponding to a relatively conserved region in flatworm SL RNAs, which includes the splice donor site and nucleotides 5′ and 3′ of the site, as probes for SL RNAs and as primers to PCR amplify and clone tandemly repeated SL RNAs genes from other flatworms (particularly turbellaria, monogenes, and tapeworms). These studies should provide additional information on the distribution and evolutionary history of *trans*-splicing in the phylum. Subsequent correlation of the presence and characteristics of the SL RNAs, their genes, and *trans*-splicing of enolase might also be informative in refining phylogenetic relationships among flatworms and perhaps in analyzing the origins and evolution of parasitism within the phylum.

The presence of *trans*-splicing in two distinct metazoan phyla (Nematoda and Platyhelminthes) suggests evolutionary conservation or alternatively, convergent evolution of *trans*-splicing under particular and as yet undetermined pressures. In contrast to other groups studied (i.e., the nematodes and kinetoplastida), flatworm spliced leaders appear to exhibit the least sequence or length conservation, yet it is clear that they are related and likely to be descended from a common ancestor. The lack of SL and SL RNA sequence conservation among the various groups known to undergo *trans*-splicing (flagellates, nematodes, and flatworms) makes it difficult to assess if *trans*-splicing in these various groups is related to a common ancestor. In addition, the lack of consistent phylogenetic data regarding early metazoan groups precludes accurately defining the evolutionary relationship and origins for flatworms and nematodes. Consequently, it is currently not possible to distinguish whether the differences as well as similarities among spliced leaders, the SL RNAs, and their genes indicate that *trans*-splicing has evolved from a common ancestor or if *trans*-splicing may have evolved independently in several groups with the observed similarities representing convergent evolution perhaps driven by chemical determinism (Weiner, 1993).

Our current hypothesis is that *trans*-splicing is also likely to be present in other lower metazoa (for example, sponges, cnidarians, ctenophores, and nemerterneans; see Fig. 1B), and we are currently attempting to exploit common features characteristic of spliced leaders, SL RNAs and their genes to detect, identify, and characterize *trans*-splicing in metazoa. These common features include: 1) metazoan SL RNAs typically contain a trimethyl-guanosine (TMG) cap structure; 2) the conserved SL RNA length is ~ 90–120 bases; 3) the organization of the SL RNA genes is in tandem arrays of 100–200 copies which may be linked to the 5S repeat; and 4) in known *trans*-splicing organisms, at least 10% of the mRNAs appear to acquire the spliced leader. The success and relative ease of characterizing nucleotide or amino acid sequences derived from the amplification of enolase mRNAs is also currently being explored as a phylogenetic tool in lower metazoa. Such studies in conjunction with the identification and distribution of spliced leaders, SL RNAs, SL RNA genes, and other aspects of *trans*-splicing in selected flatworm groups or lower metazoa might be useful in exploring the phylogeny of flatworms and lower metazoa as well as questions regarding the evolutionary origins and importance of *trans*-splicing in early metazoa. Perhaps, however, only with the development of systems to dissect and compare the importance of various elements associated with *trans*-splicing in metazoa other than nematodes or through carefully designed heterologous experiments in the *Ascaris* in vitro system will we resolve any questions regarding evolutionary origin and conservation of the mechanism and elements required for *trans*-splicing.

FUNCTIONAL OR BIOLOGICAL SIGNIFICANCE OF *TRANS*-SPLICING IN METAZOA

Although *trans*-splicing has been studied for several years, its biological and functional role, particularly in metazoa, remain unclear. Most, if not all, mRNAs in trypanosomes contain a 39-nucleotide SL sequence at their 5′ termini (Agabian, 1990). In contrast, in nematodes, trematodes, and *Euglena*, apparently only a subset of mRNAs contain the SL. As previously described, analyses of a small subset of mRNAs that possess an SL in *C. elegans* or in schistosomes suggest that these mRNAs or their encoded proteins do not fit into any discrete categories, nor is there any apparent tissue specific regulation of SL RNA synthesis. The TMG cap structure is retained on the nematode SL after it is donated to actin mRNAs (Doren and Hirsh, 1990; Liou and Blumenthal, 1990). The TMG cap or SL might endow *trans*-spliced mRNAs with specific properties, including effects on mRNA stability, translational efficiency, or regulation, a role in *cis*-splicing of precursor mRNAs, transport, or a compartmentalization or targeting signal. These potential effects, however, remain to be demonstrated, and to date no specific properties or effects of the SL or its cap on mRNAs have been demonstrated, with the possible exception of the role of *trans*-splicing as a capping mechanism required for mRNA stability in trypanosomes (see below).

The only evidence for a biological and functional role for *trans*-splicing is associated with its potential for two separable roles: 1) in the mechanism of capping of mRNAs and 2) for the resolution of polycistronic transcription units into individual mRNAs. At least in trypanosomes, a number of primary mRNA transcripts appear polycistronic and there is evidence that capping and maturation to monocistronic transcripts is the result, in part, of 5′ end processing via *trans*-splicing of the SL and 3′ processing via cleavage and polyadenylation (Agabian, 1990; Johnson et al., 1987; Muhich and Boothroyd, 1988; Tschudi and Ullu, 1988). Capping derived by *trans*-splicing also appears essential for mRNA stability in trypanosomes (Huang and Van der Ploeg, 1991; Ullu and Tschudi, 1991). Spieth et al. (1993) have recently proposed that a select set of *trans*-spliced mRNAs in *C. elegans* that acquire an alternate SL (SL-2) are processed from internal genes within operons that appear to produce polycistronic transcripts. They have suggested that the alternate SL-2 addition occurs only to internally located genes within such polycistronic transcription units and that this *trans*-splicing functions to resolve polycistronic transcription units. The potential contribution of *trans*-splicing to mRNA capping or processing of polycistronic transcription units in nematode genes that acquire the common SL or in *trans*-spliced flatworm genes, however, is not known. Experiments using transgenic transformation of *C. elegans* suggest that potential promotors for several *trans*-spliced genes appear to be located within several kilobases upstream from the *trans*-splice acceptor site. However, definitive identification and characterization of promotors or transcription initiation sites in either nematode or flatworm protein coding genes has not yet been done, and it remains to be determined if a general function of *trans*-splicing is associated with maturation of polycistronic transcription units in flatworms and the majority of *trans*-spliced nematode genes (Nilsen, 1993).

Transcription initiation sites for *trans*-spliced genes might be unusually heterogeneous in helminths producing 5′ untranslated regions of highly different lengths. *Trans*-splicing might then function to generate defined lengths of 5′ ends, and SL addition might ensure an appropriate translation intiation context (in relation to length, sequence, and/or secondary structure) for these mRNAs (Huang and Hirsh, 1992). Alternatively, *trans*-splicing in metazoa might simply serve as a capping mechanism conferring mRNAs with particular properties (transport, stability, translation, localization) derived from the

SL or TMG that remain to be identified. It has also been suggested that SL function might be associated with genomic location and could serve different roles for different mRNAs (Donelson and Zeng, 1990).

Maturation of cellular mRNAs by *trans*-splicing ranges from apparently 100% in the kinetoplastids, to a variable and smaller percentage in nematodes and flatworms, and finally to an apparent absence in higher invertebrates (fruit flies–Arthropods; sea urchins–Echinoderms) and vertebrates. Why more evolutionarily advanced metazoa exhibit progressively less *trans*-splicing is not known, but it seems reasonable to speculate that the reduction of *trans*-splicing in higher organisms is associated with the presence of alternate mechanisms of gene expression that have superceded the need or function of *trans*-splicing. Analysis of the distribution of *trans*-splicing and a systematic characterization and comparison of transcription units and promotors for *trans*-spliced and non-*trans*-spliced genes in lower metazoa seem essential to gain an understanding of the signficance of this mechanism of gene expression and its functional importance. In addition, a fundamental understanding of the properties of translation in these metazoa and the translation of *trans*-spliced mRNAs might also help to uncover the signficance of *trans*-splicing. Although much progress has been made in understanding the potential mechanism for discrimination of splice acceptor sites used for *cis*- or *trans*-splicing in nematodes, much remains to be determined concerning the temporal relationship of the processing events of *cis*- and *trans*-splicing and polyadenylation and the regulatory interplay of transcriptional and post-transcriptional processes in determining steady state levels of *trans*-spliced mRNAs in metazoan cells. Without the development of functional assay systems in flatworms or other metazoa, it is likely that only the powerful combination of genetics, DNA transformation, and in vitro transcription and splicing systems available in nematodes will continue to contribute to our understanding of the mechanisms of *trans*-splicing and provide the answers to the enigma of the function of *trans*-splicing in metazoa.

ACKNOWLEDGMENTS

This work was done in part by students participating in the molecular biology section of the Biology of Parasitism course during the summers of 1992 and 1993. Their enthusiasm and contributions to this work are gratefully acknowledged. I thank the members of my laboratory at San Francisco State University for their many and signficant contributions to this work and Karen Wassarman and Lee Niswander for their helpful comments on the manuscript. This work was supported in part by the Office of Research and Sponsored Programs at San Francisco State University and by grant A1327709 from the National Institutes of Health.

REFERENCES

Agabian N (1990): *Trans*-splicing of nuclear pre-mRNAs. Cell 61:1157–1160.

Bektesh S, Van Doren K, Hirsh D (1988): Presence of the *Caenorhabditis elegans* spliced leader on different mRNAs and in different genera of nematodes. Genes Dev 2:1277–1283.

Blair D (1993): The phylogenetic position of the aspidobothrea within the parasitic flatworms inferred from ribosomal RNA sequence data. Int J Parasitol 23:169–178.

Blumenthal T (1993): Mammalian cells can *trans*-splice. But do they? BioEssays 15:347–348.

Blumenthal T, Thomas J (1988): *Cis* and *trans* mRNA splicing in *C. elegans*. Trends Genet 4:305–308.

Boothroyd JC (1985): Antigenic variation in African trypanosomes. Annu Rev Microbiol 39:475–502.

Borst P (1986): Discontinuous transcription and antigenic variation in trypanosomes. Annu Rev Biochem 55:701–732.

Bruzik JP, Van Doren K, Hirsh D, Steitz JA (1988): *Trans* splicing involves a novel form of small nuclear ribonucleoprotein particles. Nature 335:559–562.

Conrad R, Liou RF, Blumenthal T (1993): Conversion of a *trans*-spliced gene in *C. elegans* into a conventional gene by introduction of a splice donor site. EMBO J 12:1249–1255.

Conrad R, Thomas J, Spieth J, Blumenthal T (1991): Insertion of part of an intron into the 5′ untranslated region of a *Caenorhabditis elegans* gene converts it into a *trans*-spliced gene. Mol Cell Biol 11:1921–1926.

Davis RE, Singh H, Botka C, Hardwick C, Meanawy A, Villanueva J (1994a): RNA trans-splicing in *Fasciola hepatica*: Identification of an SL RNA and spliced leader sequences on mRNAs. J Biol Chem 269:20026–20031.

Davis RE, Singh H, Hardwick C, Rajkovic A, Rottman F, Villanueva J (1994b): Organization and analysis of *trans*-spliced genes in the human parasite *Schistosoma mansoni*. Manuscript in preparation.

Davis RE, Villanueva J, Botka C, Hardwick C (1994c): *Trans*-splicing in an early clade of flatworms: Analysis of conserved features in flatworm SL RNAs. Manuscript in preparation.

Donelson JE, Zeng W (1990): A comparison of *trans*-RNA splicing in trypanosomes and nematodes. Parasitol Today 6:327–333.

Doren KV, Hirsh D (1990): mRNAs that mature through *trans*-splicing in *Caenorhabditis elegans* have a trimethylguanosine at their 5′ termini. Mol Cell Biol 10:1769–1772.

dos Reis MG, Davis RE, Singh H, Skelly P, Shoemaker CB (1993): Characterization of the *Schistosoma mansoni* gene encoding the glycolytic enzyme, triosephosphate isomerase. Mol Biochem Parasitol 59:235–242.

El-Meanawy MA, Davis RE, Rajkovic A, Rottman FM (1994): *Schistosoma mansoni*: Characterization of U1, U2, and U6 small nuclear RNAs. Manuscript submitted.

Hannon G, Maroney PA, Yu Y-T, Hannon GE, Nilsen TW (1992): Interaction of U6 snRNA with a sequence required for function of the nematode SL RNA in *trans*-splicing. Science 258:1775–1780.

Huang J, Van der Ploeg HT (1991): Maturation of polycistronic pre-mRNA in *Trypanosoma brucei*: Analysis of *trans*-splicing and poly (A) addition at nascent RNA transcripts from the hsp70 locus. Mol Cell Biol 11:3180–3190.

Huang X-Y, Hirsh D (1992): RNA *Trans*-splicing. In: Setlow JK, ed. Gen Eng 14:211–229.

Johnson PJ, Kooter JM, Borst P (1987): Inactivation of transcription by UV irradiation of *T. brucei* provides evidence for a multicistronic transcription unit including a VSG gene. Cell 51:273–281.

Laird PW (1989): *Trans*-splicing in trypanosomes—archaism or adaptation? Trends Genet 5:204–208.

LeCuyer KA, Crothers DM (1993): The *Leptomonas collosum* spliced leader RNA can switch between two alternate structural forms. Biochemistry 32:5301–5311.

Liou R-F, Blumenthal T (1990): *Trans*-spliced *Caenorhabditis elegans* mRNAs retain trimethylguanosine caps. Mol Cell Biol 10:1764–1768.

Maroney PA, Hannon GJ, Nilsen TW (1990): Transcription and cap trimethylation of a nematode spliced leader RNA in a cell-free system. Proc Natl Acad Sci USA 87:709–713.

Maroney PA, Hannon GJ, Shambaugh JD, Nilsen TW (1991): Intramolecular base pairing between the nematode spliced leader and its 5´ splice site is not essential for *trans*-splicing in vitro. EMBO J 10:3869–3875.

Muhich MJ, Boothroyd JC (1988): Polycistronic transcripts in trypanosomes and their accumulation during heat shock: Evidence for a precursor role in mRNA synthesis. Mol Cell Biol 8:3837–3846

Nilsen TW (1989): *Trans*-splicing in nematodes. Exp Parasitol 69:413–416.

Nilsen TW (1992): *Trans*-splicing in protozoa and helminths. Infect Agents Dis 1:212–218.

Nilsen TW (1993): *Trans*-splicing of nematode pre-messenger RNA. Annu Rev of Microbiol 47:413–440.

Rajkovic A, Davis RE, Simonsen JN, Rottman FM (1990): A spliced leader is present on a subset of mRNAs from the human parasite *Schistosoma mansoni*. Proc Natl Acad Sci USA 87:8879–8883.

Rhode K (1990): Phylogeny of platyhelminthes, with special reference to parasitic groups. Int J Parasitol 20:979–1007.

Spieth J, Brooke G, Kuersten S, Lea K, Blumenthal T (1993): Operons in *C. elegans*: Polycistronic mRNA precursors are processed by *trans*-splicing of SL2 to downstream coding regions. Cell 73:521–532.

Tschudi C, Ullu E (1988): Polygene transcripts are precursors to calmodulin mRNAs in trypanosomes. EMBO J 7:455–463.

Ullu E, Tschudi C (1991): *Trans*-splicing in trypanosomes requires methylation of the 5´ end of the spliced leader RNA. Proc Natl Acad Sci USA 88:10074–10078.

Ullu E, Tschudi C (1993): 2´-*O*-methyl RNA oligonucleotides identify two functional elements in the trypanosome spliced leader ribonucleoprotein particle. J Biol Chem 268:13068–13073.

Wainright PO, Hinkle G, Sogin ML, Stickel SK (1993); Monophyletic origins of the metazoa: An evolutionary link with fungi. Science 260:340–342.

Weiner AM (1993): mRNA splicing and autocatalytic introns: Distant cousins or the products of chemical determinism. Cell 72:161–164.

Molecular Approaches to Parasitology, pages 321–340
© 1995 Wiley-Liss, Inc.

Ascaris and *Caenorhabditis*: Complementary Organisms for Studying Germline Determination

Deborah L. Roussell, Michael E. Gruidl, Monique A. Kreutzer, James P. Richards, and Karen L. Bennett

Department of Molecular Microbiology and Immunology, School of Medicine, University of Missouri, Columbia, Missouri 65212

INTRODUCTION

Ascaris has many strengths for studying the specification of cell lineages. These strengths have been recognized for over 100 years. In the nineteenth century the biologist Theodor Boveri both observed and tested several aspects of *Ascaris* biology. He was first to verify Weissman's theory of the constancy of the genome in describing the phenomenon of chromatin diminution (Boveri, 1887), the selective loss of significant portions of the genome from all the cells of the early ascarid embryo that will become somatic lineages, with the genome of the germline remaining constant. The chapter in this volume by F. Müller and colleagues describes the current molecular understanding of the diminution process, with the resulting remodeling of the chromosomes and addition of new telomeres. Our chapter deals with the question of how the nematode germline cell lineage is established ("determined") by the 28–32-cell stage of the developing embryo. We have approached this question of development using the swine parasite *Ascaris lumbricoides* var. *suum* and the free-living soil nematode *Caenorhabditis elegans* as complementary organisms for molecular, biochemical, and genetic analyses.

BACKGROUND TO *ASCARIS* BIOLOGY

Ascaris offers significant biochemical advantages for germline studies. The female *A. lumbricoides* worm lays an estimated 250,000 eggs per day. These eggs are laid fertilized and uncleaved. They develop into infectious eggs containing pre-hatching larvae in the external environment. This development occurs over an extended period of time (18–30 days, depending on the ambient temperature). (Readers are referred to the chapter by Müller for a more complete description of the parasite's biology.) Investigators wishing to use synchronous stages of embryos have only to dissect uterine tissue from the female, digest the uterine wall with a hypochlorite solution, and incubate the eggs at room temperature, preferably with good aeration and gentle shaking. Often an acid or base (0.1N HCl, H_2SO_4 or NaOH) is used to discourage bacterial contamination. After an initial lag of a day or more, the eggs proceed to divide synchronously, approximately twice a day. The individuals in a population are not strictly synchronous; they may vary by one cleavage or more. Hundreds of grams of these staged embryos are easily obtained. Dissected uteri can be stored for over a year at 4°C with little loss in embryonic viability, necessitating far fewer trips to the abbatoir than needed by those researchers who require fresh adult tissue. Nuclei from early embryos, shown in Figure 1C, have been very useful in our laboratory for run-on transcription assays, establishing that even four- to eight-cell embryos are transcriptionally active and that they are already producing the spliced leader (SL1) RNA needed for the *trans*-splicing reaction (Cleavinger et al., 1989; Nilsen et al., 1989). In addition, adult tissue can be dissected and frozen at −80°C for later use in protein or RNA extractions. Thus *Ascaris* offers great advantages over *Caenorhabditis* for biochemical studies. *Caenorhabditis*, a 1 mm worm, lays only five to six hundred eggs in its 17 day life span (average of 4 days of egg laying), and, importantly, the embryos are in various early stages of development when laid, making synchronous embryonic preparations impossible. Because of the small size of all stages of the worm, individual tissue preparations are not possible with *Caenorhabditis*.

CAENORHABDITIS AS A MODEL

Caenorhabditis is amenable to both classic and molecular genetics. Because this worm is transparent throughout its entire life span, each cell division, which is invariant in the wild-type animal, has been painstakingly recorded; thus the entire cell lineage from fertilized egg to adult is known (Sulston and Horvitz, 1977; Sulston et al., 1983). Most of the *Caenorhabditis* genome of 1×10^8 bp (*Ascaris* is $\sim 3 \times 10^8$ bp after diminution) has been ordered onto a series of overlapping cosmids and more recently onto yeast artificial chromosomes (YACs) (Coulson et al., 1986, 1991), such that when one identifies a piece of genomic DNA of interest, it can usually be physically mapped with the use of a grid of ~950 overlapping YACs. Genomic clones can be more precisely mapped by sending them off to the laboratory of A. Coulson at the MRC, in Cambridge, England, where their restriction diges-

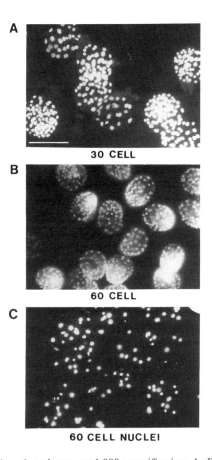

Fig. 1.   Synchronous *Ascaris* embryos at ×1,000 magnification. **A:** Diamidinophenylindole (DAPI)–stained embryos at ~30-cell stage prior to disruption. Bar = 50 μm. **B:** ~60–cell embryos. **C:** DAPI-stained isolated nuclei from the ~60-cell embryos. A Zeiss Auxioplan microscope with an epifluorescent filter was used for the photomicroscopy. In each stage, some embryos are approximately one division removed from the reported average. (Reproduced from Cleavinger et al., 1989.)

tion "fingerprints" are compared with those in the set of overlapping cosmids. The YAC grids and the cosmid physical mapping service are available to all worm researchers. Map positions of all identified genes on the growing physical map are then added to the computer networks, the Worm Community System, and ACEDB, a *C. elegans* data base. An example of one small section of the physical map is shown in Figure 2 for a region of chromosome 1 (*C. elegans* has five autosomes and an X chromosome; *A. lumbricoides* has 23 sets of

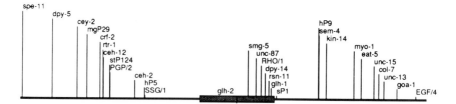

Fig. 2. The physical map of LGI, chromosome 1, of the nematode *Caenorhabditis elegans*, as displayed in ACEDB (a *C. elegans* data base). The physical map locations of the two germline helicases *glh-1* and *glh-2* are shown.

chromosomes). Two of the genes discussed in this text, *glh-1* and *glh-2*, are found ~100–200 kb apart in this region of the genome (Fig. 2). In *Caenorhabditis*, many regions of the genome have been genetically analyzed using saturation mutagenesis to identify essential genes. For example, in the region of chromosome 1 near the *dumpy-14 (dpy-14)* gene (Fig. 2), the Rose laboratory at the University of British Columbia in Vancouver has isolated 37 mutations that are lethal at some stage in the worm's development (McKim et al., 1992). The availability of lethal mutations from many regions of the genome often provides candidate mutants for newly cloned genes, as will be discussed for two of the genes we have cloned, *glh-1* and *cyclin B*.

The use of *Ascaris* and *Caenorhabditis* as complementary organisms depends on the similarity of their genes and proteins. While a good geologic record for nematode species does not exist, estimates of the evolutionary distance between the two species have been made by comparing the DNA sequences of the entire mitochondrial genomes for each. The estimates suggest a rather recent divergence of 80 million years (Okimoto et al., 1992). In the admittedly limited subset of nucleic acid and antibody probes tested in our laboratory, DNA cross hybridization and antibody reactivity is by far the rule rather than the exception (eg., Figs. 3,4).

P-GRANULES

In all higher eukaryotes thus far examined, the embryonic precursor cells that will become the adult germline contain nonmembranous granules of electron-dense material that is germline specific. These granules have been reported in nematodes (Wolf et al., 1983) and have been named P-granules because in *Caenorhabditis* they are specifically localized to the P_4 cell, the one cell of the 28 cell embryo that, as the germline precursor, is destined to produce all the eggs and sperm in the adult animal. The P_4 cell will divide once to yield the Z_2 and Z_3 cells; then later in development these two cells will

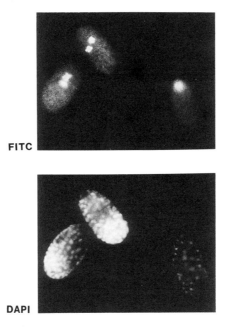

Fig. 3. *Ascaris* anti-P-granule antibodies cross-react with the P-granules of *Caenorhabditis*.
Top: Three *C. elegans* embryos reacted with the monoclonal antibody, Asc 30, followed by a
goat-antimouse fluorescein (FITC)–conjugated secondary antibody. **Bottom:** The same embryos stained with DAPI, which stains the nuclei. The youngest embryo, on the right, is at the
~28–32 cell stage. The two embryos on the left are postgastrulation, and the P$_4$ cell has already
divided to produce the two daughter germline precursor cells, Z$_2$ and Z$_3$.

proliferate mitotically and finally undergo meiotic divisions. In the fruit fly,
Drosophila melanogaster, similar germline-specific granules are called *polar
granules*, as they are found in the posteriorly localized germline precursors,
the pole cells. In mammals the material is called by the French word *nuage*,
because it looks like clouds surrounding the nuclei of the mammalian germline
precursor cells. There is evidence from *Drosophila* that these granules are more
than just markers of the germline. Mutations that result in missing or reduced
numbers of polar granules produce agametic adults, with no eggs or sperm.
These mutations have a *grandchildless* phenotype. Because the components
of the germ granules are supplied by the mother to the embryo, a homozygous
mutant *grandchildless* embryo from a heterozygous mother still has granules
and is fertile, but there are no further generations, no grandchildren, and the F$_3$
generation is sterile. Several *grandchildless* mutations in *Drosophila* (*vasa*,
oskar, *tudor*, *valois*, *staufen*, and *mago nashi*) have been reported; mutations

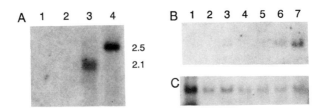

Fig. 4. Developmental expression of *glh-1*. RNAs from various nematode tissues and stages of the life cycle were analyzed using a 2.3 kb, gel-purified, and [³²P]labeled *glh-1* cDNA. **A:** Each lane contains 3 µg of poly(A)⁺ RNA from lanes 1–3, *A. lumbricoides* var. *suum* gut tissue (lane 1), male gonadal tissue (lane 2), and ovarian tissue (lane 3); and lane 4, *C. elegans* mixed stage worms. RNA sizes were estimated from the mobility of an RNA ladder (BRL, Gaithersburg, MD.) **B:** Each lane contains 10 µg of *C. elegans* total RNA: lane 1, embryonic RNA; lanes 2–6, first larval (L1), second larval (L2), dauer, third larval (L3), and fourth larval (L4) stage RNA; and lane 7, adult RNA. **C:** As a control, the Northern blot in **B** was also hybridized to a [³²P]labeled *Caenorhabditis* heat shock protein (HSP70) cloned DNA; HSP70 RNA levels are fairly constant in all but the embryonic stage when levels are higher, as previously observed (Reproduced from Roussell and Bennett, 1993, with permission of the publisher.)

in any one of these genes result in polar granules being reduced or missing (Lasko and Ashburner, 1988; Hay et al., 1988b; Kim-Ha et al., 1991; Ephrussi et al., 1991; Golumbeski et al., 1991; Schubach and Wieschaus, 1986; St Johnston et al., 1991; Boswell et al., 1991). Unfortunately, genetic screens in mutagenized *Caenorhabditis* to look for F₃ sterile animals have revealed none that show reduced or missing P-granules, although an interesting class of *maternal effect sterile* (*mes*) mutants was detected (Capowski et al., 1991). Because the main focus of our laboratory is on defining the components of the nematode P-granules, with the goal of understanding the role these granules may play in the early determination of the germline cell lineage, we began with a reverse genetics approach.

Polar and P-granules contain RNA as well as protein. Over 20 years ago A. Mahowald (1971) reported RNA staining in the polar granules; similar staining has been observed for the nematode P-granules by D. Albertson, MRC, Cambridge (personal communication). Several polar granule components including *oskar*, *staufen*, and *germ cell-less* (Kim-Ha et al., 1991; St Johnston et al., 1991; Jongens et al., 1992) localize as RNAs to the posterior of the *Drosophila* oocyte, where the polar granules are forming. Cyclin B RNA also localizes to the polar granules in the posterior of the oocyte. This concentration of cyclin B RNA in the polar granules was found, not by genetics, but by in situ hybridization in the laboratory of D. Glover (Whitfield et al., 1989). We are interested in identifying the RNAs as well as the proteins that localize to the nematode P-granules.

THE SEARCH FOR P-GRANULE GENES

The Antibody Approach

We began by producing monoclonal antibodies from protein homogenates of *Ascaris* embryos. (Such an approach had been previously reported with *Caenorhabditis* embryonic protein by S. Strome while in the laboratory of W. Wood [Strome and Wood, 1983]). The spleens from two immunized mice were fused with myeloma cells, and multiple independent hybridoma lines were carried out by the class of 1985 of the Biology of Parasitism course at the MBL while one of us (K.L.B.) was a student in the course. Once established, each line was tested for reactivity against *Ascaris* egg protein, and several of the most positive lines were successively cloned (thanks to the expertise of one of the course instructors, Dr. M. Strand of the School of Medicine, Johns Hopkins University). The antibody supernatants were later tested by immunocytochemistry for specificity of binding to the *Caenorhabditis* P-granules. Eight lines were found that bound P-granules with varying levels of background staining. The Asc 30, an IgM antibody, is shown in Figure 3 binding to three *Caenorhabditis* embryos in the top panel as detected with an FITC-conjugated secondary antibody. The nuclei of the same embryos are shown stained with DAPI at the bottom. For the youngest embryo, on the right, the P_4 cell is recognized by Asc 30. For the two older embryos on the left, the Z_2 and Z_3 cells are detected. Unfortunately, neither the bank of antibodies produced by the Wood group nor those of our own, have yet proven useful in attempts to isolate the genes encoding the cognate P-granule components recognized by the antibodies. Therefore, after several unsuccessful attempts using our monoclonal antibodies, we decided to try other approaches.

The Polymerase Chain Reaction Approach

In the last few years, genes encoding several of the components of the *Drosophila* polar granules have been reported. These include *vasa*, *tudor*, *staufen*, *germ cell-less*, and *oskar*. Of these, most are new or "pioneer" proteins; only the sequence of the predicted vasa protein indicates that it belongs to a known family of proteins, that of the RNA binding helicases (Nielsen et al., 1985; Hirling et al., 1989; Company et al., 1991). That vasa, the first germ granule component to be identified, is a putative RNA helicase fits well with the proposed role of the germ granules in binding RNAs. RNA helicases contain seven conserved motifs, two of which are necessary ATP binding sites. The function of the other conserved helicase domains is less clear, although RNA and DNA helicases differ only in that motif 1a is unique to RNA helicases and that motif 2 uniquely contains the amino acids D-E-A-D/H. This "DEAD/H box" has been shown by mutational analysis to be critical for RNA helicase function (Schmid and Linder, 1991). The known or predicted functions of various RNA helicases include binding to RNA to unwind secondary structure. The best studied RNA helicase is eIF-4A, an enzyme that binds to the cap of all mRNAS, facilitating their translation. Other helicases have roles, largely undefined, in splicing and in cell growth. One distinct subfamily of these helicases, based on sequence relatedness outside the helicase domains, includes vasa, which is expressed during *Drosophila* oogenesis (Lasko and Ashburner, 1988; Hay et al., 1988b); PL-10 from the mouse, which is expressed exclusively during spermatogenesis (Leroy et al., 1989); An3, a putative helicase that localizes to the animal pole in the frog *Xenopus* oocyte (Gururajan et al., 1991); and Ded1, a gene from the yeast *Saccharomyces* believed to participate in splicing (de Valoir et al., 1991). It is not clear how vasa functions in the polar granules, but it is possible that the protein facilitates the translation of germline-specific RNAs at some time in development. Certainly many other roles could be postulated, and the function may be specific to the germline.

We decided to clone the family of RNA helicases from *Caenorhabditis*, using the polymerase chain reaction (PCR), with primers designed from conserved helicase motifs 1a and 2, using the *C. elegans* codon bias. For ease in subsequent cloning, end-linked restriction enzyme sites were designed into these primers. Three major PCR bands were detected using *C. elegans* genomic DNA (introns are often very small in *C. elegans*) and individual cloned PCR fragments were sequenced. One of our PCR products was the *C. elegans* eIF-4A equivalent, CeIF (Roussell and Bennett, 1992). Another product, rhel-1, most closely matched the *vasa*/PL-10 subgroup and was used to isolate multiple cDNAS, coding for two genes in *Caenorhabditis*, *glh-1* and *glh-2*. The first report of the cloning and analysis of *glh-1* expression has recently been published (Roussell and Bennett, 1993); because none of the cDNAS isolated for *glh-2* are full length, information regarding this gene is still unpublished. Several unique features of the glh-1 predicted protein and its 3´ untranslated region (UTR) are discussed below.

Using similar PCR strategies, the *cyclin A* and *B* genes from *Caenorhabditis* have also been cloned in our laboratory. Cyclin A and B proteins are involved in cell cycle regulation, in the S phase for cyclin A and at the G2/M transition for cyclin A and B. In the last few years, cyclins have been the object of intense study by many laboratories. The *cyclin A* and the two *B*-like genes of *Caenorhabditis* that we have isolated are very similar to those of the cyclins from other organisms, with a conserved "cyclin box" (e.g., Tachibana et al., 1990). A unique feature of many nematode genes, including the cyclins, is that at least two of the nematode cyclin RNAs appear to be processed with the addition of the spliced leader, SL1, by *trans*-splicing (J.P. Richards and M.A. Kreutzer, unpublished results). The "destruction box," a sequence of 9–10 amino acids necessary for periodic destruction of the cyclin protein at each round of cell division (Glotzer et al., 1991), is also somewhat unusual in *C. elegans* in containing a proline, as well as other amino acid changes that are conserved between the *C.elegans cyclin A1* and *B* cDNAs. Like the *glh* genes discussed below, the 3′ UTRs of the nematode cyclin genes contain multiple potential regulatory motifs. The *Caenorhabditis glh-1* gene, as well as the three *Caenorhabditis* cyclin genes we have studied, all cross hybridize to *Ascaris* at moderate stringency. Potential cyclin genes have been cloned from an *Ascaris* ovarian cDNA library we constructed; the *Ascaris glh*-like genes have not yet been sought.

Sequence analysis of the *glh-1* cDNA, GenBank acsession No. L19948, and of the predicted glh-1 protein reveals that glh-1 contains all seven conserved helicase motifs and that the predicted protein matches vasa and PL-10 with about 43% identity and 57% similarity. In contrast, it matches eIF-4A with only 24% identity, and RNA helicases in other subfamilies match no better than eIF-4A. Thus glh-1 is most like the proteins in the vasa/PL-10 subfamily. In addition, the N terminus of the glh-1 predicted protein contains five tandem repeats of a glycine-rich sequence; vasa is the only other helicase with tandem glycine repeats of which there are also five; however, in vasa the repeats are 7 amino acids long with a charged arginine residue, while the repeats in glh-1 are 10 amino acids long and are uncharged. Other RNA helicases have glycine-rich regions, but no repeats. Southern blots probed with this 5′-most region of *glh-1* to genomic DNA only detect the *glh-1* gene. In addition, our two glh helicases are unique among RNA helicase genes in that they possess retroviral-type zinc fingers. Similar zinc fingers in the retroviral nucleic acid binding (NBP) proteins have been shown to bind RNA (Delahunty et al., 1992). A cellular sterol hormone binding protein has also been reported to have zinc fingers of this type (Rajavashisth et al., 1989). glh-1 has four of these zinc fingers in the N-terminal region of the predicted protein (Roussell and Bennett, 1993).

TISSUE AND DEVELOPMENTAL REGULATION OF *glh-1* EXPRESSION

Extensive Northern analyses of *glh-1* expression have revealed that expression of *glh-1* correlates with the presence of mitotic germ cell precursors, oocytes, and sperm, indicating it may be a germline-specific helicase (Roussell and Bennett, 1993). However, we cannot rule out the possibility of low levels of somatically derived *glh-1* message, or the possibility that the high levels of *glh-1* message detected in the germline might be coming from the somatic gonad, dependent on signals from the germline. Figure 4A shows the 2.3 kb *glh-1* message in mixed stage *Caenorhabditis* poly(A)$^+$ RNA, (lane 4); poly(A)$^+$ RNA from various dissected *Ascaris* tissues (intestine, male testis, and ovaries) were also tested, lanes 1–3. Rather stringent hybridizations for all panels of Figure 4 were carried out at 65°C, with washes to O.5 × SSPE, 65°C. A 2.1 kb *glh-1*-like message is readily detected in *Ascaris* ovarian RNA (Fig. 4, lane 3); upon very long exposure, a similar-sized message is seen in the male tissue (not shown). No message can be detected in the intestine or in the L1/L2 larval RNA tested, even upon longer exposures (not shown). Thus the *Ascaris* results indicate the *glh-1*-like gene produces an ovarian message, with the presence of *glh-1* in male tissue perhaps indicating low levels of expression in the proliferating mitotic germ cells, or in sperm. Vasa protein and RNA are also detected at low levels in *Drosophila* male tissue (Hay et al., 1988a). To look at expression of *glh-1* in *Caenorhabditis*, a developmental time course of total *Caenorhabditis* mRNA has been examined for *glh-1* expression (Fig. 4B). (The blot was kindly provided by Drs. B. Dalley and M. Golomb, University of Missouri.) *glh-1* expression is very faintly detected in the *C. elegans* L3 stage RNA (lane 5), with the signal being slightly stronger in the L4 (lane 6), and most strongly detected in the adult (lane 7). This time frame correlates with the beginning of germline proliferation in the L3, the formation of mature sperm in L4, and the switch to oogenesis in the young hermaphrodite adult, with mitotic germline proliferation continuing throughout the adult life of the worm.

There are many mutant strains in *Caenorhabditis* that manifest defects in the germline. We looked at levels of expression of *glh-1* in four mutant strains for which temperature sensitive alleles are available. Grown at the permissive temperature, 15°C, these worms are wild type; at the restrictive temperature, 25°C, their germlines are defective, while all of the somatic tissues, including the gonad, appear normal (Austin and Kimble, 1987; Beanan and Strome, 1992; Spence et al., 1990). When *glh-1* was tested with poly(A)$^+$ RNAs extracted from these strains, in each case the levels of *glh-1* varied as expected for a germline transcript. That is, in mutants with excess oocytes or sperm the levels of *glh-1* message were elevated, while in the *germline proliferation* (glp) strains *glp-1* and *glp-4*, greatly reduced, although detectable, *glh-1* levels were found (Roussell and Bennett, 1993) (Fig. 5). The worms used for extracting RNAs for the *glp* strains were older adults that were monitored by Nomarski microscopy to assure ourselves that the proliferation phenotype had not been lost in our growing large liquid cultures of the strains. The strains were provided by Drs. J. Kimble, S. Strome, and the *C. elegans* Stock Center at the University of Missouri (for details, see Roussell and Bennett, 1993). Older *glp-4* mutants slowly accumulate more germ cell precursors, but never produce eggs or sperm; *glp-1* animals prematurely enter meiosis and produce a few mature sperm. Thus the small amount of *glh-1* observed could be accounted for by the numbers of remaining germ cell precursors or sperm in these *glp* strains.

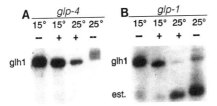

Fig. 5. Different polyadenylated forms of *glh-1* RNA in the *glp-4* and *glp-1* mutants. RNAs from *glp-4* and *glp-1* mutant worms grown at permissive (15°C) or restrictive (25°C) temperature were hybridized to excess oligo dT and digested with RNase H. Treated (+) RNA samples were compared with untreated (–) control RNAs by northern blot analysis. Each lane contains 3 μg of poly(A)$^+$ RNA from either *glp-4* mutant worms (**A**) or *glp-1* mutant worms (**B**). The gel-purified and [^{32}P]labeled hybridization probes were the 2.3 kb *glh-1* cDNA (**A**) and the 5′-most 300 bp fragment of the *glh-1* cDNA (a *glh-1* specific probe) and the esterase cDNA (control) (**B**) (McGhee et al., 1990). **B** required a longer exposure to detect the *glh-1* RNAs with the smaller, 300 bp probe. (Reproduced from Roussell and Bennett, 1993, with permission of the publisher.)

We also noticed, to our surprise, that some of the *glh-1* RNA in both of the nonpermissive *glp* mutant RNAs was of a larger size, particularly for *glp-4* (Fig. 5). The larger *glh-1* messages shown in Figure 5 could have been due to various causes, including the use of different promoters, differential splicing, or different polyadenylation states. We have established that the larger species seen in both the *glp* mutant strains is due to differences in the polyadenylation state of the *glh-1* RNA. Using oligo dT hybridization, followed by RNAse H digestion, which digests RNA in a double-stranded RNA/DNA hybrid, the *glh-1* mRNA from both *glp* animals grown at 25°C is reduced to the same-sized A$^-$ message as that seen for the *glp* animals grown at 15°C (compare lanes 2 and 3, Fig. 5A,B). The experiment was repeated (Fig. 5B) with the small *glh-1*-specific probe to assure ourselves that the differences seen were due to *glh-1* and not to cross–hybridization to *glh-2*. We also included several somatic probes as controls. The gut esterase gene (McGhee et al., 1990) (Fig. 5B), as well as two other somatic probes tested, (pharyngeal myosin [Miller et al., 1986] and vitellogenin [Spieth and Blumenthal, 1985] [results not shown]) showed no differences in adenylation state in these germline-defective RNAs.

In examining the ~150 nt 3′ UTRs of *glh-1* and *glh-2*, we noticed that each contains multiple copies of two "elements" that have been reported in other organisms to affect adenylation state and to regulate translation, (Fig. 6). These elements are the adenylation control element (ACE) and the *nos* response element (NRE) (Wharton and Struhl, 1991; Huarte et al., 1992). Neither have been rigorously defined as being sufficient for their observed function. In the oocytes of the mouse and *Xenopus*, UT-rich ACE sequences, consensus glh1   TAGAAAACCGACCAATTGATAGTGTTCGCATTTATTAAATGCTGTCAGTT.......CCCCCAATATTTATCCTGCCCTTGTTGTTGATTTTAATTGTA....

       ***   :: : : : :   :   :   ::::: :: ::: ::::: :::: ::::

glh2   TAGATGTATCTGCATATCCTTCAAATGTTGTCCATATTGTATCAGTAAATTATAATGCCCCCTTTTTATATTCTCCTTATCATG..TAAATGTTCTATT

glh1   ......TTTGTTGGTGTTGGTTGTCGTTATAGTC....CTCGCCGCA.TAACTCTGTTCAATA$_n$

      :::: :::::::   :: ::::::: :::

glh2   GATTTTTGCTGGTGTAAAACGTTTTTATAGTAGTAAATCCTCCACAGTGAATTGTAAATTGTATCAAAACAAGACATTGATTAAATTGTTCGAGACTTA$_n$

Fig. 6. The 3' untranslated regions of *glh-1* and *glh-2* are compared with one another (double dots). Both are short (*glh-1* is 138 nt before the poly(A) tail, *glh-2* is 200 nt). Each contains two potential ACE elements (boxed) and three bipartite potential NRE elements (ovals). One NRE in *glh-2* is an exact 11/11 nt match with those reported in *bicoid* and *hunchback*; the other five match 9–10/11nt. The sequence of *glh-2* is still preliminary. (Wharton and Struhl, 1991.)

A/UU$_4$AA/U, are implicated in an initial deadenylation of the targeted maternal message (which has received a long poly(A) tail in the nucleus). This deadenlyation results in storage of the message and translational repression. Later when the message is needed during oocyte maturation or during embryogenesis, the message is readenylated and translated. It is known that the poly(A) signal is needed in combination with the ACE sequence for this readenylation step. These regulatory deadenylations–readenlyations are carried out in the cytoplasm (another name for these same elements is cytoplasmic polyadenylation elements, CPES). ACE motifs have been tested in the mouse tPA gene (Huarte et al., 1992). The 3′ UTRs of *glh-1* and *glh-2* each contain two potential ACE elements, (Fig. 6), while the *cyclin* RNAs, also likely to be maternal transcripts, each have one or more potential ACE elements in their 3′ UTRs (J.P. Richards and M.A. Kreutzer, unpublished results). However, we have not yet tested these elements for function in the *glh* or *cyclin* genes; therefore, the adenylation differences shown for *glh-1* in Figure 5 may or may not be due to the presence of ACE sequences. NRE elements are less well studied; they have only been recently reported in the literature, and in both cases for *Drosophila* (Wharton and Struhl, 1991; Dalby and Glover, 1993). As first described, NRE elements are found in two maternal anteriorly localized RNAs, *hunchback* and *bicoid*, both of which have been shown to be repressed by the posterior morphogenic protein *nanos (nos)*. The RNAs of *hunchback* and *bicoid* are perceptibly shorter when *nanos* protein is present (Wharton and Struhl, 1991). Recently the posteriorly localized cyclin B RNA from *Drosophila* has also been shown to be translationally repressed; that repression is relieved when an NRE-like element is removed from the cyclin B 3′ UTR (Dalby and Glover, 1993). The *glh-1* and *glh-2* cDNAs both contain three copies of the 11 nt bipartite NRE elements, GTTGT X$_n$ATTGTA, although only one is perfect; the others are a match of 9–10/11nt (Fig. 6). Each *C. elegans cyclin* gene also contains one or more imperfect putative NRE elements (J.P. Richards and M.A. Kreutzer, unpublished results). Again, we must stress that these have not been tested, but will briefly describe below how we plan to test these potentially exciting regulators.

LOCALIZATION OF THE *glh-1* GENE PRODUCT

One piece of preliminary datum from our laboratory bears strongly on the topic of this chapter, that of identifying potential components of the nematode germline P-granules. Fusion proteins made from two different regions of the *glh-1* cDNA in the inducible expression vector pMal were injected into mice. By Western blot analysis the polyclonal antibodies from each of six mice recognize a single ~70 kD protein in *C. elegans* protein homogenates, the predicted size for *glh-1* (D.L.Roussell and M.E.Gruidl, results not shown), while preimmune sera from each mouse is negative. When the immune serum from these same mice is used for immunochemical localization in C. elegans adults and embryos, they each recognize the proliferating germ cell nuclei and oocytes in the adult, staining uniformly in the cytoplasm; more interestingly, when embryos were stained, each antibody selectively recognizes the germline precursor cells P_4 or Z_2 and Z_3. Figure 7C,E shows one of these polyclonal antibodies, in comparison to the preimmune sera in Figure 7A. DAPI staining of these embryos is shown in Figure 7B,D. The staining in each case is localized to the germline precursor. Even in the youngest two cell embryo uppermost in Figure 7E, the antibody is clearly more concentrated in the P_1 cell than in the AB cell. These results are still very preliminary because we have yet to establish whether the staining seen is due to glh-1 or glh-2, as we have not been able to produce sufficient protein to immunize with the glh-1–specific N-terminal fusion construct. With that caveat in mind, needless to say, we are very excited about the possibility that the first P granule component may be isolated.

CLOSING IN ON FUNCTION THROUGH GENETICS

The last information that bears on the possibility of continued progress in determining the potential role of P-granule components in specifying the germline comes from genetic studies in C. elegans. As mentioned in the Introduction, saturation mutagenesis in the region where glh-1 and glh-2 map has

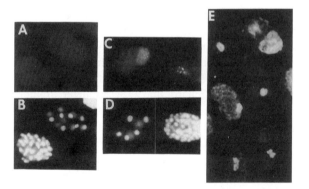

Fig. 7. Detection of glh-1 protein with anti-glh-1 polyclonal antibodies. FITC-conjugated secondary antibodies were used to detect antibodies from preimmune sera (A) or from hyperimmune sera (C,E). DAPI-stained nuclei are shown in B and D for A and C, respectively. A–D were photographed with a Zeiss Axioplan microscope. E was prepared as a digital image with a MRC-600 laser confocal microscope and transferred to film using the Universal Imaging and the Image 1 software. The confocal microscope, imaging equipment, and software are available to researchers through the Molecular Cytology Core facility, University of Missouri.

been done in Vancouver, BC. The Rose laboratory has recently been rescuing lethal mutations in the *dpy-14* region with cosmids that map to that region. They have rescued one lethal mutation, *let-545*, with the cosmid to which *glh-1* maps, T21G5 (S. McKay and A. Rose, personal communication). The phenotype of *let-545* is that of an adult sterile, with defects in germline proliferation, producing no oocytes or sperm. Many of the strong alleles of genes for the polar granule components of *Drosophila* have similar defects in oogenesis. We are currently establishing a microinjection "facility" (an inverted microscope, a microinjector, and a micromanipulator) to attempt rescue of *let-545* with genomic clones of *glh-1*. Also, another Vancouver group, that of D. Baillie, has isolated nine candidate lethal mutations that map very close to the physical map location of the *C. elegans cyclin B* gene. These candidates will also be tested, looking for rescue of their lethal phenotype by injection of the *cyclin B* genomic clone, along with the selectable *roller* (*rol-6*) marker plasmid (Mello et al., 1991). To date, no mutation in a cyclin B gene has been identified in any higher eukaryote. Again the strength of saturation genetics in *Caenorhabditis*, as well as the sharing community of research, may serve us well.

DISCUSSION

Although most of the results presented in this chapter deal with our cloned *Caenorhabditis* genes, we perceive that *Ascaris* will be a major contributor to determining the role of P-granules in development. The *Caenorhabditis* genes in both the *glh* and *cyclin* family cross-hybridize well with *Ascaris* (see Fig. 4, for example). Although not shown in this chapter, we have isolated candidate *Ascaris* genes for each of the three *Caenorhabditis* cyclins. Because in situ hybridization to nematode embryos is a technique that is only in the trial-and-error stage, we have reasoned that in situ hybridization of the *cyclins* to sectioned *Ascaris* embryos, a synchronous population, will be more interpretable than trying the same experiment with mixed-stage *Caenorhabditis* embryos. We hypothesize that the glh helicases are binding RNAs in the P-granules. We would like to express glh protein in vitro and attempt to bind in vitro-produced *cyclin* B RNA by northwestern blotting. Northwestern blotting with similar in vitro-produced RNA and protein was used to demonstrate the relationship between the *Drosophila Sxl* protein and the *tra1* RNA, two components of the fly sex determination pathway (Inoue et al., 1990). We plan to evoke more "natural" means if the in vitro experiments do not succeed. *Ascaris* offers the advantage of rather unlimited supplies of ovarian and staged early embryonic RNAs. We plan to work out the conditions of glh binding using *cyclin B* RNA, if *cyclin B* localizes to the P_4 cell. Perhaps the *Ascaris* RNAs that we propose specifically bind the germline helicases can be bound and eluted.

Although possibly requiring multiple rounds of binding and elution, with the use of nonspecific competitor RNAs to increase specific versus nonspecific binding, these *Ascaris* RNAs will then be cloned as cDNAs and identified.

The *glh-1* gene is unique among the RNA helicases in possessing four zinc fingers. We reason that these additional motifs are not likely to be required for helicase activity, but instead may confer additional specificity to the RNA binding capacity of the predicted glh-1 and glh-2 proteins. We would also like to test whether the glh-1 glycine repeats may be involved in an aggregation function as has been proposed for the glycine repeats in a family of plant cell-wall proteins, and for loricin, a member of the keratin family (Steinert et al., 1991). The anti-P-granule antibody staining shows dramatic aggregation or concentration with successive cell divisions in embryogenesis (Fig. 3), as does the anti-glh antibody (Fig. 7). Because transformation of *C. elegans* by micro-injection of RNA and DNA is a well-developed technique, questions regarding the role of various coding and noncoding regions of the *glh* and *cyclin* genes can be addressed. The use of a β-galactosidase reporter gene or an epitope tag will allow for detection of the expression and/or localization of the injected construct (Fire et al., 1990).

The role in development of the sequence elements in the 3′ UTR is especially intriguing. In both the *glh* and the *cyclin* genes, multiple potential regulatory elements are concentrated in very short untranslated regions. This may not be so surprising; many nematode messages are *trans*-spliced very close to the initiation codon. Therefore most post-translational control may need to be in the 3′ signal. We predict that signals for localization of RNAs and translational–adenylation signals will be found in these regions along with the well-known poly(A) signal found in most messages. Again, using reporter genes and also by putting these UTRs onto heterologous genes, these rather novel regulatory elements can be dissected and their functions elucidated.

The anti-glh-1 antibody data indicate that the glh protein is confined to the germline precursor cell(s) in the embryo. In the oocyte of the *C. elegans* adult, the glh protein is not confined to a region, but is found throughout the cytoplasm. In this respect, glh protein differs from vasa protein that is already posteriorly localized in the *Drosophila* oocyte. Therefore the glh protein may be asymmetrically segregated into the germline P_4 cell during the first few divisions of embryogenesis, like the P-granules that are localized by microfilaments, as the laboratory of S. Strome has shown, using the anti-P-granule antibodies and microfilament inhibitors (Hill and Strome, 1990). Alternatively, because *glh-1* and *glh-2* both have potential NRE elements and *vasa* does not, the glh maternal protein could turn over in the first few embryonic cell divisions and then the *glh* RNA could be selectively repressed in all cells but the P_4 (and later Z_2 and Z_3) cell(s). We intend to test these alternative models.

Mutations in *glh-1* and *cyclin B* genes would make many additional experiments available to us. Only one advantage will be mentioned here. From *Droso-phila* we know that the polar granules are complex, composed of several different proteins and RNAs. It is not obvious that homologs for some of the other germ granule components will be easily found in nematodes, as there are no conserved regions from which to design primers for PCR. One powerful way to isolate the genes that interact with a gene of interest is to start with the mutant and screen for intergenic suppressors, other genes that effectively reverse the mutant phenotype. These genes often code for interacting proteins. If we show by microinjection that *let-545* is a *glh-1* mutation, we would initiate such a suppressor screen with *let-545*. As a parallel alternative approach, we can immunoprecipitate the glh proteins with our anti-glh-1 polyclonal antibodies and attempt to identify the proteins that complex with the glh putative helicases.

CONCLUSION

As an approach to understanding how the germline is determined in nematodes, we have cloned and have begun to characterize two families of genes in the nematode, the *glh* and *cyclin* genes. These genes are potential components of the germline-specific P-granules. A role for glh proteins in germline specification has become more likely with our recent finding, using antibodies to glh, that the glh protein(s) segregate with the germline precursor cells in the *C. elegans* embryo. We also expect that the 3´ UTRs of each gene in these families, which appear to have multiple regulatory motifs, may post-transcriptionally coordinate their expression in development. The availability of unlimited stage- and tissue-specific RNAs from *Ascaris* could allow us to isolate other RNAs yet to have been identified that may be bound by glh zinc fingers in the P-granule "treasure chest."

ACKNOWLEDGMENTS

K.L.B. acknowledges the Captain Kidd, where good friends who started her on this project met. The work was supported by Career Advancement Award DCB-9110298 from the NSF and grant 2414 AR from the Council for Tobacco Research to K.L.B. D.L.R. and M.E.G. were supported as postdoctoral trainees by NIH training grant DHHS T32 AI-07276-03/5, awarded to the Molecular Microbiology and Immunology Department, University of Missouri.

REFERENCES

Austin J, Kimble J (1987): *glp-1* is required in the germ line for regulation of the decision between mitosis and meiosis in *C. elegans*. Cell 51:589–599.

Beanan MJ, Strome S (1992): Characterization of a germ-line proliferation mutation in *C. elegans*. Development 116:755–766.

Boswell RE, Prout ME, Steichen JC (1991): Mutations in a newly identified *Drosophila melanogaster* gene, *mago nashi*, disrupt germ cell formation and result in the formation of mirror-image symmetrical double abdomen embryos. Development 113:373–384.

Boveri T (1887): Uber differenzierung der zellkerne wahrend der furchung des eies von *Ascaris megalocephala*. Anat Anz 2:688–693.

Capowski EE, Martin P, Garvin C, Strome S (1991): Identification of grandchildless loci whose products are required for normal germ-line development in the nematode *Caenorhabditis elegans*. Genetics 129:1061–1072.

Cleavinger PJ, McDowell JW, Bennett KL (1989): Transcription in nematodes: Early *Ascaris* embryos are transcriptionally active. Dev Biol 133:600–604.

Company M, Arenas J, Abelson J (1991): Requirement of the RNA helicase-like protein PRP22 for release of messenger RNA from spliceosomes. Nature 349:487–493.

Coulson A, Kozono Y, Lutterbach B, Shownkeen R, Sulston J, Waterston R (1991): YACs and the *C. elegans* genome. Bioessays 13:413–417.

Coulson A, Sulston J, Brenner S, Karn J (1986): Toward a physical map of the genome of the nematod *Caenorhabditis elegans*. Proc Natl Acad Sci USA 83:7821–7825.

Dalby B, Glover DM (1993): Discrete sequence elements control posterior pole accumulation and translational repression of maternal cyclin B RNA in *Drosophila*. EMBO J 12:1219–1227.

Delahunty MD, South TL, Summers MF, Karpel RL (1992): Nucleic acid interactive properties of a peptide corresponding to the N-terminal zinc finger domain of HIV-1 nucleocapsid protein. Biochemistry 31:6461–6469.

de Valoir T, Tucker MA, Belikoff EJ, Camp LA, Bolduc C, Beckingham K (1991): A second maternally expressed *Drosophila* gene encodes a putative RNA helicase of the "DEAD box" family. Proc Natl Acad Sci USA 88:2113–2117.

Ephrussi A, Dickinson LK, Lehmann R (1991): *Oskar* organizes the germ plasma and directs localization of the posterior determinant *nanos*. Cell 66:37–50.

Fire A, Harrison SW, Dixon D (1990): A modular set of lacZ fusion vectors for studying gene expression in *Caenorhabditis elegans*. Gene 93:189–198.

Glotzer M, Murray AW, Kirschner MW (1991): Cyclin is degraded by the ubiquitin pathway. Nature 349:132–138.

Golumbeski GS, Bardsley A, Tax F, Boswell RE (1991): *tudor*, a posterior-group gene of *Drosophila melanogaster*, encodes a novel protein and an mRNA localized during mid-oogenesis. Genes Dev 5:2060–2070.

Gururajan R, Perry-O'Keefe H, Melton DA, Weeks DL (1991): The *Xenopus* localized messenger RNA An3 may encode an ATP-dependent RNA helicase. Nature 349:717–719.

Hay B, Ackerman L, Barbel S, Jan LY, Jan YN (1988a): Identification of a component of *Drosophila* polar granules. Development 103:625–640.

Hay B, Jan LY, Jan YN (1988b): A protein component of *Drosophila* polar granules is encoded by *vasa* and has extensive sequence similarity to ATP-dependent helicases. Cell 55:577–587.

Hill DP, Strome S (1990): Brief cytochalasin-induced disruption of microfilaments during a critical interval in 1-cell *C. elegans* embryos alters the partitioning of developmental instructions to the 2-cell embryo. Development 108:159–172.

Hirling H, Scheffner M, Restle T, Stahl H (1989): RNA helicase activity associated with the human p68 protein. Nature 339:562–564.

Huarte J, Stutz A, O'Connell ML, Gubler P, Belin D, Darrow AL, Strickland S, Vassalli JD (1992): Transient translational silencing by reversible mRNA deadenylation. Cell 69:1021–1030.

Inoue K, Hoshijima K, Sakamoto H, Shimura Y (1990): Binding of the *Drosophila* sex-lethal gene product to the alternative splice site of transformer primary transcript. Nature 344:461–463.

Jongens TA, Hay B, Jan LY, Jan YN (1992): The *germ cell-less* gene product: A posteriorly localized component necessary for germ cell development in *Drosophila*. Cell 70:569–584.

Kim-Ha J, Smith JL, Macdonald PM (1991): *oskar* mRNA is localized to the posterior pole of the *Drosophila* oocyte. Cell 66:23–35.

Lasko PF, Ashburner M (1988): The product of the *Drosophila* gene *vasa* is very similar to eukaryotic initiation factor-4A. Nature 335:611–617.

Leroy P, Alzari P, Sassoon D, Wolgemuth D, Fellous M (1989): The protein encoded by a murine male germ cell-specific transcript is a putative ATP-dependent RNA helicase. Cell 57:549–559.

Mahowald AP (1971): Polar granules of *Drosophila*. IV. Cytochemical studies showing loss of RNA from polar granules during early stages of embryogenesis. J Exp Zool 176:345–352.

McGhee JD, Birchall JC, Chung MA, Cottrell DA, Edgar LG, Svendsen PC, Ferrari DC (1990): Production of null mutants in the major intestinal esterase gene (*ges-1*) of the nematode *Caenorhabditis elegans*. Genetics 125:505–514.

McKim KS, Starr T, Rose AM (1992): Genetic and molecular analysis of the *dpy-14* region in *Caenorhabditis elegans*. Mol Gen Genet 233:241–251.

Mello CC, Kramer JM, Stinchcomb D, Ambros V (1991): Efficient gene transfer in *C.elegans:* Extrachromosomal maintenance and integration of transforming sequences. EMBO J 10:3959–3970.

Miller DM, Stockdale FE, Karn J (1986): Immunological identification of the genes encoding the four myosin heavy chain isoforms of *Caenorhabditis elegans*. Proc Natl Acad Sci USA 83:2305–2309.

Nielsen PJ, McMaster GK, Trachsel H (1985): Cloning of eukaryotic protein synthesis initiation factor genes: Isolation and characterization of cDNA clones encoding factor eIF-4A. Nucleic Acids Res 13:6867–6880.

Nilsen TW, Shambaugh J, Denker J, Chubb G, Faser C, Putman L, Bennett KL (1989): Characterization and expression of a spliced leader RNA in the parasitic nematode *Ascaris lumbricoides* var. *suum*. Mol Cell Biol 9:3543–3547.

Okimoto R, Macfarlane JL, Clary DO, Wolstenholme DR (1992): The mitochondrial genomes of two nematodes, *Caenorhabditis elegans* and *Ascaris suum*. Genetics 130:471–498.

Rajavashisth TB, Taylor AK, Andalibi A, Svenson KL, Lusis AJ (1989): Identification of a zinc finger protein that binds to the sterol regulatory element. Science 245:640–643.

Roussell DL, Bennett KL (1992): *Caenorhabditis* cDNA encodes an eIF-4A-like gene. Nucleic Acids Res 20:3783.

Roussell DL, Bennett KL (1993): glh-1: A germline putative RNA helicase from *Caenorhabditis* has four fingers. Proc Natl Acad Sci USA 90:9300–9304.

Schmid SR, Linder P (1991): Translation initiation factor 4A from *Saccharomyces cerevisiae*: Analysis of residues conserved in the D-E-A-D family of RNA helicases. Mol Cell Biol 11:3463–3471.

Schubach T, Wieschaus EF (1986): Maternal-effect mutations altering the anterior-posterior pattern of the *Drosophila* embryo. Roux's Arch Dev Biol 195:302–317.

Spence AM, Coulson A, Hodgkin J (1990): The product of *fem-1*, a nematode sex-determining gene, contains a motif found in cell cycle control proteins and receptors for cell-cell interactions. Cell 60:981–990.

Spieth J, Blumenthal T (1985): The *Caenorhabditis elegans* vitellogenin gene family includes a gene encoding a distantly related protein. Mol Cell Biol 5:2495–2501.

Steinert PM, Mack JW, Korge BP, Gan SQ, Haynes SR, Steven AC (1991): Glycine loops in proteins: Their occurrence in certain intermediate filament chains, loricrins and single-stranded RNA binding proteins. Int J Biol Macromol 13:130–139.

St Johnston D, Beuchle D, Nusslein-Volhard C (1991): *Staufen*, a gene required to localize maternal RNAs in the *Drosophila* egg. Cell 66:51–63.

Strome S, Wood WB (1983): Generation of asymmetry and segregation of germ-line granules in early *C. elegans* embryos. Cell 35:15–25.

Sulston JE, Horvitz HR (1977): Post-embryonic cell lineages of the nematode, *Caenorhabditis elegans*. Dev Biol 56:110–156.

Sulston JE, Schierenberg E, White JG, Thomson JN (1983): The embryonic cell lineage of the nematode *Caenorhabditis elegans*. Dev Biol 100:64–119.

Tachibana K, Ishiura M, Uchida T, Kishimoto T (1990): The starfish egg mRNA responsible for meiosis reinitiation encodes cyclin. Dev Biol 140:241–252.

Wharton RP, Struhl G (1991): RNA regulatory elements mediate control of *Drosophila* body pattern by the posterior morphogen *nanos*. Cell 67:955–967.

Whitfield WGF, Gonzalez C, Sanchez-Herrero E, Glover DM (1989): Transcripts of one of two *Drosophila* cyclin genes become localized in pole cells during embryogenesis. Nature 338:337–340.

Wolf N, Priess J, Hirsh D (1983): Segregation of germline granules in early embryos of *Caenorhabditis elegans:* An electron microscopic analysis. J Embryol Exp Morphol 73:297–306.

CELL BIOLOGY

Preface

The field of cell biology has been in a massive growth phase for the past 5 years or so. Not coincidentally, parasitology has also been affected by this growth and today there are several parasite systems in which sophisticated questions of cell biology are being addressed. Chief among these are issues of invasion by intracellular parasites and trafficking involved in targeting proteins to some of the novel, specialized subcellular structures in parasites and/or the infected host cell.

In this section, five chapters are presented that cover some of these topics. The first, by Jean-Francois Dubremetz, presents an overview of a system in which the questions far outnumber the answers, *Toxoplasma*.Dubremetz describes the current state of knowledge about the cell biology of this obligate intracellular parasite with an emphasis on how it invades, divides, and differentiates once inside the host.

The next chapter, by Norma Andrews, focuses on the invasion process of *T. cruzi* and what is involved on the part of the host cell and parasite. She traces the life of the parasite from the time it enters the host cell through the escape from the vacuole and then addresses what "life in the cytoplasm" may be like.

Kasturi Haldar and her colleagues discuss how *Plasmodium falciparum* deals with life in one of the most challenging environments, the erythrocyte, where the option of perverting the host cell's metabolism are limited by the absence of protein synthesis. In particular, they describe how *Plasmodium* deals with trafficking of parasite-encoded proteins once they leave the parasite itself and enter the milieu of the red blood cell.

The final two chapters deal with the signals on proteins that cause them to be targeted to particular organelles within the parasite: the glycosome of trypanosomes and the hydrogenosome of *Trichomonas*.Both of these organelles are membrane limited but apparently lie outside the secretory pathway, and thus proteins destined for them must bear an import signal (apparently neither has its own genome or protein synthetic capabilities). The chapter by Patricia Johnson and colleagues suggests a possible N-terminal signal for hydrogenosomal protein import from a detailed analysis of *Trichomonas* genes encoding such proteins.Additional experiments with the protein products reveal a possible N-terminal signal, and experiments with natural and mutated proteins in vivo and in vitro appear to confirm this target sequence. In the chapter by Jurg Sommer and C.C. Wang, elegant use is made of transfection to test the hypothesis that glycosomal proteins of trypanosomes have a C-terminal signal.

Molecular Approaches to Parasitology, pages 345–358
© 1995 Wiley-Liss, Inc.

Toxoplasma gondii: Cell Biology Update

Jean François Dubremetz

Unité 42 Inserm, 59655 Villeneuve d'Ascq, France

INTRODUCTION

Toxoplasma gondii is an obligatory intracellular parasite, as most Coccidia are. Therefore, how it invades cells and how it gets its supplies from them is a major matter of investigation. Increasing interest in toxoplasmosis due to the extension of its medical importance is bringing into the field many newcomers who need to get a general view of the parasite biology rapidly, but may not easily browse through the last 30 years of Coccidia litterature to get a good sense of what is known already or can be postulated from what has been described in related organisms and of what are the main blocks or unsolved questions that impede progress in the field. Some of these issues are discussed in the following pages.

Indeed, *T. gondii* is a Coccidia, and one must benefit from all the descriptions written in the 1960s on this protozoa and on related organisms that were better models for studying some processes such as mitosis or organelle biogenesis. Some aspects that are presently considered as critically important were overlooked at that time (such as, for exemple, the dense granules), many were observed but still await being understood (such as invasion), and some have been forgotten and were redescribed (multimembranous organelles, which are possibly the descendants of plastids) (Fig. 1).

The study of host cell invasion by *T. gondii* has long been blurred by the use of phagocytes as host cells, which hampered the interpretation of the respective contribution of both partners in the process. Internalization was for a long time viewed as phagocytosis followed by inhibition of fusion of the phagosome membrane with lysosomes. It took a while to put forward the view that the invasion process itself was the initial cause of the absence of fusion of the parasitophorous vacuole with any of the other compartments of the host cell (Joiner et al., 1990). All studies on invasion in Apicomplexa have shown very similar patterns of events, and one could think of building a "unifying theory"of invasion in the group. Being frustrated by the fact that little community has been found thus far in the protein contents of the organelles involved in the

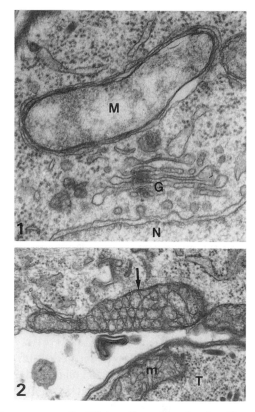

Fig. 1. Multimembranous organelle (M) in a *T. gondii* tachyzoite. The organelle has four membranes and is typically located next to the Golgi apparatus, which is itself found forming from the nuclear envelope. G, Golgi apparatus; N, nucleus. ×47,000.

Fig. 2. Modified host cell mitochondrion (arrow) found next to the parasitophorous vacuole of *T. gondii*. m, Tachyzoite mitochondrion; T, tachyzoite. ×28,000.

process, some authors presently tend to stress the differences and would give up trying to sort the basic processes out of the specific details. Even though a large variety of cells are invaded in a large variety of locations and circumstances, the similarities in the invasion are still calling for common basic functions for the organelles: The fact that the major antigens of the organelles are species or stage specific is not a reason to give up searching for similar or related molecules or activities. The basic scheme according to which micronemes are used for recognition or binding, rhoptries to build up the vacuole, and dense granules to build up the interaction machinery with the host cell is not outdated yet, and common functions can still be studied within this frame: It is important to identify common features to sort out the most basic functions that are likely to be essential.

Once inside the cell, a *T. gondii* tachyzoite may give rise to either tachyzoites or bradyzoites, depending on external factors such as the immune response in vivo. Recent studies have shown that this differentiation can be triggered in vitro, and the factors that influence the outcome of the intracellular parasites are actively sought for. This process is one example of the more general problem of differentiation in Apicomplexa where successive phases of the life cycle are triggered by external (gametocytogenesis or gametogenesis in *Plasmodium*) or internal (successive schizogonies or gametogenesis in *Eimeria*) factors and for which the molecular regulations are unknown. The tachyzoite–bradyzoite switch in *T. gondii* is probably one of the easiest to study experimentally and may therefore lead to more general conclusions if elucidated.

T. gondii is also the ideal model to study Apicomplexa cell biology (and others will claim the same for genetics). This is probably not only sentimental praise for one's favorite model, but relies on objective grounds immediately obvious when one realizes all the potential of the model and all the recent progress in its experimental handling, the last one being its transfection (Soldati and Boothroyd, 1993; Kim et al., 1993).

MOTILITY

Gliding motility of the zoites is a common feature among Apicomplexa and is indeed the basis of extracellular tachyzoite motion. Its possible link with the alignments of intramembranous particles (IMP) of the inner complex has been suggested when this structural differentiation was described and has led to a "conveyor belt hypothesis for gliding" (King, 1988). That the inner complex is found almost only in motile stages of Apicomplexa is also a strong argument for its involvement in motility. A present paradox, however, is that no membrane molecule likely to transduce the driving force is known: All surface molecules described thus far are glycosyl phosphatidyl inositol (GPI)-anchored, and the fact that most of them are released by GPI-specific phospholipase C (GPIPLC) suggests that they have no transmembrane domain. The molecular bases of gliding motility have therefore yet to be discovered.

The analogies between gliding and invasion have led to the suggestion that the driving force of invasion or the gliding of the parasite within the developing vacuole is identical to extracellular gliding motility. One observation suggests that things may be a little more complex: The alignment of IMPs has been found in the inner complex of all Apicomplexan zoites studied to date except *Plasmodium* merozoites (J.F. Dubremetz, unpublished data). These merozoites may not be motile (this is very difficult to prove because of their size), but they do invade. Therefore, IMP alignments may be the guides for gliding motility, but invasion and gliding of the moving junction is likely somehow distinct.

The slime hypothesis of gliding is supported by several observations involving different Apicomplexa leaving trails on the substrate (e.g., glass or plastic bottom of a tissue culture flask) when being translocated. This phenomenon is very poorly understood. In *Plasmodium,* the circumsporozoite protein (CSP) is supposedly shed during gliding (Stewart and Vanderberg, 1991); it may come from micronemes that would therefore need to exocytose during gliding. Indeed, an attractive hypothesis is that since micronemes are the most variable component of zoites as far as the number of organelles is concerned, the motility of zoites in vitro may somehow be correlated with the relative amount of these organelles (sporozoites of *Plasmodium*, cystozoites of *Sarcocystis* have many micronemes and are very active tachyzoites of *T. gondii*, and some *Eimeria* merozoites have few micronemes and do not glide long distances or for a long time). It is very difficult, however, to make direct correlations or to quantify motility. Against this idea is also the fact that in most zoites no surface molecules are found in micronemes, nor are any microneme molecules found on the surface in detectable amounts. The slime hypothesis also suggests that lipids of the membrane are shed, and this therefore assumes that new material must be added to the surface. Indeed, organelle exocytosis could also account for membrane addition, but there is no clear evidence for it. The possible part played by organelles in motility is therefore still to be discovered.

INVASION

The internalization of the zoite starts with the creation of a moving junction at the anterior tip of the parasite. Whether this junction actually involves molecules bridging the two plasma membranes (parasite and host) has not been shown. If any organelle has to exocytose its contents to make a junction, micronemes are the most likely candidate (Entzeroth et al., 1992), but this awaits demonstration. The membrane alteration observed in *Plasmodium knowlesi* (Aikawa et al., 1981) and *T. gondii* (Dubremetz, unpublished data) concerns the cytoplasmic face of the host cell membrane and looks more like lipid crystals than the IMPs initially described. The most likely hypothesis is that the junction freezes the communication between the two domains of a continuous bilayer (the plasmalemma of the host cell and the developing vacuole), while the parasite is providing building material for the vacuole. Lipids are likely to diffuse rapidly across this border due to their high diffusion rate, but it is not yet known whether this diffusion occurs in both leaflets of the bilayer or only in the outer one: Diffusion of the cytoplasmic layer could be restricted through the structure observed in freeze fracture. In *Plasmodium*, host cell membrane lipids seem to contribute a large part of the parasitophorous vacuole membrane (Ward et al., 1993). Surface or transmembrane proteins of the host cell do not seem to diffuse into the vacuole, as shown by several different investigations (freeze fracture, radioiodination, surface biotinylation), although this issue remains disputed and has still to be fully elucidated.

The dense granule exocytosis that occurs very soon after internalization and possibly starts even before the closure of the vacuole remains a matter of dispute as to whether it occurs by classic exocytosis (Leriche and Dubremetz, 1990) or by budding of a membranous structure at the posterior end of the tachyzoite (Sibley, personal communication). Both processes may occur simultaneously, but if so this is difficult to reconcile with the current view that only one population of dense granules exists and contains all the dense granule proteins described thus far. Analysis of the experimental triggering of dense granule release by extracellular tachyzoites (Sibley and Boothroyd, 1992) will hopefully help solve this question.

VACUOLE MEMBRANE

The membrane surrounding the intracellular parasite is known as the *parasitophorous vacuole membrane* (PVM). Proteins derived from organelles (rhoptries and dense granules) have been found associated with the PVM (reviewed by Dubremetz and Schwartzman, 1992). These observations have led to the idea that *T. gondii* could insert proteins in this membrane to interact with the host cell cytoplasm, mainly to supply its metabolic requirements. As the absence of fusion with any other compartment of the host cell excludes getting metabolites by this process, the only other way one can envision is that this membrane must have pores or channels allowing for the diffusion or the transport of metabolites to the developing parasite. Indeed, the presence of such pores allowing the diffusion of molecules up to 1,200 Da has been demonstrated recently by microinjection experiments (Schwab, Beckers, and Joiner, manuscript in submission). A similar finding using a completely different experimental approach has also been reported for *P. falciparum* (Desai et al., 1993). This porous vacuole membrane might therefore soon prove to be a major route of communication between intracellular Apicomplexa and their host cell. The proteins involved in the making of these pores are not fully characterized yet, although several candidates from the rhoptries and dense granules have been identified (Beckers, Ossorio, Dubremetz, and Joiner, manuscript in submission). Their definitive characterization will need the reconstruction of the pores in artificial membranes with purified or recombinant proteins.

Another permanent feature of the vacuole membrane is the presence on its cytoplasmic face of a continuous layer of host cell mitochondria and endoplasmic reticulum (the latter has no ribosomes on the side facing the PVM, suggesting that ribosome–mRNA complexes can no longer get access or bind to this side). Although one cannot exclude the possibility that this association is only due to space constraint, i.e., the growing vacuole pushing away the cell organelles, a specific association is more likely. Indeed, this phenomenon is specific for tachyzoite-containing vacuoles, and this basket of organelles enclosing the vacuole disappears when the latter transforms into a cyst. Another observation is that the nuclear envelope is never in contact with the PVM, although it may just be pushed away by the vacuole. But the most striking evidence for this association having a functional meaning is the morphological alteration of the host cell mitochondria associated with the PVM: their cristae are modified and sometimes fuse into a reticulated network (Fig. 2). What all of this means is unknown: One may think that the parasite relies on host cell mitochondrial metabolites and that this close association enhances their availability. Growing parasites in host cells with altered mitochondrial function may help to resolve this question.

THE TIME COURSE OF ENDODYOGENY AND MITOTIC CYCLE

Tachyzoites multiply by endodyogeny, which includes mitosis and a complex differentiation process. However, contrary to most Apicomplexa in which the zoite dedifferentiates after invasion to give rise to a schizont, *T. gondii* tachyzoites retain the complete zoite differentiation during endodyogeny. This has two major consequences: First, a tachyzoite is able to invade a host cell at any stage in its cell cycle except during cytoplasmic fission between the two daughter individuals; second, as a consequence, there is probably no correlation whatsoever between host cell invasion or host cell rupture and endodyogeny.

Indeed, although the endodyogenic cycle lasts between 6 and 12 hours depending on the strain, divided parasites can be found as early as 30 minutes after invasion in vitro, which means that they must have invaded at a late stage of endodyogeny. This observation is easy to make as parasitophorous vacuoles never fuse, and therefore the only way of finding several parasites within a single vacuole is division.

Concerning parasite release from the host cell, the best illustration of the absence of regulation by endodyogeny is the fact that tachyzoites can be released at any time in their cycle and that host cell burst proceeds much faster after multiple infection compared with single infection. The trigger is most likely related to the total parasite load the cell can stand before losing its ability to regulate its exchange balance with the outside. Indeed, as mimicked by ionophore A23187-triggered egress (Endo et al., 1982), alteration of intracellular calcium is likely to remove the inhibition of parasite motility that is typical of intravacuolar tachyzoite and to cause them to move out and search for another host cell with proper cytoplasmic ionic balance.

The most important regulatory event in endodyogeny, as is true for zoite formation in any Apicomplexa, is that the poles of the mitotic spindle will be the organizing centers for zoite development. Although mitosis has not been entirely described in *T. gondii*, all the observations reported suggest that it is identical to what occurs in *Eimeria:* Mitosis is performed via an intranuclear spindle driven by two pairs of atypical centrioles (Dubremetz, 1973). The spindle is very short in *T. gondii* and metaphase and anaphase are rapid, leading to the accumulation of kinetochores at the poles where the spindle poles transform into centrocones, specialized areas of the nuclear envelope that are physically linked to the centrioles and follow them during karyokinesis. The Golgi apparatus, which usually forms from the nuclear envelope in zoites, also divides during mitosis, and a daughter Golgi is found next to each centrocone. At a very early stage of mitosis, probably prophase, i.e., after duplication of the centrioles, the apical complex of the zoite will start forming next to each centriole pair (Fig 3). The earliest event is the formation of the apical ring from which the subpellicular microtubules will then radiate posteriorly as a basket that will gradually enclose the organelles and nucleus of the daughter tachyzoite. Very early on, the conoid forms and the inner membrane complex develops by the flattening of Golgi vesicles along the external side of the microtubular basket. The outline of the developing tachyzoite then clearly takes shape (Fig. 4). Also starting early in the development, one observes the formation of rhoptries as dense vesicles growing on the trans Golgi and later condensing their contents and growing a duct toward the conoid. As exemplified in *Eimeria* (Dubremetz, 1975), organelle biogenesis is a sequential event, and all data collected on *T. gondii* agree with this scheme: Rhoptries are made first and then micronemes at specific time points in the endogenesis. As no synchronized culture of *T. gondii* has been obtained thus far, this sequence has not been defined biochemically yet and has to be further investigated. A consequence of the endodyogeny process is that the mature tachyzoite is absolutely altruistic and is probably unable to make rhoptries and micronemes for itself: Whatever is synthesized is included in the two daughter merozoites and will only be usable after the two daughters are born by the splitting of the mother cell. The latter phenomenon is not well known: The mother tachyzoite keeps its invading organelles up to a very late stage of endogeny and what probably happens at the very end is an involution of the apical organelles of the mother whereas most of the inner complex is integrated into the developing inner complex of the daughters (Vivier and Petitprez,1969) and the plasmalemma of the mother becomes the plasmalemma of the daughters.

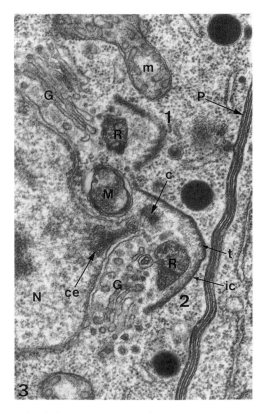

Fig. 3.   Early stage of endodyogeny in a *T. gondii* tachyzoite. Two developing apical complexes (1 and 2; oblique sections showing inner membrane complex, subpellicular microtubules, and a rhoptry precursor) are found; one of the poles of the mitotic nucleus is found in
this section and is figured by a centriole (c) on top of a centrocone (ce). This mitotic pole is
associated with apical complex 2; the other mitotic pole is associated with apical complex 1
and is not in the plane of the section. The Golgi apparatus has divided to give rise to two
organelles, each one associated with one apical complex. The multimembranous organelle
will divide between the developing parasites. ic, inner membrane complex; P, tachyzoite pel-
licle; R, rhoptry; t, subpellicular microtubule. ×41,000.

This last point is important: The surface of the parasite is then probably in
constant increase along generations, which suggests a progressive dilution of
the surface molecules with newly synthesized ones. The case of the dense
granules is unclear: Whether the mother cell can make some for its own use
and also whether they are synthesized developmentally or permanently remains to be investigated. The involution of the apical organelles at each
endodyogeny when parasites do not leave the host cell is a huge metabolic

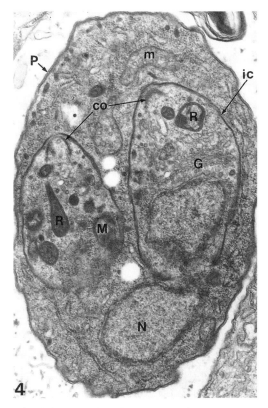

Fig. 4. Late stage of endodyogeny; the apical complex of the mother tachyzoite is not on the plane of section but would be on the top of the figure. Both daughter parasites have been sectioned through their apical complex. The inner membrane complex of both has extended backward and includes a large part of the dividing nucleus (visible only in one of the daughters). Several rhoptries are found; the multimembranous organelle has divided. The two daughters will eventually occupy most of the mother cytoplasm and will be covered with the mother plasmalemma at the end of endodyogeny, when they will separate to form two tachyzoites. co, Conoid. ×19,000.

waste; however, this makes the parasite ready to invade at any time when for some reason the host cell is destroyed. This is an advantage over most other Apicomplexa that would die when the cell is damaged before the completion of the schizogonic process. The exact fate of these organelles is unknown, and whether they are broken down to simple metabolites or whether some material could be released in the vacuole to allow the expansion of the vacuole membrane has not been investigated. In any case, the physical barrier of the developing complex excludes the integration of the rhoptries and micronemes of the mother into the daughter organisms.

Several of the rhoptry proteins are processed from higher molecular weight precursors, during their biosynthesis (Sadak et al.,1988; Soldati and Boothroyd, personal communication). The biochemical data show that this processing occurs within 30 minutes after protein synthesis, and the use of classic blocks of the Golgi trafficking (Soldati and Boothroyd, personal communication) suggest that this happens beyond the *trans* Golgi. It is therefore likely to occur during the condensing of the contents or the growth of the rhoptry duct. What is clear from the pulse chase studies is that this processing is independent of the release–reinvasion process and must occur at every round of intracellular endodyogeny.

OTHER ORGANELLES, INTRACELLULAR TRAFFICKING

Nothing is known about how new material is targetted to the surface of Apicomplexan zoites. No equivalent of the endocytic pathway is known, and there is no morphological evidence thus far of trafficking to and from the surface. In addition, the barrier of the inner complex makes it even more difficult to envision. In *T. gondii*, the exocytosis of dense granules could be a way of inserting surface molecules, since this process is probably somehow constitutive intracellularly. However, surface molecules cannot be detected on the dense granule membrane (J.F. Dubremetz, unpublished data), which decreases the likelihood of this hypothesis. The micropore, which is a lateral organelle often showing an endo- or exocytic vesicle, is the only functional candidate for all trafficking targetted at the surface, but its role has never been formally demonstrated except in *Plasmodium,* where it serves as a cytostome. Any contribution of the inner complex to the trafficking to the surface is very unlikely, as no fusion of this compartment with the plasma membrane has ever been observed, and, in addition, the IMP populations found in both membrane are clearly different and no surface molecule can be detected in the inner complex by immunoelectron microscopy.

The organelles described thus far (rhoptries, micronemes, dense granules) are the most obvious, but some components contained in low amounts but important for the parasite may still have to be identified. For example, different clear vesicles do exist in the cytoplasm of the zoite, and they may represent distinct organelles the role of which is unknown. Another organelle that has been ignored until recently may eventually be identified as derived from the plastid of a free-living protist ancestor of the phylum: The Golgi adjunct, or multimembranous organelle (it has four membranes; see Fig. 1), described in most Apicomplexa during the 1960s is the most likely candidate to contain the extrachromosomal nonmitochondrial DNA that is found in *Plasmodium* and *T. gondii* (Wilson et al., 1991). If this happens to be true, the persistence of such an organelle through evolution implies that it has an essential role in the parasite metabolism, and this will be quite interesting to elucidate.

DIFFERENTIATION

The recent development of bradyzoite-specific antibodies has shown that the expression of bradyzoite-specific proteins was far more common in in vitro grown parasites than expected but that, in most instances, the more rapid multiplication of tachyzoites led to the destruction of monolayers and prevented any further development toward the cyst stage (Soete et al, 1993). Furthermore, recent investigations have shown that the switch from tachyzoite to bradyzoites can be experimentally triggered in vitro by applying physical or chemical stress on infected cells (Soete et al., manuscript in submission).

Several observations that are relevant to the understanding of the phenomenon can be made. First, the expression of bradyzoite surface proteins by the zoites begins before cyst formation, and, in addition, the expression is sequential, one protein appearing later than the others. The starting point is therefore a vacuole containing tachyzoites, which will gradually evolve into a cyst containing bradyzoites: The transformation will occur through intermediate stages for both the zoites and the enclosing comparment. Intermediate zoites express both SAG1 (a tachyzoite-specific surface antigen) and bradyzoite-specific proteins; intermediate vacuoles have a progressively reduced network and accumulate dense material, especially at their periphery, under the PVM, that becomes the outermost limit of the cyst, as also observed in vivo (Ferguson and Hutchison, 1987). The dense material reacts strongly with antidense-granule antibodies, just as the network and PVM do; whether the cyst wall contains more than dense-granule proteins remains to be established. Bradyzoites indeed contain all the dense-granule proteins described in tachyzoites (reviewed by Cesbron-Delauw, 1994) and may contain specific dense-granule proteins in addition, but this remains to be demonstrated.

Second, bradyzoites contained in cysts seem to degenerate in vitro once the host cell floats off the monolayer (which usually means cell death); this is similar to the claim that in vivo cysts are always found within cells and cannot be free. One can therefore conclude that the cyst must interact metabolically with its host cell or at least needs the host cell cytoplasm environment to remain infectious.

Third, the most intriguing finding is the heterogeneity found in some intermediate vacuoles where the level of expression of bradyzoite molecules can be significantly different between neighboring parasites (Bohne et al., 1993; Soete et al., 1993): Knowing that all zoites within a vacuole derive from the same invader and that they grow and divide synchronously, one must conclude that very subtle differences can alter the triggering of the switch.

Fourth, we do not know to what extent the phenomenon is reversible, or, in other words, whether zoites having started expressing bradyzoite proteins can revert to pure tachyzoite within the same vacuole or have to be released and reinvade before doing so. The formation of the cyst seems to be critical in this respect, and one would guess that once the alteration of the PVM has gone far enough there must be a point of no return beyond which the metabolic interaction that is needed for tachyzoite growth cannot be restored; this has to be proven, however. In vivo, preliminary observations (Odaert and Soete, unpublished data) on reactivation suggest that release of bradyzoites from the cyst is a prerequisite to tachyzoite multiplication, as no SAG1 can ever be found in a cyst.

TOWARD EXTRACELLULAR DEVELOPMENT AND SEX IN VITRO

These are two independent goals that would greatly improve the already impressive experimental advantages of the organism to study intracellular parasitism. Being able to get rid of the host cell to multiply parasites and of the cat to make sexual recombination will indeed be the next improvements of the system. The approach toward extracellular multiplication (already achieved in *Plasmodium;* Trager and Williams, 1992) will certainly benefit from studies on the vacuole membrane permeability, as this will give a better idea of what are the actual contents of the parasitophorous vacuole; this area will also benefit from studies on the reconstitution of intracellular trafficking, as these tend to mimic better and better the composition of the cell cytoplasm, which may be close to what is found in the vacuole according to the size of the vacuolar membrane pores. Although not completely related, the synchronization of the parasite cycle will also be a major experimental breakthrough, especially if combined with extracellular development.

Sex out of the cat would relieve the geneticists from a lot of headaches due to the waste of money, time, and energy and sometimes to the social pressure associated with the use of these animals (which are actually usually very happy to get a treat of some mouse brain in addition to their usual chow and do not suffer from the infection). Gametogenesis and oocyst formation in vitro have been obtained for *Eimeria* and *Sarcocystis* and therefore there is no apparent impossibility to reach this with *T. gondii*. Experiments with the former organisms, pioneered in the 1960s (reviewed by Doran, 1973) have shown that the species requirement as well as the cell differentiation status were critical, and this will likely be true for *T. gondii* as well. However, neither *Eimeria* nor *Sarcocystis* can make tachyzoites, and the stubborn propensity of *T. gondii* to develop as tachyzoites in any cell might be a drawback in this experimental set up.

Let us be optimistic, however, and assume that the more investigators who reach the field, the sooner these limitations will be overcome and the *T. gondii* system will become even more fascinating to work with.

REFERENCES

Aikawa M, Miller LH, Rabbege J Epstein N (1981): Freeze-fracture study of the erythrocyte membrane during malarial parasite invasion. J Cell Biol 92:55–62.

Bohne W, Heeseman J, Gross U (1993): Coexistence of heterogenous populations of *Toxoplasma gondii* parasites within parasitophorous vacuoles of murine macrophages as revealed by a bradyzoite specific monoclonal antibody. Parasitol Res 79:485–487.

Cesbron-Delauw MF (1994): Dense granule organelles of *Toxoplasma gondii*: Their role in host parasite relationships. Parasitol Today 10:293–296.

Desai SA, Krogstad DJ, McCleskey EW (1993): A nutrient permeable channel on the intraerythrocytic malaria parasite. Nature 362:643–646.

Doran DJ (1973): Cultivation of Coccidia in avian embryo and cell culture. In DM Hammond, Long (eds): The Coccidia: *Eimeria, Isospora, Toxoplasma* and Related Genera. Baltimore: University Park Press, pp 183–252.

Dubremetz JF (1973): Etude ultrastructurale de la mitose schizogonique chez la coccidie *Eimeria necatrix* (Johnson 1930). J Ultrastruct Res 42:354–376.

Dubremetz JF (1975): La genèse des mérozoïtes chez la coccidie *Eimeria necatrix*. Etude Ultrastructurale. J Protozool 22:71–84.

Dubremetz JF, Schwartzman J (1992): Subcellular organelles of *Toxoplasma gondii* and host cell invasion. Res Immunol 144:31–33.

Endo T, Sethi KK, Piekarski G (1982): *Toxoplasma gondii*: Calcium ionophore A23187-mediated exit of trophozoites from infected murine macrophages. Exp Parasitol 53:179–188.

Entzeroth R, Kerckoff H, König A (1992): Microneme secretion in Coccidia: Confocal laser scanning and electron microscope study on microneme secretion of *Sarcocystis muris* using a monoclonal antibody. Eur J Cell Biol 59:405–413.

Ferguson DJP, Hutchison WM (1987): An ultrastructural study of the early development and tissue cyst formation of *Toxoplasma gondii* in the brains of mice. Parasitol Res 73:483–491.

Joiner KA, Furhman SA, Mietinnen H, Kasper LL, Mellman I (1990): *Toxoplasma gondii*: Fusion competence of parasitophorous vacuoles in Fc receptor transfected fibroblasts. Science 249:641–646.

Kim K, Soldati D, Boothroyd JC (1993): Gene replacement in *Toxoplasma gondii* with chloramphenicol acetyltransferase as selectable marker. Science 262:911–914.

King CA (1988): Cell motility of sporozoan protozoa. Parasitol Today 4:315–319.

Leriche MA, Dubremetz JF (1990): Exocytosis of *Toxoplasma gondii* dense granules into the parasitophorous vacuole after host cell invasion. Parasitol Res 76:559–562.

Sadak A, Taghy Z, Fortier B, Dubremetz JF (1988): Characterization of a family of rhoptry proteins of *Toxoplasma gondii*. Mol Biochem Parasitol 29:203–211.

Sibley LD, Boothroyd JC (1992): Calcium regulated secretion and modification of host-cell endocytic compartments by *Toxoplasma*. J Cell Biol 115:5a.

Soete M, Fortier B, Camus D, Dubremetz JF (1993): *Toxoplasma gondii*: Kinetics of bradyzoite–tachyzoite interconversion in vitro. Exp Parasitol 76:259–264.

Soldati D, Boothroyd JC (1993): Transient transfection and expression in the obligate intracellular parasite *Toxoplasma gondii*. Science 260:349–352.

Stewart MJ, Vanderberg JP (1991):Malaria sporozoites release circumsporozoite protein from their apical end and translocate it along their surface. J Protozool 38:411–421.

358 / Dubremetz

Trager W, Williams J (1992): Extracellular (axenic) development in vitro of the erythrocytic cycle of *Plasmodium falciparum*. Proc Natl Acad Sci USA 89:5351–5355.
Vivier E, Petitprez A (1969): Le complexe membranaire et son évolution lors de l'élaboration des individus-fils de *Toxoplasma gondii*..J Cell Biol 43:329–342.
Ward GE, Miller LH, Dvorak JA (1993): The origin of parasitophorous membrane lipids in malaria-infected erythrocytes. J Cell Sci 106:237–248.
Wilson RJM, Garner MJ, Feagin JE, Williamson DH (1991): Have malaria parasites three genomes. Parasitol Today 7:134–136.

Molecular Approaches to Parasitology, pages 359–369
© 1995 Wiley-Liss, Inc.

What We Talk About When We Talk About Cell Invasion: Reflections on a Trypanosome System

Norma W. Andrews

Cell Biology Department, Yale University School of Medicine, New Haven, Connecticut 06510

INTRODUCTION

Trypanosoma cruzi is an extremely versatile parasite: It has the ability to invade and replicate inside a wide variety of nucleated cells. In fact, a *T. cruzi*–resistant vertebrate cell line is still to be identified. Every cell capable of spreading on a substrate in vitro has proven to be a suitable host for the intracellular cycle of this protozoan. Therefore, a very simple and straightforward conclusion can be made at this point: If *T. cruzi* utilizes host cell resources to invade, the machinery involved must be ubiquitous, possibly related to housekeeping functions. In this chapter I discuss a few recent findings that we believe are bringing us closer to understanding how this clever parasite establishes itself inside host cells. Along the way I mention some observations the significance of which we do not fully understand yet but that our "gut feeling" tells us may be important. Also I try to put all this in a larger perspective, stressing that we have a lot to learn from paying more attention to the powerful resources mammalian cells have to offer to parasites.

CELL ENTRY

I start with the mechanism by which *T. cruzi* enters cells and then work my way back to recognition and attachment. I hope my reasons for doing this become obvious, but let me spell out something right away: In my opinion, too much time and effort has been put into receptor–ligand identification and too little into thinking about how binding leads to internalization. Host cell entry by parasites almost invariably involves the formation of a membrane-bound vacuole. This can be a big problem for a large protozoan dealing with a nonphagocytic cell. The classic approach to this problem has been to describe parasite invasion as "induced phagocytosis." The reasoning has been that upon binding to the host cell some signal is triggered that makes fibroblasts or hepatocytes behave like macrophages, extending pseudopods and engulfing the intruder. It follows that drugs like cytochalasin D, which inhibit phagocytosis by blocking actin polymerization and pseudopod extention, should prevent cell invasion. This has proven to be the case for several intracellular bacteria (Falkow, et al., 1992). However, when the experiment was done with *T. cruzi*, the results were surprising.

Schenkman and collaborators (1991) initially found that cytochalasin D had no effect on trypomastigote invasion of HeLa and MDCK cells and raised the issue that the *T. cruzi* invasion mechanism was probably distinct from classic phagocytosis. In fact, scanning electron microscopic images of the invasion process obtained a few years earlier by Victor Nussenzweig's group already suggested this: trypomastigotes were observed diving gradually into the host cell, with no sign of pseudopod extention (Schenkman et al., 1988). Further exploring these puzzling observations in my laboratory at Yale, Isabelle Tardieux found that cytochalasin D not only did not inhibit, but actually enhanced trypomastigote entry into several cell types (Tardieux et al., 1992). Thus the central question became: Where does the membrane required to form the vacuole around *T. cruzi* come from, if it is not derived from extensions of the plasma membrane, driven by actin polymerization?

At the same time we were pondering the meaning of another unexpected finding. Lysosomes in animal cells are normally clustered in the perinuclear area, associated with the microtubule organizing center. The prevailing dogma in cell biology is that material internalized by cells and destined for degradation meets lysosomes after migration to the perinuclear area, a journey that takes 15–30 minutes. Unexpectedly, when we exposed cells to trypomastigotes for short periods and then stained the fixed cells with markers for lysosomes, it became clear that lysosomes were fusing very early with the *T. cruzi*–containing vacuoles, even before the parasites were completely internalized (Hall et al., 1992). So we asked ourselves: Were these findings related? Were lysosomes the solution to the puzzle? Were they providing the membrane required to form the *T. cruzi* parasitophorous vacuole?

To test this hypothesis we decided to take advantage of experimental conditions known to change the distribution of lysosomes in mammalian cells: exposure to the fungal metabolite brefeldin A, to a membrane-permeant analog of cAMP, or to acetate buffer at pH 6.6. These agents work by different mechanisms, but they all share the capacity of inducing a dramatic migration of lysosomes from the perinuclear area to the cell periphery in a microtubule-dependent manner. The consequence of these treatments was a significant enhancement in the invasion of NRK cells by trypomastigotes, which was also microtubule-dependent. Since *T. cruzi* has a clear preference for invading at the cell margins (Schenkman et al., 1988), these findings suggested the participation of lysosomes. When the cell periphery was depleted of lysosomes, invasion was reduced. We then tested the effect of conditions that interfere not with the localization, but with the fusion capacity of lysosomes. Loading lysosomes of NRK cells with sucrose, which cannot be digested and therefore blocks lysosomal fusion with incoming vacuoles, reduced trypomastigote invasion by 50%. Entry was also significantly reduced in cells undergoing mitosis, a period in which all intracellular membrane fusion events are blocked (Warren, 1985).

We were not the first ones to show that mitotic cells are resistant to *T. cruzi* invasion. Jim Dvorak and Mark Crane published in 1981 basically the same observation from a study using synchronized HeLa cells (Dvorak and Crane, 1981). Their interpretation at the time, however, was very different. They proposed that during mitosis receptors for *T. cruzi* were not expressed on the host cell surface. Although this cannot yet be totally ruled out, when we measured the attachment rates of trypomastigotes to fixed interphase or mitotic NRK cells, we found no reduction during mitosis. We therefore believe that the explanation lies in the dynamics of intracellular organelles, particularly the lysosomes. This is a novel way of thinking about cell invasion that opens a whole new world of possibilities (cheers from the ones of us tired of pursuing boring surface receptors!).

There is another observation on *T. cruzi* invasion that has been interpreted based on differential expression of surface receptors. When polarized MDCK cells were exposed to trypomastigotes, entry was much more efficient from the basolateral domain than from the apical domain (Schenkman et al., 1988). We think that this finding can also be explained by a requirement for interaction with lysosomes. Because microtubules run vertically in polarized epithelial cells, when the cytosol of polarized MDCK cells is acidified lysosomes migrate to the basolateral domain (Parton et al., 1991). This domain is therefore the region to which lysosomes can be mobilized in these cells. The reason why invasion is poor through the apical domain could be that the elaborate cortical cytoskeleton of the brush border prevents lysosome access to the plasma membrane. In support of this interpretation, Isabelle Tardieux showed that there is a 10-fold enhancement in *T. cruzi* entry through the apical domain after the actin cytoskeleton of the MDCK cells is disrupted by cytochalasin D (Tardieux et al., 1992). This should not have occurred if the apical domain was depleted in receptors for *T. cruzi*.

What we really needed at this point was morphological evidence to support these ideas. Fortunately we were able to establish collaborations with two terrific microscopists, John Heuser (Washington University) and Paul Webster (Yale University), who helped us show that indeed there is a very early interaction of trypomastigotes with lysosomes in mammalian cells. By both light and electron microscopy it was possible to visualize parasites attached to the host cell, still completely extracellular, which were already associated with a cluster of lysosomes underneath the plasma membrane. It was also possible to catch trypomastigotes in the act of entering cells, and in this case the intracellular portion was already strongly labeled with lysosomal markers (antibodies to lgps, specific lysosome glycoproteins, or horseradish peroxidase chased into the cells for 2 hours). These striking images could mean only one thing: that the trypanosomes communicate with the host cell's intracellular environment, sending a signal that results in clustering and fusion of lysosomes at the site of invasion.

What could be the nature of this signal? A previous observation gave us a clue: the enhancement in trypomastigote invasion caused by cytochalasin D, a specific inhibitor of actin polymerization. The plasma membrane of mammalian cells is supported by the cortical cytoskeleton, a scaffold of polymerized actin (Bretscher, 1991). This is a very complex and dense network, which normally blocks the access of large organelles such as lysosomes to the plasma membrane. Several actin-binding proteins have been identified that can modulate the structure of the cortical cytoskeleton; modifications such as phosphorylation and Ca^{2+} binding control their interaction with actin filaments (Aderem, 1992). One situation in which the cortical cytoskeleton clearly has to be rearranged is during regulated secretion. For secretory granules to fuse with the plasma membrane, the actin barrier has to be locally and temporarily removed. It has actually been shown that cytochalasin D treatment stimulates degranulation in secretory cells (Aunis and Bader, 1988). We decided therefore to use regulated secretion as a model for our thinking on the cell invasion mechanism of *T. cruzi*.

The most extensively studied second messenger regulating secretion in mammalian cells is Ca^{2+}. Several examples exist showing that, keeping all other factors constant, a rise in the cytosolic free Ca^{2+} concentration triggers degranulation in several cell types, from neutrophils to neurons (De Camilli and Jahn, 1990). Work in progress in the laboratory, using protocols to buffer or deplete intracellular free Ca^{2+} in NRK cells, is suggesting that host cell Ca^{2+} transients play an important role in *T. cruzi* invasion. We are now performing experiments designed to visualize cytoplasmic Ca^{2+} transients in living cells exposed to trypomastigotes using Ca^{2+}-sensitive fluorescent dyes. Results coming soon (Tardieux et al., 1994) to a journal near you!

A frequently asked question when I talk about lysosome recruitment during *T. cruzi* invasion is: "Why lysosomes?" True, it does seem like the most dangerous way of getting into a cell. Setting aside possible eccentricities of a South American parasite, who may be deliberately choosing to go against the establishment, I have a pet idea here. This may be giving us a clue: Lysosome mobilization and fusion to the plasma membrane may not be such a difficult thing to do after all. The trypomastigotes may have learned to utilize a pathway that already exists in most cells that normally goes unnoticed because it is not part of routine cell functions. Trypomastigotes could be the tool to define this pathway, which could have very interesting implications related to the regulation of cytoskeletal rearrangements and membrane traffic. It would not be the first time, by trypanosomes overdoing something, that an important phenomenon was discovered (vide GPI anchors, RNA editing, and so forth).

ESCAPE FROM THE VACUOLE

During the first 1–2 hours of intracellular life, *T. cruzi* makes a dramatic transition. The parasitophorous vacuole is gradually disrupted, and the parasites gain access to the cytosol. This occurs while they are still at the trypomastigote stage, the flagellated invasive form. Shortly after reaching the cytoplasm trypomastigotes change into amastigotes, round forms with a short flagellum. These forms are not invasive for most nonphagocytic cells, but are very efficiently taken up by macrophages. When this happens, the amastigotes can also disrupt the phagosome and replicate in the cytosol. We suspect that amastigotes play an important role in vivo, perpetuating the infection even in the presence of an immune response (Ley et al., 1988).

We found some time ago that trypomastigotes and amastigotes secrete a protein with hemolytic activity at low pH. It was exciting when we also found, in collaboration with Victoria Ley and Victor Nussenzweig, that the *T. cruzi*–containing parasitophorous vacuoles were acidic and that neutralizing the pH of these vacuoles inhibited parasite escape. This meant that finally, after decades of speculation on how *T. cruzi* could be inducing membrane disruption, we had an activity that could explain it. When, with the help of Michael Whitlow at NYU, we measured the the lesions formed in erythrocytes by the *T. cruzi* hemolysin, we found that they were very similar to the ones formed during cell lysis by complement (~10 nm). To our surprise, the hemolytic activity copurified with a protein immunologically cross-reactive with antibodies to reduced and alkylated human C9 (the terminal component of the membrane attack complex of complement). These antibodies also recognize perforin, the lytic protein from cytotoxic lymphocytes that, like C9, lyses cells by forming transmembrane pores on their membranes (Andrews et al., 1990). This led us to name the protein Tc-TOX, as a putative *T. cruzi* toxin, and to test its pore-forming activity in a planar lipid bilayer system. We sent the purified protein to Charles Abrams and Stephen Slatin at Albert Einstein, who showed that it indeed formed channels on membranes only at pH 5.5. The channels were small, however, smaller than the 10 nm diameter measured in the molecular sieving experiments. It is not clear if the initial small pores evolve later into larger lesions, but this is a possibility. The signal in the bilayer experiments gets very noisy with time, and the interpretation is not clear. We are currently working on obtaining sequence information for Tc-TOX to understand better its mechanism of action. It has thus far proven to be a challenging task—the protein is produced in very small amounts by *T. cruzi*, and bacteria do not seem to enjoy expressing it. But stay tuned, we are not giving up!

As discussed above, we now know quite a bit more about the composition of the membrane forming the *T. cruzi* parasitophorous vacuole. We know that these vacuoles are formed in large part, if not exclusively, by host cell lysosomes. Therefore we know that lgps, lysosomal membrane glycoproteins, are present in high density on the luminal side of the vacuole. Lgps are heavily sialylated glycoproteins that account for as much as 50% of the total protein content of lysosomes (Kornfeld and Mellman, 1989). The interesting connection here was made by Lee Hall, at Yale. He realized that lgps must be among the first host proteins that *T. cruzi* encounters during its journey into cells and that this was interesting considering that one of the major surface proteins of the trypomastigote form happens to recognize sialic acid—the surface *trans*-sialidase. Several groups are actively studying this enzyme, which is part of a large family of *T. cruzi* surface glycoproteins and is capable of transferring a 2-3-sialic acid from external donors (serum glycoproteins) to terminal galactose acceptors on the surface of trypomastigotes, and back and forth (Schenkman and Eichinger, 1993). Everybody involved with this enzyme was investigating its extracellular role, since the activity was initially detected in culture supernatants, at neutral pH. But Lee noticed that there was also considerable activity between pH 5.0 and 5.5 and asked a question no one had asked before: Could the *T. cruzi* surface *trans*-sialidase be playing a role inside the vacuole, removing sialic acid from lgp? If so, would this event facilitate disruption of the vacuolar membrane? We decided to give it a shot, and it paid back. We obtained evidence supporting both hypotheses.

First, in vitro treatment with the *T. cruzi* *trans*-sialidase induced a shift of immunoprecipitated lgp to more basic pI on two-dimensional gels, indicating loss of sialic acid moieties. Second, *T. cruzi* escape from vacuoles was significantly more efficient in mutant CHO cells deficient in glycoprotein sialylation. When guinea pig erythrocytes were treated in vitro with the *T. cruzi* enzyme or with *Vibrio cholera* neuraminidase, they became more sensitive to lysis by the *T. cruzi* hemolysin. This indicated that sialic acid can act as a barrier for the pore-forming activity of Tc-TOX. Interestingly, the release of the *trans*-sialidase from the parasite's surface, an event that occurs normally at low levels through phospholipase C cleavage of the GPI anchor, is significantly enhanced when the medium is acidified. Since we know that the parasites are in an acidic compartment as soon as they enter cells, it is conceivable that the enhanced release of soluble *trans*-sialidase at low pH contributes to increase the local concentration of enzyme, resulting in desialylation of lgp (Hall et al., 1992).

At this point we come back to the issue of what is the receptor on the host cell surface that trypomastigotes bind to and what is the counter-receptor on the parasite. Evidence has accumulated recently indicating a role for sialic acid on the host cell and the *trans*-sialidase on the trypomastigote's side. Invasion is poor on cells lacking terminal sialic acid, and resialylation restores it (Ming et al., 1993; Schenkman and Eichinger, 1993). The purified *trans*-sialidase or *trans*-sialidase–specific competitive sugars inhibit trypomastigote entry (Ming et al., 1993). A complicating factor in these studies has been that inhibition is never complete; there is a low level of invasion that occurs independent of sialic acid and *trans*-sialidase. Recent evidence seems to indicate that *T. cruzi* invasion can also be mediated by host cell surface glycosaminoglycans and a heparin-binding trypomastigote surface molecule, penetrin (Ortega-Barria and Pereira, 1991).

An interesting speculation that can be made at this point is whether a sequential transfer of sialic acid between lgp on lysosomes and acceptors on the trypomastigote's surface occurs during invasion. One can imagine a scenario in which a trypomastigote binds to sialic acid or heparin-sulfate moieties on the surface of the host cell. This is followed by activation of a signal-transduction pathway (another receptor?) that triggers local rearrangement of the cortical actin cytoskeleton and mobilization of lysosomes, which start to fuse with the plasma membrane. When the first lysosome fuses, lgps from the luminal surface of lysosomes become exposed, in close proximity to the trypomastigote surface *trans*-sialidase. The resulting exchange of sialic acid stabilizes trypomastigote attachment, and at the same time promotes expansion of the vacuole, as more lysosomes approach and fuse. Videomicroscopy observation of live cells being invaded by trypomastigotes seems to support this view. The parasites initially glide back and forth on the host cell surface, but as soon as invasion starts their movement becomes unidirectional, as if intracellular structures were directing its entry into the cell. The subsequent steps, of how we believe *T. cruzi* makes the transition from lysosomes into the cytosol, have been discussed already and are summarized in Figure 1.

LIFE IN THE CYTOPLASM

Reaching the cytoplasm can be viewed as the real moment in which cell invasion occurs. While inside a vacuole, parasites are still in an extracellular-like environment. Once the vacuole is disrupted, *T. cruzi* makes intimate contact with a very different medium (free Ca^{2+} concentrations, for example, drop from 1 mM to 100 nM). It is in this medium that the trigger for replication occurs, after a mysterious lag period of ~24 hours during which the amastigotes remain dormant. It is also in this medium that the trigger for differentiation from amastigotes back to trypomastigotes occurs, shortly before cell rupture at the end of the cycle. Practi-

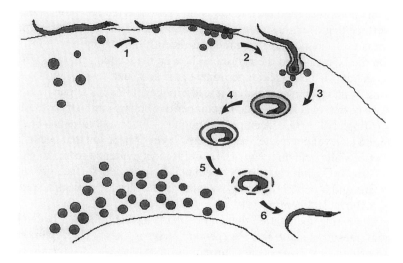

Fig. 1. Model representing the early stages of the interaction between *T. cruzi* trypomastigotes and mammalian cells. 1) Trypomastigotes attach to the cell surface. 2) Host cell lysosomes are recruited to the attachment site and start to fuse with the plasma membrane. 3) Intracellular vacuole composed of lysosomal membranes lined by lgps is formed. 4) Lgps are desialylated by the *T. cruzi trans*-sialidase. 5) The vacuolar membrane is disrupted (Tc-TOX?). 6) Trypomastigotes reach the cytosol.

cally nothing is known about the signals controlling this event; it occurs in a striking synchronous fashion, only a few hours before the trypomastigotes are released from the cell (the complete cycle takes about 4.5 days).

One of the mysteries involving the intracellular life of *T. cruzi* is the function of Ssp-4, an amastigote-specific surface glycoprotein. Ssp-4 is expressed in large amounts soon after the parasites enter the cytoplasm and is then gradually shed, a stage in which fluorescence can be detected in the cytoplasm with Ssp-4–specific monoclonal antibodies (Fig. 2A,B). Even more mysterious is the pattern in which Ssp-4 is shed intracellularly. Trypomastigotes also change into amastigotes, express Ssp-4 and shed it extracellularly. The difference is that outside of cells Ssp-4 is clearly released in a soluble form, generated by cleavage of its GPI anchor by an endogenous PIPLC (Andrews et al., 1988). Inside cells, however, a striking pattern suggesting Ssp-4 aggregation and membrane vesiculation is observed (Fig. 2C,D). We still do not know what this means; it is tempting to speculate that it is induced by a cytosolic factor interacting with the amastigote's membrane. Very interesting examples appeared recently demonstrating association of host cell cytoskeleton components with intracytoplasmic pathogens (Andrews and Webster, 1991)—something similar could be going on here.

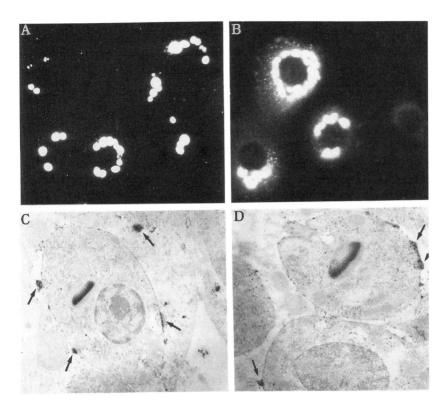

Fig. 2. Shedding of Ssp-4, the major surface glycoprotein of *T. cruzi* amastigotes, into the cytosol of host cells. **A:** Immunofluorescence, 48 hours after cell entry. **B:** Immunofluorescence, 72 hours after cell entry; **C,D:** Immunogold, 72 hours after cell entry. Arrows point to aggregates of Ssp-4. The 2C2 monoclonal antibody was used to localize Ssp-4 (Andrews et al., 1993). (C,D, electron micrographs courtesy of Dr. E.S. Robbins, New York University.)

When we were looking for phospholipase activities in *T. cruzi* we made another intriguing observation that we do not fully understand yet. As the parasites differentiate from trypomatigotes into amastigotes a very active phospholipase A_2 (PLA$_2$) is produced (Fig. 3). PLA$_2$ is known to play a central role in signal transduction mechanisms, generating arachidonic acid and subsequently oxygenated eicosanoid metabolites. These metabolites govern cellular functions as diverse as inflammation, muscle contraction, ion channel activities and neurotransmission (Pruzanski and Wadas, 1991). Why would this activity appear in *T. cruzi* only during the intracellular part of the cycle?

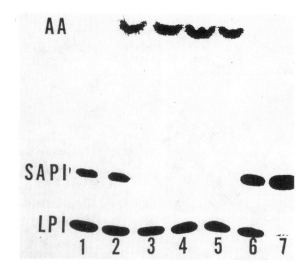

Fig. 3. Phospholipase activity in *T. cruzi* extracts. Thin layer chromatography of the products of digestion of Stearyl-arachidonyl-phosphatidylinositol (SAPI) by extracts of parasites undergoing differentiation from trypomastigotes (1) to amastigotes (5). Epimastigotes are shown in lane 6, and lane 7 is a blank with only substrate and no extract. Lyso-PI (LPI), a product of PLA_1, was detected in all samples except 7; arachidonic acid (AA), a product of PLA_2, was only detected in extracts containing amastigotes (2 = 8 hours; 3 = 24 hours; 4 = 48 hours; 5 = 72 hours).

This is the new frontier to be explored—life in the cytoplasm. Like life in another planet, most of the rules we have established with our test-tube reproductions of the extracellular environment do not apply. But fortunately we do know a bit about this foreign land. It happens to be our own cells, and all we have to do now is change our biased thinking and take advantage of the wealth of information that is out there. We predict exciting times ahead. Trypanosome products with defined functions have been identified, and now it is time for the next step, their molecular characterization. These studies may lead us to the identification of homologs in mammalian cells and trigger an explosive area of investigation.

REFERENCES

Aderem A (1992): Signal transduction and the actin cytoskeleton: The roles of MARKS and profilin. Trends Biochem Sci 17:438–443.

Andrews NW, Abrams CK, Slatin SL, Griffiths G (1990): A *T. cruzi*–secreted protein immunologically related to the complement component C9: Evidence for membrane pore-forming activity at low pH. Cell 61:1277_1287.

Andrews NW, Robbins ES, Ley V, Hong KS, Nussenzweig V (1988): Developmentally-regulated, phospholipase C-mediated release of the major surface glycoprotein of amastigotes of *Trypanosoma cruzi*. J Exp Med 167:300–314.

Andrews NW, Webster P (1991): Phagolysosomal escape by intracellular pathogens. Parasitol Today 7:335–340.

Aunis D, Bader MF (1988): The cytoskeleton as a barrier to exocytosis in secretory cells. J Exp Biol 139:253–266.

Bretscher A (1991): Microfilament structure and function in the cortical cytoskeleton. Annu Rev Cell Biol 7:337–374.

De Camilli P, Jahn R (1990): Pathways to regulated exocytosis in neurons. Annu Rev Physiol 52:625–645.

Dvorak JA, Crane M St J (1981): Vertebrate cell cycle modulates infection by protozoan parasites. Science 214:1034–1036.

Falkow S, Isberg RR, Portnoy DA (1992): The interaction of bacteria with mammalian cells. Annu Rev Cell Biol 8:333–363.

Hall BF, Webster P, Ma AK, Joiner KA, Andrews NW(1992): Desialylation of lysosomal membrane glycoproteins by *Trypanosoma cruzi*: A role for the surface neuraminidase in facilitating parasite entry into the host cell cytoplasm. J Exp Med 176:313–325.

Kornfeld S, Mellman I (1989): The biogenesis of lysosomes. Annu Rev Cell Biol 5:483–525.

Ley V, Andrews NW, Robbins ES, Nussenzweig V (1988): Amastigotes of *Trypanosoma cruzi* sustain an infective cycle in mammalian cells. J Exp Med 168:649–658.

Ming M, Chuenkova M, Ortega-Barria E, Pereira MEA (1993): Mediation of *Trypanosoma cruzi* invasion by sialic acid on the host cell and *trans*-sialidase on the trypanosome. Mol Biochem Parasitol 59:243–252.

Ortega-Barria E, Pereira MEA (1991): A novel *T. cruzi* heparin-binding protein promotes fibroblast adhesion and penetration of engineered bacteria and trypanosomes into mammalian cells. Cell 67:411–421.

Parton RG, Dotti CG, Bacallao R, Kurtz I, Simons K, Prydz K (1991): pH-induced microtubule-dependent redistribution of late endosomes in neuronal and epithelial cells. J Cell Biol 113:261–274.

Pruzanski W, Wadas P (1991): Phospholipase A_2—A mediator between proximal and distal effectors of inflammation. Immunol Today 12:143–146.

Schenkman S, Andrews NW, Nussenzweig V, Robbins ES (1988): *Trypanosoma cruzi* invade a mammalian epithelial cell in a polarized manner. Cell 55:157–165.

Schenkman S, Eichinger D (1993): *Trypanosoma cruzi trans*-sialidase and cell invasion. Parasitol Today 9:217–222.

Schenkman S, Robbins ES, Nussenzweig V (1991): Attachment of *Trypanosoma cruzi* to mammalian cells requires parasite energy, and invasion can be independent of the target cell cytoskeleton. Infect Immun 59:645–654.

Tardieux I, Nathanson MH, Andrews NW (1994): Role in host cell invasion of *Trypanosoma cruzi*-induced cytostolic free Ca^{2+} transients. J Exp Med. 179:1017–1022.

Tardieux I, Webster P, Ravesloot J, Boron W, Lunn JA, Heuser JE, Andrews NW (1992): Lysosome recruitment and fusion are early events required for trypanosome invasion of mammalian cells. Cell 71:117–1130.

Warren G (1985): Membrane traffic and organelle division. Trends Biochem Sci 10:439–443.

Molecular Approaches to Parasitology, pages 371–398
© 1995 Wiley-Liss, Inc.

The Golgi Complex in *Plasmodium falciparum*: Its Implications for a Tubovesicular Network in the Infected-Erythrocyte Cytoplasm and Secretory Export of Parasite Proteins

Kasturi Haldar, Heidi G. Elmendorf, Arpita Das, Jay L. Crary, Wen-Lu Li, Lyle Uyetake, and Sabine Lauer

Department of Microbiology and Immunology, Stanford University School of Medicine, Stanford, California 94305

INTRODUCTION

Malaria is a major infectious disease. It afflicts over 200 million people and causes 1–2 million deaths each year. The incidence of the disease is increasing largely due to the spread of *Plasmodium falciparum,* which causes the most virulent form of human malaria. This protozoan infects mature erythrocytes during its development in the blood. The cycle begins when the extracellular merozoite enters the red cell. The resulting intraerythrocytic parasite develops in a parasitophorous vacuole through morphologically distinct ring, trophozoite, and schizont stages. During schizogony, the parasite replicates mitotically to produce 16 daughter merozoites; these are released during lysis of the red cell and go on to reinvade new erythrocytes. This cycle takes 48 hours, and these parasite stages are entirely responsible for the symptoms of the disease.

Invasion is a complex, multistep process in which the merozoite attaches to and invaginates the red cell bilayer. The red cell is inherently nonendocytic. Hence, the internalization of its membrane must be induced, and secretory protein transfer from the apical organelles of the merozoite has been implicated in this uptake process (reviewed by Perkins, 1992). These organelles (comprising the rhoptries, micronemes, and dense granules), as well as the subpellicular cytoskeleton of the merozoite, disappear immediately after invasion and are not detected in the intracellular rings (Langreth and Trager, 1978).

The ring stage spans the first 24 hours of intracellular development, when there is very little increase in the size of the parasite or the parasitophorous vacuole. However, prominent membrane development occurs in the infected erythrocyte cytoplasm. Transmission electron micrographs from early studies (Aikawa, 1971) have clearly indicated that long, 0.2–0.4 μm, flattened lamellar membranes (also referred to as *cisternae* or *Maurer's clefts*) and large membrane loops, 0.1–1 μm in diameter, emerge in the infected erythrocyte cytoplasm. Later, parasite proteins were detected in these structures: A doublet of 45–47 kD has been ascribed to the cisternae while another of 28 kD (Exp1) is detected in the loops, indicating that the two membrane forms are biochemically and morphologically distinct (reviewed by Barnwell, 1990; Elmendorf and Haldar, 1993a). Lipid labeling experiments at the Biology of Parasitism course in the summer of 1992 first suggested to us that the intraerythrocytic compartments may be interconnected in live infected erythrocytes. The most recent studies using scanning electron and laser confocal microscopy confirm that they are linked in a complex reticulum of tubovesicular membranes (TVM) that extends from the parasite through the erythrocyte cytoplasm (Elford and Ferguson, 1993; Elmendorf and Haldar, 1993a; Elmendorf and Haldar, 1994). Despite this membrane growth in the erythrocyte cytoplasm, structural modifications of the erythrocyte membrane are not prominent in ring stage cells. Parasite-induced lipid import at the red cell membrane is seen at the ring stage (reviewed by Haldar, 1992; Lauer and Haldar, manuscript in preparation) but has not, as yet, been associated with any ultrastructural changes in the host cell bilayer at this stage.

At the trophozoite (~24–30 hour) and schizont (30–48 hour) stages there are prominent changes in the membrane of the erythrocyte as well as in the parasite plasma membrane (PPM) and its surrounding vacuolar membrane (PVM) (Langreth and Trager, 1978). Exogenous lipids from the extracellular medium and the erythrocyte surface are actively imported into the parasite, and prominent changes occur in the ultrastructure, transport, and adherence properties of the red cell surface. These aspects of erythrocyte modification, as well as parasite proteins exported to the red cell membrane, have been covered in several reviews (Howard, 1988; Barnwell, 1989; Cabantchik, 1990; Vial et al., 1990; Haldar, 1992) and therefore are not presented in any further detail here. The intraerythrocytic cisternae and loops that develop in the ring stages continue to be present in the trophozoite and schizont infected cell. Large vesicular structures that dominate at the ring stage appear to be replaced by longer tubular elements and smaller vesicles (Elmendorf and Haldar, 1994), suggesting a distinct function for these membranes at the later stages of growth. At schizogony the parasite undergoes mitosis and increases dra-

matically in size. Subcellular organelles within the parasite presumably replicate, and components of the apical secretory organelles are synthesised and
assembled. There is rapid enlargement of the PPM and PVM. The major protein components of the PPM, the merozoite surface proteins 1 and 2 (MSP1
and MSP2), as well as proteins that concentrate in the lumenal space between the PPM and PVM, such as Pf126, are synthesized and exported to
their correct subcellular destinations (reviewed by Haldar and Holder,
1993). Each merozoite is packaged when the parasite plasma membrane
pinches off around a daughter nucleus and a set of organelles. At the end
of the cycle, the parasitophorous vacuole lyses followed by the infected
erythrocyte membrane, and the released merozoites reinvade new host
erythrocytes within seconds.

As described above, complex events of membrane transport and assembly
occur both in the red cell and in the parasite at all stages of the asexual cycle.
The red cell is enucleated and incapable of de novo protein and lipid biosynthesis. Hence plasmodial secretory mechanisms must regulate the trafficking
of proteins and lipids between organelles in its cytoplasm as well as beyond
its PPM, to the PVM, the TVM, and the red cell. Yet very little is known of
these mechanisms or how they regulate membrane function in the infected
erythrocyte. The Golgi is a major organelle required for the sorting of proteins
and lipids in eukaryotic cells. In this chapter we will focus on the identification and localization of plasmodial Golgi activities and on their implications
for 1) the organization and function of a TVM induced by the parasite in the
cytoplasm of its host red cell and 2) secretory export of parasite proteins.

SECRETORY ACTIVITIES OF THE PARASITE
ENDOPLASMIC RETICULUM

The secretory pathway in eukaryotic cells was originally described by Palade
and coworkers as a pathway for protein transport to the secretory granules
(see Palade, 1975). In a generalization of this pathway proteins from the endoplasmic reticulum (ER)–Golgi complex are exported to a number of subcellular destinations, including the plasma membrane (reviewed by Pfeffer
and Rothman, 1987). Proteins synthesized on ribosomes in the cytoplasm that
contain an appropriate signal sequence are cotranslationally imported into the
ER. They are carried through the ER and Golgi complex by the budding
and fusion of vesicles between successive compartments. A subset may be
modified by a high mannose glycan (N-linked to the polypeptide) in the
ER with further sugar addition and modification in the Golgi (Kornfeld
and Kornfeld, 1985). Specific signals on proteins result either in their retention in the ER–Golgi complex or targetting to a further subcellular des-

tination. Thus Lys-Asp-Glu-Leu (KDEL) on the C terminus of a secretory protein results in its retention in the ER in mammalian cells (reviewed by Pelham, 1990).

Several secretory properties of the ER are detected in *Plasmodium*. Proteins exported from the parasite or concentrated in the secretory organelles of the apical complex contain appropriate hydrophobic signal sequences. These include proteins exported to the parasite plasma membrane and the vacuolar space, the vacuolar surface, and the erythrocyte cytoplasm, as well as proteins of the rhoptries, micronemes, and dense granules (reviewed by Elmendorf and Haldar, 1993a; Lingelbach, 1993; Haldar and Holder, 1993). Hence all of these proteins may be cotranslationally recruited into the lumen of the ER, which is the first step of transport in the secretory pathway. In addition, the proteins MSP1 and MSP2 of the parasite plasma membrane contain a glycosylphosphatidylinositol (GPI) anchor (reviewed by Haldar and Holder, 1993), a post-translational protein modification acquired in the lumen of the ER.

The immunoglobulin binding protein (BiP) is a prominent marker of the ER in mammalian cells. It is a chaperonin molecule required for the correct folding of proteins in the ER. Consistent with its localization in the ER, it contains a tetrapeptide sequence of KDEL on its C terminus. A putative BiP homolog has been identified in *P. falciparum,* strongly suggesting the presence of a fundamental secretory protein folding activity in the parasite ER (Kumar et al., 1991). The malarial BiP contains a C-terminal tetrapeptide sequence of SDEL (Kumar and Zheny, 1992) consistent with the XDEL motif predicted for ER retention signals in mammalian cells and yeast.

ERD2, A MARKER FOR THE GOLGI IN *PLASMODIUM*

ER retention signals are recognized by the *ERD2* gene product, which serves as a receptor required for protein retention in the endoplasmic reticulum. The function of ERD2 was originally determined from genetic evidence in yeast (Semenza et al., 1990; Lewis et al., 1990). Immunolocalization studies later indicated that ERD2 is concentrated in the *cis* Golgi network (Lewis and Pelham, 1990; Tang et al., 1993). The model proposed for ERD2 function is as follows (reviewed by Pelham, 1990). When proteins move out of the lumen of the ER into the Golgi, those with the C-terminal XDEL sequence are recognized by the ERD2 protein and recycled in a receptor–ligand complex back to the ER. Here, the complex disassociates and free ERD2 returns to the Golgi. This model is consistent with the observations that 1) the retention of resident proteins in the lumen of the ER requires their continuous retrieval from the Golgi (Pelham, 1990) and 2) overexpression of ERD2 in cells results in protein and membrane accumulation in the ER (Lewis and Pelham, 1992). The

ERD2 protein is a 26 kD polypeptide. Based on hydrophobicity and mutational analyses it is predicted to have seven transmembrane domains, resulting in most of the protein being buried in the lipid bilayer.

By PCR amplification and cloning methodologies we identified a homolog of ERD2 in *Plasmodium falciparum* (PfERD2) (Elmendorf and Haldar, 1993b). There is 40%–50% identity between ERD2 from mammalian cells, yeast, and *Plasmodium*. Importantly, in all three there is extensive identity in regions that are conserved and the proposed secondary structure is conserved. Specific residues that are important for binding to ER resident proteins in mammalian ERD2 and for recycling of the receptor to the ER are also conserved in *P. falciparum*. The *P. falciparum* protein has an additional four amino acid sequence at the C terminus. While the precise significance of this extension in either the localization of the protein or its recycling has not yet been investigated, we were able to exploit this difference to produce high-affinity antibodies to a C-terminal fragment of PfERD2. In Western blots the antibodies recognize a 26 kD parasite protein that is tightly associated with cellular membranes, consistent with the predicted size and membranous nature of ERD2s. Indirect immunofluorescence microscopy studies indicate that PfERD2 is concentrated in a "spot" in the perinuclear region within the parasite (Fig. 1A). In mammalian cells ERD2 is concentrated in the *cis* Golgi in a perinuclear location. Hence the location of PfERD2 is consistent with its concentration in a Golgi element within the parasite.

BREFELDIN A, ITS EFFECT ON PfERD2 IN THE GOLGI AND PARASITE PROTEIN SECRETION

Brefeldin A (BFA) is a heterocyclic lactone that has been found to return Golgi membranes to the ER and block protein secretion in cultured mammalian cells (reviewed by Klausner et al., 1992). When the drug is added to infected erythrocytes, it rapidly reorganizes PfERD2 in the Golgi into a more diffuse label with minor reticular elements over the body of the parasite (Fig. 1B). Removal of the drug results in a coalescence of PfERD2, indicating that the effect of the BFA is reversible and not due to nonspecific degeneration of the PfERD2 locus (Fig. 1C). The BFA diffused PFERD2 localization is similar to that of the malarial immunoglobulin binding protein (BiP), a marker for the parasite ER (Fig. 1B,D). This is consistent with the presence of a retrograde membrane transport pathway for the movement of ERD2 from the Golgi to the ER in *P. falciparum*.

BFA blocks the secretion of newly synthesized parasite proteins in ring and trophozoite-infected red cells (Crary and Haldar, 1992; Elmendorf et al., 1992). It does not affect protein synthesis, and the removal of the drug completely reverts the block in secretion. The kinetics of protein export are extremely

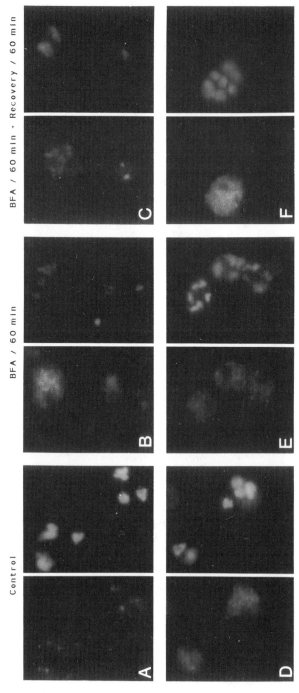

Fig. 1.   Disruption of PfERD2 localization upon treatment with brefeldin A. *P. falciparum*–infected erythrocytes were incubated at 37°C either in RPMI-1640 alone for 60 minutes (**A,D**), 5 μg/ml brefeldin A in RPMI-1640 for 60 minutes (**B,E**), or 5 μg/ml brefeldin A in RPMI-1640 for 60 minutes and then washed and reincubated in RPMI-1640 alone for an additional 60 minutes (**C,F**). Thin blood smears were made at the end of each treatment and processed as described (Elmendorf and Haldar, 1993b). Each frame contains an antibody stain in the left panel and the corresponding nuclear stain in the right panel. A–C, affinity-purified PfERD2 antibody; D–F, affinity-purified BiP antibody.

rapid. In the absence of any extracellular stimulus, newly synthesised proteins are found to be released at the PPM within 5 minutes from the onset of translation. BFA blocks transport at a site 3 minutes from translation (Crary and Haldar, 1992). The effect of BFA on the distribution of PfERD2 provides a morphological explanation for the observed block on protein export. In the export pathway, the PfERD2 site in the Golgi is expected to be encountered by newly synthesized proteins at or before 3 minutes from the onset of translation. The rapid kinetics of protein export suggest the presence of a minimal secretory apparatus within the parasite. This is consistent with a lack of prominent Golgi cisternae within the parasite and also the apparent lack of post-translational protein modifications of the secretory pathway such as sulfation (Das and Haldar, unpublished data), N-linked glycosylation, and terminal sugar modifications of N-linked glycans (Dieckmann-Schuppert et al., 1992). P. falciparum is the only organism found to be lacking in N-linked glycosylation. Although the significance of this is unknown, it presents an unfortunate hindrance in that the addition and processing of N-linked glycans cannot be used to dissect stepwise transport through the plasmodial secretory pathway.

SPHINGOMYELIN SYNTHESIS, A BIOSYNTHETIC ACTIVITY OF THE cis GOLGI IS DETECTED IN A PERINUCLEAR COMPARTMENT DISTINCT FROM THAT OF PfERD2

Sphingomyelin is universally present in higher vertebrate cells and is an important lipid component of cellular membranes. The most recent evidence indicates that it is synthesized largely in the Golgi from where it is exported by vesicular transport to the plasma membrane (reviewed by Pagano, 1990). Most of the sphingomyelin in a cell resides at its plasma membrane. Sphingomyelin from the cell surface can be internalized into endocytic vesicles and transported to the lysosomes. The fluorescent probes C6-NBD-ceramide and C5-Bodipy-ceramide have proven very useful in studying the synthesis and transport of sphingomyelin in cells. Since one of their fatty acids is a short chain these probes rapidly diffuse across aqueous space and can be delivered from exogenous liposomes or BSA–lipid complexes to cells at 0°C. Because they lack a charged head group they can also "flip" from one to the other leaflet of a lipid bilayer, and these two properties in conjunction allow them to cross all cellular membranes (Pagano, 1989; Pagano et al., 1991). When C6-NBD-ceramide is added to cultured mammalian cells it is metabolized to the fluorescent derivative of sphingomyelin and glucosylceramide in the Golgi. At 37°C, these fluorescent lipid products undergo vesicular export to the plasma membrane. However, at 20°C, a temperature at which membrane transport in the cell is greatly reduced, they remain trapped at their site of synthesis in the Golgi apparatus. BFA disrupts the observed lipid accumulation in the Golgi, consistent with the effect of this drug on the morphology of the organelle (Young et al., 1990).

NBD-ceramide is metabolized to NBD-sphingomyelin in *P. falciparum–* infected erythrocytes but not in uninfected cells (Haldar et al., 1991). When schizont-infected cells are labeled and examined by laser confocal microscopy, the fluorescent sphingomyelin staining is seen as prominent perinuclear circles (Fig. 2). Peripheral staining of the parasite plasma and vacuolar membranes is also observed but is not prominent in the optical sections shown in Figure 2. Surprisingly and unlike PfERD2, the perinuclear sphingomyelin staining is not disrupted by BFA. This strongly suggests that the two Golgi functions of PfERD2 and sphingomyelin synthase are likely to be localized in distinct compartments within the parasite.

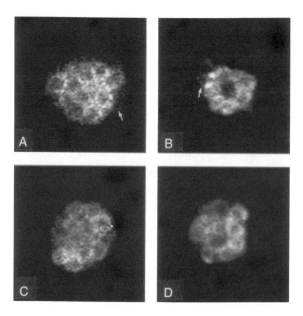

Fig. 2. C_6-NBD-sphingomyelin accumulation is brefeldin A-insensitive. *P. falciparum–* infected erythrocytes were incubated for 30 minutes at 0°C in 20 μM C_6-NBD-ceramide in 2 mg/ml defatted-BSA in RPMI-1640. Excess ceramide was removed by washing in RPMI-1640 and the incubation continued for 60 minutes at 20°C to allow conversion to C_6-NBD-sphingomyelin. Cells were then warmed to 37°C for 30 minutes in the absence (**A,B**) or presence (**C,D**) of 5 mg/ml brefeldin A, lightly fixed in 0.05% glutaraldehyde, and viewed by fluorescence confocal microscopy. Images were processed using Adobe Photoshop software. Arrows in A and B indicate the peripheral parasite membrane labeled by C_6-NBD-sphingomyelin; this peripheral membrane is not as markedly labeled in the confocal sections shown in C and D. The perinuclear staining of the daughter parasites appears as circles in a grape-like cluster.

These results have two important general implications for the organization of the Golgi in cells. The first is that even in a simple secretory apparatus, lacking *N*-linked glycosylation, the Golgi is still compartmentalized. It suggests that properties of the Golgi other than the stepwise modification of *N*-glycans need to segregated. Alternatively compartmentalization may be a natural consequence of activities such as the retrieval process of ERD2 that is then exploited by cells for other biosynthetic functions. The second implication is that ERD2 and sphingomyelin biosynthesis, both ascribed to the *cis* Golgi in mammalian cells, are clearly separated in a more primitive animal cell like *P. falciparum.*

CELL CYCLE–DEPENDENT EXPORT OF SPHINGOMYELIN SYNTHASE IN *PLASMODIUM*

Presence of the Enzyme in Merozoites, Ring, and Trophozoite-Infected Red Cells

In the asexual cycle, schizogony is a period of nuclear division and growth of the original parasite. It culminates in the formation of 10–16 merozoites (44–48 hours postinvasion) when the PPM pinches off around the daughter nuclei and a corresponding set of organelles. As indicated in the previous section, in schizonts there is a perinuclear region of sphingomyelin biosynthesis around each nucleus. When daughter merozoites form, each inherits its own perinuclear region of sphingomyelin biosynthesis, suggesting that the extracellular merozoites should contain sphingomyelin synthase (Elmendorf and Haldar, 1993b). Consistently, when merozoites were isolated, purified, and rendered completely free of other parasite stages they were found to contain high levels of sphingomyelin biosynthetic activity (Table 1) (Elmendorf and Haldar, 1994). This activity is not degraded by exogenous protease, except when the merozoites were disrupted with detergents. The detergents alone had no effect on the enzyme activity, indicating that all of the sphingomyelin synthase in the extracellular merozoite resides within the parasite (Elmendorf and Haldar, 1994).

Merozoites rapidly (within minutes) reinvade red cells and form ring stage parasites. Some merozoite components are detected in rings while others are processed and discarded (Blackman et al., 1990). When we compared levels of sphingomyelin synthesis in merozoites, rings, and trophozoites (under 30 hours of development; see Table 1) we found that equal numbers of parasites at these stages contained equal levels of enzyme activity. Furthermore, the sphingomyelin synthase activity in ring and trophozoite stage infected red cells was not decreased by cycloheximide (Table 1), indicating it was not due to de novo synthesis of the enzyme in these stages. Hence the enzyme in the

TABLE 1. Analysis of NBD-Sphingomyelin Synthesis in Merozoites, Ring, and Trophozoite-Infected Erythrocytes

	No. of cells ($\times 10^8$)	Relative fluorescence units of NBD-Sm[a]	
		15 min	30 min
Merozoites (extracellular)[b]			
Prep I	1	7	15
PrepII	2	12	23
PrepIII	2	13	27
Intracellular stages[c]			
Rings	1	6	14
	2	12	24
Trophs (<30 hours)	1	8	16
	2	14	26
Effects of cycloheximide[d]			
Rings			
+ Cycloheximide	2		29
− Cycloheximide	2		26
Trophs			
+ Cycloheximide	2		25
− Cycloheximide	2		27

[a]Each value reported is the average of three experiments.
[b]Merozoites were purified and incubated with C_6-NBD-ceramide. At the indicated times, samples were extracted and the amount of C_6-NBD-sphingomyelin synthesized was determined as described (Elmendorf and Haldar, 1994).
[c]Ring or trophozoite-infected erythrocytes were incubated with C_6-NBD-ceramide and the samples were processed identically as the merozoites.
[d]Ring or trophozoite-infected erythrocytes were either pretreated with cycloheximide or mock-treated as described in the text, incubated with C_6-NBD-ceramide for 30 minutes, and the amount of C_6-NBD-sphingomyelin was determined.

ring and trophozoite stage parasites must correspond to that present in the entering merozoite.

Export of Sphingomyelin Synthase

When cell equivalents of infected erythrocytes, parasites released from their host cells, and a fraction enriched for erythrocyte ghosts and TVM (EM/TVM membranes) were incubated with C6-NBD-ceramide, 90% of the original sphingomyelin synthase activity of infected erythrocytes was recovered from the released parasite and EM/TVM fractions; 39% was in the EM/TVM fraction while 52% was found in the released parasites (Elmendorf and Haldar, 1994). In contrast, only 5% of PfERD2 was detected in the EM/TVM fraction and 95% in the parasite. Even after accounting for the maximum levels of possible contamination, an average of 26% of the total sphingomyelin synthase activity was located in the EM/TVM fraction, indicating that the enzyme is truly exported past the parasite plasma membrane. Thus our results indicate export of a significant percentage of a Golgi enzyme beyond the parasite plasma membrane in ring and trophozite cells, but its complete intracellular retention in merozoites. The microscopy studies described in some detail in the next section show prominent sphingolipid accumulation in the TVM but not at the red cell membrane, indicating that the enzyme is exported to the TVM. Protease protection assays indicate that the exported enzyme is in the lumen of the isolated TVM (Elmendorf and Haldar, unpublished data). Here again, the results first suggesting the lumenal orientation of the enzyme in the TVM came from experiments at the Biology of Parasitism course in the summer of 1992. The sites of sphingomyelin synthase within the ring and trophozoite parasite have not been precisely defined. However, by analogy to the schizont stages and other eukaryotic cells, it is likely that the perinuclear region of sphingolipid staining corresponds to a major site of sphingomyelin biosynthesis in the ring and trophozoite's Golgi.

The stage-specific export of sphingomyelin synthase provides new insights into mechanisms of organization of this secretory enzyme in cells. In mammalians cells, subcellular fractionation studies in rat liver indicate that 87% of the sphingomyelin synthase activity is in the Golgi and 13% is at the plasma membrane. However, other studies suggest that higher levels of the enzyme may be at the plasma membrane (reviewed by Pagano, 1990). These discrepancies have raised some controversy concerning the distribution of the enzyme and the possibility that there may be two forms of sphingomyelin synthase activities in cells. We find that in the lower eukaryote *P. falciparum*, the relative distribution of the Golgi and exported forms is dependent on the cell cycle. Since the parasite sphingomyelin biosynthetic activity is entirely intracellular in merozoites, it may be ascribed to one protein whose export is mediated by a developmental reorganization of the parasite's Golgi apparatus in ring stage parasites.

MEMBRANE ORGANIZATION IN THE TVM

Presence of Reticulum

In ring and trophozoite stages, the fluorescent ceramide analogs label a perinuclear region within the parasite, the periphery of the parasite, as well as membrane compartments in the infected erythrocyte cytosol (Elmendorf and Haldar, 1994). Very low levels of label are also seen at the red cell surface. The organization of the intraerythrocytic membranes and their relationship to the parasitic surface and the red cell membrane was studied by 1) optically sectioning through the depth of the cell by laser confocal microscopy (Fig. 3) and 2) reconstructing a three-dimensional model of the surface of the parasite and its membranes in the red cell (Fig. 4).

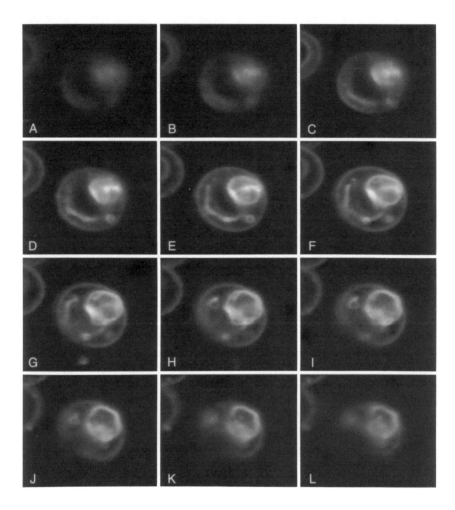

Fig. 3. Serial sections through a *P. falciparum*-infected erythrocyte labeled with C_5-DMB-ceramide. Infected erythrocytes were incubated in RPMI-1640 supplemented with 2 mg/ml defatted-BSA and 20 μM C_5-DMB-ceramide for 30 minutes at 37°C. Cells were washed to remove unincorporated label and fixed in 0.05% glutaraldehyde. (Fixation had no effects on the morphology of the membranes) (Elmendorf and Haldar, 1994). Sequential micrographs (**A–L**) were taken at 400 nm intervals along the z-axis at an excitation wavelength of 488 nm. The image depicts a single trophozoite-stage infected erythrocyte. The erythrocyte membrane is the outer circle in the micrographs. A single trophozoite parasite is the smaller, brighter circle off to the right within the erythrocyte. Note the long tubule extending outward from the surface of the parasite and the smaller vesicles attached along the length of the tubule.

Shown in Figure 3 are serial sections 400 nm apart through the depth of a trophozoite-infected red cell. In Figure 3E, the perinuclear region of staining within the parasite, the periphery of the parasite, and a long membrane extension are clearly seen in the red cell. To greater and lesser extents, all of these structures can also be seen in the previous section and subsequent ones indicating their continuity in the cell. Optical sections through ring stage parasites showed a similar perinuclear and peripheral staining of the parasite but indicated the presence of large membrane loops in the erythrocyte cytoplasm (Elmendorf and Haldar, 1994).

Intraerythrocytic structures visualized in three dimensions in ring and trophozoite stage parasites are shown in Figure 4i and ii. Several important observations emerged from these analyses: In rings, the parasites contain large membrane vesicles budding off their surface (see Fig. 4i). Despite the presence of multiple vesicular structures, the developing membranes are all connected in a TVM that is attached to the parasite. At the trophozoite stage the intraerythrocytic structure is a long tubular element extending from the parasite, with protruding ear-like vesicles (Figs. 3, 4ii). A deep indentation seen on the surface of the parasite in Figure 4ii may represent a site of an endocytic vacuole for the uptake of hemoglobin. Our results would suggest that in both ring and trohozoite-infected cells, one end of the TVM remains closely juxtaposed to the parasite's surface in the infected red cell. Scanning electron micrographs of parasites released from their red cell by Elford and Ferguson (1993) indicate that extensions of membrane tubules and vesicles are in continuum with the parasite. Together these results strongly support that in the infected red cell, even as the TVM network extends into the red cell cytosol, at one end it remains attached to the parasite.

In a time frame of seconds to minutes there is no significant movement of this TVM apparatus in the erythrocyte cytosol at either stage of parasite growth. Movement is observed only if the erythrocyte membrane lyses or swells in the process of lysis and is therefore likely to be due to a process of degeneration of the host cytosolic environment. We do detect specific sites of fluorescent sphingolipid binding in the TVM (Fig. 5). This was determined by incubating labeled infected erythrocytes with excess BSA in a process that back-extracts excess lipid from the cells. This depleted all of the label in the red cell and in some areas of the TVM. Yet other regions of the TVM remained labeled, indicating that they specifically bound the fluorescent sphingolipids (Fig. 5). We have not as yet directly examined the movement of these sphingolipid-binding domains in the reticulum.

Both the microscopy analyses and back-extraction studies indicated that the red cell membrane is not a site of sphingolipid accumulation. However, the tight apposition seen between the TVM (particularly its tubular extensions) and the erythrocyte membrane suggests that the TVM interacts with the

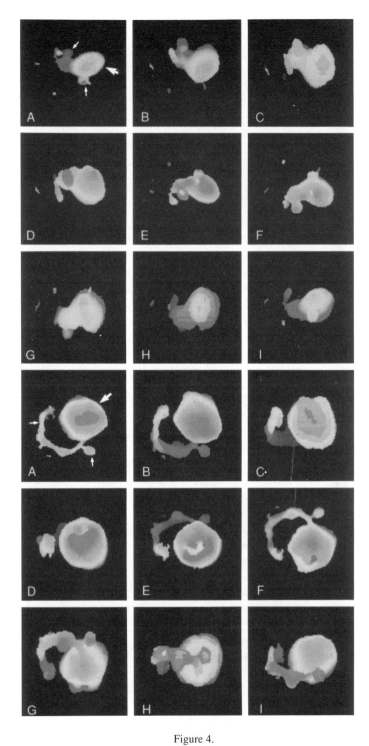

I.

II.

Figure 4.

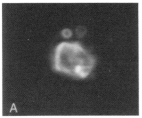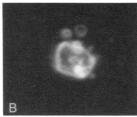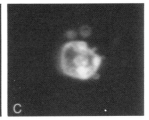

Fig. 5. Sites of specific ceramide accumulation in *P. falciparum*–infected erythrocytes labeled with C_6-NBD-ceramide. Infected erythrocytes were loaded with 20 mM C_6-NBD-ceramide at 0°C, unincorporated label removed by extensive washing, and partial metabolic conversion of probe to C_6-NBD-sphingomyelin allowed to continue at 37°C. Cells were then back-extracted three times at 0°C in the presence of 7 mg/ml defatted BSA. Visualization of cells was performed as described in Figure 3. Three consecutive sections from the center of the cell are shown.

cytoplasmic face of the red cell membrane, possibly its cytoskeleton. These interactions may contribute to the conversion of the intraerythrocytic membranes from large vesicles into tubules as the parasite matures from the ring to the trophozoite stage. The asymmetric distribution of sphingomyelin and phosphatidylcholine proposed for the Golgi apparatus in mammalian cells (shingomyelin, inner leaflet; phosphatidylcholine, outer leaflet) is proposed to force the Golgi into flattened saccules (Sheetz and Singer, 1974; Pagano, 1988). The export of parasite sphingomyelin synthase should result in synthesis of sphingomyelin in the lumen of the TVM. If this is coupled to the accumulation of a second lipid species, such as phosphatidylcholine, it could also provide a mechanism for flattening large vesicles in ring stages to tubular structures in trophozoites.

Fig. 4. Three-dimensional reconstructions of DMB-labeled parasites. **i:** Three-dimensional reconstruction of the ring-stage parasite. Twenty consecutive images taken at 400 nm intervals through the depth of the infected erythrocyte were used to recalculate the three-dimensional morphology of the parasite. The images were first processed through a Gaussian data filter to eliminate nonspecific signal and noise, and then the image intensity threshold was set to exclude signal from uninfected erythrocytes in the same sample. Sequential images **(A–L)** are shown as the model rotates around the x-axis at 40° intervals. The large arrows in A points to the body of the parasite, while the two smaller arrows point to two large vesicular structures protruding from the surface of the parasite. **ii:** Three-dimensional reconstruction of the trophozoite-stage parasite shown in serial sections in Figure 3. Images were processed as described in i. The large arrow in A points to the body of the parasite, while the two smaller arrows point to the long tubule and a smaller vesicle protruding from the tubule.

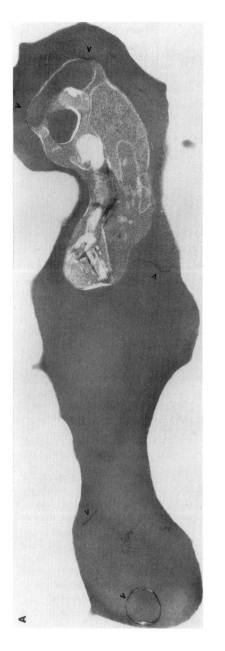

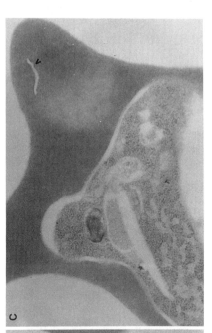

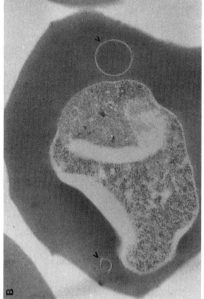

Relationship of TVM to Clefts and Loops Seen in Thin Sections

To determine the morphologies of the sphingolipid-labeled, intraerythrocytic membranes at the level of the electron microscope, lipid-labeled cells were perfused with diaminobenzidine, irradiated in the fluorescence microscope, and processed for electron microscopy. In the resulting thin sections prominent, black, photooxidation products of polymerized diaminobenzidine were seen in membranous cisternae and loops in the red cell cytoplasm (Haldar et al., 1991) (Fig. 6A), indicating that these structures corresponded to the lipid-labeled intraerythrocytic membranes seen by fluorescence microscopy (Figs. 3, 4). Regions of the vacuolar membrane were also labeled, indicating domains enriched for the fluorescent sphingolipids. In cells that lacked either the fluorescent lipid or diaminobenzidine (Fig. 6B,C), the intraerythrocytic structures were not labeled. Despite the intracellular perinuclear arc of sphingolipid labeling in cells as shown in Figures 2 and 3, no precipitate was detected within the parasite. This is probably because diaminobenzidine does not cross membranes easily and did not enter the parasite (Haldar et al., 1991).

Why does this reticulum appear as discrete cisternae and membrane loops in transmission electron micrographs? One explanation is that a thin section through a tubule or large vesicle may well appear as lamellar membranes of a cisternae or whorls of a loop. But since these two membrane morphologies have distinct protein components (the loops contain the 28 kD protein Exp1, while the cisternae concentrate a 45 kD parasite protein), they must somehow be separated in the TVM. We see specific sites of sphingolipid accumulation in the TVM and the periphery of the parasite, which suggests that they can sustain distinct lipid domains in the bilayer. Thus lipid–protein interactions in these domains could allow them to include and/or exclude specific proteins and effectively "sort" proteins in the membrane of the vacuole and the TVM. For instance, when the 45 kD protein and Exp1 are exported to the vacuolar surface–TVM, the concentration of the 45 kD protein in a domain could give rise to regions enriched for this protein but depleted of the Exp1. This sorting could be the first step in effectively creating cisternal membranes that are enriched for the 45 kD, and biochemically and morphologically distinct from

---

Fig. 6.   Localization of C6-NBD-cer in electron micrographs. Infected erythrocytes were fixed in glutaraldehyde in 250 mM sucrose, 10 mM sodium phosphate, and 50 mM sodium cacodylate, pH 7.4, labeled with C6-NBD-cer, and back-extracted to display prominent parasite-associated fluorescence. The cells were subsequently incubated with DAB, irradiated, and processed for electron microscopy. **A:** Precipitates were observed as indicated by arrowheads. **B:** Control incubations, unlabeled cells incubated with DAB and irradiated, and **C:** labeled cells irradiated in the absence of DAB did not display any specific precipitates.

the large membrane loops depleted of the 45 kD polypeptide but containing Exp1. Although such sorting events can result in the formation of the distinct compartments, they do not necessarily require a physical discontinuity of membrane between the TVM structures or the parasitophorous vacuolar membrane. There is evidence that in tubovesicular organelles of higher vertebrate cells, microdomains are capable of sorting proteins and lipids within a continuous lumen (Hopkins et al., 1990).

MEMBRANE MOVEMENT AND FUNCTION IN THE TVM

The export of sphingomyelin synthase into the TVM is of particular interest when compared with the retention of a *P. falciparum* homolog of ERD2 in a perinuclear Golgi element within the parasite (Elmendorf and Haldar, 1993b). The separation by the malaria parasite of these two Golgi activities (presumed to be contained within overlapping compartments of mammalian cells) suggests that the TVM cannot be considered to be simply a second "misplaced" parasite Golgi. The parasite instead elaborates a unique organelle, endowed as we have shown with at least one Golgi-like characteristic in its lipid-processing capabilities, but perhaps more limited in various other classic Golgi functions.

Budding

The development of the TVM appears to be due to the budding of membrane from the parasite. In earlier studies when the cisternae and loops were thought to be distinct from the vacuole, it was suggested that budding results from release of vesicular membranes from the vacuolar surface (Howard, 1988; Barnwell, 1990). Although the more recent evidence indicates that the tubovesicular elements do not disassociate from the vacuole (Elmendorf and Haldar, 1993a, 1994; Elford and Ferguson, 1993), we still need to account for processes of vesicular and tubular membrane assembly at the vacuolar surface. Most interestingly, what drives these processes in the erythrocyte cytosol?

Essentially two types of vesicles have been characterized in cells. Clathrin-coated vesicles mediate endocytosis and transport from the *trans* Golgi to the plasma membrane in the regulated pathway of protein secretion (reviewed by Pearse and Robinson, 1990). Nonclathrin-coated vesicles have been identified by Rothman and his colleagues to mediate transport in the Golgi. The formation of these vesicles requires a number of cytosolic proteins to assemble as a coat on the emerging vesicle (Orci et al., 1993). Seven major coat proteins (COPs) have been described. One, B-COP, has been sequenced and found to contain homologies to B and B´ adaptins of clathrin coats (Duden et al., 1991). This has suggested that the two types of coated vesicles may form by similar mechanisms. Compared with coated vesicle formation less is known of mechanisms of tubule formation. However, tubulation is clearly well established as a property of the Golgi that is capable of supporting protein transport and also shows an absolute requirement for cytosolic factors (Cluett et al., 1993).

The erythrocyte cytosol contains high levels of hemoglobin. Whether it contains other proteins of either host or parasite origin that could drive vesicle or tubule formation at the surface of the parasitophorous vacuole remains largely unknown. In initial studies we found that residual levels of human heavy chain clathrin are present, but are not found in association with the intraerythrocytic structures or the vacuolar or the red cell membrane (Li and Haldar, unpublished data). The export of sphingomyelin synthase by the intracellular parasite suggests that the de novo synthesis of sphingomyelin may contribute to membrane growth and possibly vesiculation at the vacuolar surface. However, it is likely that additional cytosolic factors of membrane budding are also required in the infected erythrocyte cytoplasm. Their identification could potentially define the minimal cytosolic components required to drive vesicle and/or tubule assembly in the cytoplasm of a very simple eukaryotic cell, the mature erythrocyte.

Transport Functions

The morphological similarity of the TVM cisternae as seen by transmission electron microscopy and the Golgi cisternae of mammalian cells, and a perceived need by the parasite for transport functions beyond its plasma membrane, led to the proposal that the TVM might function as a "trafficking organelle" in the erythrocyte (Howard, 1988). The possible functions of intraerythrocytic membranes in protein transport from and to the red cell surface, are of particular interest with respect to mechanisms for the uptake of macromolecules, export of potential antigens, the assembly of virulence determinants such as knobs and an understanding of basic cellular processes of the reconstitution of trafficking in the red cell membrane. However, the absence of N-linked glycosylation and the lack of either suitable markers or appropriate reagents have precluded a direct analysis of mechanisms of protein export or import at the red cell surface. Since secretory transport requires movement of proteins and lipids, we investigated lipid trafficking between the parasite, TVM, and red cell.

The intraerythrocytic parasite must support a very high level of membrane and lipid accumulation but is incapable of de novo synthesis of fatty acids (reviewed by Holz, 1977; Vial et al., 1990; Simoes et al., 1992; Haldar, 1992). It obtains fatty acids from the imported lipids, and, as shown by Grellier et al. (1991), an exogenous source of lipids appears to be essential for parasite growth in culture. These lipids must cross the red cell membrane and cytosol prior to their delivery to the parasite. Fluorescent phospholipids and sphingomyelins delivered to the red cell membrane have been detected in the TVM of the erythrocyte cytosol (reviewed by Haldar, 1992; Lauer and Haldar, unpublished data). It is particularly interesting that analogs of phosphatidylcholine (PC) are translocated across the infected erythrocyte membrane. These are not internalized in uninfected red cells. The results of three groups now indicate that this first step of import is not endocytosis, but a parasite–protein-mediated process of PC "flip flop" from the exoplasmic to the cytoplasmic face of the infected red cell membrane (Haldar et al., 1989; Grellier et al., 1991; Simoes et al., 1991). Grellier et al. (1991) first demonstrated that the internalized lipids could be detected in the intraerythrocytic membranes and proposed that these structures provided a unidirectional pathway for lipid import into the cell. In contrast, Pouvelle et al. (1991) have proposed that lipids are internalized by a parasitophorous "duct" in continuum with the red cell membrane. This duct activity has been a contentious point in the literature (Haldar and Uyetake, 1992; Sherman and Zidovetzki, 1992; Fujioka and Aikawa, 1993). While its morphology is similar to the tubules of the TVM and the latter interact with the cytoplasmic components of the red cell membrane, both biochemical and microscopic analyses support that structures of the TVM are not in bilayer continuum with the red cell surface. Thus additional corroborative evidence for "duct" activities is not yet available.

We also examined the movement of fluorescent lipid analogs from the parasite to the red cell membrane. Surprisingly while a number of fluorescent phospho- and sphingolipid analogs can be exported from the parasite to the TVM, there is no evidence that any are delivered to the erythrocyte membrane (reviewed by Haldar, 1992). Plasmodial sphingomyelin synthesized in the TVM is also not detected at the red cell surface (Haldar et al., 1991; Elmendorf and Haldar, 1993a, 1994) (Figs. 2, 5). These results strongly support the absence of bulk membrane export to the red cell surface. They imply that if forward transport from the TVM to the red cell membrane exists, the rates of inward transport from the host cell are much faster and the bulk movement of membrane is inward. The reverse happens in mammalian cells, when sphingomyelin and its fluorescent analog synthesized in the Golgi are exported out to the plasma membrane but not delivered to the ER. Although a pathway of retrograde transport (which returns the ERD2 protein) from the Golgi to the ER exists, it is not observed unless forward transport out of the Golgi is blocked by drugs such as BFA.

Finally, we have studied the biosynthetic transport of the 45 kD protein of the intraerythrocytic cisternae as a marker for the development of this compartment of the TVM. Our results indicate that the protein is synthesized and exported to the TVM by a BFA-sensitive pathway in the ring and early trophozoite stage parasites (Das, et al., 1994), consistent with the secretory development of the TVM in these stages. In contrast, although the 45 kD cisternal protein is not synthesized in late trophozoites and schizonts, it is phosphorylated and detected in both membrane-associated and soluble forms in these cells. This suggests that the protein is post-translationally modified in a stage-specific manner to alter its membrane interactions with the TVM in mature parasite-infected erythrocytes. Our lipid labeling studies indicate a stage-specific change in the morphological organization of the TVM: large secretory vesicles of membrane growth dominate in rings, while tubular structures and smaller vesicles consistent with transport and sorting morphologies in membranes are present in trophozoites. Thus independent lines of experimentation appear to be converging in support of the same hypothesis, that the TVM network assembled early in the parasite's life cycle displays stage-specific membrane properties later in the cycle.

In the late trophozoite stage and schizogony the parasite plasma membrane enlarges presumably by the biosynthetic export of proteins (such as MSP1 and 2) and lipids to this membrane. There is also concomitant increase in the size of the parasitophorous vacuole in schizonts. We propose that "retrograde" transport from the TVM supports the growth the vacuole in the mature infected erythrocytes. This eliminates the need for bulk membrane export from the parasite plasma membrane and provides an explanation of why a protein such as MSP1, an abundant marker of the plasma membrane, is not exported to the vacuolar surface. It is also consistent with 1) protein and lipid evidence for stage-specific transport functions of the TVM in mature infected erythrocytes and 2) the role of the TVM in lipid import from the infected red cell membrane.

MODELS OF TVM ASSEMBLY AND SECRETORY EXPORT IN *PLASMODIUM*

In the last MBL lecture series on The Biology of Parasitism, published 5 years ago, Howard (1988) proposed a model for protein export from the malaria parasite. We recently suggested an alternate model for secretory protein export and membrane assembly in the TVM (Elmendorf and Haldar, 1993a). In a significant departure from the earlier model we proposed that membrane compartments in the erythrocyte cytosol were not distinct from each other and the vacuole, but remained in association with the vacuolar surface as a TVM network. We now add that there is regulated export of the secretory enzyme sphingomyelin synthase into the TVM and the stage-specific changes in the organization of the TVM during the asexual cycle (Fig. 7A). In addition, the 45 kD protein of Maurer's clefts, a component protein of the TVM, is constitutively exported by a BFA-sensitive secretory pathway in the first 30 hours of development. Hence, both cell cycle regulated organization of a parasite Golgi activity and membrane protein export through the secretory pathway contribute to the development of the TVM network in the infected red cell.

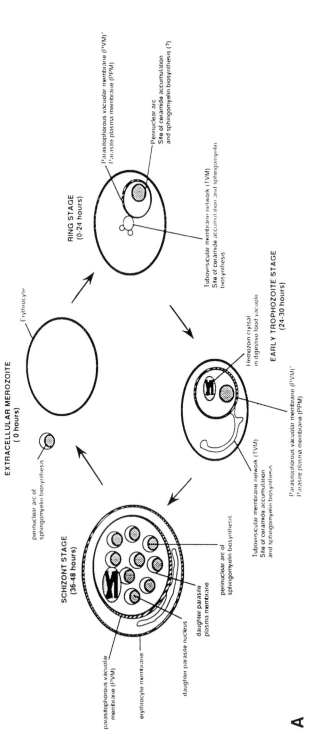

EXTRACELLULAR MEROZOITE
(0 hours)

Erythrocyte

perinuclear arc of
sphingomyelin biosynthesis

RING STAGE
(0-24 hours)

Parasitophorous vacuolar membrane (PVM)·
Parasite plasma membrane (PPM)

Perinuclear arc
Site of ceramide accumulation
and sphingomyelin biosynthesis (?)

Tubovesicular membrane network (TVM)
Site of ceramide accumulation and sphingomyelin
biosynthesis

EARLY TROPHOZOITE STAGE
(24-30 hours)

Hemozoin crystal
in digestive food vacuole

Parasitophorous vacuolar membrane (PVM)·
Parasite plasma membrane (PPM)

Tubovesicular membrane network (TVM)
Site of ceramide accumulation
and sphingomyelin biosynthesis

SCHIZONT STAGE
(36-48 hours)

parasitophorous vacuolar
membrane (PVM)

erythrocyte membrane

daughter parasite nucleus

daughter parasite
plasma membrane

perinuclear arc of
sphingomyelin biosynthesis

Tubovesicular membrane network (TVM)
Site of ceramide accumulation
and sphingomyelin biosynthesis

A

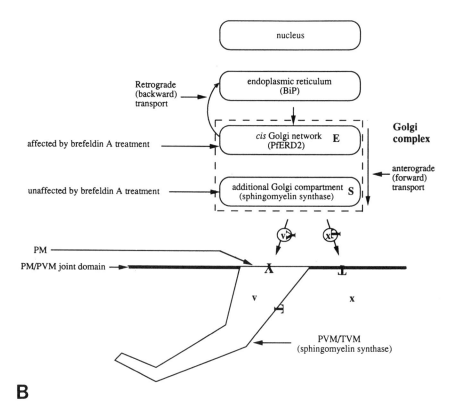

nucleus

endoplasmic reticulum
(BiP)

Retrograde
(backward)
transport

cis Golgi network E
(PfERD2)

affected by brefeldin A treatment

Golgi
complex

anterograde
(forward)
transport

additional Golgi compartment S
(sphingomyelin synthase)

unaffected by brefeldin A treatment

PM

PM/PVM joint domain →   X̄   L̄

v   x

PVM/TVM
(sphingomyelin synthase)

B

Fig. 7. **A:** Model for the stage-specific regulation of sphingomyelin synthase activity and morphology of the TVM. The life cycle of *P. falciparum* is shown starting at the left with the mature schizont stage. Following the cycle in a clockwise direction, merozoites are released and reinvade new erythrocytes. During the merozoite stage the enzyme is localized within the parasite in a perinuclear arc. After invasion, the parasite matures into ring and then trophozoite stages. Note that it is not possible to distinguish between sphingolipid staining of membrane from the parasitophorous vacuolar membrane and the parasite plasma membrane at the ring and trophozoite stages. Here the parasite induces the development of a tubovesicular network beyond its plasma membrane and exports the sphingomyelin synthase enzyme, originally present solely within the merozoite, partially outward into these membranes. The cycle is completed with the maturation of the parasite into the mitotically dividing schizont stage. As expected, the parasite appears to replicate sphingomyelin synthase as it divides, resulting in enzyme levels increased 10–15-fold in the schizont stages compared with the earlier intracellular stages (data unpublished). **B:** Model for secretory export of parasite proteins. The Golgi complex contains a compartment with PfERD2 (E). A second Golgi compartment containing sphingomyelin synthase (S) is also present. Proteins exit the ER and enter E. A retrograde pathway of PfERD2 recycling to the ER originates in this compartment. Export through the complex occurs by anterograde (forward) membrane flow. Two distinct classes of export vesicles are proposed to emerge from the Golgi complex. Contents of vesicles destined for release at the plasma membrane (PM)/parasitophorous vacuolar membrane (PVM) joint domain: X, soluble parasite proteins (such as GBP 130) targeted for the intraerythrocytic space; T, integral membrane proteins (such as Exp-1) of the PVM and tubovesicular membrane (TVM). Contents of vesicles destined for release at the plasma membrane (PM): V, soluble parasite proteins (such as Pf126/SERA) targeted for the parasitophorous vacuolar space; Y, integral membrane proteins of the PM (such as MSP 1).

We further proposed that subsequent to transport through the ER–Golgi complex, vesicles carrying proteins exported to the TVM are sorted away from those targeted to plasma membrane (Elmendorf and Haldar, 1993a). These vesicles fuse with a joint domain of the PPM and PVM: Soluble proteins in their lumen are delivered to the erythrocyte cytoplasm, while membrane proteins are delivered to the vacuolar surface and the TVM. Gormley et al. (1992) have independently proposed the presence of a joint domain of the PPM and PVM. Our hypothesis was put forth because the original model of Howard proposed that 1) vesicular transport from the PPM to the PVM led to insertion of proteins in the PVM and 2) soluble proteins delivered to the lumenal space were post-translationally transported across the vacuolar membrane into the erythrocyte cytosol. No. 1 would result in the export of parasite cytosolic proteins to the erythrocyte cytosol. This has not yet been observed, despite the identification of several, exported parasite proteins. Furthermore, the presence of signal sequences on almost all exported proteins and the BFA block to secretion also support that in the majority exported plasmodial proteins are not cytosolic but traverse the secretory pathway. Based on eukaryotic models of protein translocation, transport across the vacuolar membrane in No. 2 would require at a minimum a chaperonin, recognition mechanism, and integral membrane protein translocon (Siegel and Walter, 1989; Wickner et al., 1991; Wienhaus and Neupert, 1992). These would have to be exported by the parasite, making for a rather complicated, energy expensive solution for export. In contrast, the formation of two different classes of vesicles, targeted to different domains of the plasma membrane, is now well established in the epithelial cells (Simons and Wandingerness, 1990) and does not require export of the cellular transport apparatus beyond the PPM.

Shown in Figure 7B is a schematic representation of what is currently known of the secretory apparatus within the parasite. We have demonstrated the presence of a Golgi complex in the parasite. It has at least two compartments: one is the ERD2 site (E) and sensitive to BFA, with a retrograde pathway of membrane transport to return ERD2-ligand complexes back to the ER. A second compartment contains sphingomyelin synthase (S). It is insensitive to BFA and therefore expected to lie beyond E. Since the Golgi is a major site for the sorting of proteins and lipids in cells, it is reasonable to propose that the sorting of exported proteins into distinct vesicle classes occurs in the parasite's Golgi complex. All proteins exiting the ER within minutes encounter the BFA-sensitive ERD2 site (E) and enter the Golgi. By anterograde transport the exported proteins move forward through the Golgi complex. Delineation of further steps of intra-Golgi transport should indicate how and where in the complex these exported proteins are sorted into transport vesicles destined for the PPM, PVM, and/or the TVM.

CONCLUDING REMARKS

The current models of protein transport in eukaryotes are developed largely from studies in mammalian cells and yeast and do not deal with membrane development beyond the plasma membrane of a cell. *Plasmodium*'s development of its vacuole and membranes in the erythrocyte cytoplasm is therefore novel. While the parasite shares many common aspects of the secretory pathway with higher cells, our studies suggest that because of its specialized biological niche it also manifests prominently secretory mechanisms of the Golgi that are not apparent in these cells. It therefore provides a unique model system to study secretion and membrane development in eukaryotic cells.

ACKNOWLEDGMENTS

We thank Dr. S. Seft for assistance with confocal microscopy at the MBL; Dr. S.J. Smith, M. Feinstein, H. Deacon, and W. Jung at the Cell Sciences Imaging Facility, Beckman Center, Stanford University, for their advice and assistance with the confocal microscopy and image analysis at Stanford; and N. Ghori for assistance in electron microscopy at Stanford. We also particularly thank the students and assistants of the Biology of Parasitism, 91 and 92, and Drs. Jean Francois Dubremetz, John Boothroyd, and Rick Komuniecki for their active participation in our studies of Golgi activities and the TVM in *Plasmodium*.

REFERENCES

Aikawa M (1971): *Plasmodium*: The fine structure of malarial parasites. Exp Parasitol 30:284–320.

Barnwell JW (1989): Cytoadherence and sequestration in falciparum malaria. Exp Parasitol 69:407–412.

Barnwell JW (1990): Vesicle mediated transport of membrane and proteins in malaria-infected erythrocytes. Blood Cells 16:379–395.

Blackman MJ, Heidrich HG, Donachi S, McBride JS, Holder AA (1990): A single fragment of a malaria merozoite surface protein remains on the parasite during red cell invasion and is the target of invasion-inhibiting antibodies. J Exp Med 172:379–382.

Cabantchik ZI (1990): Properties of permeation pathways induced in human red cell membranes by malaria parasites. Blood Cells 16:421–432.

Cluett EB, Wood SA, Banta M, Brown WJ (1993): Tubulation of Golgi membranes in vivo and in vitro. J Cell Biol 120:15–24.

Crary J, Haldar K (1992): Brefeldin A inhibits protein secretion and parasite maturation in the ring stage of *Plasmodium falciparum*. Mol Biochem Parasitol 53:185–192.

Das A, Elmendorf HG, Li W-L, Haldar K (1994): Biosynthetic export and processing of a 45 kDa protein detected in membrane clefts of erythrocytes infected with *Plasmodium falciparum*. Biochem J (in press).

Dieckmann-Schuppert A, Bender S, Odenthal-Schnittler M, Bause E, Schwarz RT (1992): Apparent lack of *N*-glycosylation in the asexual intraerythrocytic stage of *Plasmodium falciparum*. Eur J Biochem 205:815–825.

396 / Haldar et al.

Duden R, Griffiths G, Frank R, Argos P, Kreis TE (1991): B-COP, a 110 kd protein associated with non-clathrin coated vesicles and the Golgi complex shows homology to B-adaptin. Cell 64:649–665.

Elford BC, Ferguson DJP (1993): Secretory processes in *Plasmodium*. Parasitol Today 9:80–81.

Elmendorf HG, Bangs JD, Haldar K (1992): Synthesis and secretion of proteins by released malarial parasites. Mol Biochem Parasitol 52:215–223.

Elmendorf HG, Haldar K (1993a): Secretory Transport in *Plasmodium*. Parasitol Today 9:98–102.

Elmendorf HG, Haldar K (1993b): Identification and localization of ERD2 in the malaria parasite *Plasmodium falciparum*: Separation from sites of sphingomyelin synthesis and implications for organization of the Golgi. EMBO J 12:4763–4773.

Elmendorf HG, Haldar K (1994): *Plasmodium falciparum* exports the Golgi marker sphingomyelin synthase into a tubovesicular network in the cytoplasm of mature erythrocytes. J Cell Biol 124:449–462.

Fujioka H, Aikawa M (1993): Morphological changes of clefts in *Plasmodium*-infected erythrocytes under adverse conditions. Exp Parasitol 76:302–307.

Gormley JA, Howard RJ, Taraschi TF (1992): Trafficking of malarial proteins to the host cell cytoplasm and the erythrocyte surface involves multiple pathways. J Cell Biol 119:1481–1495.

Grellier P, Rigomier D, Clavey V, Fuchart J-C, Schrevel J (1991): Lipid traffic between high density lipoproteins and *Plasmodium falciparum*–infected red blood cells. J Cell Biol 112:267–278.

Haldar K (1992): Lipid transport in *Plasmodium*. Infect Agents Dis 1:254–262.

Haldar K, de Amorim AF, Cross GAM (1989): Transport of fluorescent phospholipid analogues from the erythrocyte membrane to the parasite in *Plasmodium falciparum*–infected red cells. J Cell Biol 108:2183–2192.

Haldar K, Holder AA (1993): Export of parasite proteins to the erythrocyte in *Plasmodium falciparum*–infected erythrocytes. Semin Cell Biol 4:345–353.

Haldar K, Uyetake L (1992): The movement of fluorescent endocytic tracers in *Plasmodium falciparum*–infected erythrocytes. Mol Biochem Parasitol 50:161–178.

Haldar K, Uyetake L, Ghori N, Elmendorf HG, Li W-l (1991): The accumulation and metabolism of a fluorescent ceramide derivative in *Plasmodium falciparum*–infected erythrocytes. Mol Biochem Parasitol 49:143–156.

Holz GG (1997): Lipids and the malarial parasites. Bull: WHO 55:237–248.

Hopkins CR, Gibson A, Shipman M, Miller K (1990): Movement of internalized ligand–receptor complexes along a continuous endosomal reticulum. Nature 346:335–339.

Howard RJ (1988): *Plasmodium falciparum* proteins at the host erythrocyte membrane: Their biological and immunological significance and novel parasite organelles which deliver them to the cell surface. In P.T. Englund, A. Sher (eds): MBL Lecture Series in Biology, vol 9, The Biology of Parasitism. New York: Alan R. Liss, Inc., pp. 111–145.

Klausner RD, Donaldson JG, Lippincott-Schwarz J (1992): Brefeldin A: Insights into the control of membrane traffic and organelle structure. J Cell Biol 116:1071–1080.

Kornfeld R, Kornfeld S (1985): Assembly of asparagine linked oligosaccharides. Annu Rev Biochem 54:631–664.

Kumar N, Koski G, Harada M, Aikawa M, Zheng H (1991): Induction and localization of *Plasmodium falciparum* stress proteins related to the heat shock protein 70 family. Mol Biochem Parasitol 48:47–58.

Kumar N, Zheny H (1992): Nucleotide sequence of a *Plasmodium falciparum* stress protein with similarity to mammalian 78-kDa glucose regulated protein. Mol Biochem Parasitol 56:353–356.

Langreth SG, Trager W (1978): Fine structure of human malaria in vitro. J Protozool 25:443–452.

Lewis MJ, Pelham HRB (1990): A human homologue of the yeast HDEL receptor. Nature 348:162–163.

Lewis MJ, Pelham HRB (1992): Ligand induced redistribution of the human KDEL receptor from the Golgi complex to endoplasmic reticulum. Cell 68:353–364.

Lewis MJ, Sweet DJ, Pelham HRB (1990): The *ERD2* gene determines the specificity of the luminal ER protein retention system. Cell 61:1359–1363.

Lingelbach K (1993): *Plasmodium falciparum*: A molecular view of protein transport from the parasite into the host erythrocyte. Exp Parasitol 76:318–327.

Orci L, Palmer DJ, Ravazzola M, Perrelet A, Amherdt M, Rothman JE (1993): Budding from Golgi membranes requires the coatomer complex of non clathrin coat proteins. Nature 362:648–652.

Pagano RE (1988): What is the fate of diacylglycerol produced in the Golgi apparatus? TIBS 13:202–205.

Pagano RE (1989): A fluorescent derivative of ceramide: Physical properties and use in studying the Golgi apparatus of animal cells. Methods Cell Biol 29:75–85.

Pagano RE (1990): The Golgi apparatus: Insights from lipid biochemistry. Biochem Soc Trans 18:361–366.

Pagano RE, Martin OC, Kang HC, Haugland RP (1991): A novel fluorescent ceramide analogue for studying membrane traffic in animal cells: accumulation at the Golgi apparatus results in altered spectral properties of the sphingolipid precursor. J Cell Biol 113:1267–1279.

Palade GE (1975): Intracellular aspects of the process of protein synthesis. Science 189:347–358.

Pearse BMF, Robinson MS (1990): Clathrin, adaptors and sorting. Annu Rev Cell Biol 6:151–171.

Pelham HRB (1990): The retention signal for soluble proteins of the endoplasmic reticulum. Trends Biochem Sci 15:483–486.

Perkins ME (1992): Rhoptry organelles of apicomplexan parasites. Parasitol Today 8:28–32.

Pfeffer SR, Rothman JE (1987): Biosynthetic protein transport and sorting by the endoplasmic reticulum and the Golgi. Annu Rev Biochem 56:829–852.

Pouvelle B, Spiegel R, Hsiao L, Howard RJ, Morris RL, Thomas AP, Taraschi TF (1991): Direct access to serum macromolecules by intraerythrocytic malaria parasites. Nature 353:73–75.

Semenza JC, Hardwick KG, Dean N, Pelham HRB (1990): *ERD2*, a yeast gene required for the receptor mediated retrieval of luminal ER proteins from the secretory pathway. Cell 61:1349–1357.

Sheetz MP, Singer SJ (1974): Biological membranes as bilayer couples—A molecular mechanism of drug erythrocyte interactions. Proc Natl Acad Sci USA 71:4457–4461.

Sherman IW, Zidovetzki R (1992): A parasitophorous duct in *Plasmodium*-infected red blood cells. Parasitol Today 8:2–3.

Siegel V, Walter P (1989): Assembly of proteins in the endoplasmic reticulum. Curr Opin Cell Biol 1:635–638.

Simoes AP, Moll GN, Slotbloom AJ, Roelofson B, Op den Kamp JA (1991): Selective internalization of choline phospholipids in *Plasmodium falciparum* parasitized erythrocytes. Biochim Biophys Acta 1063:45–50.

Simoes AP, Roelofson B, Op den Kamp JAF (1992): Lipid compartmentalization in erythrocytes parasitized by *Plasmodium* spp. Parasitol Today 8:18–21.

Simons K, Wandinger-Ness A (1990): Polarized sorting in epithelia. Cell 62:207–210.

Tang BL, Wong SH, Qi ZL, Low SH, Hong W (1993): Molecular cloning, characterization subcellular localization and dynamics of p23, the mammalian KDEL receptor. J Cell Biol 120:325–338.

Vial HJ, Anceli ML, Phillipot JR, Thuet MJ (1990): Biosynthesis and dynamics of lipids in *Plasmodium*-infected mature mammalian erythrocytes. Blood Cells 16:531–555.

Wickner W, Driessen AJ, Hartl FU (1991) The enzymology of protein translocation across the *Escherichia coli* plasma membrane. Annu Rev Biochem 60:101–124.

Wienhues U, Neupert W (1992): Protein translocation across mitochondrial membranes. BioEssays 14:17–23.

Young WW, Lutz MS, Mills SE, Lechler-Osborn S (1990): Use of brefeldin A to define sites of glycosphingolipid synthesis: GA2/GM2/GD2 synthase is trans to the brefeldin A block. Proc Natl Acad Sci USA 87:6838–6842.

Molecular Approaches to Parasitology, pages 399–411

Cell Biology of Trichomonads: Protein Targeting to the Hydrogenosome

Patricia J. Johnson, Peter J. Bradley, and Carol J. Lahti

Department of Microbiology and Immunology and Molecular Biology Institute, University of California, Los Angeles, California 90024

INTRODUCTION

Trichomonads are flagellated protists of the group Parabasalia. Recent molecular phylogenetic studies indicate that Parabasalia are one of the earliest lineages to diverge from the main line to eukaryotic evolution (Cavalier-Smith, 1987; Sogin, 1991). The unusual features that characterize these ancient eukaryotes have attracted the attention of scientists with interests varying from energy metabolism to organelle biogenesis. Additionally, parasitic trichomonads have also received considerable attention from the medical community. *Trichomonas vaginalis* and *Tritichomonas foetus*, the two most highly studied trichomonads, parasitize the urogenital tract of humans and cattle, respectively, and manifest themselves as sexually transmitted diseases. Human trichomoniasis is one of the more common causes of vaginitis worldwide, with over 150 million cases reported each year. Three million cases are reported in the United States alone, making trichomoniasis one of the more prevalent parasitic diseases in this country.

Trichomoniasis in cattle accounts for serious financial loss in agriculture, as infection frequently results in fetal abortion. In addition to *T. vaginalis* and *T. foetus*, the avian-infective trichomonad *Trichomonas gallinae* has provided a system for studying parasites that reside in the respiratory tract. Taxonomical, structural, biochemical, and immunological aspects of trichomonads have been reviewed in a recent book edited by Honigberg (1990). Various aspects have also been discussed in previous reviews (e.g., Kulda et al., 1986; Müller, 1988; Johnson, 1993; Heine and McGregor, 1993). Readers interested in a broader knowledge of this fascinating group of primitive parasites are encouraged to consult these reviews.

THE PARASITE

The human-infective trichomonad *T. vaginalis* is the only flagellate found in the flora of the vagina. In addition to the vagina, this parasite may be found in the urethra of infected females. In males, the organism resides in the seminal vesicles and urethra and, less frequently, the prostate. *T. vaginalis* is a noninvasive, extracellular parasite; however, it does attach to the epithelial cells of the urogenital tract of the host to absorb nutrients. Many strains are low-grade pathogens, and infections may be asymptomatic. Infected women do generally present symptoms; however, the severity ranges from mild to intense inflammation. On the other hand, infections in men are typically asymptomatic. This is a clever strategy for a parasite to evolve, as a substantial fraction of infected hosts are unperturbed and thus transmit the parasite without impediment.

The life cycle of *T. vaginalis* is quite simple. The organism is transmitted from host to host by sexual intercourse. Trichomoniasis may also be acquired by newborns during delivery; however, this mode of transmission accounts for a small percentage of reported cases. *T. vaginalis* has no intermediate or reservoir hosts and no sexual stages. The parasite exists as a single form—the motile, ovoid-shaped trophozoite. No cyst stage has been reported, and the parasite is not capable of surviving outside its human host.

This ancient cell type is characterized by four anterior flagella and contains a fifth embedded in the plasma membrane. The undulating membrane formed by this fifth flagella extends about half the length of the cell and is visually identified by light microscopy. Other cellular structures typical of trichomonads include the costa, a contractile organelle that is closely associated with the undulating membrane and attached to the flagellar basal body (kinetosome), and the axostyle, an axial skeleton composed of parallel microtubules. The precise functions of these structural components are unknown. The costa is a motile organelle that may provide mechanical support for the undulating membrane. The axostyle is assumed to provide structural integrity to the cell. It extends throughout the cell, protruding at the posterior end to form a characteristic "spike" detectable by light microscopy.

The perinuclear area surrounding the single, anterior nucleus contains well-developed endoplasmic reticulum and Golgi complex. The cytoplasm is rich in glycogen granules and contains a variety of vacuoles, including lysosomes. Mitochondria and peroxisomes, two of the "hallmark" organelles of a typical eukaryotic cell, are conspicuously absent in the trichomonad cell. Trichomonads do, however, contain a redox organelle involved in carbohydrate metabolism called the *hydrogenosome* (Lindmark and Müller. 1973; Lindmark et al., 1975). The absence of mitochondria and the presence of hydrogenosomes, organelles that are both involved in carbohydrate catabolism, has generated considerable speculation regarding the relationship of these two organelles. Both organelles are thought to have an endosymbiotic origin. The major question has been whether hydrogenosomes arose by conversion of mitochondria (Cavalier-Smith, 1987; Finlay and Fenchel, 1989) or through independent endosymbiosis involving an anaerobic bacterium (Whatley et al., 1979; Müller, 1980).

THE HYDROGENOSOME

The hydrogenosome was first described in trichomonads (Lindmark and Müller, 1973; Lindmark et al., 1975) and has been most extensively analyzed in *T. vaginalis* and *T. foetus*. This organelle plays a central role in carbohydrate metabolism in these aerotolerant anaerobes. Following the breakdown of glucose to pyruvate in the cytosol, pyruvate fermentation occurs in the hydrogenosome of the trichomonad cell. Figure 1 shows a partial metabolic map of the hydrogenosome, as described by Steinbüchel and Müller (1986). Within the hydrogenosome, pyruvate is oxidatively decarboxylated and acetyl

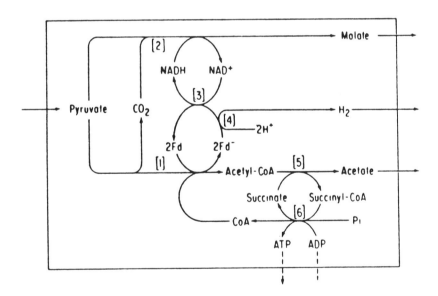

Fig. 1. Diagrammatic representation of hydrogenosomal metabolism of *Trichomonas vaginalis*. Arrows indicate the assumed direction in vivo. The broken arrow denotes a postulated adenyl nucleotide transfer. The box indicates location within the organelle but does not reflect specific intraorganellar localization. [1], pyruvate:ferredoxin oxidoreductase; [2], malate dehydrogenase (decarboxylating) (NAD); [3], NAD: ferredoxin oxidoreductase; [4], H_2: ferredoxin oxidoreductase; [5], acetate:succinate CoA transferase; [6], succinyl CoA synthetase; and Fd, ferredoxin. (Reproduced from Steinbüchel and Müller, 1986, with permission of the publisher.)

CoA is formed. This process is mediated by pyruvate:ferrodoxin oxidoreductase. Electrons are transferred from pyruvate:ferrodoxin oxidoreductase to the iron-sulfur protein ferredoxin. Ferredoxin mediates the transfer of electrons to protons to form molecular hydrogen, a process catalyzed by hydrogenase. Acetyl CoA is converted to acetate with the concomitant conversion of succinate to succinyl CoA by succinyl CoA synthetase, a reaction coupled to ATP formation via substrate-level phosphorylation. In addition to this pathway involved in pyruvate fermentation, other hydrogenosomal activities have been identified (Müller, 1988). A complete description of the metabolic properties of this organelle remains to be revealed.

Recently hydrogenosomes have been identified in a broad phylogenetic range of organisms. Hydrogenosome-like organelles (i.e., vesicles that possess hydrogenase activity) have been described in rumen-dwelling ciliates, such as *Dasytricha ruminantium* (Yarlett et al., 1981) *Isotricha* (Lloyd et al., 1989), and *Polypastron multivesiculatum* (Paul et al., 1990), as well as the rumen fungus *Neocallimastrix* (Yarlett et al., 1986; O'Fallon et al., 1991). In addition to these symbiotic organisms, hydrogenosome-like vesicles are found in free-living ciliates including *Plagiopyla* and *Sonderia* (reviewed by Fenchel and Finlay, 1991). All organisms known to contain hydrogenosomes are either anaerobic or aerotolerant anaerobes, and all appear to lack mitochondria. Given the limited number of anaerobes that have been examined to date, it is safe to predict that hydrogenosomes will be found in an even broader range of organisms. Comparative analyses of hydrogenosomes from different organisms will be valuable in understanding the origin and function of these intriguing organelles.

Biochemical analyses of trichomonad hydrogenosomes have revealed properties that are both similar to and different from mitochondria. The biochemical pathway shown in Figure 1 differs notably from that found in mitochondria. For example, the enzyme that mediates decarboxylation of pyruvate in hydrogenosomes, pyruvate:ferredoxin oxidoreductase, is markedly different from its counterpart in mitochondria, pyruvate dehydrogenase complex. Likewise, mitochondria do not possess a hydrogenase, a marker enzyme of the hydrogenosome. Interestingly, pyruvate:ferredoxin oxidoreductase and hydrogenase commonly are found in anaerobic bacteria. On the other hand, our analysis of the hydrogenosomal protein ferredoxin shows this protein to be more similar to the [2Fe-2S] ferredoxin found in mitochondria and the aerobic bacteria *Pseudomonas putida* than to its counterpart in anaerobic bacteria and other amitochondrial protists (Johnson et al., 1990). Also similar to mitochondria, ATP is produced via substrate-level phosphorylation. This reaction is mediated by succinyl CoA synthetase, a Krebs cycle enzyme that catalyzes the same reaction in hydrogenosomes and mitochondria.

Although there are marked differences between mitochondria and hydrogenosomes, the organelles are functionally similar. Both contain pathways involved in pyruvate catabolism and energy production. The similarities between hydrogenosomes and mitochondria and the fact that cells that contain hydrogenosomes invariably lack mitochondria have led to the proposal that hydrogenosomes are modified or degenerate mitochondria (Cavalier-Smith, 1987). In this regard it is noteworthy that evolutionary analysis of the ribosomal RNA of trichomonads (Leipe et al., 1993) indicates that trichomonads diverged from the main line of eukaryotic evolution prior to the advent of true mitochondria. This suggests that hydrogenosomes and mitochondria have evolved from a common progenitor organelle, as opposed to the true conversion of one organelle to the other (Johnson et al., 1993). Alternatively, hydrogenosomes and mitochondria may have arisen entirely independently. There is strong evidence that mitochondria arose via an endosymbiosis of an aerobic bacteria with a eukaryotic cell. Given the ability of hydrogenosomes to metabolize in the absence of oxygen, it has been proposed that hydrogenosomes originated through endosymbiosis of an anaerobic bacterium and a primitive eukaryotic cell (Whatley et al., 1979; Müller, 1980). To distinguish between these opposing hypotheses, a better definition of the biochemistry and biogenesis of the hydrogenosome will be necessary.

Hydrogenosomes are bounded by a double membrane (Honigberg et al., 1984); however, the inner membrane neither forms cristae nor contains detectable cytochromes or cardiolipin as found in mitochondria (Lloyd et al., 1979a; Paltauf and Meingassner, 1982). Similarly, hydrogenosomes do not appear to contain F0F1 ATPase activity (Lloyd et al., 1979b). The composition of hydrogenosomal membranes remains to be determined and should prove to be an important area of research in the future.

Interestingly, hydrogenosomes do not appear to contain genetic material or ribosomes (e.g., Müller, 1988). At first glance this might be interpreted to argue against a common origin of hydrogenosomes and mitochondria. However, we would argue that, taking into account the composition of the mitochondrial genome, it is not surprising that hydrogenosomes lack genetic material. The proteins encoded in the mitochondrial genome are primarily inner membrane components of electron transport (Attardi and Schatz, 1988). As hydrogenosomes do not possess an active cytochrome chain and the inner membrane is structurally dissimilar to that of mitochondria, the maintenance of such a genome in hydrogenosomes would seem unnecessary. If mitochondria can rid themselves of >99% of their ancestral genome, then hydrogenosomes should be able to finish the job!

BIOGENESIS OF HYDROGENOSOMES

We have begun to study the biogenesis of the hydrogenosome on the premise that this work will provide clues regarding the origin of hydrogenosomes and their relationship with classic eukaryotic organelles, such as mitochondria. Our approach has involved purification of hydrogenosomes and hydrogeno-somal proteins, as well as the genes which encode these proteins. The protein profile of *T. vaginalis* hydrogenosomes is shown in Figure 2 (HY fraction). Purified organelles, fractionated by SDS-polyacrylamide gel electrophoresis, appear to contain 15–20 prominently staining protein bands in addition to a large number of less abundant proteins. A high pH carbonate treatment allows separation of soluble (MAT) and integral (MB) membrane proteins. In addi-tion to numerous soluble proteins, the organelle contains seven to eight abun-dant, unidentified membrane proteins (Fig. 2).

Using antibodies made against total *T. vaginalis* hydrogenosomal proteins, we have screened expression libraries and isolated a number of distinct cDNAs encoding hydrogenosomal proteins. This chapter focuses on the analyses of

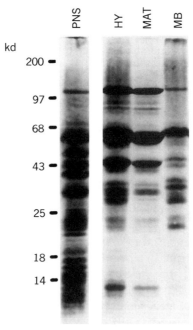

Fig. 2. Protein profile of purified hydrogenosomes of *Trichomonas vaginalis*. Organelles were gradient purified as described by Lahti et al. (1992). Postnuclear supernatants (PNS) were separated on a 45% Percoll, 0.25 M sucrose gradient to yield purified hydrogenosomes (HY). The organelles were further fractionated into soluble (MAT) and integral (MB) mem-brane fractions by sodium carbonate, high pH treatment. Proteins were electrophoresed on a 12% polyacrylamide gel. To visualize the proteins, the gel was fixed and stained with Coo-massie blue. Molecular weight markers are in kilodaltons.

two of these genes and their protein products. These are ferredoxin, a small iron-sulfur protein involved in electron transfer, and the β-subunit of succinyl CoA synthetase (β-SCS), an enzyme involved in substrate-level production of ATP (Fig. 1). The *T. vaginalis* ferredoxin gene was found to be single copy and to encode a protein of 101 amino acids. The sequence of this gene was shown to correspond to the partial sequence of the purified protein isolated from *T. vaginalis* hydrogenosomes (Johnson et al., 1990). This protein has a molecular mass of approximately 10 kD, a midpoint potential of –320 mV, and an iron-sulfur center with axial symmetry (Gorrell et al., 1984; Chapman et al., 1986). Biochemical and structural analyses showed that the *T. vaginalis* protein is a [2Fe-2S] ferredoxin, similar to those found in mitochondria and aerobic bacteria (Johnson et al., 1990). This is in contrast to the only ferredoxin reported from another anaerobic protist, *Entamoeba histolytica* (Huber et al., 1988; Reeves et al., 1980). The *E. histolytica* ferredoxin is a 2[4Fe-4S] protein similar to the ferredoxin found in the anaerobic bacteria *Clostridium pasteurianum* (Graves et al., 1985).

There are at least three distinct, but similar, genes encoding hydrogenosomal β-SCS in *T. vaginalis*. The complete sequence analysis of one of these genes revealed an open reading frame encoding a protein of 407 amino acids. The *T. vaginalis* protein, purified using immunoaffinity chromatography, has a molecular mass of approximately 43 kD (Lahti et al., 1992). The sequence of the β-SCS protein is 65% similar to the β-SCS of *Escherichia coli* and 68% similar to mitochondrial β-SCS (Buck et al., 1985; Bridger et al., 1987). The apparent molecular weight of the succinyl CoA synthetase holoenzyme of *T. vaginalis* is approximately 150 kD, consistent with a tetrametric structure composed of two α-subunits and two β-subunits (Jenkins et al., 1991).

Using the genes encoding ferredoxin and β-SCS, we have studied how these proteins are targeted and translocated into hydrogenosomes. Specifically, we have asked the following questions: 1) Are hydrogenosomal proteins made on free or membrane-bound polysomes? In other words, are these proteins post-translationally or cotranslationally translocated into the organelle? 2) Are these proteins made as larger precursors that are cleaved upon translocation? This question is pertinent, as proteins that are transported into mitochondria are typically synthesized with an N-terminal leader sequence that is cleaved upon translocation. In contrast, proteins destined for the nucleus (Kalderon et al., 1984), peroxisomes (Fujiki et al., 1984), or glycosomes (Hart et al., 1987) do not undergo post-translational processing. 3) What are the signal(s) on hydrogensomal proteins that confer specific targeting of these proteins into the organelle? 4) How does the process of translocation and the signals that confer specificity compare with those used to sort nuclear-encoded proteins into other organelles such as the mitochondria, peroxisome, nucleus, chloroplast and glycosome?

Lahti and Johnson (1991) have shown that hydrogenosomal proteins are synthesized on free polyribosomes. This was demonstrated by fractionating membrane-associated and free polyribosomes on sucrose gradients and extracting RNA from both fractions. These RNAs were tested for the presence of ferredoxin and β-SCS mRNAs, and it was found that the mRNAs encoding both proteins were found exclusively in the free polysome fraction. These data indicate that hydrogensomal proteins are synthesized on free polysomes, released in the cytoplasm, and subsequently translocated into the organelle. It can also be inferred from this that hydrogenosomes multiply by fission of pre-existing organelles. Proteins that are sorted into organelles that multiply by fission invariably are made on free polysomes. In contrast, proteins that are sorted into organelles that multiply by budding from the endoplasmic reticulum are synthesized on membrane-associated ribosomes (Gasser et al., 1982; Fujiki et al., 1984; Hart et al., 1987). These studies are consistent with morphological data that support multiplication of hydrogenosomes by fission (Kulda et al., 1986).

The complete sequence analyses of genes encoding ferredoxin and the α- and β-SCS and a comparison of the N-terminal sequence of the purified proteins isolated from *T. vaginalis* hydrogenosomes indicate that hydrogenosomal proteins are synthesized with N-terminal sequences that are cleaved from the mature proteins. N-terminal amino acid analyses demonstrated that ferredoxin (Johnson et al., 1990), and β-SCS (Lahti et al., 1992) and α-SCS (Lahti et al., 1994), isolated from hydrogenosomes lack eight to eleven amino acids that are encoded in the genes. Furthermore, size fractionation of the full-length ferredoxin protein and the mature protein found in hydrogenosomes showed that the mature protein is approximately 1 kD smaller than the unprocessed protein (Lahti and Johnson, 1991). *T. vaginalis* adenylate kinase has also been reported to have a nine-amino-acid N-terminal extension that is absent from the protein purified from hydrogenosomes (Länge et al., 1994). These observations have led to the hypothesis that the signal that targets and translocates hydrogenosomal proteins into the organelle is an N-terminal peptide (leader sequence) that is cleaved from the protein upon translocation (Johnson et al., 1990; Lahti and Johnson, 1991; Lahti et al., 1992).

N-terminal leader sequences of hydrogenosomal proteins are shown in Figure 3. These sequences contain a number of strictly conserved amino acids. For example, all seven leaders have a leucine at position 2, six of the seven have a serine at position 3, and all contain arginine at position –2 relative to the apparent cleavage site. Interestingly, the similarity of these short leader sequences and the leader sequences involved in the translocation of proteins into the matrix of the mitochondria is striking (Fig. 3). Forty percent of known mitochondrial leader sequences begin with methionine-leucine, and

Leader Sequences on Hydrogenosomal Proteins

βSCS	1	M L S A S S N F A R N
βSCS	53	M L S S S F A R N
αSCS	1	M L A G D F S R N
αSCS	2	M L S S S F E R N
αSCS	3	M L S S S F E R N
AK		M L S T L A K R F
Fd		M L S Q V C R F

Properties of Mitochondrial Leader Sequences

Overrepresentation of Arg(R), Leu(L), and Ser(S)
Arg(R) residue found at -2 or -10 from cleavage site
40% begin with Met(M) Leu(L)
16% begin with Met(M) Leu(L) Ser(S)
Rich in basic and hydroxylated residues
Form amphipathic alpha-helix

Fig. 3. N-terminal leader sequences on *Trichomonas vaginalis* hydrogenosomal proteins. Leader sequences were deduced by comparing the nucleotide sequence of the corresponding *T. vaginalis* genes and the amino acid sequences derived from direct sequence of the mature protein purified from hydrogenosomes. For details regarding the ferredoxin (Fd) leader sequence, see Johnson et al. (1990); β-succinyl CoA synthetase (β-SCS), see Lahti et al. (1992); α-succinyl CoA synthetase (α-SCS), see Lahti et al., (1994); and adenylate kinase (AK), see Länge et al., (1994). For comparison, properties of mitochondrial leader sequences are listed below.

16% begin with methionine-leucine-serine (whereas chloroplast leader sequences almost invariably begin with methionine-alanine). Also, a majority of mitochondrial leader sequences contain arginine at either -2 or -10 from the cleavage site (Hendrick et al., 1989; von Heijne, 1989). Arginine, leucine, and serine typically are overrepresented in mitochondrial leader sequences, and all three amino acids are present in each of these short hydrogenosomal leader sequences. Finally, both hydrogenosomal and mitochondrial leader sequences have the potential to form amphiphilic α-helices (von Heijne, 1986; Johnson et al., 1990).

The conservation of the primary sequence of the seven putative hydrogenosomal targeting signals studied to date appears to be greater than that observed for mitochondrial targeting signals. Also, hydrogenosomal leader sequences appear to differ markedly from those of mitochondrial proteins in length. Leader sequences of mitochondrial proteins are typically 20–80 amino acids, whereas the leaders identified thus far for hydrogenosomal proteins are 8–11 amino acids. Nevertheless, the general biochemical compositions of hydrogenosomal and mitochondrial targeting signals are similar.

To test the hypothesis that the short N-terminal leader sequence on hydrogenosomal proteins is the signal required to specifically target and translocate proteins into the hydrogenosome, we have developed an in vitro protein targeting assay (unpublished). These experiments consist of mixing Percoll gradient-purified hydrogenosomes with radiolabeled full-length hydrogenosomal proteins in the presence of an ATP regenerating system and under conditions that stabilize the organelles. Using our in vitro system and protease protection assays, we have demonstrated that radiolabeled ferredoxin can be translocated into the organelle. Translocation is accompanied by cleavage of the protein to the size predicted for the mature ferredoxin lacking the eight amino acid leader. Moreover, translocation and cleavage is strictly dependent on the presence of this eight amino acid leader sequence. Proteins lacking the leader sequence do not even bind to the outer surface of hydrogenosomes. Furthermore, protein translocation and cleavage is dependent on ATP and *T. vaginalis* cytosol. Temperature is also important, as binding and translocation are blocked at 4°C (unpublished data). These findings show that the leader sequence is necessary for translocation of proteins into the organelle, providing evidence that this is the signal that specifically targets proteins into hydrogenosomes.

CONCLUSIONS

In this chapter, we have reviewed a number of biochemical properties of the hydrogenosome, a redox organelle found exclusively in certain anaerobes that lack mitochondria. The focus of our research has been to gain an insight into the origin and biogenesis of the hydrogenosome. Our observations have allowed a number of parallels to be drawn between hydrogenosomes and mitochondria. 1) All examined hydrogenosomal proteins appear to be synthesized on free polysomes, with an N-terminal leader sequence that is absent from the mature protein, similar to that observed for nuclear-encoded mitochondrial proteins. 2) This N-terminal leader is required for translocation of the protein into hydrogenosomes in vitro and is removed in the process. 3) Translocation is an active process that is ATP and temperature dependent and requires cytosolic components. 4) The N-terminal leader of hydrogenosomal proteins is similar to presequences that direct proteins into mitochondria. These data indicate that mechanisms underlying protein targeting and biogenesis of hydrogensosomes and mitochondria are similar.

The observation that the N-terminal signal, which appears to sort proteins into the hydrogenosome, is biochemically similar to the signal that sorts nuclear-encoded mitochondrial proteins into the mitochondria is consistent with a common origin of these organelles. Furthermore, data that suggest trichomonads evolved from the main line of eukaryotic evolution prior to the appearance of true mitochondria allow speculation that hydrogenosomes and mitochondria evolved from a common progenitor organelle, as opposed to the popular theory that hydrogenosomes are derived from mitochondria. In light of the significant metabolic differences between hydrogenosomes and mitochondria, a progenitor organelle that evolved into a hydrogenosome in anaerobic cells and a mitochondrion in aerobic cells seems more probable than the conversion of a bona fide mitochondria into hydrogenosomes. On the other hand, the similarities of hydrogenosomes and mitochondria may reflect convergent evolution, and the two organelles may have evolved independently. Clearly, additional data were needed to resolve the conflicting hypotheses regarding the relationship of these organelles. Further biochemical analysis of trichomonad hydrogenosomes, as well as a comparative analysis of hydrogenosomes found in diverse phylogenetic organisms, should provide additional insight into the origin and classification of this intriguing organelle.

ACKNOWLEDGMENTS

This research was supported by Public Health Service grant AI 27857 from the National Institutes of Health and by a Burroughs-Wellcome New Investigator in Molecular Parasitology Award (to P.J.J.).

REFERENCES

Attardi G, Schatz G (1988): Biogenesis of mitochondria. Annu Rev Cell Biol 4:289–333.
Bridger WA, Wolodico WT, Henning W, Upton C, Majumdar R, Williams SP (1987): The subunits of succinyl coenzymeA synthetase: Function and assembly. Bioch Soc Symp 54:103–111.
Buck D, Spencer ME, Guest JR (1985): Primary structure of the succinyl CoA synthetase of *Escherichia coli*. Biochemistry 24:6245–6552.
Cavalier-Smith T (1987): The simultaneous symbiotic origin of mitochondria, chloroplasts and microbodies. Ann NY Acad Sci 503:55–72.
Chapman A, Cammack R, Linstead DJ, Lloyd D (1986): Respiration of *Trichomonas vaginalis*. Eur J Biochem 156:193–198.
Fenchel T, Finlay BJ (1991): The biology of free-living anaerobic ciliates. Eur J Protistol 26:201–215.
Finlay BJ, Fenchel T (1989): Hydrogenosomes in some anaerobic protozoa resemble mitochondria. FEMS Microbiol Lett 65:311–314.
Fujiki Y, Rachubinski RA, Lazarow PB (1984): Synthesis of a major integral membrane polypeptide of rat liver peroxisomes on free polysomes. Proc Natl Acad Sci USA 81:7127–7131.
Gasser SM, Daum G, Schatz G (1982): Import of proteins into mitochondria. J Biol Chem 257:13034–13041.
Gorrell TE, Yarlett N, Müller M (1984): Isolation and characterization of *Trichomonas vaginalis* ferredoxin. Carlsberg Res Commun 49:259–268.
Graves MC, Mullenbach GT, Rabinowitz JC (1985): Cloning and nucleotide sequence determination of the *Clostridium pasteurianum* ferredoxin gene. Proc Natl Acad Sci USA 82:1653–1657.

Hart DT, Baudhuim P, Opperdoes FR, de Duve C (1987): Biogenesis of the glycosome in *Trypanosoma brucei:* The synthesis, translocation and turnover of glycosomal polypeptides. J Eur Mol Biol Org 6:1403–1411.

Heine P, McGregor JA (1993): *Trichomonas vaginalis*—A reemerging pathogen. Clin Obst Gynecol 36:137–144.

Hendrick JP, Hodges PE, Rosenberg LE (1989): Survey of amino terminal proteolytic cleavage sites in mitochondrial precursor proteins: Leader peptides cleaved by two matrix proteases share a three amino acid sequence motif. Proc Natl Acad Sci USA 86:4056–4060.

Honigberg BM (1990): Trichomonads Parasitic in Humans. New York: Springer-Verlag.

Honigberg BM, Volkmann D, Entzeroth R, Scholtyseck E (1984): A freeze-fracture electron microscope study of *Trichomonas vaginalis* (Donne) and *Tritichomonas foetus* (Reidmuller). J Protozool 31:116–131.

Huber M, Garfinkel L, Gitler C, Mirelman D, Revel M, Rozenblatt S (1988): Nucleotide sequence analysis of an *Entamoeba histolytica* ferredoxin gene. Mol Biochem Parasitol 31:27–33.

Jenkins TM, Gorrell TE, Müller M, Weitzman PDJ (1991): Hydrogenosomal succinate thiokinase in *Tritichomonas foetus* and *Trichomonas vaginalis*. Biochm Biophys Res Commun 179:892–896.

Johnson PJ, d'Oliveira CE, Gorrell TE, Müller M (1990): Molecular analysis of the hydrogenosomal ferredoxin of the anaerobic protist *Trichomonas vaginalis*. Proc Natl Acad Sci USA 87:6097–6101.

Johnson PJ (1993): Metronidazole and drug resistance. Parasitol Today 9:183–186.

Johnson PJ, Lahti CJ, Bradley PJ (1993): Biogenesis of the hydrogenosome in the anaerobic protist, *Trichomonas vaginalis*. J Parasitol 79:664–670.

Kalderon D, Roberts BL, Richardson WD, Smith AE (1984): A short amino acid sequence able to specify nuclear location. Cell 39:499–509.

Kulda J, Nohynkova E, Ludvik J (1986): Basic structure and function of the trichomonad cell. Acta Univ Carolinae-Biol 30:181–198.

Lahti CJ, d'Oliveira CE, Johnson PJ (1992): Beta-succinyl coenzyme A synthetase from *Trichomonas vaginalis* is a soluble hydrogenosomal protein with an amino terminal sequence that resembles mitochondrial presequences. J Bacteriol 174:6822–6830.

Lahti CJ, Johnson PJ (1991): *Trichomonas vaginalis* hydrogenosomal proteins are synthesized on free polyribosomes and may undergo processing upon maturation. Mol Biochem Parasitol 46:307–310.

Lahti CJ, Bradley PJ, Johnson PJ (1994): Molecular characterization of the α-subunit of *Trichomonas vaginalis* hydrogenosomal succinyl CoA synthetase. Mol Biochem Parasitol 66:309–318.

Länge S, Rozario C, Müller M (1994): Primary structure of the hydrogenosomal adenylate kinase of *Trichomonas vaginalis* and its phylogenetic relationships. Mol Biochem Parasitol 66:297–308.

Leipe DD, Gunderson JH, Nerad TA, Sogin ML (1993): Small subunit ribosomal RNA[+] of *Hexamita inflata* and the quest for the first branch in the eukaryotic tree. Mol Biochem Parasitol 59:41–48.

Lindmark DG, Müller M (1973): Hydrogenosome, a cytoplasmic organelle of the anaerobic flagellate *Tritichomonas foetus,* and its role in pyruvate metabolism. J Biol Chem 248:7724–7728.

Lindmark DG, Müller M, Shio H (1975): Hydrogenosomes in *Trichomonas vaginalis*. J Parasitol 61:552–554.

Lloyd D, Hillman K, Yarlett N, Williams AG (1989): Hydrogen production by rumen holotrich protozoa: Effects of oxygen and implications for metabolic control by in situ conditions. J Protozool 36:205–213.

Lloyd D, Lindmark DG, Müller M (1979a): Respiration of *Tritichomonas foetus:* Absence of detectable cytochromes. J Parasitol 65:466–469.

Lloyd D, Lindmark DG, Müller M (1979b): Adenosine triphosphatase activity of *Tritichomonas foetus.* J Gen Microbiol 115:301–307.

Müller M (1980): The hydrogenosome. Symp Soc Gen Microbiol 30:127–142.

Müller M (1988): Energy metabolism of protozoa without mitochondria. Annu Rev Microbiol 42:465–488.

O'Fallon JV, Wright RW, Calza RE (1991): Glucose metabolic pathways in the anaerobic rumen fungus *Neocallimastric frontalis.* Biochem J 274:595–599.

Paltauf F, Meingassner JG (1982): The absence of cardiolipin in hydrogenosomes of *Trichomonas vaginalis* and *Tritrichomonas foetus.* J Parasitol 68:949–950.

Paul RG, Williams AG, Bulter RD (1990): Hydrogenosomes in the rumen entodiniomorphid ciliate *Polyplastron multivesiculatum.* J Gen Microbiol 136:1981–1989.

Reeves RE, Guthrie JD, Lobelle-Rich P (1980): *Entamoeba histolytica:* Isolation of ferredoxin. Exp Parasitol 49:83–88.

Sogin ML (1991): Early evolution and the origin of eukaryotes. Curr Opin Genet Dev 1:457–463.

Steinbüchel A, Müller M (1986): Anaerobic pyruvate metabolism of *Tritrichomonas foetus* and *Trichomonas vaginalis* hydrogenosomes. Mol Biochem Parasitol 20:57–65.

von Heijne G (1986): Mitochondrial targeting sequences may form amphiphilic alpha helices. J Eur Mol Biol Org 5:1335–1342.

von Heijne G, Steppuhn J, Herrmann RG (1989): Domain structure of mitochondrial and chloroplast targeting peptides. Eur J Biochem 180:535–545.

Whatley JM, John P, Whatley FR (1979): From extracellular to intracellular: The establishment of mitochondria and chloroplasts. Proc R Soc Lond Ser B 204:165–187.

Yarlett N, Hann AC, Lloyd D, Williams A (1981): Hydrogenosomes in the rumen protozoan *Dasytricha ruminantium* Schuberg. J Biochem 200:365–372.

Yarlett N, Orpin CG, Munn EA, Yarlett NC, Greenwood CA (1986): Hydrogenosomes in the rumen fungus *Neocallimastrix patriciarum.* Biochem J 236:729–739.

Molecular Approaches to Parasitology, pages 413–426
© 1995 Wiley-Liss, Inc.

Import of Proteins Into the Glycosomes of *Trypanosoma brucei*

Jürg M. Sommer and C.C. Wang

*Department of Pharmaceutical Chemistry, University of California,
San Francisco, California 94143*

INTRODUCTION

The parasitic hemoflagellate *Trypanosoma brucei* causes sleeping sickness in humans and nagana in domestic livestock of Africa. It is characterized by a dimorphic life cycle that includes an insect (procyclic) form, carried by the tsetse fly, as well as a bloodstream form in the mammalian host. In the bloodstream form, several biosynthetic pathways, including the tricarboxylic acid cycle and the cytochrome-dependent electron transport chain, are completely suppressed (Vickerman et al., 1988). Without a fully functional mitochondrion, it depends entirely on glycolysis and substrate-level phosphorylation for its energy production. Although the glucose supply in the host's bloodstream is abundant, the energy production under these conditions is rather inefficient, resulting in two ATP and two pyruvate molecules generated from each glucose molecule (Fairlamb and Opperdoes, 1986). However, by compartmentalizing the first seven glycolytic enzymes and two glycerol-metabolizing enzymes into a membrane-bound microbody organelle, named the *glycosome* by Opperdoes and Borst (1977), the parasite has found an ingenious way to increase the rate of glycolysis. The extraordinarily high concentration of enzymes (340 mg/ml) and glycolytic intermediates in the millimolar range (Visser et al., 1981) inside the 60 or so glycosomes per cell (Tetley and Vickerman, 1991) allow glycolysis to proceed at a rate 50 times that found in an ordinary mammalian cell (Fairlamb and Opperdoes, 1986). Inhibition of the glycolytic pathway would be clearly deleterious to the bloodstream form of *T. brucei,* and attempts at specific inhibition of glycosomal enzyme activities may ultimately lead to new chemotherapeutic agents (Willson et al., 1992). As an alternative strategy, an understanding of the specific steps in the assembly of this unique organelle could provide a more suitable target for drug interference. The biogenesis of the glycosome has thus been studied in considerable detail over the past few years. Below we review some of the key features of the glycosome and the current knowledge on glycosomal protein import.

BIOGENESIS OF THE GLYCOSOME

Glycosomes appear to be present in all trypanosome species, as well as in *Leishmania, Crithidia, Phytomonas,* and *Trypanoplasma* (Opperdoes and Michels, 1993). All of these organisms belong to the order Kinetoplastida, characterized by the presence of a single mitochondrial structure per cell, including the prominent kinetoplast, which accommodates the unique organization of their mitochondrial DNA. The glycosome, on the other hand, contains no nucleic acids, and its matrix is surrounded by a single phospholipid bilayer membrane, forming a globular organelle with a diameter of 0.2–0.3 μm (Opperdoes et al., 1984). Morphologically, the glycosomes resemble other microbodies such as the peroxisomes and glyoxysomes. But the lack of catalase and other peroxidases in the glycosomes of *T. brucei* distinguishes them from peroxisomes and led to some controversy over their evolutionary origin (Borst, 1986). However, their kinship to peroxisomes has recently been substantiated through the ability to import peroxisomal proteins into glycosomes in vivo (Sommer et al., 1992) (see below) and the detection of catalase in glycosomes of lower trypanosomatids (Soares and De, 1988) and in other kinetoplast species, as well as *Phytomonas* (Sanchez et al., 1992), *Crithidia,* and *Trypanoplasma* spp. (Opperdoes et al., 1988). In addition, some of the enzymes required for β-oxidation of fatty acids and ether lipid biosynthesis, typically associated with peroxisomes, have also been localized to the glycosomes in a number of kinetoplastids (Opperdoes, 1984; Hart and Opperdoes, 1984). There is little doubt today that glycosomes and peroxisomes are members of the same family of intracellular organelles. Thus, if the study of glycosomal biogenesis is to result in the identification of useful target(s) for antitrypanosomal chemotherapy, it must focus on certain subtle differences between peroxisomal and glycosomal assembly.

Glycosomal proteins in *T. brucei* are encoded by nuclear genes. In many cases, there is also a cytoplasmic isozyme present, which is predominantly expressed in the insect stage of the life cycle (Michels et al., 1986; Parsons and Hill, 1989). The genes encoding glycosomal and cytoplasmic versions of the same enzyme are often arranged in tandem repeats and expressed as polycistronic transcripts (Gibson et al., 1988), followed by individual *trans*-splicing and polyadenylation. The rate of transcription of these genes is thus usually similar in the bloodstream and insect forms of the parasite, and any cell type-specific regulation of expression must occur post-transcriptionally. With the exception of glyceraldehyde-3-phosphate dehydrogenase (Michels et al., 1991), multiple glycolytic isozymes in *T. brucei* have probably arisen by duplication of a gene coding for a cytoplasmic enzyme. Subsequently, one of the proteins acquired a glycosomal targeting signal. In many cases, the cytoplasmic isozyme has been retained and is highly homologous to the glycosomal protein. In addition, there is strong evidence of more recent gene conversion events between gene copies encoding the glycosomal and cytoplasmic isozymes (Le Blancq et al., 1988; Alexander et al., 1990). This has led in some instances to virtually identical protein sequences except for minor differences, such as a unique 38 amino acid C-terminal extension in the glycosomal isozyme of *Crithidia fasciculata* 3-phosphoglycerate kinase (PGK) (Swinkels et al., 1988). Such extensive similarities between the two differently localized proteins should thus facilitate the identification of glycosomal targeting signals.

The translocation of proteins into the glycosome occurs post-translationally, within 3–5 minutes after protein synthesis (Clayton, 1988; Hart et al., 1987). No proteolytic modification has been detected upon import of any of the glycosomal proteins studied to date. During the purification of glycolytic proteins from *T. brucei* it became apparent that all of the major glycosomal enzymes, except glucosephosphate isomerase (PGI), displayed isoelectric points several pH units higher than those of their cytosolic or mammalian and yeast counterparts (Misset et al., 1986). Structural modeling using coordiantes of homologous enzymes from other organisms revealed that in each case some of the excess positive charges are distributed in two "hot spots," approximately 40Å apart, each consisting of one or more basic amino acid residues within 7Å of each other (Wierenga et al., 1987). A similar surface constellation of basic amino acids was also found in PGI, even through it has an isoelectric point of 7.5 (Marchand et al., 1989). Since the presence of these "hot spots" is a major difference between the glycosomal and cytoplasmic enzymes, they were postulated to be involved in the glycosomal protein import (Wierenga et al., 1987). However, it was subsequently found that in several homologous glycosomal proteins from other species these hot spots did not exist (Kendall et al., 1990; Swinkels et al., 1988). Clearly, the hot spots could not be a general requirement for glycosomal protein import.

IMPORT OF FOREIGN PROTEINS INTO THE GLYCOSOME

After the initial observation that firefly luciferase expressed in mammalian cells was imported into peroxisomes (Keller et al., 1987) and that the import depended on the C-terminal tripeptide SKL of luciferase (Gould et al., 1989), it soon became apparent that this SKL-dependent targeting mechanism was conserved among the peroxisomes of mammals, plants, insects, and yeasts (Gould et al., 1990). Of the *T. brucei* glycosomal enzymes with known amino acid sequences, glyceraldehyde-3-phosphate dehydrogenase ends in AKL, glucose-6-phosphate isomerase in SHL, and phosphoenolpyruvate carboxykinase in SRL (Table 1), which are expected to function as peroxisomal targeting signals. An antibody raised against the C-terminal SKL sequence specifically labeled the glycosomes in *T. brucei* thin sections and recognized a handful of glycosomal

TABLE 1. Glycosomal Protein Targeting Signals

Protein	Species	Signal	Reference
Glyceraldehyde-phosphate dehydrogenase	T. brucei	C-terminal AKL	Michels et al. (1986)
	T. cruzi	C-terminal ARL	Kendall et al. (1990)
	L. mexicana	C-terminal SKM	Hannaert et al. (1992)
	T. borelli	C-terminal AKL	Opperdoes and Michels (1993)
Glucosephosphate isomerase	T. brucei	C-terminal SHL	Marchand, et al. (1989)
	L. mexicana	C-terminal AHL	Opperdoes and Michels (1993)
Phosphoenolpyruvate carboxykinase	T. brucei	C-terminal SRL	Sommer et al. (1994)
	T. cruzi	C-terminal ARL	Sommer et al. (1994)
Phosphoglycerate kinase (gPGK)	T. brucei	C-terminal SSL	Sommer et al. (1993)
	C. fasciculata	C-terminus	Swinkels et al. (1988)
Phosphoglycerate kinase (56PGK)	T. brucei	Unknown; internal?	Alexander and Parsons (1991)
	C. fasciculata	Unknown; internal?	Swinkels et al. (1992b)
Triosephosphate isomerase	T. brucei	Unknown; internal?	Swinkels et al. (1986)
Fructose-biphosphate aldolase	T. brucei	N-terminal?	Clayton (1985)

proteins on a Western blot, indicating the presence of a few, as yet unknown, glycosomal proteins ending in SKL (Keller et al., 1991). Fung and Clayton (1991) showed that after transient in vivo expression of a chloramphenicol acetyltransferase (CAT) protein with an added C-terminal SKL sequence, the CAT activity was associated with the glycosomal fraction, suggesting that the C-terminal SKL is a glycosomal targeting signal. To demonstrate that this C-terminal tripeptide indeed functions as a signal for glycosomal import, we expressed firefly luciferase in stable transformants of *T. brucei,* where the exact localization could be verified by immunoelectron microscopy (Sommer et al., 1992).

The expression of foreign genes in trypanosomes, and in kinetoplastids in general, has only recently become possible, following the identification of suitable promoters (Lee and van der Ploeg, 1990). In *T. brucei,* either the PARP (procyclic acidic repetitive protein) or the VSG (variant surface glycoprotein) promoters can be used for this purpose. To produce stable transformants, three marker genes are currently available that confer drug resistance to neomycin (G418), hygromycin B, or phleomycin (Lee and van der Ploeg, 1991; Jefferies et al., 1993). Until recently, the lack of a replicating vector required insertion of the plasmid DNA into the genome for the production of stable transformants (Patnaik et al., 1993). Using the PARP promoter, we were able to express luciferase in a tandem array with the *neo* or *hyg* gene by including a splice signal in front of each gene, and stable transformants were obtained by targeted insertion of this construct into the tubulin locus. The majority of transformants obtained in this way did indeed express high levels of luciferase, and its import into the glycosome was confirmed by immunoelectron microscopy (Sommer et al., 1992). Site-directed mutagenesis of the C-terminal tripeptide indicated that import of luciferase into the glycosomes was indeed dependent on the SKL sequence. However, many of our mutations in the SKL sequence retained sufficient information to target luciferase to the glycosomes of *T. brucei* (Fig. 1). The efficiency of import of the mutant luciferase proteins was expressed as the percent of pelleted (glycosomal) luciferase activity following digitonin solubilization of the plasma membrane and centrifugation (Visser and Opperdoes, 1980). Immunoelectron microscopy showed that partial activity found in the pellet fraction corresponded to a partial import into the glycosome. Accordingly, the serine residue in the C-terminal SKL sequence of luciferase could be replaced with the small neutral, polar amino acids alanine, asparagine, cysteine, glycine, proline, or threonine, as well as histidine, while resulting in at least 50% of the protein being imported into the glycosome. The lysine residue could be substituted with an amino acid capable of hydrogen bonding, either arginine, asparagine, glutamine, histidine, methionine, or serine, but not threonine or the acidic amino acids aspartate and glutamate. A positively charged side chain was not needed at this position for glycosomal import, although this appeared to be a requirement for import into mamma-

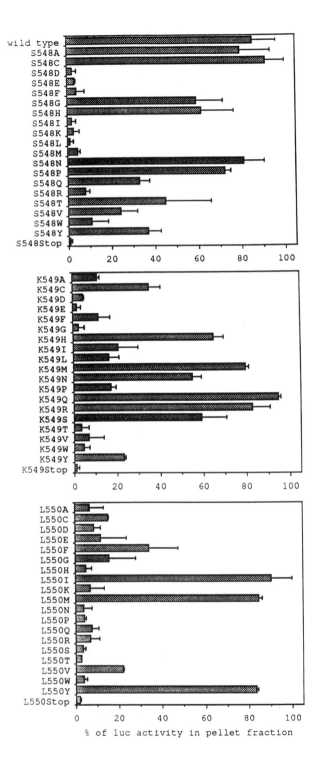

% of luc activity in pellet fraction

lian peroxisomes (Gould et al., 1989). The C-terminal leucine could only be replaced with one of the hydrophobic amino acids isoleucine, methionine, or tyrosine. Thus, the amino acids that can make up a glycosomal targeting signal at the C terminus of luciferase consist of {A/C/G/H/N/P/S/T} {H/K/M/N/Q/R/S} {I/L/M/Y}.

However, it should be pointed out that not all possible combinations of these three families of amino acids have been tested, nor are all of them expected to form functional targeting signals. It was found for peroxisomal import that certain combinations of two substituting amino acids can abolish the import completely (Swinkels et al., 1992a). In general, many more substitutions are tolerated in the glycosomal targeting signal than for peroxisomal import in mammalian cells. In particular, we found two tripeptide sequences, SSL and SKI, that allowed protein import into the glycosomes but were shown not to act as peroxisomal targeting signals in mammalian cells (Gould et al., 1989; Blattner et al., 1992). The reason for this increased degeneracy in the glycosomal tripeptide targeting signal is not clear, but in light of the perplexing problem of localizing most of the glycolytic enzymes to the glycosome during the course of evolution, a lowering of the stringency for glycosomal import may have facilitated the acquisition of targeting signals for those proteins originally located in the cytoplasm.

THE TARGETING SIGNAL FOR IMPORT OF GLYCOSOMAL 3-PHOSPHOGLYCERATE KINASE

A serine-serine-leucine (SSL) sequence is located at the C terminus of *T. brucei* glycosomal 3-phosphoglycerate kinase (gPGK), at the end of a 20 amino acid extension found on gPGK, but not on the otherwise 93% identical cytoplasmic PGK (cPGK). The SSL sequence is unable to target luciferase or the CAT protein to the mammalian peroxisome (Gould et al., 1989; Blattner et al., 1992). It also appears that gPGK is not targeted to the peroxisome when expressed in *Saccharomyces cerevisiae* (Michels and Opperdoes, 1991), suggesting that it does not contain a universally functional peroxisomal targeting signal. However, as mentioned above, a C-terminal SSL results in import of luciferase into the glycosomes. When the entire 20 amino acid extension of gPGK was appended to the CAT protein, this fusion protein was recovered in the glycosomal fraction (Fung and Clayton, 1991) and became associated with

---

Fig. 1. Import of mutant luciferase into the glycosomes of *T. brucei*. Bars correspond to the percentage ± SD of luciferase activity recovered in the pellet fraction following digitonin solubilization and centrifugation of tranformants expressing luciferase proteins with single amino acid changes in the C-terminal SKL sequence.

the glycosome, as detected by indirect immunofluorescence microscopy (Blattner et al., 1992).

The gPGK protein is predominantly expressed in the bloodstream form of *T. brucei*. In the procyclic form an alternate glycosomal PGK (56PGK) is expressed, encoded by the "A gene" of the PGK gene cluster (Alexander and Parsons, 1991). The 56PGK is highly homologous to gPGK, except for its lack of a C-terminal extension and the presence of a unique 80 amino acid insertion in the N-terminal half of the protein. Since the 56PGK protein ends in the tripeptide DKE, which is unlikely a targeting signal for glycosomal import, it may contain an N-terminal or internal signal. We explored the possibility that such a signal may have been conserved between the gPGK and 56PGK. It is known that some peroxisomal proteins contain multiple, independently functioning targeting signals or internal sequences required in addition to a C-terminal tripeptide signal (Kragler et al., 1993; Distel et al., 1992). It is thus not unlikely that *T. brucei* gPGK may contain glycosomal targeting information in addition to the C-terminal SSL sequence. By expressing a fusion protein in which the C-terminal SKL tripeptide of luciferase was replaced with the entire gPGK protein, we showed that the glycosomal import of this fusion protein was still dependent on the C-terminal SSL sequence (Sommer et al., 1993). Thus, there is probably no independently functioning internal signal that could target gPGK to the glycosomes. Additional experiments confirmed that the SSL tripeptide at the C terminus of luciferase, or another reporter protein, bacterial β-glucuronidase (GUS), is sufficient to direct these proteins into the glycosome, as indicated by immunoelectron microscopy. The inclusion of the entire 20 amino acid C-terminal extension of gPGK at the end of luciferase or GUS increased the efficiency of import somewhat, but there appears to be little sequence specificity immediately preceding the SSL sequence, and the amino acid extension on gPGK may simply result in a more efficient presentation of the C-terminal tripeptide to the import machinery (Sommer et al., 1993).

The results from our gPGK gene fusion experiments also showed that the hot spots, which are present on the surface of gPGK, are not required for import into the glycosome (Sommer et al., 1993). However, we cannot rule out the possibility that the excess positive charges in glycosomal proteins may increase the efficiency of import by initial targeting of gPGK to the glycosomal membrane. An in vitro assay that measures the association of newly synthesized gPGK with purified glycosomes demonstrated a specific affinity for gPGK, but not cPGK (Sommer et al., 1990). This interaction was partially urea and protease resistant. However, the analysis of chimeric proteins made from portions of gPGK and cPGK indicated that this in vitro interaction was not dependent on the C-terminal SSL sequence, but rather on regions containing some of the excess basic charges (K. Alexander, J. Sommer, C.C. Wang and M. Parsons, unpublished data). Since our current in vivo protein targeting assay cannot measure the rate of import, additional experiments will be required to determine what, if any, effect the extra basic amino acids might have on glycosomal protein import.

While the function of the hot spots in *T. brucei* glycosomal proteins remains a mystery, they could be responsible for the antitrypanosomal activity of Suramin, a drug that has been used in the treatment of early stages of African sleeping sickness (Voogd et al., 1993). At physiological pH, Suramin contains two clusters of negatively charged sulfonyl groups. Several of the glycosomal enzymes, including hexokinase, glucosephosphate isomerase, aldolase, glycerolphosphate dehydrogenase, glycerol kinase, and PGK are inhibited at a much lower Suramin concentration than their cytoplasmic or mammalian counterparts, possibly as a result of direct interaction of Suramin with the excess basic amino acids (Willson et al., 1993). Suramin enters the trypanosome by endocytosis of drug-bound serum proteins (Fairlamb and Bowman, 1980). However, this highly charged molecule is not expected to cross the glycosomal membrane, and we find it unlikely that Suramin would inhibit the activity of glycosomal enzymes inside the glycosome. On the other hand, Suramin may bind to newly synthesized glycosomal proteins in the cytoplasm. This interaction could inhibit translocation of the proteins across the glycosomal membrane by preventing their unfolding in a way that has been well documented for the inhibition of import of methotrexate-bound dihydrofolate reductase fusion proteins into the mitochondria (Eilers and Schatz, 1986). It is also interesting to note that Suramin at a concentration of 10 μM inhibits the in vitro import of acyl-CoA oxidase into purified rat liver peroxisomes (Imanaka et al., 1992). In this case, inhibition occurs through the interaction of Suramin with the peroxisome, rather than the imported protein, as indicated by Suramin pretreatment of the peroxisomes. Clearly, the effects of Suramin on glycosomal protein import need to be investigated in more detail.

OTHER GLYCOSOMAL TARGETING SIGNALS

Two microbody proteins have been identified that contain cleavable N-terminal sequences. The watermelon malate dehydrogenase has a 37 amino acid presequence (Gietl, 1990), and the human and rat 3-ketoacyl-CoA thiolase presequences range from 26 to 36 amino acids (Swinkels et al., 1991; Osumi et al., 1991). In the case of thiolase, these N-terminal sequences have been shown to target a reporter protein to the peroxisome (Swinkels et al., 1991; Osumi et al., 1991). An amino acid motif consisting of RLXXXXX{Q/H}L, where X may be almost any amino acid, is likely to be involved in the targeting, since it is also conserved at the N termini of thiolases from three yeast species. It is not yet clear, however, if this sequence represents a widely used peroxisomal import signal. Protein database searches revealed that this motif is also occasionally found in mitochondrial presequences. It has recently been shown that a single amino acid change in the N-terminal signal of peroxisomal thiolase can mistarget this protein to the mitochondria (Osumi et al., 1992). It is thus possible that the peroxisomal thiolase has diverged from an ancestral mitochondrial thiolase by means of modifying the N-terminal signal for localization to the peroxisome. Among the *T. brucei* glycosomal enzymes, aldolase has a similar motif at the N terminus (Clayton, 1985). It is tempting to speculate that this sequence is the glycosomal targeting signal, since aldolase lacks an obvious C-terminal signal. However, this has not yet been demonstrated experimentally.

The RLXXXXX{Q/H}L motif can also be found at internal locations in several peroxisomal proteins, including most of the known plant catalases, human serine-pyruvate aminotransferase, and *T. brucei* glucose-6-phosphate isomerase. However, this sequence occurs at random in one of every 100 proteins, and the finding of such sequences in peroxisomal proteins may thus not be significant. Further experimental studies will be required to determine the exact nature of internal targeting signals in both glycosomes and peroxisomes.

MEMBRANE PROTEINS, CYTOSOLIC FACTORS, AND ENERGY REQUIREMENTS FOR GLYCOSOMAL PROTEIN IMPORT

Two integral glycosomal membrane proteins of 24 and 26 kD have been identified that are present in both bloodstream and procyclic forms of *T. brucei* (Aman and Wang, 1987). However, their function is unknown, and a possible involvement in protein translocation has not been demonstrated. In the yeast *Pichia pastoris,* a peroxisomal membrane-associated protein of 65 kD has recently been shown to bind specifically to peptides ending in SKL (McCollum et al., 1993). Most likely, this protein is part of the import machinery for peroxisomal proteins with a C-terminal tripeptide signal. Additional SKL-binding proteins may also be present in the cytoplasm (Wendland and Subramani, 1993), possibly acting as shuttle proteins to deliver peroxisomal proteins to the import machinery. Other cytoplasmic factors may also include "chaperonins" required for the unfolding of the peroxisomal precursor proteins (Wendland and Subramani, 1993). In vivo, the peroxisomal import process requires ATP hydrolysis, but not GTP (Soto et al., 1993). The energy requirement for in vivo glycosomal protein import has not been investigated, but it is unlikely to differ significantly from that of peroxisomal import.

CONCLUSION

The study of glycosomal protein import in *T. brucei* has confirmed that these organelles are indeed sufficiently related to the peroxisomes of higher eukaryotes to share at least one import mechanism. Few, but significant differences exist in the specificities of the mammalian and the trypanosomal import machineries for the C-terminal targeting signal. Further experiments are required to test whether the N-terminal targeting signal of peroxisomal thiolase and the related sequence at the N terminus of *T. brucei* aldolase are able to target proteins to the glycosomes and to define the nature of the presumably internal targeting signals of several other glycosomal proteins. The extra basic amino acids found in glycosomal proteins are apparently not required for protein import. They could be essential for allowing a high concentration of glycolytic intermediates in the glycosome by neutralizing the negative charges of these substrates (Opperdoes and Michels, 1993), but also for facilitating the targeting of proteins to the negatively charged glycosomal membrane. The most likely targets of the trypanocidal drug Suramin could be the cytoplasmic glycerolphosphate oxidase and NAD^+-dependent glycerolphosphate dehydrogenase, originally proposed by Fairlamb and Bowman (1980). However, a possible interference of Suramin with glycosomal protein unfolding in the cytoplasm prior to translocation into the glycosome cannot be ruled out at this time.

REFERENCES

Alexander K, Parail AC, Parsons M (1990): An allele of *Trypanosoma brucei* cytoplasmic phosphoglycerate kinase is a mosaic of other alleles and genes. Mol Biochem Parasitol 42:293–296.

Alexander K, Parsons M (1991): A phosphoglycerate kinase-like molecule localized to glycosomal microbodies: Evidence that the topogenic signal is not at the C-terminus. Mol Biochem Parasitol 46:1–10.

Aman RA, Wang CC (1987): Identification of two integral glycosomal membrane proteins in *Trypanosoma brucei*. Mol Biochem Parasitol 25:93–92.

Blattner J, Swinkels B, Dorsam H, Prospero T, Subramani S, Clayton C (1992): Glycosome assembly in trypanosomes: Variations in the acceptable degeneracy of a COOH-terminal microbody targeting signal. J Cell Biol 119:1129–1136.

Borst P (1986): How proteins get into microbodies (peroxisomes, glyoxysomes, glycosomes). Biochim Biphys Acta 866:179–203.

Clayton CE (1985): Structure and regulated expression of genes encoding fructose biphosphate aldolase in *Trypanosoma brucei*. Eur J Biochem 153:403–406.

Clayton CE (1988): Most proteins, including fructose bisphosphate aldolase, are stable in the procyclic trypomastigote form of *Trypanosoma brucei*. Mol Biochem Parasitol 28:43–46.

Distel B, Gould SJ, Voorn BT, Van der Berg M, Tabak HF, Subramani S (1992): The carboxyl-terminal tripeptide serine-lysine-leucine of firefly luciferase is necessary but not sufficient for peroxisomal import in yeast. New Biol 4:157–165.

Ellers M, Schatz G (1986): Binding of a specific ligand inhibits import of a purified precursor protein into mitochondria. Nature 322:228–232.

Fairlamb AH, Bowman IB (1980): Uptake of the trypanocidal drug Suramin by bloodstream forms of *Trypanosoma brucei* and its effect on respiration and growth rate in vivo. Mol Biochem Parasitol 1:315–333.

Fairlamb AH, Opperdoes FR (1986): Carbohydrate metabolism in African trypanosomes with special reference to the glycosome. In M.J. Morgan (ed): Carbohydrate Metabolism in Cultured Cells. New York, Plenum, pp. 183–224.

Fung K, Clayton C (1991): Recognition of a peroxisomal tripeptide entry signal by the glycosomes of Trypanosoma brucei. Mol Biochem Parasitol 45:261–264.

Gibson WC, Swinkels BW, Borst P (1988): Post-transcriptional control of the differential expression of phosphoglycerate kinase genes in Trypanosoma brucei. J Mol Biol 201:315–325.

Gietl C (1990: Glyoxysomal malate dehydrogenase from watermelon is synthesized with an amino-terminal transit peptide. Proc Natl Acad Sci USA 87:5773–5777.

Gould SJ, Keller GA, Hosken N, Wilkinson J, Subramani S (1989): A conserved tripeptide sorts proteins to peroxisomes. J Cell Biol 108:1657–1664.

Gould SJ, Keller GA, Schneider M, Howell SH, Garrard LJ, Goodman JM, Distel B, Tabak H, Subramani S (1990): Peroxisomal protein import is conserved between yeast, plants, insects and mammals. EMBO J 9:85–90.

Hannaert V, Blaauw M, Kohl L, Allert S, Opperdoes FR, Michels PA (1992): Molecular analysis of the cytosolic and glycosomal glyceraldehyde-3-phosphate dehydrogenase in Leishmania mexicana. Mol Biochem Parasitol 55:115–126.

Hart DT, Baudhuin P, Opperdoes FR, C. dD (1987): Biogenesis of the glycosome in Trypanosoma brucei: The synthesis, translocation and turnover of glycosomal polypeptides. EMBO J 6:1403–1411.

Hart DT, Opperdoes FR (1984): The occurrence of glycosomes (microbodies) in the promastigote stage of four major Leishmania species. Mol Biochem Parasitol 13:159–172.

Imanaka T, Lazarow PB, Takano T (1992): Suramin prevents import of acyl-CoA oxidase into rat liver peroxisomes. Biochim Biophys Acta 1134:197–202.

Jefferies D, Tebabi P, Le RD, Pays E (1993): The ble resistance gene as a new selectable marker for Trypanosoma brucei: Fly transmission of stable procyclic transformants to produce antibiotic resistant bloodstream forms. Nucleic Acids Res 21:191–195.

Keller GA, Gould S, Deluca M, Subramani S (1987): Firefly luciferase is targeted to peroxisomes in mammalian cells. Proc Natl Acad Sci USA 84:3264–3268.

Keller GA, Krisans S, Gould SJ, Sommer JM, Wang CC, Schliebs W, Kunau W, Brody S, Subramani S (1991): Evolutionary conservation of a microbody targeting signal that targets proteins to peroxisomes, glyoxysomes, and glycosomes. J Cell Biol 114:893–904.

Kendall G, Wilderspin AF, Ashall F, Miles MA, Kelly JM (1990): Trypanosoma cruzi glycosomal glyceraldehyde-3-phosphate dehydrogenase does not conform to the 'hotspot' topogenic signal model. EMBO J 9:2751–2758.

Kragler F, Langeder A, Raupachova J, Binder M, Hartig A (1993): Two independent peroxisomal targeting signals in catalase A of Saccharomyces cerevisiae. J Cell Biol 120:665–673.

Le Blancq SM, Swinkels BW, Gibson WC, Borst P (1988): Evidence for gene conversion between the phosphoglycerate kinase genes of Trypanosoma brucei. J Mol Biol 200:439–447.

Lee MG, van der Ploeg LH (1990): Homologous recombination and stable transfection in the parasitic protozoan Trypanosoma brucei. Science 250:1583–1587.

Lee MG, van der Ploeg LHT (1991): The hygromycin B-resistance-encoding gene as a selectable marker for stable transformation of Trypanosoma brucei. Gene 105:255–257.

Marchand M, Kooystra U, Wierenga RK, Lambeir AM, Van BJ, Opperdoes FR, Michels PA (1989): Glucosephosphate isomerase from Trypanosoma brucei. Cloning and characterization of the gene and analysis of the enzyme. Eur J Biochem 184:455–464.

McCollum D, Monosov E, Subramani S (1993): The pas8 mutant of Pichia pastoris exhibits the peroxisomal protein import deficiencies of Zellweger syndrome cells—The PAS8 protein binds to the COOH-terminal tripeptide peroxisomal targeting signal, and is a member of the TPR protein family. J Cell Biol 121:761–774.

Michels PA, Marchand M, Kohl L, Allert S, Wierenga RK, Opperdoes FR (1991): The cytosolic and glycosomal isoenzymes of glyceraldehyde-3-phosphate dehydrogenase in *Trypanosoma brucei* have a distant evolutionary relationship. Eur J Biochem 198:421–428.

Michels PA, Poliszczak A, Osinga KA, Misset O, Van BJ, Wierenga RK, Borst P, Opperdoes FR (1986): Two tandemly linked identical genes code for the glycosomal glyceraldehyde-phosphate dehydrogenase in *Trypanosoma brucei*. EMBO J 5:1049–1056.

Michels PAM, Opperdoes FR (1991): The evolutionary origin of glycosomes. Parasitol Today 7:105–109.

Misset O, Bos OJ, Opperdoes FR (1986). Glycolytic enzymes of *Trypanosoma brucei*. Simultaneous purification, intraglycosomal concentrations and physical properties. Eur J Biochem 157:441–453.

Opperdoes FR (1984): Localization of the initial steps in alkoxyphospholipid biosynthesis in glycosomes (microbodies) of *Trypanosoma brucei*. FEBS Lett 169:35–39.

Opperdoes FR, Baudhuin P, Coppens I, De RC, Edwards SW, Weijers PJ, Misset O (1984): Purification, morphometric analysis, and characterization of the glycosomes (microbodies) of the protozoan hemoflagellate *Trypanosoma brucei*. J Cell Biol 98:1178–1184.

Opperdoes FR, Borst P (1977): Localization of nine glycolytic enzymes in a microbody-like organelle in *Trypanosoma brucei:* The glycosome. FEBS Lett 80:360–364.

Opperdoes FR, Michels PA (1993): The glycosomes of the Kinetoplastida. Biochimie 75:231–234.

Opperdoes FR, Nohynkova E, Van Schaftingen E, Lambeir AM, Veenhuis M, Van Roy J (1988): Demonstration of glycosomes (microbodies) in the Bodonid flagellate *Trypanoplasma borelli* (Protozoa, Kinetoplastida). Mol Biochem Parasitol 30:155–163.

Osumi T, Tsukamoto T, Hata S (1992): Signal peptide for peroxisomal targeting: replacement of an essential histidine residue by certain amino acids converts the amino-terminal presequence of peroxisomal 3-ketoacyl-CoA thiolase to a mitochondrial signal peptide. Biochem Biophys Res Commun 186:811–818.

Osumi T, Tsukamoto T, Hata S, Yokota S, Miura S, Fujiki Y, Hijikata M, Miyazawa S, Hashimoto T (1991): Amino-terminal presequence of the precursor of peroxisomal 3-ketoacyl-CoA thiolase is a cleavage signal peptide for peroxisomal targeting. Biochem Biophys Res Commun 181:947–954.

Parsons M, Hill T (1989): Elevated phosphoglycerate kinase mRNA but not protein in monomorphic *Trypanosoma brucei:* Implications for stage-regulation and post-transcriptional control. Mol Biochem Parasitol 33:215–227.

Parsons M, Smith JM (1989): Trypanosome glycosomal protein P60 is homologous to phosphoenolpyruvate carboxykinase (ATP). Nucleic Acids Res 17:6411.

Patnaik PK, Kulkarni SK, Cross GA (1993): Autonomously replicating single-copy episomes in *Trypanosoma* show unusual stability. EMBO J 12:2529–2538.

Sanchez MM, Lasztity D, Coppens I, Opperdoes FR (1992): Characterization of carbohydrate metabolism and demonstration of glycosomes in a *Phytomonas* sp. isolated from *Euphorbia characias*. Mol Biochem Parasitol 54:185–199.

Soares MJ, De SW (1988): Cytoplasmic organelles of trypanosomatids: A cytochemical and stereological study. J Submicrosc Cytol Pathol 20:349–361.

Sommer JM, Cheng QL, Keller GA, Wang CC (1992): In vivo import of firefly luciferase into the glycosomes of *Trypanosoma brucei* and mutational analysis of the C-terminal targeting signal. Mol Biol Cell 3:749–759.

Sommer JM, Nguyen TT, Wang CC (1994): Phosphoenolpyruvate carboxykinase of *Trypanosoma brucei* is targeted to the glycosomes by a C-terminal sequence. FEBS Lett (in press).

Sommer JM, Peterson G, Keller GA, Parsons M, Wang CC (1993): The C-terminal tripeptide of glycosomal phosphoglycerate kinase is both necessary and sufficient for import into the glycosomes of *Trypanosoma brucei*. FEBS Lett 316:53–58.

Sommer JM, Thissen JA, Parsons M, Wang CC (1990): Characterization of an in vitro assay for import of 3-phosphoglycerate kinase into the glycosomes of *Trypanosoma brucei*. Mol Cell Biol 10:4545–4554.

Soto U, Pepperkok R, Ansorge W, Just WW (1993): Import of firefly luciferase into mammalian peroxisomes in vivo requires nucleoside triphosphates. Exp Cell Res 205:66–75.

Swinkels BW, Evers R, Borst P (1988): The topogenic signal of the glycosomal (microbody) phosphoglycerate kinase of *Crithidia fasciculata* resides in a carboxy-terminal extension. EMBO J 7:1159–1165.

Swinkels BW, Gibson WC, Osinga KA, Kramer R, Veeneman GH, van Boom JH, Borst P (1986): Characterization of the gene for the microbody (glycosomal) triosephosphate isomerase of *Trypanosoma brucei*. EMBO J 5:1291–1298.

Swinkels BW, Gould SJ, Bodnar AG, Rachubinski RA, Subramani S (1991): A novel, cleavable peroxisomal targeting signal at the amino-terminus of the rat 3-ketoacyl-CoA thiolase. EMBO J 10:3255–3262.

Swinkels BW, Gould SJ, Subramani S (1992a): Targeting efficiencies of various permutations of the consensus C-terminal tripeptide peroxisomal targeting signal. FEBS Lett 305:133–136.

Swinkels BW, Loiseau A, Opperdoes FR, Borst P (1992b): A phosphoglycerate kinase-related gene conserved between *Trypanosoma brucei* and *Crithidia fasciculata*. Mol Biochem Parasitol 50:69–78.

Tetley L, Vickerman K (1991): The glycosomes of trypanosomes: number and distribution as revealed by electron spectroscopic imaging and 3-D reconstruction. J Microsc 162:83–90.

Vickerman K, Tetley L, Hendry KA, Turner CM (1988): Biology of African trypanosomes in the tsetse fly. Biol Cell 64:109–119.

Visser N, Opperdoes FR (1980): Glycolysis in *Trypanosoma brucei*. Eur J Biochem 103:623–632.

Visser N, Opperdoes FR, Borst P (1981): Subcellular compartmentation of glycolytic intermediates in *Trypanosoma brucei*. Eur J Biochem 118:521–526.

Voogd TE, Vansterkenburg ELM, Wilting J, Janssen LHM (1993): Recent research on the biological activity of Suramin. Pharmacol Rev 45:177–203.

Wendland M, Subramani S (1993): Cytosol-dependent peroxisomal protein import in a permeabilized cell system. J Cell Biol 120:675–685.

Wierenga RK, Swinkels B, Michels PA, Osinga K, Misset O, Van BJ, Gibson WC, Postma JP, Borst P, Opperdoes FR (1987): Common elements on the surface of glycolytic enzymes from *Trypanosoma brucei* may serve as topogenic signals for import into glycosomes. EMBO J 6:215–221.

Willson M, Callens M, Kuntz DA, Perié J, Opperdoes FR (1993): Synthesis and activity of inhibitors highly specific for the glycolytic enzymes from *Trypanosoma brucei*. Mol Biochem Parasitol 59:201–210.

Willson M, Périé JJ, Melacaze F, Opperdoes F, Callens M (1992): Biological properties of amidinium sulfinic and sulfonic acid derivatives: Inhibition of glycolytic enzymes of *Trypanosoma brucei* and protective effect on cell growth. Eur J Med Chem 27:799–808.

IMMUNE RESPONSE

Preface

The final section brings us full circle, back to the host–parasite interaction, but this time focusing in on the nature of the *host's* response to infection. As with the field of immunology of infectious diseases in general, there is a great emphasis here on the nature of the cells and cytokines that modulate the immune response. This is not to say that antibodies and other immune mechanisms are not important; only that in recent years there has been a remarkable change in our understanding of how the immune response is regulated. The chapters that follow reflect these most recent findings.

Alan Sher starts off with a chapter in which he covers various parasite systems and attempts to synthesize a coherent scheme to explain the nature of the very different responses and outcomes seen with each. Steve Reed picks up the story with two parasites, *Leishmania* and *Trypanosoma cruzi,* focusing on the particular roles of TGF-β and IL-10. The possible use of cytokines in therapy is also discussed.

Rich Locksley and Steve Reiner use *Leishmania* as a model to look at what distinguishes susceptible from resistant mice. They show that the nature of the response in the two strains is radically different and that the major difference is the degree to which Th1 versus Th2 cells are stimulated. They conclude with some thoughts on how genetic engineering might be used in the future to produce a parasite that preferentially elicits a protective Th1 response.

The next chapter, by Fred Finkelman, William Gause, and Joe Urban, examines the different situation with nematode infections where a Th2 response can be protective and a Th1 response damaging to the host. The implications of these results for vaccine design, including the possible coadministration of the appropriate cytokines as a form of adjuvant on vaccination, are discussed.

The chapter by John Mansfield redresses the imbalance that molecular biologists have brought to the subject of immunity to African the trypanosomes: antibodies and antigenic variation are probably only a small part of the total response.

The final two chapters deal with the nature of the immune response during infection with organisms from different helminth phyla. Both the chapter on the immunology of schistosomiasis by Ed Pearce and filariasis by Tom Nutman emphasize the integration of basic immunology with the potential for recombinant vaccines. This is one of the most exciting areas of current parasite immunology research and where, for many, the ultimate prize lies.

Molecular Approaches to Parasitology, pages 431–442
© 1995 Wiley-Liss, Inc.

Regulation of Cell-Mediated Immunity by Parasites: The Ups and Downs of an Important Host Adaptation

Alan Sher

Laboratory of Parasitic Diseases, National Institute of Allergy and Infectious Diseases, Bethesda, Maryland 20892

INTRODUCTION

Parasites are highly successful organisms that have cleverly outwitted the valiant attempts of not only their hosts but also of many parasitologists to eradicate them by immunological means. Clearly, a major step in each parasite's evolution was its adaptation to the immune systems of its vertebrate definitive and, in some cases, invertebrate intermediate hosts. The study of these adaptations is one of the most unique and fascinating aspects of the immuno-parasitology field. Initially, much of the work on immune adaptation focused on mechanisms by which parasites evade or inactivate specific host effector responses (e.g., Porter and Knight, 1974). In the past decade, the emphasis has shifted toward understanding how parasites might directly regulate the induction of these responses, a trend that reflects the current fascination with the interaction of parasites with the regulatory cytokine network (e.g., Sher and Coffman, 1992). This chapter focuses on the mechanisms by which parasites regulate host immune responses for their own benefit. In particular, I discuss the relationship of these changes to the biological strategy of different parasites and argue that the immunoregulatory pattern characteristic of a given infection is determined during the initial contact between host and parasite.

HOW TO DEAL WITH HOST IMMUNITY: DIFFERENT PARASITES HAVE DIFFERENT BIOLOGICAL STRATEGIES

Given the enormous selective force of host resistance, the concept that parasites have learned to regulate host immune responses for their own benefit makes good evolutionary sense. Indeed, parasite infection-associated host immunological alterations (e.g., immunosuppression in visceral leishmaniasis,

African trypanosomiasis, filariasis) have been well documented in both experimental models and humans for several decades. Nevertheless, it is only recently that immunoparasitologists have had the knowledge and tools to determine whether such immunological changes reflect the regulation of responses specifically affecting parasite survival. As discussed below, the elucidation of the important role played by T cell–mediated immunity and its regulation by cytokines were two important developments which set the stage for this analysis.

Since the primary goal of most parasites is to evade host resistance, an obvious biological strategy would be to *downregulate* host protective responses. Such a strategy should clearly be followed by parasites that need to establish long-term chronic infections but that themselves are not highly virulent. Helminths and certain species of persistent protozoa (e.g., *Toxoplasma cruzi, Leishmania donovani*) are important members of this group; however, less immediately obvious is that some highly virulent parasites (e.g., *Toxoplasma gondii, Leishmania major* in resistant host strains) may actually *upregulate* vertebrate defenses in order to regulate their own numbers, thereby ensuring the survival of the host niche (this point is further discussed in the following chapters by Reed and by Locksley and Reiner). Such organisms (typically protozoa) are usually driven into a quiescent phase by the protective responses they promote, re-emerging only after passage to another nonimmune definitive or intermediate host or as a consequence of immunosuppression. A third approach taken by parasites such as malaria blood stages and African trypanosomes is to allow the immune system to regulate their numbers but to maintain active infection by directly evading the lethal effects of the response.

At a more detailed level, it is likely that many parasites combine the above biological strategies during different stages of their life cycles. For example, cutaneous *Leishmania spp.* may initially suppress innate defense mechanisms to gain entry into macrophages and then stimulate them to regulate their own growth. Regardless of the strategy(ies) employed, the end result is the same: the persistence of both parasite and host for a sufficient period to ensure transmission.

If, indeed, this concept is correct and each parasite has a pre-determined blueprint for interacting with the host immune response, then by what mechanisms does the parasite trigger these biologically important immunoregulatory changes?

THE IMPORTANCE OF CELL-MEDIATED DEFENSE MECHANISMS

Although humoral immunity plays a major role in acquired resistance to a variety of different parasites, there are surprisingly few examples in which humoral responses are actively regulated during parasitic infection, and these usually involve alterations in antibody isotype rather than overall levels (e.g.,

Khalife et al., 1986). Instead, most regulation appears to occur at the level of T-cell–mediated immune responses as evidenced by changes in lymphocyte proliferation, cytokine production, and effector cell activation. These alterations, which are readily detectable in both infected humans and experimental hosts, are likely to reflect the need to regulate cell-mediated effector mechanisms that have a major impact on parasite survival.

The concept of cell-mediated immunity was carefully described in the first edition of this book (James and Scott, 1988). Briefly, T cells (usually of the Th1 CD4$^+$ or CD8$^+$ phenotype) are stimulated by antigen to secrete lymphokines (notably IFN-γ and TNF-α) which activate effector cells to mediate immune killing. The most important cytokine-activated cell for parasite killing appears to be the macrophage. In nearly every system studied, the production of reactive nitrogen oxide (NO) species appears to be the mechanism by which these cells kill parasites or inhibit their growth (James and Nacy, 1993). The high toxicity of NO and its ability to cross biological membranes freely make it an extremely potent mediator of microbial immunity. Its production must therefore be tightly regulated, both endogenously by the host to prevent self-injury and by parasites recognized by T-cell–mediated defenses in order to produce chronic infections. This regulation can occur either at the level of the T cell producing the activating lymphokines (sometimes through an effect on accessory cells) or at the level of the macrophage effector cell itself and is mediated by another group of cytokines produced exogenously by T cells or endogenously by macrophages (Fig. 1).

T CELL SUBSETS AND REGULATORY CYTOKINES

The regulatory cytokines that control host cell-mediated immunity are produced in response to as yet poorly defined parasite stimuli; however, a considerable amount of information has been gathered about the cellular source of these molecules and how they interact with their target effectors (Table 1). The discovery in the mid-1980s that CD4$^+$ T cells can be divided into two major subsets (Th1 and Th2) based on their cytokine secretion pattern has provided a major framework for understanding the specificity of the regulatory response (Mosmann and Coffman, 1989). Th1 cells produce IFN-γ, IL-2, and lymphotoxin, three cytokines that are crucial for cell-mediated immunity, while Th2 cells produce a series of cytokines, IL-4, IL-5, IL-6, IL-10, and IL-13, that are important for antibody production and can have strong downregulatory activity. Thus, an attractive hypothesis is that Th1-dependent cell-mediated responses are cross-regulated by the cytokine products of Th2 cells (Mosmann and Coffman, 1989; Sher et al., 1992).

The concept of Th1-Th2 cross-regulation, while correct in its overall outlines, must now be tempered by the realization that many of the same regula-

STEP #1:   (LYMPHOKINE INDUCTION)   STEP #2: (MACROPHAGE ACTIVATION)

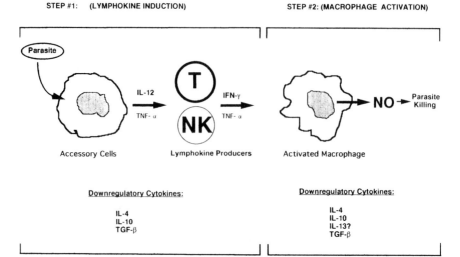

Accessory Cells   Lymphokine Producers   Activated Macrophage

Downregulatory Cytokines: Downregulatory Cytokines:

IL-4   IL-4
IL-10   IL-10
TGF-β   IL-13?
                                            TGF-β

Fig. 1.   Mechanisms by which macrophages become activated to kill parasites. Parasites interact with accessory cells (often themselves macrophages) and induce a series of monokines (IL-12, TNF-α, IL-1) that promote the differentiation and triggering of Th1 CD4$^+$, CD8$^+$ lymphocytes, and NK cells, which, in turn, secrete the lymphokines IFN-γ and TNF-α necessary for macrophage activation. In the case of CD4$^+$ and CD8$^+$ cells, lymphokine production requires specific recognition of parasite antigens by T-cell receptors; however, NK cells offer an alternative pathway in which lymphokine production can be stimulated nonspecifically in the absence of T cells and antigen recognition. The end result of macrophage activation in the mouse and other species is the production of toxic metabolites. Of these, nitrogen oxides (NO) appear to be primarily responsible for the killing of parasite targets.

Parasites that in their interaction with accessory cells stimulate high levels of monokine (and in particular) IL-12 synthesis upregulate this pathway of cell-mediated immunity. In contrast, other parasites stimulate the production of cytokines (IL-4, IL-10, IL-13?, TGF-β) that downregulate the process, inhibiting either lymphokine production and/or the ability of lymphokines to activate macrophages. Because some cytokines (e.g., IL-10) appear to act dually at the level of both lymphokine production and macrophage activation, they may be particularly efficient at suppressing cell-mediated immune responses.

tory cytokines produced by Th2 cells can also be derived from non-T cells (Table 1). For example, IL-10, an important downregulatory cytokine originally thought to be synthesized exclusively by Th2 lymphocytes, is now known to be produced in high levels by macrophages and B cells as well (Moore et al., 1993). A further complexity is that some of the cytokines with downregulatory activity can, under different settings, upregulate cell-mediated immunity, and vice versa. Thus, IL-4, which is a powerful deactivator of IFN-γ–activated macrophages, can itself under certain circumstances function as a macrophage activator (Crawford et al., 1987).

TABLE 1. Cytokines That Regulate Cell-Mediated Immunity

Activity	Name	Major cellular sources	Principle mechanisms of action
Upregulatory	IFN-γ	Th1, CD8⁺ T cells, NK cells	Activates effector cell microbicidal functions; limits proliferation of Th2 cells
	IL-2	Th1, CD8⁺ T cells, B cells(?)	T-cell growth factor
	TNF-α	T cells, macrophages	Costimulus for macrophage and NK cell activation
	IL-2	Macrophages, B cells, neutrophils	Stimulates differentiation of Th1 and CD8⁺ cells, NK cell IFN-γ production
Downregulatory	IL-4	Th2 cells, mast cells, basophils	Promotes Th2 differentiation; inhibits macrophage activation
	IL-10	Th2 cells, B cells, macrophages, mast cells	Inhibits IFN-γ production from T and NK cells; blocks monokine synthesis, macrophage effector function
	TGF-β	Many cell types	Inhibits lymphocyte proliferation, monokine synthesis, macrophage and NK cell effector function
	IL-13	Th2 cells, others(?)	Inhibits monokine synthesis, activation of bone marrow–derived macrophages

While the induction of cell-mediated immunity is still thought to be largely the domain of the Th1-derived cytokines, an important new, non-T-cell–derived cytokine has recently been characterized that is a potent upregulator of the entire process. This cytokine, IL-12, produced by macrophages (and probably B cells and neutrophils), promotes the expansion of both Th1 CD4⁺ and CD8⁺ cells and the induction of IFN-γ synthesis from natural killer (NK) cells. It thus is even more potent than IFN-γ itself in inducing host resistance (Scott, 1993). The induction of IL-12 is likely to be a major mechanism by which parasites upregulate cell-mediated responses against themselves (see below). In the following sections, I present two examples from studies on murine experimental models of how parasites manipulate host cytokine responses, albeit in different directions, to their own advantage.

SCHISTOSOMA MANSONI: A MODEL DOWNREGULATORY PARASITE

Schistosomes are blood-dwelling helminths that produce chronic infections often lasting decades. Clearly, it is in this parasite's interest to downregulate cell-mediated immunity, particularly since in vitro studies have shown that this parasite can be highly susceptible to damage by cytokine-activated macrophages and endothelial cells (James and Nacy, 1993). Indeed, early immunologic studies documented suppressed lymphocyte proliferative responses to parasite antigens in chronically infected humans as well as mice.

The discovery of CD4⁺ subsets and regulatory cytokines has provided a new basis by which to analyze the phenomenon of downmodulation in schistosomiasis. Schistosomes, like other helminths, induce strong Th2 cytokine responses to both parasite antigens and mitogen. The major stimulus for this response is the schistosome egg (Fig. 2), and studies in the mouse model have shown that the deposition of eggs during infection results in a switch from a predominantly Th1 cytokine pattern to a Th2 pattern (see Pearce, this volume). Importantly, Th1 cytokine responses to parasite antigens, mitogen, and foreign antigens (myoglobin, vaccinia virus) become downregulated during this phase (Sher et al., 1992). Thus, the switch from a Th1 to a Th2 response seen during schistosome infection appears, in its broad outlines, to be a manifestation of cytokine cross-regulation.

The major cytokine implicated in the downregulation of Th1 responses in murine schistosome infection is IL-10 (Sher et al., 1992). Produced by CD4⁺ cells in response to antigenic stimulation at the same time during infection when IFN-γ and IL-2 responses are downmodulated, IL-10 has also recently been shown to be produced by B cells and macrophages obtained from the same animals (D. Harn, M. Stadecker, personal communications). More importantly, neutralization of IL-10 causes an upregulation of splenic Th1 responses in vitro, removing most of the observed suppression (Sher et al., 1992).

In addition to inhibiting the production of IFN-γ and IL-2 by CD4⁺ cells, IL-10 could also downregulate cell-mediated immunity at the level of mac-

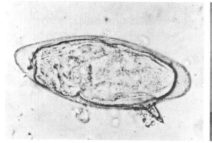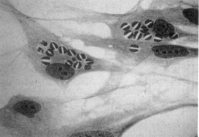

Fig. 2.   Examples of downregulatory and upregulatory parasites studied by our group. Schistosome eggs (left) induce cytokines that suppress cell-mediated immunity, whereas tachyzoites of *T. gondii* (shown during intracellular growth within fibroblasts, right) promote the development of this protective response.

rophage effector cells (Fig. 1). Thus, IL-10 has been shown to block the activation of macrophages for killing of schistosomula in vitro by suppressing the production of NO (Oswald et al., 1992). Moreover, this inhibition is dramatically enhanced when IL-10 is combined with small amounts of IL-4 or TGF-β, two other downregulatory cytokines produced during patent schistosome infection (James and Nacy, 1993; Sher et al., 1992). The end result of IL-10 production is therefore a dual inhibition in the production of macrophage-activating cytokines and the ability of these cytokines to activate macrophages (Fig. 1).

While the concept that IL-10 is the central downmodulator of cellular responses in schistosomiasis is attractive and the evidence compelling, we still have not formally shown that the production of this downregulatory cytokine promotes parasite survival. Studies in genetically engineered IL-10 knockout mice offer the best approach and are now in progress. A major implication of this hypothesis is that helminth-induced Th2 responses serve to protect worms from the immune response. This is seemingly in contradiction to the protective role postulated for Th2-controlled immune responses (IgE, eosinophilia, mastocytosis) in both human schistosomiasis (Capron, 1992) and other murine worm infections (Urban et al., 1992). Nevertheless, regardless of whether these Th2-dependent phenomena play a role in protecting the host against superinfection (concomitant immunity), the simultaneous downregulation of cell-mediated immunity by the same cytokines would be of definite advantage to the parasite.

TOXOPLASMA GONDII: AN UPREGULATORY PARASITE

In common with *S. mansoni, Toxoplasma gondii* needs to persist in its hosts long enough to ensure maintenance of transmission; however, *T. gondii* in its intermediate hosts (e.g., rodents, birds, humans) has adopted a different biological strategy for persistence (Frenkel, 1988; Gazzinelli et al., 1993a). Because of the high virulence of the replicative tachzoite stage (Fig. 2) and its ability to promiscuously infect a wide range of nucleated host cells, *T. gondii* has decided to utilize host cell-mediated immunity to control its own numbers, thereby ensuring host survival. This response leads to encystment of the parasite in tissues and to a state of dormancy in which the parasite is waiting for the intermediate host to be eaten by the definitive host, the cat (a somewhat misguided strategy, when the intermediate host is a human!). Human AIDS provides an unfortunate but striking testimony to the importance of host cell-mediated immunity in maintaining the normal biology of toxoplasma infection. In a large proportion of patients doubly infected with HIV and *T. gondii*, the progressive loss in T-cell function leads to uncontrolled cyst rupture and an acute infection that, if left untreated, causes a fatal encephalitis (Frenkel, 1988; Luft and Remington, 1993).

Infection with *T. gondii* offers a superb example of cytokine-dependent host resistance. As originally demonstrated by Jack Remington and his colleagues, depletion of IFN-γ with neutralizing monoclonal antibodies in mice leads to uncontrolled acute infection and results in reactivation of dormant (cyst stage) infection when given chronically. TNF-α has also recently been shown to play a major role in resistance against *Toxoplasma*. This dual requirement for IFN-γ and TNF-α is consistent with the concept that activated macrophages are the key effectors of immunity, since these cytokines can function to prime and trigger macrophage function (Fig. 2). Also consistent with this hypothesis is the observation that mice infected with *T. gondii* show nonspecific resistance to a variety of other pathogens known to be susceptible to cell-mediated immunity (Gazzinelli et al., 1993a).

In hosts with established immunity against *Toxoplasma*, both CD8⁺ and CD4⁺ T cells contribute the IFN-γ involved in resistance, with CD8⁺ cells often playing the dominant role (Gazzinelli et al., 1993a). Recently, NK cells were implicated as an alternative source of this cytokine. Thus, in β_2-microglobulin "knockout mice," which fail to make CD8⁺ lymphocytes, NK cells become the major effectors of IFN-γ-dependent immunity against *T. gondii* after vaccination (Denkers et al., 1993). Moreover, the parasite, in the absence of T cells, is able to stimulate NK cells in vitro to produce the cytokine by means of a reaction requiring macrophage accessory cells (Sher et al., 1993). In this pathway, *T. gondii* products stimulate the macrophage to secrete both TNF-α and IL-12, which act synergistically in stimulating NK cells to synthesize IFN-γ (Fig. 1) (Gazzinelli et al., 1993b). As discussed below, this ability of the parasite to stimulate IL-12 production is likely to be an important factor in its upregulation of the entire cell-mediated response.

PARASITE-INDUCED IL-12 AS THE INITIATOR OF THE CELL-MEDIATED RESPONSE

In addition to its role in triggering IFN-γ synthesis by NK cells, IL-12 has recently been shown to influence the development of IFN-γ–producing Th1 cells both directly and indirectly through the action of NK cell-derived IFN-γ (Scott, 1993). The potent regulatory effect of IL-12 in initiating cell-mediated immunity against parasites is evidenced by recent experiments in which rIL-12 administered during the first few days of infection was able to alter the course of murine infection with *L. major*, causing otherwise susceptible BALB/c mice to develop a Th1 response that heals their infections (Heinzel et al., 1993; Sypek et al., 1993). Conversely, anti-IL-12 has been shown to make resistant mice more susceptible to infection with *L. major* (Sypek et al., 1993), *T. gondii*, and other intracellular pathogens (unpublished data from several groups). These findings indicate that the ability to stimulate IL-12 production early in infection may dictate the nature of the subsequent Th response.

What then are the parasite factors that determine whether IL-12 will be induced? Since macrophages appear to be the major source of this cytokine, the ability to infect cells of the macrophage lineage would appear to be an important factor in IL-12 production. Nevertheless, certain macrophage-dwelling parasites, including *Leishmania spp.* (Reiner et al., 1994), appear to be relatively poor IL-12 inducers. A more likely explanation, then, is that specific substances produced by pathogens direct IL-12 synthesis. An example of such a molecule is bacterial lipopolysaccharide (LPS), which stimulates macrophages to synthesize a number of monokines including IL-12. Nevertheless, it is clear that both *Listeria* and *Toxoplasma* stimulate IL-12 production by means of molecules distinct from LPS. In the case of *T. gondii*, these substances are heat-labile factors released by the parasite into culture fluid that can trigger macrophages in the absence of intracellular infection and independently of LPS receptors (Sher et al., 1993). What are these factors? What is the structural basis of their activity? Are they produced solely to upregulate cell-mediated immunity, or is this function secondary to some other, more important, biological purpose? We hope that ongoing structural work on *T. gondii* and other parasite-produced IL-12–inducing factors will provide answers to these fascinating questions, which seem to be central to an understanding of the regulation of cell-mediated immunity.

THE INITIATION OF Th2 RESPONSES BY PARASITES: THE REMAINING BLACK BOX

While we are beginning to have a clear picture of how certain intracellular parasites preferentially stimulate Th1 responses, the factors dictating the selection of Th2 responses by helminths and certain protozoa are still poorly understood. IL-4 has been shown to be required for the induction and maintenance of Th2 responses in vitro (Le Gros et al., 1990), and it is thus likely to be a major determinant of Th2 selection in vivo. Nevertheless, while we are reasonably certain that the initiation factors (IL-12, TNF-α, and others) for cell-mediated responses come from accessory cells (macrophages in particular), IL-4 is not known to be produced by any conventional antigen-processing cell. Nevertheless, there are other non-B-cell, non-T-cell, nonmacrophage-monocyte sources of this cytokine. For example, there is an as yet poorly defined population of Fcϵ receptor-positive cells in spleens of mice that can be triggered by interactions with the receptor to secrete high quantities of IL-4 (Paul et al., 1993). Interestingly, these cells increase in number during helminth infection (Williams et al., 1993); however, during a normal immune response, stimulation of the Fcϵ receptor positive cells would have to occur by binding of antigen to specific IgE molecules occupying the receptors and thus would require prior immune recognition. Thus far, attempts to define other nonsensitized cells that are nonspecifically triggered by helminths or allergens to produce IL-4 have been unsuccessful. One possibility is that naive CD4$^+$ cells themselves may be directly induced to produce IL-4 in response to exposure to these stimuli (Scott et al., 1990).

CONCLUDING REMARKS: LESSONS ON IMMUNOMODULATION FROM THE STUDY OF HOST–PARASITE INTERACTIONS

The current intellectual excitement over the analysis of mechanisms by which different host–parasite encounters trigger different and often polar T-cell responses is well deserved and presents a major new experimental approach for elucidating the fundamentals of T-subset selection. Moreover, the knowledge gained from these studies could have important practical implications for immune intervention in parasitic disease as well as other immunologically based disorders. As discussed below, the current "frenzy" of research on the immunobiology of IL-12 presents some fascinating examples of the potential of this technology.

As noted above, schistosome eggs induce strong Th2 responses that appear to play an important role in granuloma formation—the major pathological lesion of the disease schistosomiasis. Thus, neutralization of IL-4 has been shown to ablate granuloma formation in the lungs, while antibody-mediated depletion of IFN-γ, the major cytokine cross-regulating IL-4, has been shown to have an opposing, enhancing effect on this process (Wynn et al., 1993, 1994). These findings suggest that IFN-γ may have a downregulatory effect on schistosome pathology. If so, IL-12, through its promotion of IFN-γ production by NK and T cells, should suppress egg granuloma formation, and indeed our recent findings indicate that rIL-12 causes a dramatic reduction in granuloma size associated with the conversion of the egg-specific cytokine response from Th2 to Th1. Thus, IL-12 could potentially be used to alleviate diseases dependent on Th2 responses. Even more important than helminth-induced pathology in this context is allergic disease, and recent studies (see Finkelman et al., this volume) indicate that IL-12 can cause a marked suppression of serum IgE antibodies and eosinophils induced by nematode infection. These exciting findings suggest that IL-12 could be used clinically in the treatment of atopic individuals, and studies by a number of groups have been initiated to test this hypothesis.

More obvious is the potential use of IL-12 in the upregulation of cell-mediated immunity. As noted above, injected IL-12 causes *Leishmania* infections to heal in normally susceptible BALB/c mice, and this resistance is associated with a shift from a Th2 to Th1 response (Heinzel et al., 1993; Sypek et al., 1993). Recently, Scott and colleagues (Afonso et al., 1993) have used IL-12 as an immunomodulator in vaccination against this parasite. By combining the cytokine with parasite antigen, they have converted the normally nonprotective subcutaneous vaccination route into a highly protective regimen. As mentioned, IL-12 can induce the production of IFN-γ by NK cells as well as by T cells, and this property suggested to us that IL-12 might be used to induce cell-mediated immunity in T-deficient hosts. Indeed, when injected with the cytokine, *T. gondii*–infected SCID mice (which lack both B and T lymphocytes) were able to control their infections partially. The resistance induced by this treatment was shown to depend on both NK cells and IFN-γ and, thus, is likely to be due to the induction of IFN-γ secretion from that non-T-cell source (Gazzinelli et al., 1993b). The latter observation suggests that IL-12 might be used to control opportunistic infections (such as that caused by *T. gondii*) in AIDS patients or other immunocompromised individuals.

Clearly, the study of how parasites interact with and regulate the host cytokine network has already provided fundamental insights into the immune response and is contributing to the development of strategies for immunologic intervention in human disease. Moreover, the investigation of cytokine regulation in host–parasite systems should also be of basic interest to parasitologists concerned with host adaptation. Indeed, it is tempting to predict that the elucidation of the mechanisms and molecules developed by protozoa and helminths to control immune responses will become a major topic in the biology of parasitism in coming years.

ACKNOWLEDGMENTS

I am grateful to my colleagues at the NIH, both present (R. Gazzinelli, I. Oswald, E. Denkers, T. Wynn, M. Williams, I. Eltoum, J. Actor, R. Seder, W. Paul, J. Berzofsky, A. Cheever, and S. James) and past (E. Pearce, P. Scott, M. Kullberg) for their major contributions to the concepts discussed in this chapter.

REFERENCES

Afonso LCC, Scharton TM, Vieira LQ, Wysocka M, Trinchieri G, Scott P (1993): The adjuvant effect of interleukin 12 in a vaccine against *Leishmania major*. Science 263:235–237.

Capron AR (1992): Immunity to schistosomes. Curr Opin Immunol 4:419–424.

Crawford F, Finbloom D, Ohara J, Paul W, Meltzer MS (1987): B cell stimulatory factor 1 (interleukin-4) activates macrophages for increased tumoricidal activity and expression of Ia antigens. J Immunol 139:135–141.

Denkers E, Gazzinelli RT, Martin D, Sher A (1993): Emergence of NK1.1[+] cells as effectors of IFN-γ–dependent immunity to *Toxoplasma gondii* in class I–deficient mice. J Exp Med 178:1465–1472.

Frenkel JK (1988): Pathophysiology of toxoplasmosis. Parasitol Today 4:273–278.

Gazzinelli RT, Denkers E, Sher A (1993a): Host resistance to *Toxoplasma gondii*: A model for studying the selective induction of cell-mediated immunity by intracellular parasites. Infect Agents Dis 2:139–150.

Gazzinelli RT, Hieny S, Wynn TA, Wolf S, Sher A (1993b): Interleukin 12 is required for the T-lymphocyte–independent induction of interferon γ by an intracellular parasite and induces resistance in T-cell–deficient hosts. Proc Natl Acad Sci USA 90:6115–6119.

Heinzel FP, Schoenhaut DS, Rerko RM, Rosser LE, Gately MK (1993): Recombinant interleukin 12 cures mice infected with *Leishmania major*. J Exp Med 177:1505–1509.

James SL, Nacy C (1993): Effector functions of activated macrophages against parasites. Curr Opin Immunol 5:518–523.

James SL, Scott P (1988): Induction of cell-mediated immunity as a strategy for vaccination against parasites. In P.T. Englund and A. Sher (eds): The Biology of Parasitism. New York: Alan R. Liss, pp. 249–264.

Khalife J, Capron M, Capron A, Grzych JM, Butterworth AE, Dunne DW, Ouma JH (1986): Immunity in human schistosomiasis mansoni: Regulation of protective immune mechanisms by IgM blocking antibodies. J Exp Med 164:1626–1640.

Le Gros G, Ben-Sasson SZ, Seder R, Finkelman FD, Paul WE (1990): Generation of interleukin 4 (IL-4)–producing cells in vivo and in vitro: IL-2 and IL-4 are required for in vitro generation of IL-4–producing cells. J Exp Med 172:921–929.

Luft BJ, Remington JR (1993): Toxoplasmic encephalitis in AIDS. Clin Infect Dis 15:211–222.

Moore KW, O'Garra A, de Waal Malefyt R, Vieira P, Mosmann TR (1993): Interleukin-10. Annu Rev Immunol 11:165–190.

Mosmann TR, Coffman RL (1989): TH1 and TH2 cells: Different patterns of lymphokine secretion lead to different functional properties. Ann Rev Immunol 7:145–173.

Oswald IP, Wynn TA, Sher A, James SL (1992): Interleukin-10 inhibits macrophage microbicidal activity by blocking the endogenous production of TNF-α required as a costimulatory factor for IFN-γ-induced activation. Proc Natl Acad Sci USA 89:8676–8680.

Paul WE, Seder RA, Plaut M (1993): Lymphokine and cytokine production by FcåRI⁺ cells. Adv Immunol 53:1–29.

Porter R, Knight J (1974): Parasites in the Immunized Host: Mechanisms of Survival (Ciba Foundation Symposium #25). Amsterdam: Elsevier.

Reiner SL, Zheng S, Wang ZE, Stowring L, Locksley RM (1994): Leishmania promastigotes evade interleukin 12 (IL-12) induction by macrophages and stimulate a broad range of cytokines from CD4⁺ T cells during initiation of infection. J Exp Med 79:447–456.

Scott DE, Gause WC, Finkelman FD, Steinberg AD (1990): Anti-CD3 antibody induces rapid expression of cytokine genes in vivo. J Immunol 145:2183–2188.

Scott P (1993): IL-12: Initiation cytokine for cell-mediated immunity [comment]. Science 260:496–497.

Sher A, Coffman RL (1992): Regulation of immunity to parasites by T cells and T cell–derived cytokines. Annu Rev Immunol 10:385–409.

Sher A, Gazzinelli RT, Oswald IP, Clerici M, Kullberg M, Pearce EJ, Berzofsky JA, Mosmann TR, James SL, Morse HC (1992): Role of T-cell derived cytokines in the downregulation of immune responses in parasitic and retroviral infection. Immunol Rev 127:183–204.

Sher A, Oswald IP, Hieny S, Gazzinelli RT (1993): Toxoplasma gondii induces a T-independent IFN-γ response in natural killer cells that requires both adherent accessory cells and tumor necrosis factor-α. J Immunol 150:3982–3989.

Sypek JP, Chung CL, Mayor SE, Subramanyam JM, Goldman SJ, Sieburth DS, Wolf SF, Schaub RG (1993): Resolution of cutaneous leishmaniasis: Interleukin 12 initiates a protective T helper type 1 immune response. J Exp Med 177:1797–1802.

Urban JF Jr, Madden KB, Svetic A, Cheever A, Trotta PP, Gause WC, Katona IM, Finkelman FD (1992): The importance of Th2 cytokines in protective immunity to nematodes. Immunol Rev 127:205–220.

Williams ME, Kullberg MC, Barbieri S, Caspar P, Berzofsky JA, Seder R, Sher A (1993): Fcå receptor-positive cells are a major source of antigen induced interleukin-4 in spleens of mice infected with Schistosoma mansoni.. Eur J Immunol 23:1910–1916.

Wynn T, Eltoum I, Cheever AW, Lewis FA, Gause WC, Sher A (1993): Analysis of cytokine mRNA expression during primary granuloma formation induced by eggs of Schistosoma mansoni. J Immunol 151:1430–1440.

Wynn TA, Eltoum I, Oswald IP, Cheever AW, Sher A (1994): Endogenous interleukin 12 (IL-12) regulates granuloma formation induced by eggs of Schistosoma mansoni and exogenous IL-12 both inhibits and prophylactically immunizes against egg pathology. J Exp Med 179:1551–1559.

Molecular Approaches to Parasitology, pages 443–453
© 1995 Wiley-Liss, Inc.

Cytokine Control of the Macrophage Parasites *Leishmania* and *Trypanosoma cruzi*

S. G. Reed

Infectious Disease Research Institute, Seattle, Washington 98109

INTRODUCTION

Macrophage pathogens use a variety of mechanisms to escape destruction by potentially inhospitable host cells. Among these are exiting of the host cell phagolysosome, as *Trypanosoma cruzi* is capable of doing, or inhibiting phagolysosome formation, as in the case of *Toxoplasma gondii*. *Leishmania* appear to use chemical means to resist destruction while replicating within a phagolysosome. In spite of these elaborate escape mechanisms, which are only beginning to be understood, macrophages activated by cytokines are able to kill each of these parasites. Thus, as discussed in the chapter by Reiner and Locksley, T-cell products such as interferon-γ (IFN-γ), granulocyte macrophage colony-stimulating factor (GM-CSF), and tumor necrosis factor-α (TNF-α) may stimulate potent macrophage killing mechanisms, resulting in the complete or partial elimination of intracellular parasites. However, other cytokines are able to antagonize the macrophage activation processes, and these must also be considered in the evaluation of host responses to infection. Cytokines that inhibit macrophage activation, including transforming growth factor-β (TGF-β), interleukin (IL)-10, and IL-4, are important and perhaps essential for the survival of certain intracellular protozoan parasites in mammalian hosts. The regulation of these cytokines thus provides another level at which parasites may confound the immune system to promote their own intracellular survival. Furthermore, neutralization of these cytokines may be an effective therapeutic approach for certain of these pathogens. As another approach, cytokines associated with healing responses, IFN-γ and IL-12, have proven effective in both clinical and experimental treatment of protozoan parasites. Thus, important questions regarding protozoal pathogenicity include delineating mechanisms by which macrophage-activating and -inactivating cytokines are regulated by pathogens.

THE DISEASES

Leishmanial infections are worldwide in distribution, occurring in Africa, North and South America, Europe, and Asia. The clinical manifestations of the leishmaniases are varied and include visceral, cutaneous, diffuse cutaneous, and mucosal diseases. Classic visceral leishmaniasis is characterized by fever, hepatosplenomegaly, pancytopenia, and hypergammaglobulinemia and is complicated by serious infections and internal bleeding. Mortality rates are 5%–7% in visceral leishmaniasis patients who are provided standard therapy, but may reach 30% during epidemic conditions such as in Sudan, where as many as 40,000 people have recently died.

American cutaneous leishmaniasis is characterized by ulcerated lesions at the site of primary inoculation of one of several *Leishmania* species by the sandfly. There are an estimated 15–20 million cases of cutaneous leishmaniasis worldwide. Mucosal leishmaniasis is a late sequela, occurring in 1%–3% of patients with cutaneous disease. It is characterized by granulomatous lesions of the nasal septum, with occasional involvement of adjacent structures (pharynx, palate, larynx, lips). Mucosal disease is chronic, difficult to treat, often disfiguring, and fatal if the upper airway is compromised. Diffuse cutaneous leishmaniasis is characterized by multiple chronic nodular skin lesions containing many parasites and by anergy to *Leishmania* antigens. It is often refractory to therapy.

T. cruzi is a hemoflagellate protozoan parasite of humans and other mammals, primarily in Latin America. An estimated 18 million persons are infected with this parasite, and an estimated 95 million are at risk of infection. It is the leading cause of infectious heart disease in Latin America. The course of infection is varied and complex, as a result of multiple aspects of the host immune responses to antigens of *T. cruzi*, as well as genetic characteristics of both host and parasite. Human *T. cruzi* infection occurs as a result of reduviid insect vector transmission, congenital transmission, or blood transfusion. In Brazil, blood transfusion exceeds vector transmission in importance and is now responsible for the majority of new infections. In other countries, such as Bolivia, Ecuador, and Argentina, thousands of new cases occur each year by both routes, and acute Chagas' disease is relatively common.

Both *Leishmania* and *T. cruzi* infections continue to be serious threats to major populations, largely because of the lack of effective vaccines and nontoxic therapeutic agents. However, understanding the nature of infections caused by these parasites has benefited from recent advances in cytokine biology. Several important aspects of the molecular basis of the immune responses responsible for either survival or destruction of these protozoa in macrophages have recently been delineated.

CYTOKINE CONTROL OF *LEISHMANIA* AND *T. CRUZI* INFECTIONS

Leishmania and *T. cruzi* are protozoan parasites that replicate within mammalian macrophages. In the case of *Leishmania*, the macrophages are the exclusive host cell, while *T. cruzi* replicates within virtually any nucleated cell type. Macrophages produce and respond to a variety of cytokines. Several of these potent biological mediators have now been shown to control closely the course of infection with macrophage pathogens. The separation of CD4$^+$ T cells into subsets based on cytokine profiles has been essential for the characterization of response patterns during infectious diseases. Th1 cells produce IFN-γ, TNF-α, IL-2, and GM-CSF and are involved in cell-mediated immunity, while Th2 cells produce IL-4, IL-5, IL-10, and relatively less GM-CSF. A macrophage cytokine, IL-12, also has important regulatory influence on Th1/Th2 development. Another cytokine, TGF-β, produced by macrophages and a variety of other cell types, has diverse effects, which include downregulation of immune responses. During infections with intramacrophage protozoal pathogens several cytokines are now known to be associated with disease, while others are strongly linked to healing (Reed and Scott, 1993). The disease-promoting cytokines include TGF-β, IL-10, and IL-4; the healing-associated cytokines include IFN-γ, GM-CSF, and IL-12.

We began studies of cytokine therapy of parasitic infections before recombinant cytokines were available. An early success in treating a parasitic infection with cytokines was our report of using liposome-encapsulated cytokines from activated spleen cells to treat visceral leishmaniasis in mice (Reed et al., 1984). The studies were later repeated using liposome-encapsulated IFN-γ, with identical results (Reed, 1988a). Even more dramatic results were obtained using rIFN-γ to treat experimental *T. cruzi* infections (Reed, 1988b). IFN-γ cured mice of an otherwise fatal infection and prevented the immune depression that accompanied untreated infections. This observation led to the first use of IFN-γ to treat human *T. cruzi* infection (Grant et al., 1989). More recently, we treated *T. cruzi*–infected mice with liposome-encapsulated IFN-γ. A 10-fold reduction in the amount of IFN-γ needed to cure mice of acute infections was achieved with the use of encapsulated IFN-γ. We later established a role for endogenous IFN-γ in the control of *T. cruzi* infection by demonstrating that neutralizing anti-IFN-γ mAb could make genetically resistant mice susceptible to acute infection (Silva et al., 1992). In these animals, a nonlethal infection became lethal in the presence if neutralizing anti-IFN-γ. Similar results have been obtained by others in genetically resistant mice infected with *Leishmania*. Other studies have focused on the use of colony-stimulating factors to treat *Leishmania* or *T. cruzi* infections in vitro.

We reported that GM-CSF was an effective inhibitor of *T. cruzi* in both mouse and human macrophages and that GM-CSF, M-CSF, and IL-3 induced the inhibition of *Leishmania* in human monocytes and macrophages (Ho et al., 1990, 1992). Thus, Th1 cytokines are effective at limiting parasite replication in macrophages and appear to mediate in vivo resistance as well.

Although macrophage activators, particularly IFN-γ, can effectively treat *T. cruzi* infections in vitro and in vivo, treating *Leishmania* infections with macrophage activators has proven more difficult. IFN-γ and GM-CSF are effective in vitro, and limited therapeutic success has been achieved in vivo in experimental visceral leishmaniasis. However, in experimental cutaneous leishmaniasis, treatment with IFN-γ has not been successful. This failure may be due in part to the high level of macrophage-inactivating cytokines produced during infection. These include TGF-β, IL-10, and IL-4, all of which are capable of blocking the effects of macrophage activators.

Extensive reviews on Th1 and Th2 cytokines and their roles in infection have been published. Relatively less is known about the roles of TGF-β in infectious diseases or immune regulation, so this growth factor/cytokine will be discussed in more detail. TGF-β represents a family of related polypeptides that regulates the growth and differentiation of a variety of cell types. Members of this family include TGF-β types 1–5. TGF-β1 is a disulfide-linked homodimer containing two identical 112 amino acid subunits. This potent modulator of cell behavior is synthesized by several types of normal and transformed cells in culture and has been purified from various tissues. Placenta, kidney, blood platelets, and bone are particularly enriched in TGF-β. TGF-β was first characterized functionally for its effects on cell replication. It may be stimulatory or inhibitory depending on the cell type targeted. In the last decade, pleiotropic effects of TGF-β have been demonstrated. It stimulates bone formation, induces muscle cells to produce cartilage-specific extracellular matrix molecules, and inhibits growth of early hematopoietic progenitor cells, endothelial cells, and many human cancer cell lines.

TGF-β exhibits potent downregulatory effects on the immune system. Macrophages, B cells, and T cells all synthesize and release TGF-β. Among the inhibitory effects of TGF-β on immune function are to decrease IL-2 receptor induction, IFN-γ–induced class II expression, IL-1–induced thymocyte proliferation, B-cell differentiation, and the production of cytotoxic and lymphokine activated killer cells. TGF-β also blocks IFN-γ or LPS-induced macrophage activation by decreasing both oxidative and nitrogen oxide mediated responses.

The biological effects of TGF-b are mediated by binding to multiple high-affinity cell surface receptors, some or all of which are present on different cell types. Three size classes of TGF-β receptors having molecular weights of 53–70 kD (type I receptor), 80–120 kD (type II receptor), and 250–350 kD (type III receptor) have been cloned and characterized. Sequence analysis of the type III receptor predicts an 853 amino acid protein containing a single *trans*-membrane domain, a 41 amino acid cytoplasmic domain with no apparent signaling motif, and a large extracellular domain. The type III binding molecule may function as a receptor companion molecule, presenting TGF-β to neighboring type I or II receptor clusters. Type I and type II receptors are glycoproteins and display signal transduction motifs. Sequence analysis of cDNA clones encoding the type II receptor predicts a 565 amino acid *trans*-membrane protein with a cytoplasmic serine/threonine kinase domain. A putative TGF-β type I receptor has recently been cloned from murine cells, and recent experiments demonstrate that both type I and II receptor interactions are required for signal transduction. Other potential TGF-β receptor molecules include a type IV receptor as well as a type V receptor, which exhibits TGF-β stimulated serinethreonine autophosphorylation activity. Other TGF-β–binding proteins include a 38 kD protein and endoglin, a protein on the surface of endothelial cells. In addition, the proteoglycan decorin binds to and antagonizes the effects of TGF-β in vivo. The complexity of the TGF-β receptor structures and signaling processes no doubt accounts for many of the pleiotropic and in some cases paradoxical effects exhibited by TGF-β, including its ability to modulate gene transcription.

TGF-β is synthesized and secreted in a biologically latent, high molecular weight form that cannot bind to TGF-β receptors. Analysis of cDNA clones encoding TGF-β indicate that the mature 112 amino acid chain of TGF-β is derived from the C terminus of a 390 amino acid prepro–TGF-β by proteolytic cleavage following a dibasic Arg-Arg sequence immediately preceding the N-terminal Ala residue of the mature growth factor. The precursor for TGF-β contains a typical hydrophobic signal peptide and three *N*-linked glycosylation sites. Latent TGF-β (LTGF-β) consists of a noncovalent complex in which the 24 kD (active TGF-β) homodimer is noncovalently associated with a dimer of the 95 kD precursor called the *latency-associated peptide* (LAP), which is bonded by disulfide linkage to a structurally distinct 135 kD binding protein.

The nature of the activation mechanism of LTGF-β is essentially unknown. LTGF-β can be activated in vitro by transient acidification (pH 2.0) or alkalization (pH 12.0), which disrupts the noncovalent interaction between activate TGF-β and LAP, releasing mature active TGF-β. Proteases such as plasmin have also been suggested to active LTGF-β, and there is evidence that cell–cell contact is also a requirement in cocultures of endothelial cells and pericytes. Retinoid-induced activation of LTGF-β by endothelial cells has been demonstrated to be dependent not only on enhanced plasmin levels but also on the expression of transglutaminase.

EFFECTS OF MACROPHAGE INACTIVATING CYTOKINE ON PARASITIC INFECTIONS

Because TGF-β is produced by macrophages and has potent inhibitory effects on macrophage function, it was a natural candidate for a molecule capable of promoting infection by intracellular parasites. Initial studies demonstrated that biologically active TGF-β was secreted by mouse spleen cells during *T. cruzi* infection (Silva et al., 1991). A role for TGF-β in the pathogenesis of *T. cruzi* infection was suggested by the observation that genetically resistant mice were made susceptible to acute infection by the administration of rTGF-β. At least one important mechanism by which TGF-β appears to be exacerbating infection with *T. cruzi* is by antagonizing macrophage activators, such as IFN-γ (Tsunawaki et al., 1988). It was demonstrated that TGF-β could effectively antagonize the effects of IFN-γ both in vitro and in vivo (Silva et al., 1991). These experiments demonstrated that, even in the presence of a protective IFN-γ response, the effects of such a response could be negated by TGF-β.

Because of the potent effects of TGF-β on macrophage function, we examined the role of this cytokine in the regulation of infection with *Leishmania*, a parasite that replicates exclusively in macrophages. We found that active TGF-β was produced by macrophages following in vitro or in vivo infection with *L. amazonensis*. As was the case in experimental *T. cruzi* infection, rTGF-β was capable of rendering a genetically resistant mouse strain susceptible to disease. In vitro, leishmanial killing by activated macrophages was inhibited by TGF-β (Barral-Netto et al., 1992). In a related study, we examined the effects of TGF-β on the course of *L. braziliensis* infection in mice. This parasite normally does not cause disease in mice. However, we demonstrated that this avirulent parasite was capable of causing disease in mice that were treated with rTGF-β. This study also demonstrated a correlation between the amount of TGF-β induced by a particular parasite strain and degree of virulence displayed in vivo. Of particular interest, administration of rTGF-β was capable of activating quiescent *L. braziliensis* infections, demonstrating that the parasite is able to infect mice, although causing mild or no disease, and that local TGF-β could activate the disease process. Finally, we demonstrated an increase in IL-10 production in draining lymph nodes of TGF-β–treated mice, demonstrating that TGF-β could convert a Th1 response to a Th2 response (Barral et al., 1993). Establishing a role for endogenous TGF-β production in the mediation of leishmaniasis was the observation that the development of a leishmanial lesion was inhibited by neutralizing anti-TGF-β mAb (Barral-Netto et al., 1992).

The production of biologically active TGF-β is a characteristic of both *Leishmania* and *T. cruzi* infections and is a potent mediator of intracellular survival of these organisms. Furthermore, TGF-β can influence the T-cell cytokine pattern developing during infection. These observations indicate that the induction of host cell–derived TGF-β may be an early event that influences the outcome of infection.

ACTIVATION OF TGF-β BY PROTOZOAN PARASITES

Mouse or human macrophages infected with *T. cruzi* produced high amounts of biologically active TGF-β. This was of considerable interest because the mechanisms of TGF-β activation in biological systems is not understood. We performed a series of experiments that demonstrated that a dominant *T. cruzi* enzyme, a cysteine protease, was capable of activating TGF-β. For these studies, we cultured CHO cells transfected with a mammalian TGF-β gene with [^{35}S]Met and Cys, labeling residues in both the latent and active regions. The labeled latent molecule was incubated with either native cysteine protease, purified on affinity columns, or recombinant cysteine protease, provided by James McKerrow. It was demonstrated that both native and recombinant cysteine proteases were able to cleave latent TGF-β with a resulting accumulation of a 25 kD product corresponding to active TGF-β. In addition, we demonstrated that specific inhibitors of the parasite cysteine protease blocked the enzyme activity, while other inhibitors did not.

To determine whether biologically active TGF-β was produced from the latent precursor following treatment with trypanosome cysteine protease, two approaches were used. In the first, we infected monolayers of the rTGF-β–expressing CHO cell line with *T. cruzi*. Infection of these cells led to a time-dependent increase in biologically active TGF-β. Nontransfected CHO cells infected with *T. cruzi* produced negligible amounts of TGF-β. This demonstrated an infection-associated activation of the latent rTGF-β. In the second approach, the addition of recombinant cysteine protease to recombinant latent TGF-β resulted in the production of biologically active TGF-β. The finding that parasite enzymes may actively regulate the processing of LTGF-β adds a new dimension to understanding how parasites may influence host immune responses. That they possess the ability to activate as well as to induce host TGF-β may indicate how important this cytokine is to parasite survival. Questions related to the mechanisms by which parasite enzymes act on TGF-β will be an area of considerable interest for future study.

REGULATION OF PROTOZOAN INFECTION BY INTERLEUKIN-10

Another potent macrophage inactivator is IL-10. This cytokine, originally named *cytokine synthesis inhibitory factor*, is produced by T cells, B cells, and macrophages. In addition to its ability to diminish IFN-γ production by T cells, IL-10 has been shown in several systems to block the effects of IFN-γ on macrophages. The ability to downregulate macrophage activation is perhaps the most important role of IL-10 in infectious diseases. We observed that susceptible, but not resistant, mice produced biologically active IL-10 following infection with *T. cruzi* (Silva et al., 1992). These studies have been expanded to determine the cell source of the IL-10 and the kinetics of IL-10 production in resistant and susceptible mice following infection. The key observations arising from these studies are that splenic and peritoneal macrophages, B cells, and T cells produce IL-10 following intraperitoneal infection with *T. cruzi*. IL-10 production is seen as early 48 hours following infection. Of particular interest was the finding that genetically susceptible mice not only produced higher levels of IL-10 during infection but also produced higher levels of IFN-γ than genetically resistant mice. This observation appears to contradict the demonstrated importance of IFN-γ in mediating resistance to *T. cruzi* infection. However, the intensity of IFN-c production may reflect the futile efforts of the host immune system to control infection, which cannot be accomplished because of the increased levels of TGF-β and IL-10 that acts to block IFN-γ effects.

One consequence of inhibiting macrophage function is the resulting effect on macrophage-dependent T-cell activation. For example, IL-10 inhibits T-cell activation, and recent data suggest that the inhibition of T-cell activation by IL-10 is mediated by the downregulating IL-12, an important cytokine in promoting Th1 responses. Of particular interest are the ability of IL-12 to antagonize the effects of IL-10 on T-cell activation and the cross-regulation between these cytokines. Similarly, TGF-β and IL-4 may promote Th2 development by inhibiting IL-12 and possibly other cytokines involved in Th1 development. Furthermore, IL-12 increases production of IFN-γ by natural killer cells, leading to decreased IL-10 production by macrophages as well as further increased production of IL-12 by macrophages. Thus the interaction of the key macrophage cytokines IL-12, IL-10, and TGF-β is critical for regulating intracellular pathogens and Th1/Th2 responses (Reed and Scott, 1993).

CYTOKINES AND CYTOKINE ANTAGONISTS AS THERAPEUTICS

In experimental *L. major* infections a dominant Th1 response is associated with healing while a predominant Th2 response is associated with disease progression. Of particular interest is the observation that a non-T-cell cytokine, IL-12, can promote the development of Th1 cells. IL-12 has recently been implicated in the resolution of leishmaniasis through mechanisms that initiate a Th1 response and protective immunity. Although it is not known what factors are responsible to drive Th1 or Th2 responses selectively, it is clear from in vitro and in vivo studies that cytokines can influence these patterns. In addition, both the form of an immunizing antigen and the antigen dose may influence the Th1/Th2 patterns that develop (Yang et al., 1993; Bretscher et al., 1992). A recent study has also demonstrated the importance of genetic factors in determining Th1 and Th2 response patterns.

Recent work has begun to elucidate the role of cytokines in the immune regulation of human leishmaniasis. Attempts to correlate Th1 cytokines with various clinical forms of leishmaniasis have suggested that IL-2 and IFN-γ are associated with a controlled infection or healing response in cutaneous leishmaniasis. A predominance of Th2 cytokine patterns has been noted in lesions of patients with diffuse cutaneous leishmaniasis. We have performed cytokine evaluations in patients with several forms of leishmaniasis to determine the possible roles of different cytokines on healing and pathogenesis. In visceral and cutaneous leishmaniasis, we have found an accumulation of mRNA for IL-10 and IL-4 in lesion sites, as well as in lymph node tissue (Ghalib et al., 1993). Of interest, IL-10 mRNA was increased in lymph nodes from patients with acute visceral leishmaniasis as compared to those from the same patients following therapy. Unexpectedly, however, IFN-γ mRNA was also abundant in acute patient tissues in spite of the inability of these individuals to control the infections. The coexpression of IFN-γ and IL-10 is similar to our observations in mice infected with *T. cruzi*. Again, it appears that the production of IL-10 and not the absence of IFN-γ is a more important factor in determining susceptibility to disease. Abundant mRNA for IFN-γ was present in both pre- and post-treatment lymphnodes. IL-4 mRNA was also found to be increased in most pretreatment, but not post-treatment, samples. Of the cytokines thus far examined, IL-10 was most clearly associated with pathology in visceral leishmaniasis.

In vitro studies further supported an important role for IL-10 in the regulation of T-cell responses in human leishmaniasis. Recombinant IL-10 completely blocked leishmania-driven proliferation of peripheral blood mononuclear cells (PBMC) from treated patients, and neutralizing anti-IL-10 mAb restored leishmania-driven responses in PBMC from acutely infected patients. Of particular interest, acute patient PBMC, traditionally believed to be nonresponsive to antigens of *Leishmania*, were found to produce IL-10 mRNA in specific response to the parasite. IL-10 is effective in blocking the intracellular killing of protozoa by macrophages and it is likely that this is an important consequence of increased IL-10 in visceral leishmaniasis.

Other studies have examined the association between TGF-β and human cutaneous leishmaniasis. We established that active TGF-β was produced by human monocytes infected with leishmania and that exogenous TGF-β added to human monocyte cultures exacerbated in vitro infection and blocked IFN-γ–induced parasite killing. Plasma from patients with cutaneous, diffuse cutaneous, or mucosal leishmaniasis all had elevated levels of active TGF-β as compared with endemic and nonendemic area controls. In vitro stimulation of cutaneous or mucosal leishmaniasis patient PBMC, but not normal PBMC, with leishmania lysate elicited the production of active TGF-β. In addition, TGF-β was detected in active cutaneous leishmaniasis lesions, but not in normal skin. These data indicate a regulatory role for TGF-β in human leishmaniasis. Further studies are underway to elucidate the roles of TGF-β in pathology and disease progression in human leishmaniasis.

Knowledge of the mechanisms of parasite survival in macrophages opens the possibility for several different strategic approaches for immunotherapy. The application of cytokine biology to infectious diseases has included the use of IFN-γ to treat a variety of parasitic infections in vitro. In addition, IFN-γ has been used in vivo to treat *T. cruzi*, leishmaniasis, and other infections in mice. These promising results have led to the clinical application of IFN-γ for the treatment of both cutaneous and visceral leishmaniasis (Badaro et al., 1990, 1993a). IFN-γ, in combination with antimony, has also been used to treat refractory diffuse cutaneous leishmaniasis (Badaro and Johnson, 1993). The results to date have indicated that IFN-γ can significantly improve standard antimonial therapy. IFN-γ has also been used to treat human *T. cruzi* infection, although no trials have been performed. GM-CSF has also been used effectively to inhibit both *Leishmania* and *T. cruzi* in human macrophage cultures. More recently, GM-CSF has been implicated as a potent stimulator of Th1 responses. For these and other reasons, GM-CSF has begun to be used as a therapeutic agent for visceral leishmaniasis. We have recently completed a study demonstrating that GM-CSF, in combination with antimony, improved the therapeutic results over those seen with antimony alone (Badaro et al., 1993b).

Although cytokine therapies appear to have promise, abundant evidence from both human and animal studies has indicated the importance of cytokines that inhibit macrophage function and/or Th1 development in disease progression. Cytokine antagonists, used alone or in combination with cytokines or chemotherapeutics, may represent the ideal approach for the treatment of parasitic infections. The categories of antagonists include anticytokine or cytokine receptor antibodies, soluble cytokine receptors, mutant cytokines, and peptides that may compete for receptor binding. Another approach, based on our findings of TGF-β activation by a parasite enzyme, may be to block protease activity, thus reducing the amounts of active TGF-β. Indeed, such inhibitors have shown some promise in limiting *T. cruzi* replication in vitro.

CONCLUSION

The delineation of cytokine responses during parasitic infections and the availability of recombinant cytokines and cytokine antagonists have opened exciting new possibilities for the treatment of these diseases. Parasite infection models have contributed significantly to the understanding of cytokine regulation, and this understanding can now be applied to developing improved therapeutics for patients who have benefited little from modern technologies. New therapeutic strategies based on blocking these cytokines may now be investigated.

REFERENCES

Badaro R, Carvalho SJ, Badaro F, Nascimento C, Sobel J, Saito Y, Johnson, Jr., WD, Jones TC (1993a): Cytokines in the management of leishmaniasis. In R. van Furth (ed): Hemopoietic Growth Factor and Mononuclear Phagocytes. pp. 111–112.

Badaro R, Falcoff E, Badaro FS, Carvalho EM, Pedral-Sampaio D, Barral A, Carvalho JS, Barral-Netto M, Brandely M, Silva L, Bina JC, Teixeira R, Falcoff R, Rocha H, Ho JL, Johnson WD,Jr. (1990): Treatment of visceral leishmaniasis with pentavalent antimony and interferon gamma. N Engl J Med 322:16–21.

Badaro R, Johnson, Jr., WD (1993): The role of g-IFN in the treatment of visceral and diffuse cutaneous leishmaniasis. J Infect Dis Suppl. 1:513–517.

Badaro R, Nascimento C, Carvalho JS, Badaro F, Russo D, Ho JL, Reed SG, Johnson, Jr., WD, Jones TC (1993b): Recombinant human granulocyte-macrophage colony-stimulating factor reverses neutropenia and reduces secondary infections in visceral leishmaniasis. J Infect Dis 170:413–418.

Barral A, Barral-Netto M, Yong EC, Brownell CE, Twardzik DR, Reed SG (1993): Transforming growth factor-b as a virulence mechanism for *Leishmania braziliensis*. Proc Nat Acad Sci USA 90:3442–3446.

Barral-Netto M, Barral A, Brownell CE, Skeiky YAW, Ellingsworth LR, Twardzik DR, Reed SG (1992): Transforming growth factor-b in *Leishmania* infection: An important parasite escape mechanism. Science 257:545–548.

Bretscher PA, Wei G, Menon JN, Bielefeldt-Ohmann H (1992): Establishment of stable, cell-mediated immunity that makes "susceptible" mice resistant to *Leishmania major*. Science 257:539–542.

Ghalib HG, Piuvezam MR, Skeiky YAW, Siddig M, Hashim FA, El-Hassan AM, Russo DM, Reed SG (1993): Interleukin 10 production correlates with pathology in human *Leishmania donovani* infections. J Clin Invest 92:324–329.

Grant IH, Gold JVW, Wittner M, et al. (1989): Transfusion associated acute Chagas' disease acquired in the United States. Ann Intern Med 111:849–51.

Ho JL, Reed SG, Sobel J, Arruda S, He SH, Wick EA, Grabstein KH (1992): Interleukin-3 induces antimicrobial activity against *Leishmania amazonensis* and *Trypanosoma cruzi* and tumoricidal activity in human peripheral blood-derived macrophages. Infect Immun 60:1984–1993.

Ho JL, Reed SG, Wick EA, Giordano M (1990): Granulocyte-macrophage and macrophage colony-stimulating factors augment the intracellular killing of *Leishmania mexicana amazonensis*. J Inf Dis 162:224–230.

Reed SG (1988): Liposome encapsulated lymphokine for the treatment of experimental visceral leishmaniasis. In G Gregoriadis (ed): Liposomes as Drug Carriers. London: J. Wiley and Sons, pp. 337–44.

Reed SG (1988): In vivo administration of recombinant interferon-gamma induces macrophage activation, and prevents acute disease, immune suppression, and death in experimental *Trypanosoma cruzi* infection. J Immunol 140:4342–4347.

Reed SG, Barral-Netto M, Inverso JA (1984): Treatment of experimental visceral leishmaniasis with lymphokine encapsulated in liposomes. J Immunol 132:3116–3119.

Reed SG, Scott P (1993): T cell and cytokine responses in leishmaniasis. Cur Opin Immunol 5:524–531.

Silva JS, Morrissey PJ, Grabstein KH, Mohler KM, Anderson D, Reed SG (1992): IL-10 and regulation of experimental *Trypanosoma cruzi* infections. J Exp Med 175:169–174.

Silva JS, Twardzik DR, Reed SG (1991): Regulation of *Trypanosoma cruzi* infections in vitro and in vivo by transforming growth factor-beta (TGF-b). J Exp Med 174:539.

Tsunawaki S, Sporn M, Ding A, Nathan C (1988): Deactivation of macrophage by transforming growth factor-b. Nature 334:260.

Yang X, Gieni RS, Mosmann TR, HayGlass KT (1993): Chemically modified antigen preferentially elicits induction of Th1-like cytokine synthesis patterns in vivo. J Exp Med 178:349–353.

Molecular Approaches to Parasitology, pages 455–466
© 1995 Wiley-Liss, Inc.

Murine Leishmaniasis and the Regulation of CD4$^+$ Cell Development

Richard M. Locksley and Steven L. Reiner

Departments of Medicine and Microbiology/Immunology, UCSF Medical Center, San Francisco, California 94143-0654

INTRODUCTION

Leishmania are dimorphic protozoa that exist as flagellated promastigotes within the sandfly vector and as obligate intracellular amastigotes within the mammalian host. These organisms live only within macrophages, where they replicate by binary fission. Building on the preceding chapters by Reed and Sher, here we discuss the detailed nature of the host's immune response to *Leishmania* and ways in which this response might be influenced through use of recombinant organisms. The potential of such strategies for creating effective vaccines is briefly mentioned.

ANTIGEN PRESENTATION

The intracellular compartment within which amastigotes proliferate is an acidic environment that has been characterized using biochemical markers as a late endolysosomal vacuole (Russell et al., 1992). Immunohistochemical studies have colocalized major histocompatibility (MHC) class II molecules within the amastigote-filled compartment (Russell et al., 1992). Replication of amastigotes within an MHC class II compartment would be expected to result in the stabilization of large numbers of MHC molecules by parasite antigens on the surface of the infected macrophage (Germain and Hendrix, 1991). The observation that mice rendered MHC class II deficient through targeted gene disruption are incapable of restricting *Leishmania major* inoculation, despite the presence of normal CD8$^+$ T-cell populations (Locksley et al., 1993), provides further support for the marked CD4 T cell dependence of this infection (Locksley and Scott, 1991). Conversely, mice with targeted disruption of the β$_2$-microglobulin gene have normal CD4$^+$ cells but no CD8$^+$ T cells and are capable of healing when challenged with *L. major* (Wang et al., 1993). Thus *Leishmania*, despite their intracellular location, primarily target antigens to the MHC class II pathway, in contrast to the use of the MHC class I pathway by most intracellular organisms, such as viruses, and other intracellular parasites, including *Trypanosoma cruzi*. An illustration of these two antigen presentation pathways is depicted in Figure 1.

TH1 VERSUS TH2 RESPONSE

The capacity to resolve *Leishmania* infection in both mice (Heinzel et al., 1989) and humans (Holaday et al., 1993) requires the development of CD4[+] T cells that generate interferon (IFN)-γ, a critical cytokine required for the priming of macrophages to a microbicidal state. As best studied using *L. major* infec-

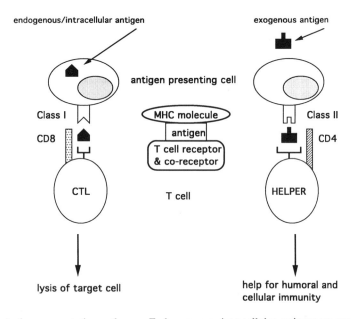

Fig. 1. Antigen presentation pathways. Endogenous or intracellular antigens are processed into octa- or nano-peptides that bind class I MHC molecules for presentation to CD8[+] lymphocytes. The cytolytic (CTL) activity of the T cell mediates destruction of the parasitized or transformed cell. Exogenous antigens are usually processed into longer peptides (12–24 amino acid residues) that are bound to MHC class II molecules during the intersection of phagocytic and lysosomal compartments. Presentation of these antigens to CD4[+] T cells results in the release of lymphokines, soluble mediators of helper activity for humoral and cellular immunity. *Leishmania* have adapted to survive within the highly acidic late endosomal compartment, which is a site of class II MHC stabilization by peptides. Thus, despite their exclusive intracellular presence in the mammalian host, immunity to these organisms depends on the quality of the CD4[+] and not the CD8[+] T-cell responses.

tion of inbred strains of mice, resistant strains, including C57BL/6, C3H/HeN, and B10D.2, infected subcutaneously develop a small nodule at the site of inoculation that resolves over 3–4 weeks, coincident with the appearance of Th1 cells, effector CD4$^+$ T cells that generate the cytokines IFN-γ, lymphotoxin, and, in lesser amounts, interleukin (IL)-2 (Mosmann and Coffman, 1989). In contrast, susceptible BALB/c mice develop progressive enlargement of the local subcutaneous lesion, disseminate the parasite to the spleen, and uniformly die over 12–16 weeks (Fig. 2). These mice generate an aberrant CD4$^+$ T-cell response to this intracellular organism, with the appearance of Th2 cells, effector CD4$^+$ T cells that generate the cytokines IL-4 and IL-10 (Heinzel et al., 1991). These cytokines have been demonstrated to suppress the capacity of macrophages to release proinflammatory cytokines such as tumor necrosis factor (TNF)-α, chemokines, and IL-12, to inhibit the ability of macrophages to provide accessory cell support for Th1 cells for the generation of cytokines, including IFN-γ, and to interfere with macrophage activation mediated by IFN-γ (Lehn et al., 1989; Tripp et al., 1993; Oswald et al., 1992; de Waal Malefyt et al., 1991). The demonstration that effector cytokines mediate different aspects of the host immune response and are expressed by distinct subsets of CD4$^+$ T cells constitutes a major advance in our understanding of the impact of infectious diseases (Fig. 3). The *L. major* experimental model remains one of the

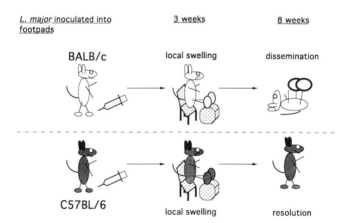

Fig. 2. The murine leishmaniasis model. Mice inoculated in the hind footpads with *L. major* experience local swelling and parasite replication until the third week following infection. At that time susceptible animals, typified by the BALB/c strain, develop progressive lymphoid and visceral dissemination that mimics human visceral leishmaniasis caused by *L. donovani*. Resistant animals, such as the C57BL/6 strain, control parasite replication locally and resolve swelling over the ensuing few weeks. Despite solid and lifelong immunity, organisms can be recovered indefinitely from resistant animals following culture of spleen and lymphoid organs.

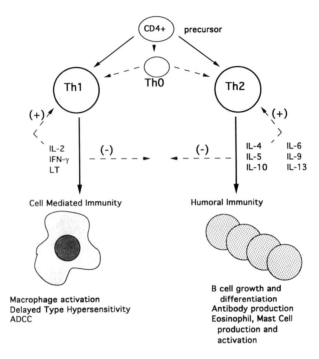

Fig. 3. CD4[+] T-helper subsets. The dichotomous responses of inbred strains of mice to infection with *L. major* has become the best characterized in vivo correlate of the two types of T-helper cells that arise in response to repeated antigenic stimulation. The Th1 and Th2 subsets can arise from a common Th0 precursor but have differing patterns of cytokine production and helper function, as well as mutually cross-inhibitory properties. The macrophage-activating activities mediated by Th1 cells are required for control of *Leishmania*.

best-characterized systems for examining the polarization of CD4[+] T-cell subsets in response to infectious agents. Intense interest has been focused on the signals that mediate differentiation of these disparate immunologic responses.

Although BALB/c mice respond aberrantly to *L. major*, this response is not due to the inability to generate protective Th1 cells. As first demonstrated using sublethal irradiation (Howard et al., 1981), a number of interventions, including administration of monoclonal antibodies to CD4 (Titus et al., 1985), IL-4 (Sadick et al., 1990), or IL-2 (Heinzel et al., 1993a), or administration of recombinant IL-12 (Heinzel et al., 1993b; Sypek et al., 1993), have the capacity to cure simultaneously infected BALB/c mice; in each case, such interventions are associated with the development of Th1 responses. These interventions must be administered within the first week of infection; later time points have proven ineffective (Fig. 4). Such studies suggest that the signals that mediate

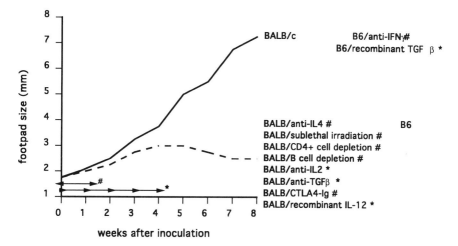

Fig. 4. Interventions that reverse the disease phenotype of leishmaniasis. A number of interventions are capable of reversing the genetic phenotype of healer or susceptible strains of mice. All must be administered within the first week or two of infection, suggesting that once CD4$^+$ subsets have been committed reversal is difficult through immunomodulation alone.

the generation of effector Th1 or Th2 cells must be present during the initial presentation of antigen to naive T cells. Once generated, Th1 and Th2 cells remain committed; transfer of parasite-specific T-cell lines into immunodeficient SCID mice was capable of reconstituting both immunity and exacerbation to subsequent infection, dependent on the Th1 or Th2 phenotype of the donor cells (Holaday et al., 1991).

The developmental lineage of mature CD4$^+$ cells has been best characterized using mice transgenic for single T-cell receptor (TCR) molecules. By virtue of allelic exclusion, animals into which a mature, rearranged, TCR transgene has been introduced develop a population of peripheral CD4$^+$ T cells that predominantly express the donated transgene. Examination of the development of these cells into Th1 and Th2 cells can be accomplished in vitro and the effects of various cytokines or antigen-presenting cell (APC) populations tested. Such analyses have demonstrated the critical roles for IL-4 in the differentiation of Th2 cells and for IL-12 in the differentiation of Th1 cells (Seder et al., 1992; Hsieh et al., 1993b). IL-10 modulates the capacity of Th1 cells to develop when macrophages, but not B cells, serve as APC (Hsieh et al., 1992). Although dendritic cells comprise the optimal APC for CD4$^+$ T-cell development in vitro, purified dendritic cells alone are incapable of inducing Th1 cell development in the absence of certain cytokines—IL-1, IL-12, and TNF-α—that can be supplied by macrophages (Hsieh et al, 1993a). Thus, effective Th1-cell development probably requires both optimal APC presentation to naive, or Thp, CD4$^+$ cells in addition to cytokines provided by macrophages within the vicinity of the inflammatory focus. Of these macrophage-dependent cytokines, IL-12 is necessary, but may not be sufficient, in the absence of additional cytokine signals. The requisite signals for Th2 development remain less well characterized. IL-4 is required for Th2 development in vitro (Seder et al., 1992) and in vivo (Le Gros et al., 1990), and mice rendered IL-4 deficient by targeted gene knockout are incapable of generating Th2 responses (Kopf et al., 1993). Unclear, however, is whether IL-4 is alone sufficient for Th2 development and the cellular source of the initial IL-4 produced during in vivo immune responses. Administration of exogenous recombinant IL-4 to normally resistant mice caused transient Th2-like responses in the draining lymph node cells of mice infected with *L. major* (Chatelain et al., 1992), but was incapable of sustaining Th2 development; such mice heal according to their underlying genetic phenotype (Sadick et al., 1991). Mice transgenic for constitutive IL-4 expression were rendered incapable of restricting local control of the parasite, but visceralization and death were not demonstrated, and lesion growth was substantially slower than occurs in susceptible BALB/c mice (Leal et al., 1993). Further, the demonstration of IL-4 in any cell other than a CD4$^+$ T cell remains to be demonstrated in leishmaniasis (Heinzel et al., 1991), raising questions regarding the source of IL-4 required for the development of a Th2 population. Mast cells are a potential source of IL-4, and adoptive transfer of mast cells to mast cell–deficient mice did retard, but not prevent, the resolution of *L. major* infection (R.G. Titus, personal communication). No differences in the course of *Leishmania* infection could be demonstrated when *L. amazonensis* was used in mast cell–deficient mice (Katakura et al., 1993). These various experiments, although not conclusive, suggest that IL-4 is required but not sufficient for Th2 cell development.

Experiments using mice transgenic for single TCR (Seder et al., 1992; Hsieh et al., 1993b), as well as limiting dilution analysis (Rocken et al., 1992), have established the capacity of Th1 and Th2 cells to develop from the same precursor CD4$^+$ population. Such findings have important implications for vaccine development, since they suggest that underlying genetic predisposition, rather than responses to different antigens, underlies the susceptibility to infectious diseases. This has been studied using the *L. major* model by characterizing the responding CD4$^+$ T-cell populations during both healing and progressive disease (Reiner et al., 1993). As assessed using flow cytometric analysis of Vβ usage, Northern and Southern analyses of TCR usage, and direct sequencing of *L. major*–specific Th1 and Th2 clones, comparable populations of CD4$^+$ T cells comprise both lineages. Interestingly, a restricted population bearing the Vα8/Vβ4 TCR heterodimer was predominantly represented in both Th1 and Th2 lineages, suggesting that the early CD4$^+$ cell response may be oligoclonal (Reiner et al., 1993). The close relationship between these populations is consistent with the earlier studies in TCR transgenic mice, demonstrating the capacity of naive CD4$^+$ T cells to differentiate to either Th1 or Th2 cells under the appropriate conditions (Seder et al., 1992; Hsieh et al., 1993b).

THE ROLE OF MACROPHAGES

The interactions of *L. major* with macrophage populations from both susceptible and resistant mice have been investigated in vitro in an attempt to localize the genetic defect to the macrophage. Macrophages from either phenotype supported comparable growth of amastigotes in vitro and could be comparably activated with lymphokines (Strect et al., 1987). Transcriptional activation of a number of cytokines, including IL-10, IL-12, TNF-α, MIP-1α and TGF-β has also been examined in bone marrow macrophage populations from BALB/c and C57BL/6 mice following infection with *L. major* promastigotes in vitro. In contrast to a number of stimuli, including antigens of *Toxoplasma gondi* (Gazzinelli et al., 1993), *Listeria* (Hsieh et al., 1993b), and bacterial endotoxin (Hsieh et al., 1993a), *Leishmania* enter macrophages relatively quietly; none of these cytokines was induced during invasion and conversion to the amastigote forms, except for TNF-α, which was slightly but consistently elevated (Reiner et al., 1994). Induction of TNF-α was also noted using assays detecting the generation of the secreted protein (Green et al., 1990). The release of bioactive TGF-β has been demonstrated following the invasion of macrophages by *L. braziliensis* and *L. amazonensis* (Barral-Netto et al., 1992), suggesting that post-transcriptional changes in secretion and activation may be involved. However, no differences were noted whether macrophages were used from genetically resistant or susceptible mice. Mature metacyclic promastigotes of *L. major* utilize the macrophage CR1 (CD35) receptor (Da Silva et al., 1989), suggesting that cross-linking CR1 is insufficient to trigger activation of cytokine gene transcription in resting macrophages. Taken together, these data have been unable to show any fundamental differences in the response of macrophages from resistant or susceptible mice to *L. major* in vitro. It still remains possible that differences in other, perhaps undiscovered, cytokines or in the regulation of adhesion molecules required in antigen presentation to CD4$^+$ T cells underlies the genetic susceptibility phenotype. it is difficult, however, to reconcile the capacity of anti-CD4$^+$ or sublethal irradiation, interventions that would not be predicted to affect the endogenous macrophage population, with their capacity to enable susceptible BALB/c mice to develop a healer phenotype.

THE ROLE OF CYTOKINES

In contrast to their silent entry into macrophages, *L. major* promastigotes stimulate a vigorous cytokine response in CD4$^+$ T cells draining the site of inoculation that is maximal after 4 days (Reiner et al., 1994). Both IL-2 and IL-4 are expressed in the CD4$^+$ population, as well as variable amounts of IL-10 and IFN-γ, consistent with activation of a Th0 population. None of these cytokines are expressed in significant amounts following infection of T-cell–deficient SCID animals or normal mice pretreated with anti-CD4 monoclonal antibodies to deplete CD4$^+$ T cells, suggesting that CD4$^+$ T cells are required for expression of these early cytokines. Interestingly, most of the IFN-γ transcripts appear in the CD4$^-$ population, consistent with expression in natural killer (NK) cells. Although IL-12 is a major inducer of IFN-γ expression in NK cells (Chan et al., 1991), no IL-12 transcripts could be identified during the initial 4 days after infection, consistent with the data using invasion of macrophages in vitro. In humans, IL-13 has been demonstrated to induce IFN-γ expression in NK cells in a synergistic manner with IL-2 (Minty et al., 1993). Examination of CD4$^+$ T cells from *L. major*–infected mice in both resistant and susceptible strains revealed induction of IL-13 mRNA, suggesting that *Leishmania* may induce a T-cell–dependent, IL-12–independent pathway for IFN-γ expression through the induction of IL-2 and IL-13 in CD4$^+$ T cells. Importantly, these cytokine responses in the CD4$^+$ populations were comparable between susceptible and resistant strains, suggesting that the early cytokine response, as defined using these reagents, could not account for the disparate outcomes of disease.

Between days 4 and 7 after infection, susceptible mice demonstrated striking downregulation of mRNA for IL-4 and IL-2 to baseline levels, whereas susceptible BALB/c mice failed to substantially downregulate the levels of these transcripts. By 14 days, the CD4$^+$ subsets begin to demonstrate the highly polarized expression of Th1 and Th2 cells in the healer and nonhealer strains, respectively (Reiner et al., 1993). These data suggest that the failure to downregulate the early burst of IL-2 and IL-4 that occurs after 4 days may underlie the susceptibility of BALB/c mice. Whether the defect truly lies at the level of the T cell or reflects aberrant signals received from APC, however, remains unknown. The data do suggest that the inability of immunologic interventions, such as anti-IL-4 or anti-CD4 antibodies, to reverse the susceptibility phenotype when administered 7 or more days after infection may reflect the finding that the critical developmental pathways that result in commitment to the Th1 or Th2 lineage occur between the fourth and seventh days.

FUTURE APPROACHES

The finding that *Leishmania* have evolved to evade induction of IL-12 in host macrophages is undoubtedly critical to the survival of the organism. Indeed, administration of exogenous recombinant IL-12 at the time of infection allows susceptible BALB/c mice to heal and establish a Th1 cytokine phenotype (Heinzel et al., 1993b; Sypek et al., 1993). Several novel approaches can be suggested to take advantage of these findings. First, engineering *Leishmania* that induce IL-12 might be predicted to constitute an effective vaccine for leishmaniasis. Such organisms would establish strong IFN-γ responses at the time of infection and should be rapidly destroyed. At the same time, memory T cells of the protective Th1 phenotype should be established. The capacity to transfect biologically active cytokines into *Leishmania* has been established, although, in the case of IFN-γ, such engineered organisms were not capable of inducing a protective Th1 response when introduced into susceptible mice (Tobin et al., 1993). Although transfected IFN-γ was capable of activating macrophages from within, IL-12 is a heterodimer that might not be efficiently secreted or get from the infected vacuole to the extracellular space in order to achieve activation of target NK and T cells. Such obstacles might be circumvented by the second strategy, which takes advantage of the capacity of certain organisms, such as *Listeria* (Hsieh et al., 1993b) and *Toxoplasma* (Gazzinelli et al., 1993), to induce IL-12 release from macrophages. Although further evidence is required, available data have demonstrated that the molecules from these microorganisms that induce IL-12 release are protease sensitive, suggesting they are proteins. A *Listeria* or *Toxoplasma* library could be established in the appropriate transfection plasmids (Tobin et al., 1993) and used to transfect *Leishmania*, generating a library of promastigotes. These organisms in turn would be inoculated onto isolated macrophages, taking advantage of the observation that wild-type *Leishmania* do not induce IL-12 p40 transcription in these cells (Reiner et al., 1994). Pools of inoculated transfectants would be screened for IL-12p40 induction, thus allowing for the identification of the IL-12–inducing molecule. Although a number of potential problems might occur, such as a role for attached carbohydrate or glycan moieties or the requirement for more than one molecule, success would not only identify microbial products that induce IL-12 that might be important adjuvants for stimulating the cellular immune response, but would also generate potential *Leishmania* vaccines, e.g., organisms engineered to mediate their own destruction while establishing protective Th1-mediated immunity.

ACKNOWLEDGMENTS

The authors are grateful for the numerous insightful comments offered by the faculty and students of the Biology of Parasitism course at Woods Hole and for support from the NIH and the Burroughs Wellcome Fund.

REFERENCES

Barral-Netto M, Barral A, Brownell CE, Skeiky YAW, Ellingsworth LR, Twardzik DR, Reed SG (1992): Transforming growth factor-β in leishmanial infection: A parasite escape mechanism. Science 257:545–548.

Chan SH, Perussia B, Gupta JW, Kobayashi M, Pospisil M, Young HA, Wolf SF, Young D, Clark SD, Trinchieri G (1991): Induction of interferon γ production by natural killer cell stimulatory factor: Characterization of the responder cells and synergy with other inducers. J Exp Med 173:869–880.

Chatelain R, Varkila K, Coffman RL (1992): IL-4 induces a Th2 response in *Leishmania* major-infected mice. J Immunol 148:1182–1187.

Da Silva RP, Hall BF, Joiner KA, Sacks DL (1989): CR1, the C3b receptor, mediates the binding of infective *Leishmania major* metacyclic promastigotes to human macrophages. J Immunol 143:617–622.

de Waal Malefyt R, Abrams J, Bennett B, Figdor CG, deVries JE (1991): Interleukin 10 (IL-10) inhibits cytokine synthesis by human monocytes: An autoregulatory role of IL-10 produced by monocytes. J Exp Med 174:1209–1220.

Gazzinelli RT, Hieny S, Wynn TA, Wolf S, Sher A (1993): Interleukin 12 is required for the T-lymphocyte–independent induction of interferon γ by an intracellular parasite and induces resistance in T-cell–deficient hosts. Proc Natl Acad Sci USA 90:6115–6119.

Germain RN, Hendrix LR (1991): MHC class II structure, occupancy and surface expression determined by post-endoplasmic reticulum antigen binding. Nature 353:134–139.

Green SJ, Crawford RM, Hockmeyer JT, Meltzer MS, Nacy CA (1990): *Leishmania major* amastigotes initiate the L-arginine dependent killing mechanism in IFN-γ stimulated macrophages by induction of TNF-α. J Immunol 145:4290–4298.

Heinzel FP, Rerko RM, Hatam F, Locksley RM (1993a): Interleukin 2 is necessary for progression of leishmaniasis in susceptible murine hosts. J Immunol 150:3924–3931.

Heinzel FP, Sadick MD, Holaday BJ, Coffman RL, Locksley RM (1989): Reciprocal expression of gamma-interferon or interleukin-4 during the resolution or progression of murine leishmaniasis. Evidence for expansion of distinct helper T-cell subsets. J Exp Med 169:59–72.

Heinzel FP, Sadick MD, Mutha SS, Locksley RM (1991): Production of interferon-α, IL-2, IL-4 and IL-10 by CD4+ lymphocytes in vivo during healing and progressive murine leishmaniasis. Proc Natl Acad Sci USA 88:7011–7015.

Heinzel FP, Schoenhaut DS, Rerko RM, Rosser LE, Gately MK (1993b): Recombinant interleukin 12 cures mice infected with *Leishmania major.* J Exp Med 177:1505–1509.

Holaday BJ, Pompeu M, Evans T, deBraga D, Texeira M, Sousa A, Sadick MD, Vasconcelos AW, Abrams JS, Pearson RD, Locksley RM (1993): Correlates of *Leishmania*-specific immunity in the clinical spectrum of infection with *Leishmania chagasi.* J Infect Dis 167:411–417.

Holaday BJ, Sadick MD, Wang ZE, Reiner SL, Heinzel FP, Parslow TG, Locksley RM (1991): Reconstitution of *Leishmania* immunity in SCID mice using Th1- and Th2-like cell lines. J Immunol 147:1653–1658.

Howard J, Hale C, Liew FY (1981): Immunological regulation of experimental cutaneous leishmaniasis. IV. Prophylactic effect of sublethal irradiation as a result of abrogation of suppressor T cell generation in mice genetically susceptible to *Leishmania tropica.* J Exp Med 153:557–568.

Hsieh CS, Heimberger AB, Gold JS, O'Garra A, Murphy KM (1992): Differential regulation of T helper phenotype development by interleukins 4 and 10 in an αβ T-cell–receptor transgenic system. Proc Natl Acad Sci USA 89:6065–6069.

Hsieh CS, Macatonia SE, O'Garra A, Murphy KM (1993a): Pathogen-induced Th1 phenotype development in CD4$^+$ αβ-TCR transgenic T cells is macrophage dependent. Int Immunol 5:371–382.

Hsieh CS, Macatonia SE, Tripp CS, Wolf SF, O'Garra A, Murphy KM (1993b): Development of Th1 CD4$^+$ T cells through IL-12 produced by *Listeria*-induced macrophages. Science 260:547–549.

Katakura K, Saburo S, Hamada A, Matsuda H, Watanabe N (1993): Cutaneous leishmaniasis in mast cell-deficient W/W^v mice. Infect Immun 61:2242–2244.

Kopf M, Le Gros G, Bachmann M, Lamers MC, Bluethmann H, Kohler G (1993): Disruption of the murine IL-4 gene blocks Th2 cytokine responses. Nature 362:245–248.

Leal LMCC, Moss DW, Kuhn R, Muller W, Liew FY (1993): Interleukin-4 transgenic mice of resistant background are susceptible to *Leishmania major* infection. Eur J Immunol 23:566–569.

Le Gros G, Ben-Sasson SZ, Seder R, Finkelman FD, Paul WE (1990): Generation of interleukin 4 (IL-4)–producing cells in vivo and in vitro: IL-2 and IL-4 are required for in vitro generation of IL-4–producing cells. J Exp Med 172:921–929.

Lehn M, Weiser WY, Engelhorn S, Gillis S, Remold RG (1989): IL-4 inhibits H$_2$O$_2$ production and antileishmanial capacity of human cultured monocytes mediated by IFN-γ. J Immunol 143:3020–3024.

Locksley RM, Reiner SL, Hatam F, Littman DR, Killeen N (1993): Helper T cells without CD4: Control of leishmaniasis in CD4-deficient mice. Science 261:1448–1451.

Locksley RM, Scott P (1991): Helper T-cell subsets in mouse leishmaniasis: Induction, expansion and effector function. Immunoparasitol Today 12:A58–A61.

Minty A, Chalon P, Cerocq JM, Dumont X, Guillemot JC, Kaghad M, Labit C, Leplatois P, Liauzun P, Miloux B, et al. (1993): Interleukin 13 is a new human lymphokine regulating inflammatory and immune responses. Nature 362:248–250.

Mosmann TR, Coffman RML (1989): Th1 and Th2 cells: Different patterns of lymphokine secretion lead to different functional properties. Annu Rev Immunol 7:145–173.

Oswald IP, Gazzinelli RT, Sher A, James SL (1992): IL-10 synergizes with IL-4 and transforming growth factor-β to inhibit macrophage cytotoxic activity. J Immunol 148:3578–3582.

Reiner SL, Wang ZE, Hatam F, Scott P, Locksley RM (1993): Th1 and Th2 cell antigen receptors in experimental leishmaniasis. Science 259:1457–1460.

Reiner SL, Zheng S, Wang ZE, Stowring L, Locksley RM (1994): *Leishmania* promastigotes evade IL-2 induction by macrophages and stimulate a broad range of cytokines from CD4$^+$ cells during initiation of infection. J Exp Med 179:447–456.

Rocken M, Saurat JH, Hauser C (1992): A common precursor for CD4$^+$ T cells producing IL-2 or IL-4. J Immunol 148:1031–1038.

Russell DG, Xu S, Chakraborty P (1992): Intracellular trafficking and the parasitophorous vacuole of *Leishmania mexicana*–infected macrophages. J Cell Sci 103:1193–1210.

Sadick MD, Heinzel FP, Holaday BJ, Pu RT, Dawkins RS, Locksley RM (1990): Cure of murine leishmaniasis with anti-IL-4 monoclonal antibody. Evidence for a T cell-dependent, IFN-γ–independent mechanism. J Exp Med 171:115–127.

Sadick MD, Street N, Mosmann TR, Locksley RM (1991): Cytokine regulation in murine leishmaniasis: Interleukin 4 is not sufficient to mediate progressive disease in resistant C57BL/6 mice. Infect Immun 59:4710–4714.

Seder RA, Paul WE, Davis MM, de St. Groth BF (1992): The presence of interleukin 4 during in vitro priming determines the lymphokine-producing potential of CD4$^+$ T cells from T cell receptor transgenic mice. J Exp Med 176:1091–1098.

Strect H, Bogdan C, Tingle A, Rollinghoff M (1987): Murine cutaneous leishmaniasis: Comparative study on the capacity of macrophages from healer and non-healer mouse strains to control *L. tropica* replication. Zbl Bakt Hyg 263:594–604.

Sypek JP, Chung CL, Mayor SEH, Subramanyam JM, Goldman SJ, Dieburth DS, Wolf SF, Schaub RG (1993): Resolution of cutaneous leishmaniasis: Interleukin 12 initiates a protective T helper type 1 immune response. J Exp Med 177:1797–1802.

Titus RG, Milon G, Marchal G, Vassalli P, Cerottini JC, Louis JA (1985): Therapeutic effect of anti-L3T4 monoclonal antibody GK1.5 on cutaneous leishmaniasis in genetically susceptible BALB/c mice. J Immunol 135:2108–2114.

Tobin JF, Reiner SL, Hatam F, Zheng S, Leptak CL, Wirth DF, Locksley RM (1993): Transfected *Leishmania* expressing biologically active IFN-γ. J Immunol 150:5059–5069.

Tripp CS, Wolf SF, Unanue ER (1993): Interleukin 12 and tumor necrosis factor α are costimulators of interferon γ production by natural killer cells in severe combined immunodeficiency mice with listeriosis, and interleukin 10 is a physiologic antagonist. Proc Natl Acad Sci USA 90:3725–3729.

Wang ZE, Reiner SL, Hatam F, Heinzel FP, Bouvier J, Turk CW, Locksley RM (1993): Targeted activation of CD8[+] cells and infection of β-microglobulin deficient mice fail to confirm a primary protective role for CD8[+] cells in experimental leishmaniasis. J Immunol 151:2077–2086.

Molecular Approaches to Parasitology, pages 467–476
© 1995 Wiley-Liss, Inc.

Cytokine Control of Protective Immunity Against Nematode Infections

Fred D. Finkelman, William C. Gause, and Joseph F. Urban, Jr.

Departments of Medicine (F.D.F.) and Microbiology and Immunology (W.C.G.), F. Edward He'bert School of Medicine of the Uniformed Services University of the Health Sciences, Bethesda, Maryland, 20814; Helminthic Diseases Laboratory, Livestock and Poultry Sciences Institute, Agricultural Research Service, U.S. Department of Agriculture, Beltsville, Maryland 20705 (J.F.U.)

INTRODUCTION

As already discussed in detail in preceding chapters, the control of parasitic infections by the immune system is dependent on the production of cytokines that limit parasite reproduction and survival. A parasite-specific immune response in which inappropriate cytokines are secreted will fail to induce the effector mechanisms that protect the host and can actually enhance parasite dissemination. For example, BALB/c mice, which respond to *Leishmania major* infection with considerable T-cell production of interleukin (IL)-4, rather than interferon (IFN)-γ, develop generalized disease more rapidly than do T-cell–deficient mice, while most other mouse strains, which produce considerably more IFN-γ than IL-4 in response to *L. major* infection, control the disease (Locksley et al., 1991). The requirement for IFN-γ to induce macrophage nitrous oxide (NO) production, which is needed to kill ingested leishmania amastigotes, and the ability of IL-4 to block the induction of NO synthetase explain how the BALB/c cytokine response leads to disease dissemination (Liew et al., 1990).

The great morphological and physiological differences among parasites would suggest that a single effector mechanism, or set of effector mechanisms, would not be able to control all parasite infections. Inasmuch as cytokines induce or block different effector mechanisms, this same consideration would suggest that the cytokines that protect or exacerbate disease would differ in hosts infected with different parasites. This hypothesis is supported by evidence that mice infected with intestinal nematode parasites demonstrate a relationship between cytokine expression and protective immunity that is opposite to that seen in mice infected with *L. major*: IL-4 contributes to protective immunity, while IFNs enhance parasite survival and fecundity.

INFLUENCE OF IL-4 ON IMMUNITY TO NEMATODE PARASITE INFECTION

The influence of IL-4 on worm survival and fecundity has been studied in mice infected with each of four different nematode parasites that inhabit the gut: *Heligmosomoides polygyrus*, *Nippostrongylus brasiliensis*, *Trichinella spiralis*, and *Trichuris muris*. IL-4 contributes to protective immunity in mice infected with each of these parasites; however, the extent to which IL-4 is required for a protective immune response differs considerably in mice infected with the different parasites. Dependence on IL-4 for protective immunity is most easily illustrated in mice infected with *H. polygyrus* or *Trichuris muris*. BALB/c mice given a primary inoculation with *H. polygyrus* develop an intestinal infection that lasts for several months (Urban et al., 1991a). IL-4 gene expression by gut-associated lymphoid tissue becomes elevated by 4 days after infection, but remains high during the the next 10 days (Svetic' et al., 1993). Treating mice during a primary infection with anti-IL-4 receptor (IL-4R) mAb has no effect on worm survival, but increases worm fecundity. In contrast, treating mice during a primary infection with a long-lasting IL-4 preparation terminates infection (J.F. Urban, Jr., and F.D. Finkelman, manuscript in preparation). During a challenge (second) infection, in which levels of IL-4 gene expression are considerably greater than during a primary infection, and in which host CD4$^+$ T cells limit worm fecundity and survival, anti-IL-4R mAb increases worm survival and fecundity to levels that are characteristic of a primary infection (Urban et al., 1991b). Thus, increasing IL-4 levels in mice infected with this parasite protects the host, while inhibiting IL-4 activity abolishes protective immunity.

Studies by Else and Grencis (1991) with *Trichuris muris*–infected mice provide consistent data. Most mouse strains, such as BALB/k, eliminate *Trichuris muris* from the gut before it develops into the mature, egg-laying stage. These mouse strains generate a Th2 response (considerable IL-4 and IL-5, little IFN-γ) to *Trichuris muris*. A few strains, however, such as AKR and B10.BR, develop a chronic fecund infection when inoculated with *Trichuris muris* ova. These mouse strains generate a predominantly Th1 response (considerable IFN-γ, little IL-4 or IL-5) (Else and Grencis, 1991). Treatment of mice of the normally resistant strains with anti-IL-4R mAb leads to the development of a chronic, fecund infection, while IL-4 treatment of mice of the normally susceptible strains causes worms to be expelled before they become fecund (Else et al., 1994).

Protective immunity to *N. brasiliensis* is less IL-4–dependent than is protective immunity to *Trichuris muris* or *H. polygyrus*. *N. brasiliensis*, unlike *H. polygyrus* or *Trichuris muris*, completes its life cycle by producing fertile ova and is expelled from the gut of infected BALB/c mice within 10 days of inoculation. While worm expulsion during a primary infection is CD4$^+$ T cell dependent (Katona et al., 1988), it occurs normally in mice treated with anti-IL-4R mAb and in transgenic mice that lack a functional IL-4 gene (Kühn et al., 1991; J.F. Urban, Jr., and F.D. Finkelman, unpublished data). This does not necessarily mean, however, that IL-4 is uninvolved in effector mechanisms that protect against this parasite. It is possible that more than one effector mechanism is activated in *N. brasiliensis*–infected mice and that each is sufficient, by itself, to cause worm expulsion, so that elimination of one effector mechanism has no apparent effect. This hypothesis is supported by observations that IL-4 treatment causes congenitally athymic *N. brasiliensis*–inoculated mice, which normally develop a chronic infection, to expel the parasite. IL-4 has a similar effect in anti-CD4 mAb-treated, *N. brasiliensis*–inoculated normal mice (J.F. Urban, Jr., and F.D. Finkelman, manuscript in preparation).

An IL-4 contribution to protective immunity is also apparent in BALB/c mice infected with *Trichinella spiralis*. Although there is currently no evidence that IL-4 limits adult worm survival in mice infected with this parasite, it appears to play a role in limiting fecundity, which increases in mice treated with anti-IL-4R mAb and decreases when mice are treated with IL-4 (J.F. Urban, Jr., and F.D. Finkelman, manuscript in preparation). These observations stand in contrast to a previous report that parasite adults survive longer in mouse strains that generate a Th2 response to *Trichinella spiralis* infection than in those that generate a Th1 response (Pond et al., 1989). It is notable that this report studied cytokine responses by spleen cells and that mesenteric lymph node cells, which probably better reflect the immune status of the gut, generate a Th2 response in both mouse strains (Kelly et al., 1991).

MECHANISM OF ACTION OF IL-4 IN LIMITING NEMATODE INFECTIONS

IL-4 is required for the generation of an IgE response in mice and contributes to the stimulation of intestinal mucosal mastocytosis (Finkelman et al., 1990; Madden et al., 1991). These considerations made it seem likely that IL-4 would contribute to worm expulsion primarily by stimulating the production of specific IgE antibody that would bind to mucosal mast cells in the intestine and induce them to degranulate when cross-linked by parasite antigens. Against this hypothesis, however, are the observations that suppression of an IgE response with an anti-IgE mAb fails to block protective immunity in mice given a challenge infection with *H. polygyrus* (Katona et al., 1992) and that protective immunity is relatively intact in W/W^v mice, which lack the ability to generate a mucosal mast cell response (J.F. Urban, Jr., and F.D. Finkelman, unpublished data). Inasmuch as IL-4 can act as an autocrine growth factor for Th2 cells and contribute to their production of other cytokines

(Lichtman et al., 1987), it was also possible that the IL-4 requirement for *H. polygyrus* expulsion might relate primarily to its stimulation of the production of other Th2 cytokines. This also now seems to be unlikely, as IL-4 can induce anti-CD4 mAb-treated mice to expel this parasite. Studies of the kinetics of IL-4 effects during a primary *H. polygyrus* infection indicate that it substantially decreases adult worm fecundity within 1 day after the initiation of treatment, although treatment for several days is required to cause worm expulsion. The rapidity of the IL-4 effect suggests that it works directly either to damage the parasite or to make the host gut inhospitable to the parasite, perhaps by limiting parasite nutrition. We presently favor the latter possibility, because 1) in vitro studies fail to show any toxic effect of IL-4 on *H. polygyrus* and 2) an antimouse IL-4R mAb, which would not be expected to bind to a putative parasite IL-4R, blocks the in vivo ability of IL-4 to decrease worm fecundity (J.F. Urban, Jr., and F.D. Finkelman, manuscript in preparation). There is not yet, however, any direct evidence that IL-4 has an effect on the host gut that limits parasite nutrition.

The observations that IL-4 is required for *H. polygyrus* expulsion during a second infection while no requirement seems to exist for either IgE or mucosal mast cells does not prove that the IgE–mast cell effector mechanism is uninvolved in protective immunity to this parasite. Just as IL-4 is sufficient, but not necessary, to expel *N. brasiliensis* during a primary infection, the IgE–mast cell mechanism may be one of several mechanisms by which IL-4 contributes to worm expulsion. Consistent with this possibility, studies of *Trichinella spiralis*–infected rats have demonstrated a protective effect of IgE from immune animals, but have also shown that IgG antibodies can provide protection (Ahmad et al., 1991). Furthermore other Th2-associated responses have been shown to provide redundant host protection against worm infection: IL-5 that is produced by mice that have been given a second infection with *Strongyloides venezuelensis* contributes to the killing of this parasite during larval migration through the lungs, but blocking of this cytokine fails to increase the time required to expel adults from the gut (Korenaga et al., 1991). We favor a model that suggests that host responses to a class of parasites are somewhat stereotyped and include the induction of a range of effector mechanisms that should be capable of limiting the growth or fecundity of most members of the class. For some parasite species within the class a single effector mechanism may protect the host while others contribute nothing to the limitation of infection; for other parasite species several redundant mechanisms may each be capable of limiting infection; for still others none of the available mechanisms may be capable of protecting the host. Such a model could explain why IgE and mast cells, which have the potential to do considerable damage to the host, are retained in evolution and expressed in circumstances in which they do not seem necessary.

EFFECTS OF INTERFERONS AND IL-12
ON NEMATODE INFECTIONS

The frequent antagonism between IL-4 and IFN-γ led us to test whether the latter cytokine, which is required to protect hosts against a variety of intracellular parasites, might exacerbate nematode infections. Most studies have been performed in mice infected with *N. brasiliensis*. As mice normally expel this parasite by 10 days after inoculation and expulsion is CD4[+] T cell dependent (Urban et al., 1991a), it is relatively easy to determine whether treatment with IFN or any other agent interferes with expulsion. Our studies have revealed that treatment with IFN-γ leads to a large increase in worm fecundity. Adult worm expulsion is delayed, but not prevented, even if IFN-γ administration is continued on a daily basis (Urban et al., 1994). Agents that induce the production of IFN-γ have a similar effect. Treatment of mice with IL-12, which induces natural killer (NK) cells and T cells to secrete IFN-γ and blocks the secretion of IL-4 (Kobayashi et al., 1989; Manetti et al., 1993), blocks expulsion of *N. brasiliensis* adults for an even longer period of time than does exogenously administered IFN-γ (J.F. Urban, Jr., and F.D. Finkelman, manuscript in preparation). Heat-killed *Brucella abortus*, which induces an IFN-γ response (possibly by stimulating IL-12 production) also enhances *N. brasiliensis* fecundity and survival (Urban et al., 1994). These effects of both IL-12 and *B. abortus* are IFN-γ dependent, as they are completely inhibited by anti-IFN-γ mAb. Thus, endogenously produced IFN-γ, as well as exogenous IFN-γ, can inhibit protective immunity to *N. brasiliensis*. These observations suggest that simultaneous infection with two parasites that induce and are controlled by antagonistic cytokines might make the host more susceptible to both parasites. Initial studies of mice that have been simultaneously infected with *N. brasiliensis* and the intestinal protozoan parasite *Eimeria papillata*, which, like other *Eimeria* species, induces and is controlled by an IFN-γ response (Rose et al., 1989), are consistent with this hypothesis. Treatment with anti-IFN-γ mAb ameliorates the *N. brasiliensis* infection, but exacerbates the *Eimeria* infection (J.F. Urban, Jr., and F.D. Finkelman, unpublished data). This observation contrasts with the failure of gut infections with *N. brasiliensis* to interfere with footpad infections with *L. major* (R. Locksley, personal communication). Most likely, the compartmentalization of cytokine responses is sufficiently tight that adverse effects are generally observed only when two parasites infect the same or overlapping organ systems. It is likely, however, that this occurs in humans in developing countries with sufficient frequency to have a substantial negative impact on the control of multiple infectious diseases.

The mechanism by which IFN-γ interferes with protective immunity to nematode parasites is not known. IFN-γ blocks the proliferation of Th2 cells

(Gajewski and Fitch, 1988), inhibits peripheral blood and tissue eosinophilia and the pulmonary inflammation that develops in response to the lung stage of *N. brasiliensis*, and delays the development of IgE and mucosal mast cell responses (Urban et al., 1994). It is unlikely that IFN-γ inhibition of IL-3, IL-4, IL-5, or IL-9 production is solely responsible for its negative effect on protective immunity, since treatment of mice with antibodies against any of these cytokines has no effect on worm expulsion and little, if any, effect on fecundity (J.F. Urban, Jr., and F.D. Finkelman, unpublished data). It is also unlikely that a simple toxic effect on the host fully accounts for the negative effects of IFN-γ on worm expulsion. First, administration of exogenous IFN-γ can enhance protective immunity against other parasites (Suzuki et al., 1988). Second, with continued IFN-γ treatment, the host, instead of succumbing to accumulated toxic effects, eventually generates a Th2 response (increased IL-3, IL-4, and IL-5 gene expression with the generation of large IgE and mast cell responses) and expels the parasite (Urban et al., 1994). It is possible that the escape from the negative effect of IFN-γ would not occur if larger doses of IFN-γ could be administered, as worm expulsion is delayed for a longer period of time by treatment with IL-12 than by treatment with sublethal doses of IFN-γ (J.F. Urban, Jr., and F.D. Finkelman, manuscript in preparation). IL-12 treatment, by stimulating the production of IFN-γ at sites where T cells and NK cells are concentrated, may allow higher and more prolonged levels of IFN-γ to be maintained in these important sites than can be achieved when IFN-γ itself is injected.

The effects of IFN-γ on worm fecundity and expulsion are closely mimicked by IFN-α (Urban et al., 1994). This indicates that the mechanism by which IFN-γ enhances worm fecundity and survival is likely to be an action that is shared by IFN-γ and IFN-α, such as inhibition of Th2 responses (Finkelman et al., 1991), rather than one that distinguishes the two cytokines, such as the stimulation of inducible NO synthetase production by macrophages (an effect of IFN-γ that is not shared by IFN-α).

CONTROL OF CYTOKINE RESPONSES IN PARASITE-INFECTED MICE

The opposite effects of IL-4 and IFN-γ responses on protective immunity in mice infected with intracellular parasites or gut-dwelling nematodes suggest that it is imperative for hosts to have a way to make the appropriate cytokine responses to particular parasites. This conclusion is supported by the deleterious effects of making the wrong cytokine response to a pathogen (e.g., the IL-4 response made by BALB/c mice infected with *L. major* or the IFN-γ response made by B10.BR mice infected with *Trichuris muris*). We have suggested that important characteristics that are expressed by groups of parasites have been selected as triggers for appropriate cytokine responses. For example, bacterial lipopolysaccharide (LPS) and double-stranded RNA, among other triggers, stimulate the production of IL-12 and IFN-α, which in turn enhance IFN-γ production and inhibit IL-4 production (Kobayashi et al., 1989; Manetti et al., 1993; Finkelman et al., 1991). The selection of LPS and double-stranded RNA as triggers for the Th1 responses that are appropriate for mice infected with gram-negative bacteria or viruses makes sense in evolutionary terms: Pathogens would be expected to cease the expression of molecules that stimulate hosts to make cytokine responses that are deleterious to the pathogen unless, like gram-negative bacterial LPS and viral double-stranded RNA, they serve critical functions for the pathogen. Less is known about the mechanisms through which nematodes trigger a Th2 response. To date, the only cytokine that is known to trigger the production of a Th2 response is IL-4 itself (Swain et al., 1990; LeGros et al., 1990). The ability of IL-4 to enhance IL-4 production by differentiating CD4$^+$ T cells and the ability of basophils to secrete IL-4 (Seder et al., 1991) has raised the possibility that nematode-produced substances might induce basophils to secrete IL-4, which could then influence T-cell differentiation. This hypothesis is supported by the observations that parasite-derived molecules can induce basophils to degranulate (Helm et al., 1993) and that proteases, which must be produced in large quantity by nematodes to facilitate penetration of host tissues as well as parasite transition from one larval stage to the next, stimulate rapid IL-4 secretion as well as in vivo IgE responses (Finkelman and Urban, 1992). Against this hypothesis, however, is the failure to find evidence of increased IL-4 gene expression in the gut-associated lymphoid tissues of *H. polygyrus*–infected mice prior to its increased expression by CD4$^+$ T cells several days after host inoculation. This is in contrast to the increased IL-5 and IL-9 gene expression in the fundic region of the stomach and in Peyer's patches of the upper intestine within 3–6 hours after inoculation (Svetic' et al., 1993). While this observation is not inconsistent with the possibility that infective *H. polygyrus* larvae trigger the release of stored IL-4 without stimulating an increase in IL-4 gene transcription, it suggests that there may be molecules other than IL-4 that can trigger T cells to secrete this cytokine. Investigation of the effects of nematode extracts and secretions on T-cell differentiation in the presence of IL-4 antagonists may be useful for distinguishing between these possibilities.

PRACTICAL IMPLICATIONS

Gastrointestinal roundworm parasites, including those within the genera *Necator, Ancylostoma, Ascaris, Trichuris,* and *Strongyloides,* infect approximately 1 billion people worldwide and are believed to cause approximately 1 million deaths annually (Walsh, 1984). Chronic malnutrition induced by these infections causes great morbidity, including colitis, rectal prolapse, anorexia, growth retardation, and impaired cognitive function, and increases the susceptibility of infected individuals to other infections (Grencis et al., 1993). Although primary health care and effective public sanitation can successfully eliminate human gastrointestinal parasitism, immunological intervention may promote control in situations in which gastrointestinal parasitism remains endemic and intractable.

Successful immunization procedures may be more cost-effective than other forms of therapy, and immune elimination of gastrointestinal parasites avoids the often severe immunopathological consequences of destruction of tissue parasites by pharmacological agents. Our observations of cytokine effects on host immunity to nematodes demonstrate, however, that host protection is only likely to be induced if a vaccine induces a strong immune response that is specific in two distinct ways: It must recognize antigenic determinants on the parasite, and it must be characterized by the production of those cytokines that limit the ability of the parasite to survive and reproduce rather than those cytokines that enhance parasite survival and reproduction. As different cytokines enhance or inhibit the ability of the host to control different parasites, it will be necessary to determine which cytokines play critical roles in the control of specific parasites and to devise vaccination techniques that elicit the desired cytokine response.

Preliminary studies with IFN-α and IL-12 suggest that these cytokines, or agents that induce their production, may be useful adjuvants for vaccination against parasites that are controlled by an IFN-γ response (Gajewski and Fitch, 1988; Heinzel et al., 1993). For parasites that are controlled by an IL-4 response, such as nematodes, effective vaccination may be enhanced by IL-4 itself or by still to be discovered cytokines that we hypothesize are also involved in the triggering of a Th2 response. The successful use of IL-4, in a long-acting formulation (Finkelman et al., 1993), as a treatment of mice that have established *H. polygyrus*, and *N. brasiliensis*, even when T cells are deficient, suggests that cytokines will be useful for the treatment of human disease. One considerable potential benefit of cytokine treatment of established disease relative to anthelmintic treatment might be the induction of a memory immune response that is able to limit reinfection. Studies are currently being performed in rodent models to investigate this possibility.

ACKNOWLEDGEMENTS

We thank our many collaborators in the experiments that we have described: Kathryn Else, Maurice Gately, Richard Grencis, Ildy Katona, Kathleen Madden, Suzanne Morris, William Paul, Antonela Svetic′, and Paul Trotta. This work was supported in part by Naval Medical Research and Development

Command contracts number N0007592WR00024 and N0007592WR00035, U.S. Department of Agriculture CRIS 1265-31320-009, National Institutes of Health Grants AI-26150 and AI-21328, and a grant from Hoffmann-La Roche, Inc.

REFERENCES

Ahmad A, Wang CH, Bell RG (1991): A role for IgE in intestinal immunity: Expression of rapid expulsion of *Trichinella spiralis* in rats transfused with IgE and thoracic duct lymphocytes. J Immunol 146:3563.

Else KJ, Finkelman FD, Maliszewski CR, Grencis RK (1994): Cytokine mediated regulation of chronic intestinal helminth infection. J Exp Med 179:347–351.

Else KJ, Grencis RK (1991): Cellular immune responses to the murine nematode parasite *Trichuris muris*. I. Differential cytokine production during acute or chronic infection. Immunology 72:508.

Finkelman FD, Holmes J, Katona IM, Urban JF, Beckman MP, Park LS, Schooley KA, Coffman RL, Mosmann TR, Paul WE (1990): Lymphokine control of in vivo immunoglobulin isotype selection. Annu Rev Immunol 8:303.

Finkelman FD, Madden KB, Morris SC, Holmes JM, Boiani N, Katona IM, Maliszewski CR (1993): Anti-cytokine antibodies as carrier proteins: Prolongation of in vivo effects of exogenous cytokines by injection of cytokine–anti-cytokine antibody complexes. J Immunol 151:1235.

Finkelman FD, Svetic A, Gresser I, Snapper C, Holmes J, Trotta P, Katona IM, Gause WC (1991): Regulation by interferon-α of immunoglobulin isotype selection and lymphokine production in mice. J Exp Med 174:1179.

Finkelman FD, Urban JF Jr (1992): Cytokines: Making the right choice. Parasitol Today 8:311.

Gajewski TF, Fitch FW (1988): Anti-proliferative effect of IFN-γ in immune regulation. I. IFN-γ inhibits the proliferation of Th2 but not Th1 murine helper T cell clones. J Immunol 140:4245.

Grencis RK, Else KJ, Bancroft AJ, Bundy DAP (1993): *Trichuris* update '93. Parasitol Today 9:309.

Heinzel FP, Shoenhaut DS, Rerko RM, Rosser LE, Gately MK (1993): Recombinant interleukin 12 cures mice infected with *Leishmania major*. J Exp Med 177:1505.

Helm BA, Moreira DM, Rhodes N (1993): A possible link between the nature of mast cell triggering agents and the induction of an immunoglobulin E response, abstracted. FASEB J 150:178A.

Katona I, Madden K, Thyphronitis G, Urban J Jr, Finkelman F (1992): Suppression of a *Heligmosomoides polygyrus*–induced IgE response by an anti-IgE mAb, abstracted. 8th International Congress of Immunology. Budapest, Hungary, 1992, p. 462.

Katona IM, Urban JF Jr, Finkelman FD (1988): The role of L3T4+ and Lyt2+ T cells in the IgE response and immunity to *Nippostrongylus brasiliensis*. J Immunol 140:3206.

Kelly EAB, Cruz ES, Hauda KM, Wassom EL (1991): IFN-γ and IL-5–producing cells compartmentalize to different lymphoid organs in *Trichinella spiralis*-infected mice. J Immunol 147:306.

Kobayashi M, Fitz L, Ryan M, Hewick RM, Clark SC, Chan S, Loudon R, Sherman F, Perussia B, Trinchieri G (1989): Identification and purification of natural killer cell stimulatory factor (NKSF), a cytokine with multiple biological effects on human lymphocytes. J Exp Med 170:827.

Korenaga M, Hitoshi Y, Yamaguchi N, Sato Y, Takatsu K, Tada I (1991): The role of interleukin-5 in protective immunity to *Strongyloides venezuelensis* infection in mice. Immunol 72:502.

Kühn R, Rajewsky K, Müller W (1991): Generation and analysis of interleukin-4 deficient mice. Science 254:707.

Le Gros G, Ben-Sasson SZ, Seder R, Finkelman FD, Paul WE (1990): Generation of interleukin 4-producing cells in vivo and in vitro: IL-2 and IL-4 are required for in vitro generation of IL-4 producing cells. J Exp Med 172:921.

Lichtman AH, Kurt-Jones EA, Abbas AK (1987): B cell stimulatory factor 1 and not interleukin 2 is the autocrine growth factor for some helper T lymphocytes. Proc Natl Acad Sci USA 84:824.

Liew FY, Li Y, Millott S (1990): Tumor necrosis factor-α synergizes with IFN-γ in mediating killing of *Leishmania major* through the induction of nitric oxide. J Immunol 143:4306.

Locksley R, Heinzel F, Loladay B, Mutha S, Reiner S, Sadick M (1991): Induction of Th1 and Th2 CD4 subsets during murine L. *major* infection. Res Immunol 142:2832.

Madden KB, Urban JF Jr, Ziltener HJ, Schrader JW, Finkelman FD, Katona IM (1991): Antibodies to IL-3 and IL-4 suppress helminth-induced intestinal mastocytosis. J Immunol 147:1387.

Manetti R, Parronchi P, Giudizi MG, Piccinni M-P, Maggi E, Trinchieri G, Romagnani S (1993): Natural killer cell stimulatory factor (Interleukin 12 (IL-12)) induces T helper type 1 (Th1)-specific immune responses and inhibits the development of IL-4-producing Th cells. J Exp Med 177:1199.

Pond L, Wassom DL, Hayes CE (1989): Evidence for differential induction of helper T cell subsets during *Trichinella spiralis* infection. J Immunol 143:4232.

Rose ME, Wakelin D, Hesketh P (1989): Gamma interferon controls *Eimeria vermiformis* primary infection in BALB/c mice. Infect Immun 7:1599.

Seder RA, Paul WE, Dvorak AM, Sharkis SJ, Kagey-Sobotka A, Niv Y, Finkelman FD, Barbieri SA, Galli SJ, Plaut M (1991): Mouse splenic and bone marrow cell populations that express high affinity Fcϵ receptors and produce IL-4 are highly enriched in basophils. Proc Natl Acad Sci USA 88:2835.

Suzuki Y, Orellana MA, Schreiber RD, Remington JS (1988): Interferon-gamma: The major mediator of resistance against *Toxoplasma gondii*. Science 240:516.

Svetic' A, Madden KB, di Zhou X, Lu P, Katona IM, Finkelman FD, Urban JF Jr, Gause WC (1993): A primary intestinal helminthic infection rapidly induces a gut-associated elevation of Th2-associated cytokines and IL-3. J Immunol 150:3434.

Swain SL, Weinberg AD, English M, Huston G (1990):0 IL-4 directs the development of Th2-like helper effectors. J Immunol 145:3796.

Urban JF Jr, Katona IM, Finkelman FD (1991a): *Heligmosomoides polygyrus*: CD4$^+$ but not CD8$^+$ T cells regulate the IgE response and protective immunity in mice. Exp Parasitol 73:500.

Urban JF Jr, Katona IM, Paul WE, Finkelman FD (1991b): Interleukin 4 is important in protective immunity to a gastrointestinal nematode infection in mice. Proc Natl Acad Sci USA 88:5513.

Urban JF Jr, Madden KB, Cheever AW, Trotta PP, Katona IM, Finkelman FD (1993): Interferon inhibits inflammatory responses and protective immunity in mice infected with the nematode parasite, *Nippostrongylus brasiliensis*. J Immunol 151:7086.

Walsh JA (1984): In K.J.S. Warreen, A.A.F Mahmoud (eds): *Tropical and Geographical Medicine*. New York: McGraw-Hill, pp. 1073–1085.

Molecular Approaches to Parasitology, pages 477–496
© 1995 Wiley-Liss, Inc.

Immunobiology of Trypanosomiasis: A Revisionist View

John M. Mansfield

Laboratory of Immunology, Department of Animal Health & Biomedical Sciences, University of Wisconsin, Madison, Wisconsin 53706

INTRODUCTION

The central immunological paradigm of African trypanosomiasis is one in which host antibody responses to parasite antigen are pitted against trypanosome antigenic variation, with the parasites evading destruction. This paradigm now is undergoing expansive if not dramatic re-evaluation, as recent discoveries from this and other laboratories concerning trypanosome–macrophage–T-cell interactions have focused attention on events other than antibodies and antigenic variation. The purpose of this chapter is to present some of these new findings in an historical context and to demonstrate how the results are changing our understanding of the disease process of African trypanosomiasis.

THE PARADIGM

The rather static paradigm that has persisted now for several decades is that infected hosts make B-cell responses to the trypanosome variant surface glycoprotein (VSG), an immunodominant surface antigen that covers the parasite plasma membrane; this immune response results in control of parasitemia. However, trypanosomes have the remarkable ability to undergo transcriptional switching of VSG genes, thereby displaying antigenically distinct VSG surface coats to the host immune system and escaping immune elimination (Cross, 1990; Mansfield, 1990). This interplay of host VSG-specific immunity and trypanosome antigenic variation leads to the archetypal fluctuating parasitemias associated with chronic African trypanosomiasis. What the paradigm has not addressed, however, is the biological relevance of such responses in the context of genetically based resistance to disease and the host or parasite factors that may modulate or regulate such responses. The findings and speculations presented below address these issues and largely are from my own research;

as such, results are presented here as part of a personal, but probably very representative, odyssey in the field of trypanosome immunology.

HERESY: GENETICS STUDIES REVEAL MECHANISMS OF RESISTANCE TO TRYPANOSOMES THAT ARE NOT LINKED TO VSG SPECIFIC ANTIBODY RESPONSES

The odyssey had its beginnings in two separate (we thought) major questions that were being addressed in our laboratory: First, are VSG specific B-cell responses and the subsequent control of parasitemia linked functionally and genetically to the expression of host resistance? Second, what cellular and molecular factors regulate host B-cell responses to VSG determinants? An emphasis on VSG-specific B-cell responses in our work, and in the work of many others, was not unexpected, since it was generally accepted that the VSG antibody response is critical to host survival and that the VSG molecule itself displays biological properties that may influence host immune function (Levine and Mansfield, 1984; Morrison and Murray, 1985; Musoke and Barbett, 1977; Tizard et al., 1978; Mathias et al., 1990). In addressing the first major question, some important background information must be presented (reviewed by Mansfield, 1990): 1) There are demonstrable, genetically based differences in the abilities of infected animals to control infection with African trypanosomes; 2) there are demonstrable, genetically based differences among animals in terms of their abilities to make VSG-specific B-cell responses that control parasitemias; and 3) there are demonstrable associations between the ability to mount strong VSG-specific B-cell responses that control parasitemia and the ability to display relative resistance.

To begin, experimental immunogenetic studies in this laboratory and elsewhere have demonstrated that non-MHC-linked "background" genes of the host determine relative resistance to infection in inbred mice when infections are initiated with genetically homogeneous trypanosome populations (Levine and Mansfield, 1981, 1984; DeGee and Mansfield, 1984; DeGee et al., 1988; Clayton, 1978; Morrison and Murray, 1979). Several model systems of human and animal trypanosomiasis have evolved from such studies, including the one used in this laboratory. We have observed a spectrum of relative resistance among inbred mouse strains infected with clones of the LouTat 1 serodeme of *Trypanosoma brucei rhodesiense* (Levine and Mansfield, 1981, 1984). At one end of the spectrum are relatively resistant mice (e.g., B10.BR mice; $H-2^k$) that survive for up to 70 days postinfection and exhibit many of the hallmarks of human trypanosomiasis, including fluctuating parasitemias. At the other end of the spectrum are relatively susceptible mice (e.g., C3H mice; $H-2^k$) that survive for less than 21 days postinfection and exhibit uncontrolled parasitemias. Also, many mouse strains (e.g., CBA mice; $H-2^k$) exhibit an intermediate form of resistance in which mice survive for 30–40 days postinfection with variable control of parasitemia. Our early observations on the immune status of resistant and susceptible mice revealed that resistant animals mounted very strong VSG-specific antibody responses during infection while the susceptible animals made no detectable, or very low, VSG antibody responses when infected. Thus, there was an apparent association between resistance status and immune responsiveness to VSG, and the link seemed obvious: Those animals that made more rapid and stronger VSG-specific antibody responses were those that were better able to control parasitemias; such control of the parasite burden ultimately determined how long the infected animal lived.

Closer scrutiny, however, revealed something quite unexpected. For example, in bone marrow cell transplantation studies in which semiallogeneic radiation chimeras were constructed between resistant and susceptible animals, we found a functional *dissociation* between the ability of chimeras to control parasitemia with VSG-specific B-cell responses and their ability to survive for a prolonged period of infection (DeGee and Mansfield, 1984). In the same study, we also observed that the cells or factors responsible for expression of resistance were both donor (bone marrow) derived and of recipient origin (radiation resistant). We confirmed these results by classic genetics analyses (DeGee et al., 1988). In these experiments, a genetic basis for resistance was shown by intergenic crosses between resistant and susceptible mouse strains in which susceptibility was found to be the dominant phenotype; multiple genes appeared to encode resistance traits, but no known linkage groups were identified. In contrast, host B-cell responses to epitopes of the trypanosome VSG surface coat and subsequent elimination of the predominant variant type were genetically dominant traits encoded by genes that were not linked to the genes encoding resistance. Finally, an examination of recombinant inbred mice in which the progenitor strains were resistant and susceptible strains confirmed that relative resistance and the ability to make VSG antibody responses were distinct elements. Taken together, the results revealed that control of parasitemia by VSG-specific antibody responses, *alone,* is an event not functionally or genetically linked to long-term survival following infection and that radiation-resistant cells or factors may play an important supplementary role in host resistance. The unexpected observations made in this laboratory have since been confirmed in separate approaches in several other laboratories (Greenblatt et al., 1985; Seed and Sechelski, 1989), and it is clear that host genes regulating VSG-specific B-cell responses are distinct from genes controlling cellular aspects of resistance during infection.

These results were quite surprising because of the weight of dogma regarding the demonstrated role for antibody to the VSG antigen in clearing parasites from the circulation of infected hosts and the suspected biological role of the VSG. While our findings seemed to suggest that the VSG molecule and antibody responses to it should be of little consequence in the infected host, this suggestion was tempered by several realizations: First, an important observation from all our studies was that the most resistant animals are those that inherit both the resistance phenotype *and* the ability to control parasitemias by making VSG-specific antibodies; and, second, once an animal is infected, supplemental or compensatory antibody-independent resistance mechanisms must play an additional role in controlling the infection. Thus, our results encouraged us to look for additional immune mechanisms that might be important in resistance, specifically those mechanisms associated with radiation-resistant cells that might result in extravascular (e.g., tissue) control of parasite growth or survival.

CONUNDRUM: A SEARCH FOR IMMUNE REGULATORY MECHANISMS GOVERNING VSG-SPECIFIC ANTIBODY RESPONSES

The second major question addressed the nature of regulatory elements controlling VSG-specific B-cell responses during infection; once again our results gave rise to unexpected answers. More importantly, the answers led to discoveries that since have tied together the two apparently different focuses of our work. First, as mentioned above, some animals are vigorous B-cell responders to VSGs and others are weaker responders or are unable to make a response at all after infection. We were interested not only in the regulatory events that permitted one mouse strain to respond but also in the events that inhibited the VSG response in a different strain. We began by addressing the former problem, in which we were seeking information on host immune regulatory events that controlled the vigorous stimulation of VSG-specific antibodies in infected responder animals. An early consideration was that perhaps the three-dimensional architecture of closely packed VSG homodimers in a surface coat structure would present patterns of repeating identical epitopes to the host immune system that might mimic the B-cell stimulatory activity of repeating epitopes on classic T-helper-cell–independent antigens. This was, in fact, found to be the case, since both athymic and thymus intact mice made significant VSG-specific B-cell responses when infected; furthermore, immunization of mice with soluble VSG molecules revealed that only the T-cell–sufficient mice were able to make B-cell responses to epitopes of these molecules (Mansfield et al., 1981; Reinitz and Mansfield, 1990). Thus, there was a clear difference in the ability of athymic mice to recognize epitopes presented in the context of a surface coat VSG multiplex on viable cells versus VSG epitopes presented as monomers or homodimers in the absence of a surface coat superstructure.

Several additional interesting features emerged from the experiments with athymic and thymus intact animals. First, the B-cell responses of T-cell–sufficient mice to the VSG surface coat displayed by viable trypanosomes were always much greater than the B-cell responses of T-cell–deficient mice; part of this difference was attributed to higher antibody titers in the T-dependent responses and to the presence of IgG in addition to IgM in this response. Thus, there were quantitative and qualitative differences in the VSG-specific B-cell responses of mice with T cells compared with the responses of mice without T cells. Second, if we preserved the VSG surface architecture but killed the trypanosomes by mild fixation techniques and injected these cells into mice, only the mice with T cells could make a VSG antibody response. Since some T-independent antigens provide a critical second signal to B cells in addition to the display of repeated epitopes, we suspected that viable trypanosomes must release B-cell costimulatory factor(s) that help stimulate the T-independent response. Third, not all variants of the LouTat 1 serodeme exhibited the capacity to induce a T-independent B-cell response in infected animals; whether this was due to an altered surface coat three-dimensional structure or to other features of these variants such as the lack of production of B-cell costimulatory factors was not determined. Fourth, in both thymus intact and athymic mice we always detected significant levels of antibody in preinfection or preimmune sera to VSG determinants. This latter observation melded with related observations of Müller et al. (1994) in which they demonstrated that "naturally occurring" VSG specific antibody was not only present in the sera of uninfected mice (including germ-free mice), humans, and cattle but that this antibody was reactive with several VSG molecules in a variant-specific manner. Furthermore, when the naturally occurring antibody was affinity purified on VSG substrates, the eluted antibody was found to cross-react with host cell antigens. Thus, variant-specific antibody to trypanosome VSG molecules *pre-exists* in the potential mammalian host, and this antibody may represent naturally occurring autoantibody to cellular determinants. This finding has raised the question of why trypanosomes would retain variant surface antigens for which pre-existing antibody is present in a potential host. The current speculation is that CD5[+] B cells may be the source of this cross-reactive autoantibody and that the trypanosome may benefit directly or indirectly from the early stimulation of such B cells during an infection (Müller et al., 1994).

Overall, therefore, these aggregate results revealed that while part of the B-cell stimulatory response could be attributed to a T-independent configuration of exposed surface coat VSG epitopes and perhaps to the presence of self–VSG cross-reactive B cells, much of the response was apparently T dependent. Since there was this indirect evidence for Th cell responses to the VSG molecule during infection, we and other investigators looked intently for VSG-specific T cells in infected animals but failed to find convincing evidence (Paulnock et al., 1989; Flynn et al., 1992). Thus, given the lack of direct evidence for such Th cell responses, we examined other possibilities for regulation of host B-cell responses during infection. One such possibility was regulation within the context of an idiotypic network. To this end, we made a series of monoclonal antibodies to the VSG and characterized not only the partial epitope specificity of the antibodies but also the idiotypic specificities associated with V_H regions of these antibodies (Theodos et al., 1990). Subsequently, we demonstrated that antibodies with the same VSG epitope specificity as the monoclonals were produced during infection and that a subset of such antibodies exhibited the same idiotypic specificities as the model monoclonals. We then analyzed the levels of defined VSG antibody-associated idiotype in serum and tried to correlate modulations in the levels of such idiotypes with anti-idiotypic regulatory responses of infected mice. While we did not detect anti-idiotypic responses during the period of upregulation of VSG-specific responses, we were able to detect anti-idiotypic responses that seemed to be expressed in concert with the period of idiotypic downregulation during infection (Theodos and Mansfield, 1990).

Therefore, while downregulation of VSG-specific B-cell responses may be associated with elements of an anti-idiotypic response during infection, the host elements responsible for upregulation of T-dependent components of this immune response were not detectable despite the indirect evidence for participation of Th cells. Yet, additional indirect evidence for Th-cell responses to trypanosome VSG could be obtained from sequence analyses of VSG molecules that also suggested stimulation of VSG-specific T cells. One of the unusual characteristics of trypanosome VSG molecules is that they exhibit a highly conserved tertiary structure plus conserved secondary structural elements, as shown by x-ray crytallographic studies and by an examination of molecules for certain structural motifs; these conserved structural features exist despite evidence for extensive variation in the primary amino acid sequences of such molecules (Metcalf et al., 1987; Freymann et al., 1990; Down et al., 1991). Earlier, we had examined the primary sequence of the LouTat 1 VSG molecule in relationship to many other VSG molecules and found that a consensus sequence could be obtained (Reinitz et al., 1992). The conserved elements were suspected to be important in maintaining the tertiary structure of the molecules, as suggested by Wiley and coworkers (see Freymann et al., 1990). Our sequence analysis also revealed the presence of highly *non*conserved regions within VSG molecules that perhaps represented sub-sequences associated with potential variant-specific B- and T-cell epitopes of the molecule. Of interest was the observation, based on comparisons with VSG crystal structure data, that many of these potential epitope sites were probably buried within the VSG molecule as it normally is displayed on the trypanosome membrane. One type of evolutionary pressure that may generate or maintain such internal variable sites could be VSG-specific Th-cell responses rather than B-cell responses, since these sites would not be exposed to antibodies on viable organisms with an intact surface coat, but that potentially could be processed from the shed VSG to induce Th-cell responses. More recently Wiley, Turner, and colleagues (see Blum et al., 1993) capitalized on newer information that classifies VSGs into subfamilies based on N-terminal motifs, as well as on information generated from additional VSG crystal structure data, to derive a much more complete and appropriate VSG consensus sequence. A prominent feature of their analysis is the presence of many potential nonexposed variable region sequences that may be associated with Th-cell reactivity; they formally propose that the selective pressure to maintain such sites may be to avoid recognition by Th cells to common VSG determinants during infection. A final bit of indirect structural evidence is that we have subjected several of our LouTat 1 serodeme VSG sequences, as well as other VSG sequences, to analyses that predict T-cell epitope motifs based on primary and secondary structural features. These analyses reveal that VSG molecules are rich in potential T-cell epitope reactive sites.

BREAKTHROUGH: DIRECT EVIDENCE FOR VSG SPECIFIC T HELPER CELLS IN TRYPANOSOME INFECTED ANIMALS

Thus, several discrete lines of information from immunological studies of infected or immunized mice as well as structural analyses of VSG molecules predicted that trypanosome-infected animals may make Th-cell responses to the surface coat antigen of trypanosomes in a variant-specific manner. The inability to demonstrate such responses in the peripheral lymphoid organs of infected animals, however, was discouraging. In a desperate intellectual leap we reasoned that *if* VSG-specific T-cell responses were being induced, perhaps such responses might be suppressed during infection; one of the prime candidates for such suppression could be the suppressor macrophages that are well known to be associated with depression of mitogen- and antigen-specific T-cell responses in trypanosomiasis (Mansfield et al., 1981; Wellhausen and Mansfield, 1979, 1980; Askonas, 1985; Darji et al., 1992; Borowy et al., 1990). Support for this line of reasoning came from earlier studies in which we and others had shown that animals could be immunized, in the absence of infection, to produce VSG-specific T-cell responses; alternatively, animals could be drug-cured of active infection to reveal the emergence of VSG-specific T-cell responses in peripheral lymphoid organs (Paulnock et al., 1989). As it turned out, our reasoning was only partially correct, and the breakthrough in this puzzle occurred quite by accident.

We were examining macrophages from LouTat 1–infected mice for activation-specific gene markers when we included some left-over peritoneal cells with spleen and lymph node cells in (yet another) assay for VSG-specific stimulation of T cells. The results of this experiment were identical to many other earlier tests for VSG-specific stimulation in that proliferative responses to the VSG molecule were not evident in any cell population, including the peritoneal cells. Similarly, no IL-2 or IL-4 responses to VSG were detected in the spleen or lymph node cells. The surprising result, however, was that peritoneal T cells made a strong cytokine secretory response to VSG; this response was mediated entirely by a CD4$^+$ T-cell subpopulation in an antigen-specific manner, was characterized by IL-2 but not IL-4 production, and occurred within several days of exposure to a specific variant type (Schleifer et al., 1993). An additional functional feature of the peritoneal T-cell response to VSG was the secretion of high levels of IFN-γ. Cytokine responses were not detectable in other lymphoid tissues of infected animals, with one exception: spleen and lymph node CD4$^+$ T cells were subsequently also found to produce IFN-γ, but not IL-2 or IL-4, in response to VSG. This response was found to be more variable than the peritoneal T-cell response and also varied somewhat depending on the infecting variant antigenic type and the duration of infection.

Thus, we demonstrated directly for the first time the existence of VSG-specific T-helper cells in trypanosome-infected animals (Schleifer et al., 1993). The surprising results were that these T-cell responses largely were compartmentalized to the peritoneum, with perhaps a reactive subpopulation in other lymphoid organs, and that these T cells made a cytokine secretory but not a proliferative response to specific antigen. It is important to emphasize that neither the route of infection nor the VSG isotype was important in determining these patterns. For example, we have examined individual mice infected with one LouTat serodeme variant type, which make a T-cell response to the VSG of that type, for the emergence of other known LouTat variants, and we have tested them for evidence of T-cell responses to the new variants. The same patterns of T-cell responsiveness and apparent compartmentalization to newly arising variants were observed as to the infecting variant type. Furthermore, intrinsic molecular characteristics of VSG molecules per se did not selectively induce immune response patterns of this type. For example, if mice were immunized with VSG instead of being exposed to VSG by infection, a different pattern emerged. Immunized mice produced VSG-specific Th cells in all lymphoid tissues that responded to specific VSG with both proliferative and cytokine secretory responses (IL-2, IFN-γ, and IL-4).

The membrane phenotype and MHC restriction profiles of T cells from infected animals were also compared with VSG-reactive T cells derived from immunized mice (Schleifer et al., 1993). As noted above, the VSG responsive T-cell populations of infected mice segregated with the CD4$^+$ but not CD8$^+$ T cells. When VSG-specific T-cell lines derived from infected and immunized mice were compared, all lines expressed the Thy 1$^+$, CD4$^+$, CD8$^-$, CD3$^+$, α/β

TCR$^+$, γ/δ TCR$^-$ membrane phenotype. The cytokine profiles were different, however: T lines derived from infected mice all secreted high levels of IL-2 and IFN-γ but not IL-4, while the T lines from immunized mice were mixed, with some secreting IL-2 and IFN-γ but not IL-4, some secreting IL-4 but not IL-2 and IFN-γ, and one line secreting IL-2, IFN-γ, and IL-4. Thus, T cells and T lines derived from infected mice appeared to represent exclusively a Th1-cell subset specific for VSG determinants. In contrast, T cells and lines from immunized mice represented a more diverse T-cell response in which both Th1- and Th2-cell subsets with VSG reactivity were generated. A number of VSG-specific T clones representing the Th1 phenotype have also been derived and studied with respect to their MHC restriction in terms of antigen recognition. The T-cell clones, like all of the T lines and also T cells from infected or immunized mice, were dependent on antigen-presenting cells (APC); all of the T clones tested to date are I-A^k restricted (B10.BR mice [H-2^k] were the source of the T-cell lines and clones generated). Thus, VSG-stimulated T cells represent classic Th cells that are antigen specific and MHC Class II restricted (Schleifer et al., 1993).

NEW QUESTIONS

Overall, these exciting results have provided a springboard for new investigations into antigen-specific T-cell stimulation and regulation in trypanosomiasis, control of B-cell immunoglobulin isotype expression, and examinations of VSG epitopes involved in T-cell recognition. The results have also led to new questions concerning the immunobiology of African trypanosomiasis. Several of these questions are explored here.

First, the apparent anatomical compartmentalization of VSG-reactive Th cells is puzzling. One factor that may account for the peritoneal localization of these T cells is preferential uptake or processing of the VSG molecule by B-cell or macrophage APC at this site. We know that APC derived from spleen and lymph nodes, as well as the peritoneum, can process and present appropriate VSG determinants in an MHC II–restricted manner to T cells in vitro, but we do not yet know if this occurs naturally in the course of infection. Also, if CD5$^+$ B cells, which are found in relatively high numbers in the peritoneum, play an early role in recognition of VSG molecules during infection (Müller et al., 1994), it may be that these cells preferentially are serving as APC for the T cells or may be producing factors important for Th1 cell maturation at that site; however, one such CD5 B cell factor may be IL-10, which we have not found to be upregulated in infection and which would have effects different from those that we have seen in terms of both macrophage activation (see below) and Th1 maturation. Alternatively, early activation of other peritoneal B cells or macrophages by trypanosome constituents at this site may provide for elements responsible for both early T-cell stimulation and Th1 maturation (see below). Another possibility is that activated T cells are retained within the peritoneum by adhesin or selectin interactions with other cell(s) present at that site. A third possibility is that there is some unique component of trypanosome biology involving the peritoneum. Support for this suggestion is derived from the work of Albright et al. (1990), who have determined with the nonpathogenic mouse trypanosomes that the peritoneum may be a specialized site for trypanosome replication. While there is yet no evidence for such site-specific cell division in the African trypanosomes, there may be some other special biological interaction of trypanosomes with host cells in the peritoneum that remains unseen. Overall, the question of anatomical compartmentalization of emerging parasite antigen-specific Th1-cell responses is being addressed along the lines of research discussed here.

Another question relates to the role of VSG-specific Th 1-subtype cells in promoting the T-dependent B-cell responses to VSG determinants. The cytokines produced by these T cells are IL-2 and IFN-γ without evidence, even at the transcriptional level by RT-PCR analysis, for IL-4 production (Schleifer et al., 1993; Schopf et al., 1994). We also have examined mice for the production of other cytokines associated with the Th2-cell type, such as IL-5, and have detected no evidence for such activity. The levels of IFN-γ produced during infection are quite high, sufficient that very high levels can be detected in the sera of infected mice, as we have shown (DeGee et al. 1985), and there are always detectable background IFN-γ transcripts seen in the cells from infected mice. Presumably the IFN-γ is derived from peritoneal and spleen CD4 T cells responding to VSG and other trypanosome antigens, but some may be produced by CD8 T cells that are suspected as serving as antigen *non*specific targets for the hypothetical trypanosome T-cell-activating factor described by Kristensson and colleagues (see Olsson et al., 1993). Given the high levels of IFN-γ and the absence of detectable IL-4 in our experimental system, we would expect that the predominant IgG isotypes of VSG-specific antibodies to be IgG2a and IgG3, but not IgG1 or IgE, based on the known isotype switching patterns associated with specific cytokines. Once again, the trypanosome provides a surprise: The predominant patterns were very high levels of VSG-specific IgG1 and IgG3 with no detectable IgG2a; there also is no detectable IgE (Schopf et al., 1994). This isotype pattern appears largely to be independent of the VSG type displayed by infecting trypanosomes, with the exception that some variants provoke somewhat lower IgG3 levels and a level of detectable IgG2b. We believe that we have ruled out cryptic Th2 responses to the VSG that might account for the IgG1 levels observed; there is evidence from other biological systems for IL-4 *in*dependent IgG1 production that may be applicable in our system as well. However, the unexpected absence of an IgG2a response in the presence of high IFN-γ levels may be indicative of suppression of the IgG2a switch mechanism. One potential explanation for these immunoglobulin isotype patterns may be alternative isotype switch patterns initiated by cytokines or monokines released from other cell types as the result of interaction with trypanosome constituents. For example, previous work by Diffley (see Mathias et al., 1990) has revealed that VSG transcriptionally upregulates IL-1 expression in macrophages; we have confirmed this and show, additionally, that IL-6 is also upregulated in macrophages exposed to trypanosomes or their extracts. Furthermore, Romani and her colleagues have demonstrated that animals immunized with nonviable trypanosomes make high levels of IL-6 (see Perito et al., 1992); it is possible that some of the IL-6 is macrophage derived. Taken together, we suspect that IL-1, IL-6, and perhaps other cytokines such as TNFα produced directly or indirectly by trypanosome-stimulated cells may be responsible for inducing B-cell growth and promoting alternative immunoglobulin switch patterns seen during this disease. This speculation is supported by results from mice that have been immunized with nonviable trypanosomes or trypanosome extracts and mice immunized with VSG: Despite the induction of VSG-specific Th1 and Th2 cells under these circumstances, the immunoglobulin isotype patterns of VSG-specific antibodies are very similar to those obtained during infection in which a more limited T-cell response is obtained (Schopf et al., 1994).

Another major question arising from these studies is what mechanism induced by infection permits VSG-stimulated T cells to make a cytokine response but inhibits the proliferative response. This question was answered by re-evaluating results from earlier studies on suppressor macrophages that we had published years ago (Mansfield et al., 1981; Paulnock et al., 1989; Wellhausen and Mansfield, 1979, 1980). As mentioned above, suppressor macrophages are a well-known feature of African trypanosomiasis and are associated with the depression of antigen-nonspecific T-cell responses in infected animals. In preliminary tests, we asked whether macrophages from infected mice could inhibit the responses of VSG-specific T cells from immunized mice or the VSG-specific T-cell lines. Tests showed that the addition of macrophages from infected but not uninfected mice to cell cultures resulted in the suppression of T-cell proliferative responses to VSG, but that the same cells did not affect, or in some cases enhanced, the T-cell cytokine responses to VSG. Thus, infected macrophages were able to transfer to immune T cells the effects seen when stimulating cell cultures from infected mice: inhibition of proliferation but induction of cytokine secretion.

This discovery prompted us to re-examine some of the cell biological features of trypanosome-infected mouse macrophages. As we and others had reported previously, infected macrophages express many macrophage activation characteristics, including elevated expression of MHC class II antigens, IL-1 and IL-6 production, upregulation of TNFα and prostaglandin (PG) secretion

(Mathias and Diffley, 1990; Paulnock et al., 1989; Grosskinsky and Askonas, 1981; Fierer et al., 1984; Grosskinsky et al., 1983). These results are not surprising given the levels of IFN-γ induced by trypanosome infection and the known activating effects of this cytokine on macrophages. We also found that the inducible nitric oxide synthase (iNOS) gene was transcriptionally upregulated in macrophages isolated from infected mice and that these cells were releasing significant amounts of nitric oxide (NO) compared with uninfected macrophages (Schleifer and Mansfield, 1993). Since NO has a number of important effector and chemical messenger functions that influence brain, blood vessel, immune system, and other physiological functions, we asked whether this molecule might play a direct or indirect role in the observed T-cell suppression in trypanosomiasis. Of interest was the fact that others had recently demonstrated a suppressive effect of macrophage-derived NO on T-cell responses to mitogens and antigens (Mills, 1991; Albina et al., 1991), in which the principal effect was on T-cell proliferation (Fu and Blankenhorn, 1992). Furthermore, IFN-γ is one of the key cytokines in upregulating the iNOS gene and inducing NO synthesis, and we knew that trypanosome-infected mice made strong IFN-γ responses.

Suspecting parallels, then, between those model systems of suppression and our model system of trypanosome-induced suppressor macrophages, we inhibited NO synthesis by treatment of infected cells and suppressor cell cultures with L-arginine analogs such as L-NMMA and AG. The results showed that NO production was depressed in treated cells and that both immunosuppression and suppressor cell effects were partially inhibited by treatment with the analogs as well as with other NO preventive agents. Furthermore, we demonstrated that the principal effect of treatment was on restoration of the proliferative responses of T cells to mitogen, superantigen, anti-CD3, and trypanosome VSG, with only minor enhancing effects on the existent cytokine responses of the cultures. Thus, NO was revealed to be responsible for at least part of the suppression and the suppressor cell effect in trypanosomiasis (Schleifer and Mansfield, 1993). However, we also suspected that PG may play a supplementary role in macrophage-induced suppression since we found that infected macrophages were secreting elevated levels of these compounds and since others had shown earlier that such activated macrophages produced PG (Darji et al., 1992; Fierer et al., 1984). Even though treatment of infected cell cultures with PG inhibitors such as indomethacin alone had no demonstrable effect, as we had shown previously (Wellhausen and Mansfield, 1980), we found that the simultaneous inhibition of both NO *and* PG synthesis using appropriate inhibitors resulted in complete abolition of the suppressor cell activity, thus revealing an epistatic effect mediated by NO and PG (Schleifer and Mansfield, 1993). IFN-γ was found to be the major factor responsible for induction of iNOS transcription, NO and PG secretion, and suppressor cell effects in our study, with TNFα perhaps playing a highly variable but supplementary role at different times of infection. However, despite the fact that we could reverse suppression in the early weeks of trypanosome infection by inhibiting NO and PG synthesis, we found that such treatments did not affect suppression in later stages of the disease. Therefore, other suppressive elements may be induced in long-term or chronic disease. During the tenure of our study, a short communication by Sternberg and McGuigan (1992) appeared that described the ability of L-arginine analogs partially to restore the mitogen responses of suppressed T cells in trypanosome-infected mice; thus, our work both confirmed and complemented their results by demonstrating that not only was NO involved in suppression of T-cell responses in trypanosomiasis but also that this molecule interacted with effects of PG early in infection. The role of IFN-γ in inducing the suppressor cell effects seen was also clearly elucidated in our work, thus making a complete picture in terms of activation of the suppressor cell phenotype during early infection. At the moment we are investigating the means by which NO may selectively inhibit the proliferative but not the cytokine secretory responses of VSG-specific T cells, including analyses of guanylate cyclase activation, ADP ribosyltransferase activity, and effects on ribonucleotide reductase.

T CELLS AND MACROPHAGES: A CELLULAR BASIS FOR RESISTANCE?

The studies described above are the first to define a molecular basis for immunosuppression in African trypanosomiasis. It is now clear that trypanosome antigen-stimulated $CD4^+$ Th1 cells (and, potentially, $CD8^+$ T cells stimulated by an uncharacterized trypanosome factor) produce IFN-γ that serves to activate macrophages and induce the suppressor cell mechanism. One of the products of activated macrophages, NO, is known not only to be involved in T-cell suppression but also to have potent antimicrobial effects on both intra- and extracellular microorganisms. Given that not only does one observe high IFN-γ levels and elevated numbers of activated macrophages in trypanosomiasis but also the release of NO by macrophages in many host tissues, we asked whether NO might not play a role supplementary to the VSG-specific B-cell response in providing resistance to trypanosomes. We again recalled the surprising results of our earlier transplantation and genetics studies, described above, in which we determined that VSG-specific antibody alone was insufficient to provide relative resistance to trypanosomes and in which we suggested that a radiation-resistant cell (macrophage?) may provide a supplementary tissue-based resistance mechanism.

Therefore, we initiated a series of experiments to determine whether one of the major products of activated macrophages in disease, NO, exhibited any trypanocidal or trypanostatic effects. Our approach was twofold: In one we cocultured viable trypanosomes with VSG-reactive T cells plus infected macrophages and examined the cell cultures for NO levels and trypanosome survival; in the other approach, we cocultured trypanosomes with a macrophage cell line in the presence or absence of rIFN-γ. Both experimental approaches revealed that LouTat 1 trypanosomes were exquisitely sensitive to NO and died in culture a short period of time after NO was present (Filutowicz and Mansfield, 1994). The addition of either L-NMMA or anti-IFN-γ to cultures not only inhibited NO release but also prevented the cytotoxic effect on trypanosomes. Thus, NO induction in macrophages by T-cell products may represent a major tissue-associated resistance mechanism in trypanosomiasis that controls extravascular parasites and supplements the ability of VSG-specific antibodies to control bloodstream parasites.

However, like all investigations in trypanosomiasis, discordant results soon appeared. In a recent paper by Vincendeau and colleagues (1992), NO is shown to be cytostatic but not cytotoxic for trypanosomes. In contrast Sternberg and McGuigan (1992) relate unpublished results that NO has no effect on trypanosomes. We believe, in fact, that *each* set of observations is correct, as explained below. Our laboratory is involved in studies unrelated to the central topics of this chapter in which we are cloning and characterizing trypanosome virulence genes (Inverso et al., 1988; Uphoff et al., 1994). The model system that we have developed is one in which two trypanosome populations, LouTat 1 and LouTat 1A, are compared and contrasted. One trypanosome clone, LouTat 1, produces chronic infections and kills the infected host approximately 2 months postinfection. The other trypanosome, LouTat 1A, is a subclone of LouTat 1 that will kill the same infected host strain in approximately 72 hours postinfection. Both organisms express the same VSG gene and surface coat, but there are a number of defined chromosomal, protein, RNA, and gene activation, as well as functional, differences. With respect to the latter, we have found that LouTat 1 is highly susceptible to the cytotoxic effects of NO, yet LouTat 1A appears to be completely resistant (Filutowicz and Mansfield, 1994). One potential subcellular target for NO is mitochondrial respiration; one major difference between LouTat 1 and LouTat 1A is that only LouTat 1 differentiates into the intermediate and short stumpy trypanosome forms that have a functional mitochondrion. The differences in trypanosome susceptibility to NO observed in the three sets of studies, then, may reflect similar functional variability. Thus, biological variation among trypanosomes that is independent of VSG gene expression may play a key role in susceptibility to different host resistance mechanisms.

Of course, a major and somewhat critical new question now emerges. That is, does macrophage activation by cytokines from parasite antigen-stimulated T cells result in a level of resistance that is independent of the effects of VSG-specific B-cell responses? Our current work is aimed at testing this hypothesis by determining whether these events are functionally and genetically linked to host resistance in animals that do not make VSG-specific antibodies. While preliminary results are supportive, we fully expect that the trypanosome will once again provide abundant surprises.

OVERVIEW

In order to leave the reader with a more cogent view of our results and the speculations leading from them, we present the themes shown in Figures 1 and 2 as an overview of innate and immune events that may be important in resistance to trypanosomes. In Figure 1, we suggest that trypanosome antigens such as the VSG are taken up and processed by APC such as macrophages to present relevant peptides in the context of class II MHC molecules to responder Th cells of the Th1 subtype. The subsequent stimulation of T cells leads to the secretion of IL-2 and IFN-γ, with the major biological effect being macrophage activation. The activated macrophages secrete NO (and

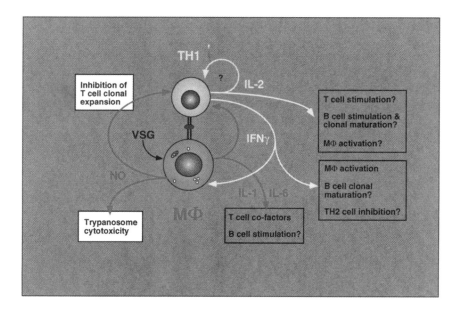

Fig. 1.   Possible outcomes of exposure to trypanosome antigens.

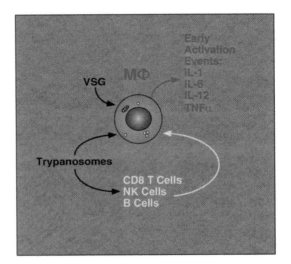

Fig. 2. Possible early events in trypanosomiasis.

PG, among other activation-associated factors), which has two principal biological effects: cytotoxic effects on trypanosomes and inhibition of T-cell proliferation. The effects of the various cytokines and monokines depicted here impinge not only on T cells and trypanosomes but also are envisioned to impact on B-cell activation and clonal differentiation, which ultimately results in the patterns of parasite antigen-specific B-cell regulation seen.

One might predict that these events would occur in a cyclical manner, whenever trypanosomes or their shed products are present in high concentrations in the blood and other tissues. The results of such T-cell stimulation and macrophage activation would affect parasites directly, via NO-mediated cytotoxicity occurring primarily in extravascular tissue sites or, indirectly, via B-cell costimulation and regulation to produce VSG-specific antibodies that would control parasites in the blood.

Of course, the events depicted in Figure 1 cannot be expected to occur de novo upon infection. Rather, the events are perceived to be those occurring after the infection has produced sufficient activated Th cells capable of secreting levels of IFN-γ that can maintain macrophage activation. Clearly, something must promote this cycle of events very early in infection; otherwise, one would be able to detect significant T-cell proliferation at some point during exposure to the first infecting variant type, which we do not. And, one should detect some level of early Th2-cell stimulation by parasite antigens, which, again, we do not. In Figure 2, then, we present what we believe to be the early events in trypanosomiasis. We suggest that trypanosome-derived products directly induce several key cytokines in critical target cells. We envision that target macrophages (or perhaps B cells or other cells) are stimulated upon exposure to trypanosomes to upregulate a subset of genes; these include IL-1, IL-6, TNFα, and, perhaps more importantly, IL-12. IL-12 is known to have several important biological functions, among them the induction of Th1-cell subsets and the early regulation of IFN-γ expression. Thus, it may be that early exposure of macrophages to trypanosome stimulatory factor(s) sets into motion a sequence of events culminating in early or enhanced IFN-γ secretion by Th0 or Th1 cells; the early production of IFN-γ subsequently serves to promote or maintain activation associated events in macrophages. An alternative scenario may be that IL-12 induces IFN-γ production in natural killer cells. In any event, we recently have been able to detect the transcriptional upregulation of both the IL-12p40 gene and the IFN-γ gene in cells from WT and SCID mice infected for only 24 hours (unpublished observations); currently we are determining which cell types are responsible for these potentially very important early cytokine responses and whether the results are critical for evolution of the Th1-cell and macrophage activation responses that become established.

CONCLUSION

I have presented here a highly personal view of parasite-induced events in trypanosomiasis that is based largely on experimental observations in my laboratory and that perhaps does not consider all alternative models. The events depicted in Figures 1 and 2 are those we suspect are involved in determining a level of host resistance that is directed at trypanosomes in the extravascular tissue spaces and associated with macrophage activation. This type of resistance mechanism is perceived to be independent of the control of parasites in blood by VSG-specific antibody responses and is one that impinges on clonal events during T-cell activation. While the new paradigms that are emerging enlarge upon our understanding of trypanosome immunology, they now also raise new and exciting questions that address fundamental issues in immunology.

ACKNOWLEDGMENTS

The studies described in this chapter were supported by grants from the National Institutes of Health. The work was conducted by postdoctoral fellows, students, and research technicians; the most recent contributions of Kathy Schleifer, Lisa Schopf, and Hanna Filutowicz are highlighted. This chapter was presented, in part, as a lecture in the Biology of Parasitism course at Woods Hole, MA, in the summer of 1993. Elements in this chapter have also appeared in condensed form in a recent review by the author (Mansfield, 1994).

REFERENCES

Albina JE, Abate JA, Henry WL Jr (1991): Nitric oxide production is required for murine resident peritoneal macrophages to suppress mitogen-stimulated T cell proliferation. Role of IFNγ in the induction of the nitric oxide-synthesizing pathway. J Immunol 147:144.

Albright JW, Pierantoni M, Albright JF (1990): Immune and nonimmune regulation of the population of *Trypanosoma musculi* in infected host mice. Infect Immun 58:1757.

Askonas BA (1985): Macrophages as mediators of immunosuppression in murine African trypanosomiasis. Curr Top Microbiol Immunol 117:119.

Blum JL, Down JA, Gurnett AM, Carrington M, Turner MJ, Wiley DC (1993): A structural motif in the variant surface glycoproteins of *Trypanosoma brucei*. Nature 362:603.

Borowy NK, Sternberg JM, Schreiber D, Nonnengasser C, Overath P (1990): Suppressive macrophages occurring in murine *Trypanosoma brucei* infection inhibit T-cell responses in vivo and in vitro. Parasite Immunol 12:233.

Clayton CE (1978): Trypanosoma brucei: Influence of host strain and parasite antigenic type on infections in mice. Exp Parasitol 44:202.

Cross GAM (1990): Cellular and genetic aspects of antigenic variation in trypanosomes. Annu Rev Immunol 8:83.

Darji A, Lucas R, Magez S, Torreele E, Palacios J, Sileghem M, Bajyana Songa E, Hamers R, De Baetselier P (1992): Mechanisms underlying trypanosome-elicited immunosuppression. Ann Soc Belg Med Trop 72 (Suppl 1):27.

De Gee AL, Levine RF, Mansfield JM (1988): Genetics of resistance to the African trypanosomes. VI. Heredity of resistance and variable surface glycoprotein-specific immune responses. J Immunol 140:283.

De Gee AL, Mansfield JM (1984): Genetics of resistance to the African trypanosomes. IV. Resistance of radiation chimeras to *Trypanosoma rhodesiense* infection. Cell Immunol 87:85.

De Gee AL, Sonnenfeld G, Mansfield JM (1985): Genetics of resistance to the African trypanosomes. V. Qualitative and quantitative differences in interferon production among susceptible and resistant mouse strains. J Immunol 134:2723.

Down JA, Garman SC, Gurnett AM, Turner MJ, Wiley DC (1991): Crystallization and preliminary x-ray analysis of an intact soluble-form variant surface glycoprotein from the African trypanosome, *Trypanosoma brucei*. J Mol Biol 218:679.

Fierer J, Salmon JA, Askonas BA (1984): African trypanosomiasis alters prostaglandin production by murine peritoneal macrophages. Clin Exp Immunol 58:548.

Filutowicz H, Mansfield JM (1994): Macrophage-mediated cytotoxicity for the African trypanosomes: Role of IFN-gamma and nitric oxide. Submitted for publication.

Flynn JN, Sileghem M, Williams DJL (1992): Parasite-specific T-cell responses of trypanotolerant and trypanosusceptible cattle during infection with *Trypanosoma congolense*. Immunology 75:639.

Freymann D, Down J, Carrington M, Roditi I, Turner M, Wiley D (1990): 2·9 Å resolution structure of the N-terminal domain of a variant surface glycoprotein from *Trypanosoma brucei*. J Mol Biol 216:141.

Fu Y, Blankenhorn EP (1992): Nitric oxide-induced anti-mitogenic effects in high and low responder rat strains. J Immunol 148:2217.

Greenblatt HC, Potter TA, Rosenstreich DL (1985): Genetic control of natural resistance to *Trypanosoma rhodesiense:* Transfer of resistance with bone marrow or spleen cells. J Infect Dis 151:911.

Grosskinsky CM, Askonas BA (1981): Macrophages as primary target cells and mediators of immune dysfunction in African trypanosomiasis. Infect Immun 33:149.

Grosskinsky CM, Ezekowitz RA, Berton G, Gordon S, Askonas BA (1983): Macrophage activation in murine African trypanosomiasis. Infect Immun 39:1080.

Inverso JA, De Gee AL, Mansfield JM (1988): Genetics of resistance to the African trypanosomes. VII. Trypanosome virulence is not linked to variable surface glycoprotein expression. J Immunol 140:289.

Levine RF, Mansfield JM (1981): Genetics of resistance to African trypanosomes: Role of the H-2 locus in determining resistance to infection with *Trypanosoma rhodesiense*. Infect Immun 34:513.

Levine RF, Mansfield JM (1984): Genetics of resistance to the African trypanosomes. III. Variant-specific antibody responses of H-2-compatible resistant and susceptible mice. J Immunol 133:1564.

Mansfield JM (1990): Immunology of African trypanosomiasis. In D.J. Wyler (ed): Modern Parasite Biology: Cellular, Immunological and Molecular Aspects. New York: W.H. Freeman, p. 222.

Mansfield JM (1994): T-cell responses to the trypanosome variant surface glycoprotein: A new paradigm? Parasitol Today 10:267.

Mansfield JM, Levine RF, Dempsey WL, Wellhausen SR, Hansen CT (1981): Lymphocyte function in experimental African trypanosomiasis. IV. Immunosuppression and suppressor cells in the athymic nu/nu mouse. Cell Immunol 63:210.

Mathias S, Perez R, Diffley P (1990): The kinetics of gene expression and maturation of IL-1a after induction with the surface coat of *Trypanosoma brucei rhodesiense* or lipopolysaccharide. J Immunol 145:3450.

Metcalf P, Blum M, Freymann D, Turner M, Wiley DC (1987): Two variant surface glycoproteins of *Trypanosoma brucei* of different sequence classes have similar 6 Å resolution x-ray structures. Nature 325:84.

Mills CD (1991): Molecular basis of "suppressor macrophages": Arginine metabolism via the nitric oxide synthetase pathway. J Immunol 146:2719.

Morrison WI, Murray M (1979): *Trypanosoma congolense:* Inheritance of susceptibility to infection in inbred strains of mice. Exp Parasitol 48:364.

Morrison WI, Murray M (1985): The role of humoral immune responses in determining susceptibility of A/J and C57BL/6 mice to infection with *Trypanosoma congolense*. Parasite Immunol 7:63.

Muller N, Mansfield JM, Seebeck T (1994): Trypanosome variant surface glycoproteins are recognized by self-reactive CD5+ B cells in uninfected hosts. Submitted for publication.

Musoke AJ, Barbet AF (1977): Activation of complement by variant-specific surface antigen of *Trypanosoma brucei*. Nature 270:438.

Olsson T, Bakhiet M, Hojeberg B, Ljungdahl A, Edlund C, Andersson G, Ekre H-P, Fung-Leung W-P, Mak T, Wigzell H, Fiszer U, Kristensson K (1993): CD8 is critically involved in lymphocyte activation by a *T. brucei brucei*–released molecule. Cell 72:715.

Paulnock DM, Smith C, Mansfield JM (1989): Antigen presenting cell function in African trypanosomiasis. In L.B. Schook, J.G. Tew (eds): Antigen Presenting Cells: Diversity, Differentiation, and Regulation. New York: Alan R. Liss, Inc., p. 135.

Perito S, Calabresi A, Romani L, Puccetti P, Bistoni F (1992): Involvement of the Th1 subset of CD4+ T cells in acquired immunity to mouse infection with *Trypanosoma equiperdum*. Cell Immunol 143:261.

Reinitz DM, Aizenstein BD, Mansfield JM (1992): Variable and conserved structural elements of trypanosome variant surface glycoproteins. Mol Biochem Parasitol 51:119.

Reinitz DM, Mansfield JM (1990): T-cell–independent and T-cell–dependent B-cell responses to exposed variant surface glycoprotein epitopes in trypanosome-infected mice. Infect Immun 58:2337.

Schleifer KW, Filutowicz H, Schopf LR, Mansfield JM (1993): Characterization of T helper cell responses to the trypanosome variant surface glycoprotein. J Immunol 150:2910.

Schleifer KW, Mansfield JM (1993): Suppressor macrophages in African trypanosomiasis inhibit T cell proliferative responses by nitric oxide and prostaglandins. J Immunol 151:5492.

Schopf LR, Filutowicz H, Mansfield JM (1994): Regulation of B cell responses to the variant surface glycoprotein molecule in trypanosomiasis. III. Ig isotype profiles and Th cell cytokine patterns suggest alternative switch mechanisms. Submitted for publication.

Seed JR, Sechelski JB (1989): African trypanosomes: Inheritance of factors involved in resistance. Exp Parasitol 69:1.

Sternberg J, McGuigan F (1992): Nitric oxide mediates suppression of T cell responses in murine *Trypanosoma brucei* infection. Eur J Immunol 22:2741.

Theodos CM, Mansfield JM (1990): Regulation of B cell responses to the variant surface glycoprotein molecule in trypanosomiasis. II. Down-regulation of idiotype expression is associated with the appearance of lymphocytes expressing antiidiotypic receptors. J Immunol 144:4022.

Theodos CM, Reinitz DM, Mansfield JM (1990): Regulation of B cell responses to the variant surface glycoprotein (VSG) molecule in trypanosomiasis. I. Epitope specificity and idiotypic profile of monoclonal antibodies to the VSG of *Trypanosoma brucei rhodesiense*. J Immunol 144:4011.

Tizard I, Nielsen KH, Seed JR, Hall JE (1978): Biologically active products from African trypanosomes. Microbiol Rev 42:664.

Uphoff T, Inverso JA, Mansfield JM (1993): Virulence regulation is not linked to the VSG molecule or the VSG gene transcription site in African trypanosomes. Submitted for publication.

Vincendeau P, Daulouede S, Veyret B, Darde ML, Bouteille B, Lemesre JL (1992): Nitric oxide-mediated cytostatic activity on *Trypanosoma brucei gambiense* and *Trypanosoma brucei brucei*. Exp Parasitol 75:353.

Wellhausen SR, Mansfield JM (1979): Lymphocyte function in experimental African trypanosomiasis. II. Splenic suppressor cell activity. J Immunol 122:818.

Wellhausen SR, Mansfield JM (1980): Characteristics of the splenic suppressor cell–target cell interaction in experimental African trypanosomiasis. Cell Immunol 54:414.

Molecular Approaches to Parasitology, pages 497–510

The Immunology of Schistosomiasis

Edward J. Pearce

*Department of Microbiology, Immunology, and Parasitology, College of
Veterinary Medicine, Cornell University, Ithaca, New York 14853*

INTRODUCTION

Despite the availability of safe chemotherapy, more than 200 million people
and countless domestic animals continue to be infected with schistosomes. In
the majority of cases, human disease is due to one of three species: *Schistosoma
haematobium, S. japonicum,* or *S. mansoni* (Jordan and Webbe, 1982). Infection with these parasites is initiated when cercariae, aquatic larval stages, penetrate the skin and transform into schistosomula, which subsequently enter
the vasculature and migrate via the lungs to the hepatic portal system
(*S. mansoni* and *S. japonicum*) or the urogenital venules (*S. haematobium*). In
these sites, schistosomes reach sexual maturity at 4–6 weeks after infection,
and female parasites begin to lay eggs shortly thereafter (Jordan and Webbe,
1982). While some of the eggs pass through the intestinal or bladder wall, are
excreted, and continue the life cycle, many are swept by the blood flow into
the liver where they become trapped in the sinusoids. The granulomata that
subsequently form around the eggs precipitate most of the serious complications of schistosomiasis, including increased hepatic portal blood pressure
(due to a presinusoidal block in blood flow), the development of portosystemic
collaterals, and eventual periportal (clay pipestem or Symmers') fibrosis. The
importance of understanding the immunology of schistosomiasis is clear when
it is considered that granuloma formation (and thus disease severity), parasite
egg production, resistance to infection, and drug efficacy are all dependent on
the immune response to the parasite.

T-HELPER CELL RESPONSES DURING INFECTION AND THEIR ROLE IN GRANULOMA FORMATION

Because of the central role of the egg-granuloma in the pathology of
schistosomiasis, much work has been directed toward understanding the gen-
esis of the lesion, in terms of both which components of the host immune

system are responsible for its formation and which egg antigens induce the activation of the relevant immune mediators.

For many years, based largely on the work of Warren and his colleagues (1967), the granuloma was considered to be a classic cell-mediated immune response. Consistent with this argument is the fact that granuloma formation largely fails to occur in infected mice that lack CD4$^+$ cells. However, in the mid-1980s, Mosmann and Coffman from their study of murine CD4$^+$ T helper (Th) cell clones described the existence of subsets of Th cells, termed Th1 and Th2, which could be distinguished on the basis of the cytokines they produced when activated (Mosmann and Coffman, 1989). The functions of the secreted cytokines indicated that Th1 cells (which make IL-2 and IFN-γ) would be responsible for macrophage activation and cell-mediated immunity (CMI) whereas Th2 cells (which make IL-4, -5, -6, and -10) would provide B cells with help and, of special relevance for schistosomiasis and other helminth infections, control IgE production (IL-4) and eosinophilia (IL-5). It was immediately obvious that the existence in vivo of similar Th subsets would provide an explanation for why CD4$^+$ cells could be responsible for many apparently mutually exclusive immune responses such as delayed-type hypersensitivity and strong antibody responses. Moreover, in terms of the granuloma, the findings indicated that an egg-specific Th1 response was likely to mediate lesion formation.

This premise was tested by the straightforward approach of assessing which cytokines were produced by parasite antigen-stimulated murine Th cells at week 8 of infection, the time of peak granuloma formation (Gryzch et al., 1991; Pearce et al., 1991). Inconsistent with the hypothesis, but compatible with the eosinophilia and elevated IgE levels that characterize schistosomiasis in mice (as well as other hosts), the predominant cytokines produced were IL-4, -5, and -10, with relatively little IL-2 or IFN-γ, suggesting that the granuloma was unlikely to be a classic delayed-type hypersensitivity response mediated by a Th1 cell. Interestingly, a time course study of splenic cell responses throughout infection revealed that the Th2 cytokines were produced in quantity only following the onset of egg production (Gryzch et al., 1991). The use of RT-PCR and/or Northern hybridization to examine cytokine gene expression in the livers of infected mice has revealed a grossly similar expression pattern to that expected from analyses of secreted cytokines (Henderson et al., 1991; Wynn et al., 1993); at 8 weeks postinfection, the upregulation of transcription of the IL-4 and IL-5 genes is greater by a considerable margin than the upregulation of expression of IFN-γ; IL-1α, -1β, -2, -6, -10; TNF-α; or GM-CSF.

To assess directly the role of a particular cytokine in granuloma formation, the most frequently used approach has been to inject neutralizing cytokine-specific mAbs into mice at the time of granuloma formation and determine histologically their effect on lesion development (most of the data from these kinds of studies were recently reviewed by Cheever, 1993, and Wynn et al., 1994). Such studies have used both infected mice and animals injected intravenously with isolated eggs so as to permit the development of pulmonary granulomas (this "lung model," pioneered over 30 years ago by von Lichtenberg, allows synchronous granuloma development and for the effect of pre-existing antiworm responses to be circumvented). At this time the effects of neutralizing MIP-1α, IFN-γ, IL-2, IL-4, IL-5, IL-10 and IL-12 have been published. In the lung model, neutralization of IFN-γ or IL-2 results in an enhanced Th2 response and larger granulomas, whereas neutralization of IL-2 and IL-4 results in the development of significantly smaller granulomas. In acutely infected mice, neutralization of MIP-1α, IL-4, or IL-2 results in smaller hepatic granulomas and, in the case of the latter, less fibrosis as well. Anti-IL-5 treatment in infected mice results in granulomas that are eosinophil free but in terms of size and fibrosis indistinguishable from normal lesions.

A role for IL-2 in granuloma formation is also strongly suggested by the observations that a passively transferred egg antigen specific Th1 cell clone facilitated larger pulmonary circumoval granuloma formation in murine recipients, though the participation of eosinophils in these lesions suggests the rapid promotion by IL-2 of a Th2 response (Chikunguwo et al., 1991). A role for IL-2 in the induction of Th2 responses was also evident both in the lung model and in infected mice where anti-IL-2 inhibited the upregulation of IL-4 (lung model only) and IL-5 production. Additionally, IL-2 is able to promote larger granuloma formation in acutely infected CD4$^+$ cell–depleted mice and in chronically infected mice with modulated granulomas. Consistent with the effects of neutralizing these cytokines, exogenous rIFN-γ and rIL-12 inhibit granuloma formation in the lung model (Wynn et al., 1994).

CMI DOWNREGULATION FOLLOWING THE ONSET OF EGG PRODUCTION

Surprisingly, IL-2 and IFN-γ, cytokines characteristic of Th1 cells, were produced in significantly lower amounts by antigen-stimulated Th cells from mice carrying egg-laying infections than by those from mice with prepatent infections (Gryzch et al., 1991; Pearce et al., 1991). The same was true even when the cells were stimulated with the potent T-cell mitogen Con A. These data indicate that 1) schistosome eggs induce Th2 responses; and 2) either eggs or, more likely, the Th responses they induce downregulate the ability of the infected animals to mount Th1 responses. This downregulation is now known to be due in part to the production of IL-10, which, in addition to working synergistically with IL-4 to counteract CMI effector functions, restricts Th1 cell cytokine production (see Oswald et al., 1992). IL-10 appears to work, at least in part, by preventing the upregulation of the CD28 ligand B7 on macrophages, thereby preventing them from activating Th1 cells (which require a costimulatory signal through CD28 to expand clonally (Linsley and Ledbetter, 1993). In keeping with this interpretation is the observation that macrophages isolated from granulomas, when pulsed with the appropriate antigen, fail to activate Th1 clones, but rather push them toward an anergic state (Flores Villanueva et al., 1994). The activation, without costimulation, of parasite antigen-specific naive Th cells throughout the acute to chronic transition during infection could also account for the reduced or "modulated" immune responsiveness evident in mice carrying older (>16 weeks) infections.

The possibility that the schistosome infection–associated lesion in CMI could deleteriously affect the ability of infected animals to mount CMI responses to unrelated antigens has been tested experimentally using schistosome-infected mice immunized with a model nonschistosome antigen, sperm whale myoglobin (Kullberg et al., 1992), or infected with the intracellular pathogen vaccinia (Actor et al., 1993). In both cases, Th1 responses specific for the nonschistosome antigens were significantly and markedly lower than those observed in uninfected mice that had been sensitized in the same way. In the case of vaccinia, cytotoxic T-cell responses were also significantly depressed, and, indeed, clearance of the virus was impaired. One implication of these data is that schistosomiasis is a risk factor for susceptibility to diseases that require CMI for control.

EARLY EGG-INDUCED IMMUNE RESPONSES

The most detailed examinations of egg-induced responses have utilized model systems in which isolated eggs are injected into either the lungs (Wynn et al., 1993, 1994) or footpads (Vella and Pearce, 1992) of normal mice. These studies have revealed a complex early evolution of the response that is somewhat compatible with the model of Th-cell differentiation that proposes that Th subsets develop via a Th0-like intermediate stage; Th0 cells produce both Th1 and Th2 cytokines upon stimulation. It is now clear that one of the first cytokines to be produced in response to eggs, both within the tissue in which eggs are deposited and by cells from the lymph nodes draining the deposition site, is, surprisingly, IFN-γ; TNF-α and IL-1β are also produced locally at this early time point. Subsequently, within 2 days, IL-2, IL-4, IL-5, IL-10, and IFN-γ are simultaneously produced both locally and in the draining lymph node. In the footpad system, IFN-γ production within the draining lymph node is subsequently downregulated such that by day 7 only small amounts of this cytokine are detectable in the supernatants of antigen- or mitogen-stimulated cells; in the lung model, IFN-γ mRNA continues to be evident in pulmonary granulomas at this time. Examination of cytokine gene transcription in the lungs of nude mice injected with eggs revealed a pattern of mRNAs similar to that observed in intact mice, except that IL-4 and IL-5 were not upregulated. Consistent with this, the ability to produce IL-4 and IL-5, but also IL-2 and IFN-γ was severely impaired when cell populations from lymph nodes draining footpads injected with eggs were depleted of CD4$^+$ cells. Taken together, these data indicate that the initial immune response to eggs at the site of deposition involves the contribution of cytokines from non-Th cells, with a subsequent development of a specific Th2-like response. Understanding the interplay of egg molecules with the front line cells of the immune system, such as macrophages, mast cells, and NK cells, and how these cells influence the final skewing of the Th response in the Th2 direction is very likely key for an understanding of egg immunogenicity (Reiner and Locksley, 1993; Wynn et al., 1994).

ANTIFECUNDITY/TRANSMISSION BLOCKING IMMUNE RESPONSES

Some of the most intriguing aspects of the interaction between schistosomes and the immune system are the sensitivity to the immunologic environment of egg production, viability, and excretion. The immune dependence of egg passage into the intestinal lumen was first described in the 1970s by Doenhoff and his colleagues, who showed that thymectomized, antithymocyte-treated, infected mice passed far fewer eggs with their feces than did infected immunocompetent mice (Doenhoff et al., 1979). Stool egg numbers could be normalized by the administration to the T-cell–depleted animals of antisera or lymphoid cells from infected T-cell–replete mice. Since the immunodeficient animals failed to mount a normal granulomatous response to parasite eggs, it was proposed that lesion formation was a prerequisite for the eggs to leave the vasculature and cross the intestinal wall; the ability of immune sera and cells to facilitate (to some extent) granuloma formation and at the same time allow egg excretion was consistent with this. Following these early discoveries, there was a lull in work on the effect of the immune response on egg production, export, and viability until the early 1990s, when two fascinating observations on the subject were reported. The first of these was that immunization with the experimental vaccine Sm28-glutathione-S-transferase (GST) not only rendered experimental animals partially resistant to infection but also resulted in surviving female parasites being less fecund than female schistosomes parasitizing unimmunized animals (Capron, 1992; Capron and Dessaint, 1992; Grezel et al., 1993; Xu et al., 1993). Moreover, eggs produced by these parasites were less viable. These effects seem largely due to the specific antibody response, since mAb specific for Sm28-GST can, in passive transfer experiments, reduce the fecundity of, and the viability of eggs produced by, established female parasites. The second new finding was that in infected SCID mice, which fail to form circumoval granulomas or excrete eggs (as expected from Doenhoff's studies), rudimentary granuloma formation and egg passage into the intestinal lumen could be restored by the injection of recombinant TNF-α (Amiri et al., 1993). Remarkably, TNF-α also stimulated increased egg production by female worms (Amiri et al., 1993).

At the time of writing, the way in which the immune response controls egg production and excretion is not well understood, but clearly is operating at several levels. It is reasonable to assume that the reason the T-cell–depleted mice of Doenhoff's experiments failed to excrete eggs is that they were unable to produce TNF-α. Presumably, in such a case, immune serum was able successfully to reconstitute the ability of T cell depleted mice to excrete eggs due to its TNF-α content. The direct effect of TNF-α in stimulating females to produce eggs is assumed to be receptor mediated. Since TNF-α analogs have been described in invertebrates, it is possible that mammalian TNF-α affects schistosomes by interacting with a receptor for the parasite analog. Since full sexual maturity in female schistosomes is male dependent, it is tempting to speculate that a TNF-α–receptor interaction is an integral part of intersexual signalling. The exact mechanism by which anti-GST antibodies affect egg production and viability remains to be determined, but it appears to be related to their ability to recognize epitopes within amino acids 190–211 at the C terminus and residues 10–43 at the N terminus (which together comprise at least part of the active site) and inhibit enzyme activity (Xu et al., 1993). Interestingly, an Sm28-GST–specific mAb that is able to reduce worm burdens in passively immunized animals, but not affect fecundity or egg viability, recognizes a distinct internal epitope (amino acids 115–131) within the antigen, indicating that this molecule has more than one crucial function for schistosome survival.

An important corollary of the observations that egg production and excretion are sensitive to immune status is that fecal egg counts may be a poor measure of infection intensity. The implications of this are discussed below.

HUMAN IMMUNE RESPONSES

Following the recent advances made in the murine system, detailed analysis of human Th cell responses during schistosomiasis especially from the point of view of which cytokines are contributing to the different clinical forms of the disease, is a priority of several laboratories. However, at present little is published in this area (but see Roberts et al., 1993).

Most of what is known of cellular immune responses during human schistosomiasis is based on proliferative assays that measure T-cell mitosis in response to stimulation with appropriate antigen. Though technically simple, these kinds of analyses have revealed a complex regulatory idiotypic network that seems to play a role in the control of pathogenesis in chronic schistosomiasis.

Chronic *S. mansoni* infection in humans is a spectral disease, with the majority of patients being asymptomatic (a state termed *intestinal* [INT]) and a minority (less than %10, termed *hepatosplenic* [HS]) exhibiting severe symptoms including hepatosplenomegaly, ascites, and, upon liver biopsy, periportal fibrosis. Acute disease, which is debilitating, is only seen when people from outside an endemic area become infected and is largely unknown among residents of an endemic area. Whereas peripheral blood mononuclear cells (PBMC) from INT patients respond poorly to soluble egg antigen (SEA), those from ambulatory HS proliferate strongly, more like those from acutely infected individuals. In other words, hyper-responsiveness is associated with more severe disease. Downregulation of the T-cell proliferative response to SEA is associated with an ability of PBMC from INT patients to respond to anti-SEA antibodies in their own sera; in contrast, egg-specific antibodies from HS and acute patients fail to express the appropriate regulatory idiotype (Colley, 1990; Montesano et al., 1989). How the stimulation of T cells by egg-specific antibodies regulates the immune response is unclear, but conceivably it could be due either to preferential stimulation of a subset of cells capable of making downregulatory cytokines such as IL-10 (which inhibits human T-cell proliferation) or through the induction in the responding T-cell population of an anergic (nonresponsive) state due to a lack during idiotype–anti-idiotype stimulation of an appropriate costimulatory signal.

More details of the mechanisms operating in this situation should be forthcoming now that a mouse model of HS has been developed (Henderson et al., 1993). This new model utilizes male CBA/J mice, 20% of which, when infected with *S. mansoni,* go on to develop a disease that is very similar to that seen in HS patients. Previously the mouse was considered to be an inadequate model for the study of HS. Remarkably, CBA/J mice with HS, like HS patients, fail to express a regulatory idiotype (defined by a mAb, E5) present on anti-SEA egg antibodies from INT patients, whereas the 80% of infected mice that do not develop HS do express this idiotype.

Typically, in areas endemic for schistosomiasis, the distribution of infection intensity is overdispersed, such that younger people (less than 15 years old) excrete more eggs (and are therefore considered to be more heavily infected) than individuals who are older. Following treatment and re-exposure to cercariae, young people generally regain heavy infections whereas older people tend not to become reinfected, or at least are reinfected at very low intensity. Such a pattern, which has been independently confirmed for *S. mansoni* in both East Africa and in South America and for *S. heamatobium* in West Africa (and which does not appear to be due to differences in water contact between children and adults), is considered to be indicative of the development with age of protective immunity (reviewed by Butterworth, 1992).

The demonstration of an immune subpopulation of people living in endemic areas has opened the way for detailed field studies of protective immune responses. To date, the tack being taken by most investigators working in this area has been to perform qualitative and quantitative analyses of antischistosome immune responses in immune and nonimmune individuals and to look for responses that correlate with the resistant state. Such an approach has revealed that levels of IgE specific for antigens of either immature or mature worms (but not parasite eggs) correlate significantly with persistent low egg output following treatment (reviewed by Butterworth, 1992). These results have been received with excitement as corroboration of the long-held belief that IgE is important for immunity to schistosomes (Butterworth, 1992; Hagan, 1993).

While there is no doubt that a role for IgE in immunity to schistosomes is inherently attractive, there remains room for alternative interpretations of the results described above. In light of the recent discovery that immune status can markedly effect egg output, there is now legitimate concern as to whether fecal egg counts are truly representative of infection intensity or rather reflect an active antifecundity immune response or an immunocompromised state. Perhaps the best available method for circumventing this problem is to measure circulating antigen, which can be an indicator of adult parasite burden. A hint that low fecal egg counts in infected people could be due to an antifecundity response is provided by the observation that the only immune response other than IgE that has been correlated with "resistance" following reinfection is the IgA response to Sm28-GST, and IgA antibodies specific for this antigen, from resistant patients, inhibit fecundity and egg viability in vitro (Grzych et al., 1993).

Another issue that confounds the interpretation of the reinfection after treatment studies is that of the contribution of portacaval anastomoses to resistance to infection. In infected mice, which, like infected people, develop portosystemic collateral circulation, resistance to secondary infection is largely due to challenge infection parasites bypassing the liver via the anastomoses and thus failing to establish in their appropriate niche (see Wilson and Sher, 1993). Presumably, such a phenomenon could be contributing to age-related immunity in infected people. This issue should be addressable through the use of ultrasound to detect portal fibrosis and associated vascular abnormalities.

As a last note on the subject, one of the most puzzling aspects of the human immunity story is the length of time it takes for people to develop a protective immune response; perhaps this reflects the lingering effects of immunoregulatory signals received in utero or a necessity for sexual maturation before the expression of the appropriate immune responses can occur.

VACCINE DEVELOPMENT

A major focus of research on schistosomiasis continues to be the development of a usable vaccine. One of the most intriguing aspects of schistosome biology is that even in the best case vaccine-induced immunity never seems to be complete, since some parasites of a challenge infection invariably survive to maturity. This observation suggests some degree of population heterogeneity and possibly antigenic variation, which allows a particular subset of parasites to survive the vaccine-induced response. This issue was addressed experimentally in a heroic study wherein mice vaccinated with irradiated cerceriae were challenge infected and eggs produced by surviving parasites used in an attempt to breed a "survivor" population (Lewis et al., 1985). The putative survivability trait was selected for over many generations, but the final generation remained as susceptible to the vaccine-induced immunity as did the original. Thus the issue of why some parasites always survive remains unsolved. Nevertheless, it is now generally accepted that a vaccine that induces only partial resistance to infection, especially if it is also able to effect fecundity and egg viability (and therefore act to prevent transmission), will be of value in controlling infection intensity and therefore disease severity.

As discussed in detail below, most of the recombinant vaccines being studied today were originally identified as important antigens in animals protectively vaccinated with ill-defined crude antigen inocula or radiation-attenuated infections. The attenuated vaccine has proved additionally useful as a model for identifying immune effector mechanisms that can operate against schistosomes. For example, based on the study of resistance to infection in different strains of mice with known immune defects, it was determined that immunity as a result of immunization with the attenuated vaccine is due largely to CMI (reviewed by James and Sher, 1990). This was confirmed recently, when vaccinated and challenged mice treated with mAb anti-IFN-γ were shown to be as susceptible to infection as unvaccinated mice (Smythies et al., 1992). In this model, mAb anti-IFN-γ was most effective at ablating resistance when given at the time of challenge infection migration through the pulmonary capillary bed, consistent with previous observations that it is at this point during both a primary and challenge infection that parasites are susceptible to elimination. Amazingly, there appears to be little evidence in this system that parasites of a challenge infection are *directly* killed by the immune response (this may explain the failure to select a "survivor population"; see above). Rather, the anamnestic immune infiltrate that develops as the challenge schistosomula traverse the lungs appears to block the migration of the parasites and causes them to leave the vasculature and make a terminal trip into the alveolar spaces, where they eventually die. The exact role played by IFN-γ in this process remains to be elucidated.

Many defined experimental vaccines have been developed. The three discussed here, Sm28-GST, rIrV-5, and triose phosphate isomerase (TPI), are probably the most promising currently available. Interestingly, they were initially developed through quite different routes.

Sm28-GST was originally identified as a 28 kD antigen recognized by immune serum from rats protectively immunized with the excretory–secretory products of schistosomula. The sequence of the gene encoding this protein revealed the protein to be a GST. Direct immunization with rGST in mice, rats, monkeys, hamsters and cattle, in some cases using several different adjuvants, including those that might be expected to promote Th1 or Th2 responsiveness (BCG and Alum, respectively), induces significant protective immunity (Capron and Dessaint, 1992; Grezel et al., 1993). Interestingly, and unexpectedly, the most profound host-protective effect of the Sm28 GST vaccine is its ability to reduce the fecundity of surviving parasites of a challenge infection and decrease the viability of those eggs that are produced; this aspect is discussed in detail above. Originally, antigen-specific IgE was considered to be the dominant immune effector mechanism induced by immunization with the Sm28-GST. However, recent vaccination studies have revealed that Sm28-GST–specific IgA may also play a significant role (Grezel et al., 1993; Grzych et al., 1993). Additionally, as alluded to above, there is now a tie-in between the anti-Sm28-GST IgA response and resistance to reinfection in humans (Grzych et al., 1993). Those patients living in infected areas who fail to become heavily reinfected following drug treatment have significantly higher levels of IgA specific for Sm28-GST and, moreover, for a synthetic peptide representing amino acids 115–131 of this antigen (a multimer of which is able to induce protective immunity in experimental animals, see Capron, 1992; Capron and Dessaint, 1992), than do those who become reinfected. In in vitro assays, IgA from the putatively immune patients, but not the susceptible individuals, could also inhibit egg production and viability, suggesting that resistant patients may possess a degree of antifecundity immunity. While inhibition of enzyme activity is necessary for IgA-mediated effects on egg production and survival, effector mechanism(s) through which IgA is able to effect parasite attrition are less obvious, though an IgA-dependent eosinophil-mediated cytotoxicity against schistosomula has been demonstrated.

rIrV5 is the designation given to a recombinant protein encoded by a clone,

IrV5, isolated from an adult schistosome cDNA library on the basis of its recognition by an antiserum that specifically recognized antigens that showed a greater or unique immunogenicity in mice multiply vaccinated with irradiated cercariae than in chronically infected mice (Soisson et al., 1992). The significance of this is that antibodies from mice vaccinated several times with irradiated cercariae, in contrast to those from infected mice, can passively immunize naive recipients against infection. It has been assumed that this difference is due to the recognition by the former of protective antigens.

Multiple vaccinations with rIrV5 in the absence of adjuvant are able to confer up to 80% resistance to infection in mice, which makes this particular antigen the most effective immunoprophylactic for schistosomiasis currently available. Using sera from animals vaccinated with rIrV5, the native antigen homologous to clone IrV5 has been identified as a 200 kD surface antigen of schistosomula. Consistent with the molecular weight of the native protein, the sequence of IrV5 has been found to share a high degree of similarity to myosin II heavy chain sequences from other species. In addition to its potential as a vaccine, an intriguing characteristic of the IrV5-encoded myosin-like protein is its localization to the outer face of the parasite's tegumental membrane; to date no other myosins have been localized to a cell surface.

TPI was first identified as a 28 kD antigen recognized by a mAb raised against a detergent extract of schistosomula (Shoemaker et al., 1992). The mAb was particularly interesting since in passive immunizations it could partially protect naive mice against infection. As is the case for Sm28-GST, the antibody inhibited the activity of the enzyme, suggesting that the protective effect of the mAb could be the result of its being inhibitory for enzyme function.

A concern with each of the antigens described above is that they have mammalian homologs and therefore presumably present a risk of inducing autoimmune responses if used as vaccines. While this outcome seems unlikely, given the apparent absence of autoimmunity in animals vaccinated with these antigens, there is an effort, at least in the case of TPI, to determine whether the least homologous regions of antigens retain the ability to induce protective immunity. This recent concern with the induction of autoimmunity by parasite proteins that share functional and sequence homology with host molecules has renewed interest both in the development of defined subunit vaccines comprised of nonhomologous peptides (Reynolds et al., 1994) and in experimental vaccine antigens that (though relatively ineffective compared with, for example, rIrV5) are unique to the parasite, such as paramyosin, a protein found only in invertebrates (James and Sher, 1990).

CONCLUSION

After years of being able merely to infer that a particular type of immune response is important for an observed effect on schistosome-induced pathology or parasite survival, a point has been reached where the technology is available to obtain definitive answers. For example, using mAbs that specifically neutralize cytokines, it is now clear that the schistosome granuloma is dependent on cytokines produced by both Th1 and Th2 cells and is not simply the product of one Th subset as opposed to another. The immediate future holds the even more exciting prospect of being able to utilize genetically altered mice to address the pertinent issues. The challenge now is to take the findings from animal models into the field and determine their relevance to human disease.

REFERENCES

Actor J, Shirai M, Kullberg M, Buller M, Sher A, Berzofsky J (1993): Helminth inection results in decreased virus-specific CD8$^+$ cytotoxic T-cell and Th1-cytokine responses as well as delayed virus clearance. Proc Natl Acad Sci USA 90:948.

Amiri P, Locksley RM, Parslow T, Sadick M, Rector E, Ritter D, McKerrow J (1993): Tumour necrosis factor-α restores granulomas and induces egg-laying in schistosome-infected SCID mice. Nature 356:604.

Butterworth AE (1992): Vaccines against schistosomiasis: Where do we stand? Trans R Soc Trop Med Hyg 86:1.

Capron A (1992): Immunity to schistosomes. Curr Opin Immunol 4:419.

Capron A, Dessaint J-P (1992): Immunologic aspects of schistosomiasis. Annu Rev Med 43:209.

Cheever AW (1993): Schistosomiasis: Infection versus disease and hypersensitivity versus immunity. Am J Pathol 142:699.

Chikunguwo SM, Kanazawa T, Dayal Y, Stadecker MJ (1991): The cell mediated response to Schistosoma antigens at the clonal level. In vivo function of cloned murine egg-specific CD4$^+$ T helper type 1 lymphocytes. J Immunol 197:3921.

Colley DG (1990): Occurrence, roles and uses of idiotypes and anti-idiotypes in parasitic diseases. In J. Cierny, J. Hiernaux (eds): Idiotypic Network and Diseases. Washington DC: ASM Press, pp 71–101.

Doenhoff MJ, Musallam R, Bain J, McGregor A (1979): Studies on the host–parasite relationship in Schistosoma mansoni–infected mice: The immunological dependence of parasite egg excretion. Immunology 35:771.

Flores Villanueva PO, Harris TS, Ricklon DE, Stadecker MJ (1994): Macrophages from schistosomal egg granulomas induce unresponsiveness in specific cloned Th1 lymphocytes in vitro and down-regulate schistosomal granulomatous disease in vivo. J Immunol 152:1847.

Grezel D, Capron M, Grzych J-M, Fontaine J, Lecocq J-P, Capron A (1993): Protective immunity induced in a rat by a single dose of the Sm28GST recombinant antigen:effector mechanisms involving IgE and IgA antibodies. Eur J Immunol 23:454.

Grzych J-M, Grezel D, Xu C-B, Neyrinck J-L, Capron M, Ouma J, Butterworth A, Capron A (1993): IgA antibodies to a protective antigen inhuman schistosomiasis. J Immunol 150:527.

Gryzch JM, Pearce EJ, Cheever A, Claulada ZA, Caspar P, Hieny S, Lewis FA, Sher A (1991): Egg deposition is the major stimulus for the production of Th2 cytokines in murine *Schistosomiasis mansoni*. J Immunol 146:1322.

Hagan P (1993): IgE and protective immunity. Parasitol Immunol 15:1.

Henderson GS, Conary JT, Summar M, McCurley TL, Colley DG (1991): In vivo molecular analysis of lymphokines involved in the murine immune response during *Schistosoma mansoni* infection. I. IL-4 mRNA, not IL-2 mRNA, is abundant in the granulomatous livers, mesenteric lymph nodes and spleens of infected mice. J Immunol 146:1322.

Henderson GS, Nix NA, Montesano MA, Gold D, Freeman GL, McCurley TL, Colley D (1993): Two distinct pathological syndromes in male CBA/J inbred mice with chronic *Schistosoma mansoni* infections. Am J Pathol 142:703.

James SL, Sher A (1990): Cell mediated immune response to schistosomiasis. Curr Top Microbiol Immunol 155:21.

Jordan P, Webbe J (1982): Schistosomiasis. London: Heinemann.

Kullberg MC, Pearce EJ, Hieny SE, Sher A, Berzofsky JA (1992): Infection with *Schistosoma mansoni* alters Th1/Th2 cytokine responsesto a non-parasite antigen. J Immunol 148:3264.

Lewis FA, Hieny S, Sher A (1985): Evidence against the existenceof subpopulations of specific *Schistosoma mansoni* subpopulations which are resistant to irradiated vaccine-induced immunity. Am J Trop Med Hyg 34:86.

Linsley P, Ledbetter J (1993): The role of CD28 receptor during T cell responses to antigen. Annu Rev Immunol 11:191.

Lukacs N, Kunkel S, Stieter R, Warmington K, Chensue S (1993): The role of macrophage inflammatory protein 1a in *Schistosoma mansoni* egg induced granulomatous inflammation. J Exp Med 177:1551.

Montesano MA, Lima MS, Oliveira RC, Gazzinelli G, Colley DG (1989): Immune responses during human schistosomiasis. XVI. Idiotypic differences in antibody preparations from patients with different clinical forms of infection. J Immunol 142:2501.

Mosmann TR, Coffman RL (1989): Th1 and Th2 cells: Different patterns of lymphokine secretion lead to different functional properties. Annu Rev Immunol 7:145.

Oswald IP, Gazzinelli RT, Sher A, James SL (1992): IL-10 synergizes with IL-4 and transforming growth factor-β to inhibit macrophage cytotoxic activity. J Immunol 148:3578.

Pearce EJ, Caspar P, Gryzch JM, Lewis FA, Sher A (1991): Downregulation of Th1 cytokine production accompanies induction of Th2 responses by a helminth, *Schistosoma mansoni*. J Exp Med 173:159.

Reiner SL, Locksley RM (1993): The worm and the protozoa: Stereotyped responses or distinct antigens. Parasitol Today 9:258.

Reynolds SR, Dahl CE, Harn DA (1994): T and B epitope determination and analysis of multiple antigenic peptides for the *Schistosoma mansoni* experimental vaccine triosephosphate isomerase. J Immunol 152:193.

Roberts M, Butterworth AE, Kimani C, Kaman T, Fulford AJC, Dunne DW, Ouma JH, Sturrock RF (1993): Immunity after treatment of human schistosomiasis: Association between cellular responses and resistance to reinfection. Infect Immun 61:4984.

Sher A, Fiorentino D, Casper P, Pearce EJ, Mossman TR (1991): Production of IL-10 by CD4[+] T lymphocytes correlates with down regulation of Th1 cytokine synthesis. J Immunol 147:2713.

Sher A, Gazzinelli R, Oswald I, Clerici M, Kullberg M, Pearce E, Berzofsky J, Mosmann T, James S, Morse H, Shearer G (1992): Role of T cell derived cytokines in the down-regulation of immune responses in parasitic and retroviral infections. Immunol Rev 127:183.

Shoemaker C, Gross A, Gebremichael A, Harn D (1992): cDNA cloning and functional expression of the *Schistosoma mansoni* protective antigen triose-phosphate isomerase. Proc Natl Acad Sci USA 89:1842.

Smythies LE, Coulson P, Wilson RA (1992): Monoclonal antibody to IFN-g modifies pulmonary inflammatory responses and abrogates immunity to *Schistosoma mansoni* in mice vaccinated with attenuated cercariae. J Immunol 149:3654.

Soisson L, Masterson C, Tom TD, McNally MT, Lowell G, Strand M (1992): Induction of protective immunity in mice using a 62kDa recombinant fragment of a *Schistosoma mansoni* surface antigen. J Immunol 149:3612.

Vella AT, Pearce EJ (1992): CD4⁺ Th2 response induced by *Schistosoma mansoni* eggs develop through an early, transient, Th0-like stage. J Immunol 148:2283.

Warren KS, Domingo EO, Cowan RBT (1967): Granuloma formation as a manifestation of delayed hypersensitivity. Am J Pathol 52:307.

Wilson RA, Sher A (1993): Vaccines against schistosomes: An alternative view. Trans R Soc Trop Med Hyg 87:238.

Wynn TA, Eltoum I, Cheever AW, Lewis FA, Gause WC, Sher A (1993): Analysis of cytokine mRNA expression during primary egg granuloma formation induced by eggs of *Schistosoma mansoni*. J Immunol 151:1430.

Wynn TA, Eltoum I, Oswald IP, Cheever AW, Sher A (1994): Endogenous interleukin 12 (IL-12) regulates granuloma formation induced by eggs of *Schistosoma mansoni* and exogenous IL-12 both inhibits and prophylactically immunizes against egg pathology. J Exp Med 179:1551.

Xu C-B, Verwaerde C, Gras-Masse H, Fontaine J, Bossus M, Trottein F, Wolowczuk I, Tartar A, Capron A (1993): *Schistosoma mansoni* 28-kDa glutathione S-transferase and immunity against parasite fecundity and egg viability. J Immunol 150:940.

Molecular Approaches to Parasitology, pages 511–523
© 1995 Wiley-Liss, Inc.

Immune Responses in Lymphatic-Dwelling Filarial Infections

Thomas B. Nutman

Laboratory of Parasitic Diseases, National Institutes of Health, Bethesda, Maryland 20892

INTRODUCTION

Although eight filarial species commonly infect humans, four are responsible for the pathology associated with most of these infections: *Brugia malayi, Wuchereria bancrofti, Onchocerca volvulus,* and *Loa loa.* Taken together, these human filarial parasites infect an estimated 140 million persons worldwide. Infection with the lymphatic-dwelling nematodes *Wuchereria bancrofti, Brugia malayi,* and *Brugia timori* affects more than 100 million individuals in Africa, Asia, many southern and western Pacific islands, the Caribbean Islands, and South America. The prevalence of these particular filarial infections is expected to increase as urbanization and poor sanitary conditions in endemic areas result in expansion of mosquito breeding sites.

For all filarial parasites, infections of the human host is initiated by the deposition of third stage larvae (L3) in the skin after a bite of an infective arthropod. The larvae mature and develop into subcutaneous or lymphatic-dwelling adult worms over a period of months to years. Mature female worms produce and subsequently release microfilariae into the bloodstream (in the case of lymphatic filariases) where they are available for uptake by the intermediate arthropod host. Like most every helminth parasite, the lymphatic dwelling filarial parasites do not replicate within the human host, but they are capable of persisting over extremely long periods of time. Because complex parasitic life cycles can only be maintained by sequential passage through generally inflexible choices of intermediate and definitive hosts, filarial parasites have adapted to optimize transmission by prolonging infection. This is critical if passage through a series of hosts depends on infrequent events such as uptake by the occasional biting arthropod.

Perhaps because of this evolutionary pressure, chronicity is the hallmark of filarial infection. For example, adult filariae may survive in host tissue for as long as 30 years, producing microfilariae throughout. In response to the evolutionary pressure for chronic infection, a range of strategies has evolved along with the parasites to maintain long-term viability in their host. Adaptations for chronicity can be so successful among filarial parasites that naturally acquired protective immunity may only be observed rarely in areas highly endemic for this infection.

The range of clinical manifestations of lymphatic filariasis is broad, and the diversity of clinical responses to filarial infection is considered to reflect the intensity and type of immune response to the parasite or parasite products (King and Nutman, 1991). A spectrum of clinical outcomes occurs following exposure to lymphatic-dwelling filariae (Fig. 1). In areas endemic for these lymphatic-dwelling parasites, cross-sectional studies have shown that most individuals in filarial endemic regions are asymptomatic and microfilaria positive. This group is generally considered to be immunologically hyporesponsive to the parasite. Because they are unable to clear their microfilariae, they serve as the reservoir for continued transmission of the parasite. In contrast, patients with pathology associated with infection (elephantiasis, adenolymphangitis, tropical pulmonary eosinophilia) are characteristically microfilaria negative. A third group, also microfilaria negative, has no evidence of infection; these individuals have not been sufficiently exposed to the parasite to acquire infection, have an occult infection, or have developed immunity to the parasite.

While the various clinical manifestations of lymphatic-dwelling filarial infections cannot be described in detail here, it is important to indicate

POSSIBLE OUTCOMES OF EXPOSURE TO FILARIAL PARASITES

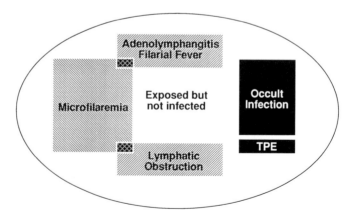

Fig. 1. A diagram of the possible outcomes of infection with lymphatic-dwelling filarial parasites in an endemic population.

some of the major features in that the immune response to the parasite appears extremely important in determining the nature of these clinical manifestations.

1. Asymptomatic microfilaremia. This form of lymphatic filariasis is one in which individuals are entirely asymptomatic despite having very large numbers of circulating microfilariae. Recently, it has been shown that such patients have lymphatic abnormalities when assessed by nuclear imaging techniques (Witte et al., 1993) and can also have clinically silent renal abnormalities (e.g., microscopic hematuria) (Dreyer et al., 1992).

2. Acute and chronic lymphatic pathology. The initial clinical manifestations of lymphatic filarial infection are most frequently fever and/or retrograde lymphangitis of the extremities. These signs usually last for a period of one to several weeks and are most common in the second and third decades of life. They may occur with increasing frequency in some persons and eventually result in persistent lymphedema of the extremities and general lymphatic incompetence. Such persons with chronic disease are usually amicrofilaremic, although microfilaremia has been observed in residents of endemic areas where transmission is high.

3. Tropical pulmonary eosinophilia (TPE). This clinical manifestation of filarial infection differs from those with other forms of the infection and appears to be related to an immediate hypersensitivity response to the filarial antigens. TPE is characterized by recurrent nocturnal cough and wheezing, reticulonodular densities on chest radiographs, peripheral blood eosinophilia $>3,000/mm^3$, extreme elevations of serum IgE and specific antifilarial antibodies, and dramatic improvement following antifilarial chemotherapy (Ottesen and Nutman, 1992).

PATHOLOGY ASSOCIATED WITH LYMPHATIC FILARIAL INFECTION

The principal pathological changes in lymphatic filariasis result from inflammatory damage to the lymphatics referable to adult and not to microfilarial stages (von Lichtenberg, 1987; Jungmann et al., 1992). Adult worms live in afferent lymphatics or sinuses of lymph nodes and induce local changes that result in lymphatic dilation and thickening of the vessel walls. Plasma cells, eosinophils, and macrophages infiltrate in and around the affected vessels and with endothelial and connective tissue proliferation lead to tortuosity of the lymphatics and damaged or incompetent lymph valves. The overlying skin shows lymphedema and chronic stasis changes with brawny edema. These consequences of filarial infection relate not to simple lymphatic obstruction by resident adult worms but rather to the host immune response to the parasite. Local immune responses directed toward the adult are believed to cause the granulomatous and proliferative processes that precede total lymphatic obstruction. It is said that as long as the worm remains viable, the vessel remains patent, although without normal function. Death of the worm, however, leads to an enhanced granulomatous reaction. Fibrosis and lymphatic obstruction progress, and, despite collateralization of the lymphatics, lymphatic function remains compromised.

PATHOGENESIS

Based on a large number of studies comparing the immune responses of individuals with lymphatic pathology and no circulating microfilariae with those asymptomatic individuals with microfilaremia, the diversity of clinical responses to filarial infection was considered solely to reflect the type of immune response and the nature of such a response to the parasite or parasite products (King and Nutman, 1991). Indeed, those asymptomatic microfilaremic individuals have been shown to be relatively immunologically hyporesponsive to the parasite, as they have relatively low serum levels of antifilarial IgG and poor ability to mount B- and T-cell responses to parasite antigens in vitro (reviewed by Ottesen, 1992). Nevertheless, more recently, the role of the parasite (particularly the adult stage) itself has been examined and thought to contribute directly to the lymphatic pathology.

The Role of the Parasite in the Induction of Pathology in Lymphatic Filariasis

With immunodeficient mice (nu/nu or SCID) infected with brugian parasites, several model systems have indicated that lymphatic dilation and proliferation of lymphatic endothelial cells occurs and leads to significant lymphedema in the absence of an intact immune (T- or B-cell–mediated) response (Vincent et al., 1984; Nelson et al., 1991). Reconstitution of these mice with immunologically competent cells from filarial sensitized animals causes marked inflammatory responses directed at the parasite that leads first to granuloma formation and then to complete lymphatic obstruction (Vickery et al., 1991). In studies of humans who are asymptomatic and microfilaria positive, there is evidence, obtained with newly described lymphatic imaging techniques (lymphoscintigraphy, high resolution ultrasound, MRI), that, even in immunologically unresponsive individuals, significant lymphatic abnormalities can be seen (Case et al., 1992; Witte et al., 1993). Furthermore, in a study of filarial-based hydrocele (an early form of lymphatic obstruction) formation, this abnormality was found to occur with almost equal frequency in those with low parasite-specific immune responses compared with those who were immunologically responsive to the parasite (Lammie et al., 1993).

Pathology Reflects the Host Immune Response

In a large number of studies comparing those individuals with asymptomatic microfilaremia and those with lymphatic pathology, a generalization has emerged suggesting that asymptomatic microfilaria-positive individuals have an inability to mount specific immune responses to parasite antigens (i.e., are relatively hyporesponsive) while those with lymphatic pathology respond vigorously to parasite antigen. It is important to realize that by avoiding the host's immune responses microfilaremia can persist, and the chances of the parasite's continued transmission are maximized. Microfilaremic individuals have selectively impaired T- and B-cell responses to filarial antigens, in contrast to the relatively strong cellular and humoral responses seen in individuals who are symptomatic and amicrofilaremic. This impairment is manifested by altered delayed-type hypersensitivity responses to intradermal application of filarial antigens (Weller et al., 1980), by a marked reduction in T-cell proliferation (Ottesen et al., 1977; Piessens et al., 1980; Nutman et al., 1987a; Lammie et al., 1988), and by reduced cytokine (IL-2 and IFN-γ) production (Nutman et al., 1987a). Microfilaremic patients also have altered B-cell responses, as indicated by both their relatively low serum levels of parasite-specific IgG (Ottesen et al., 1982) and their impaired immunoglobulin production to parasite antigens in vitro (Nutman et al., 1987b). This B-cell hyporesponsiveness, however, does not extend to all immune responses, as the frequencies of polyclonal IgE- and IgG4 secreting lymphocytes and serum antifilarial IgG4 are usually elevated in these patients (King et al., 1992). This lack of immune responsiveness in microfilaria-positive individuals is specific only for those responses directed to parasite antigens, as responses to nonparasite antigens and nonspecific stimuli (mitogens, and so forth) remain completely intact.

Previous studies have postulated the presence of parasite-derived suppressive factors or a subpopulation of suppressor cells. Recently it was proposed that individuals with microfilaremia have developed a state of immune tolerance based on the observation of decreased frequencies of antigen reactive T cells using a limiting dilution analysis (King et al., 1992). However, the examination of the relative frequencies of antigen-driven Th2 and Th1 CD4$^+$ subsets in these two clinical manifestations of lymphatic filariasis provide a more compelling framework for understanding the nature of the response to this infection. Although the microfilaremic patients have markedly lower frequencies of antigen-specific CD4$^+$ cells capable of producing IFN-γ (King et al., 1992), a finding that parallels the impaired antigen-driven proliferation and IFN and IL-2 previously seen, these patients have frequencies of IL-4–producing CD4$^+$ cells that are similar to those with chronic lymphocyte obstruction, a finding indicating a shift toward a predominantly Th2 response (King et al., 1993). This shift is supported by the observation that microfilaremic patients have markedly elevated serum levels of polyclonal IgE and IgG4 antibodies (two humoral responses associated with Th2-like responses). The mechanism for this shift to a Th2 response may result not only from an expansion of Th2-reactive clones but also from the downregulation of Th1-like responses. The addition of neutralizing antibody to IL-10 to in vitro cultures of PBMCs from microfilaremic patients restored their ability to proliferate, but had no effect on those individuals with chronic pathology (King et al., 1993).

Although the long-held view that there is a correlation between clinical outcome and immunological responsiveness to parasite products is most likely a valid view, the nature or quality of the immune response much more than the magnitude of the response is probably the major determinant of clinical outcome. Very clearly, in the asymptomatic microfilaremic individuals, the inflammatory responses are being controlled relatively vigorously by counter-regulatory cytokines (such as IL-10 or TGF-β) whereas those with lymphatic pathology respond to the parasite and its products in a manner that is proinflammatory and pathology inducing.

DETERMINANTS OF THE IMMUNE RESPONSE AND/OR CLINICAL OUTCOME

Although there are many hypotheses to explain the relationship between the immune response and clinical outcome, the major possibilities include: 1) genetic differences predisposing to a particular outcome; 2) pre- or neonatal exposure to parasites or parasite products, leading to a modulated immune response; and 3) the nature of the antigen exposure or the antigens themselves, leading to varying clinical outcomes.

Genetic Susceptibility

Epidemiological studies in areas where filariasis is endemic have revealed differential susceptibilities to infection within both the entire population and the families studied (Subrahmanyam et al., 1978). Although the cause of differential susceptibility to clinical expression has only been addressed in a few human studies, the data have implicated, in part, the major histocompatibility complex (MHC). In this regard, in Sri Lankans and southern Indians with elephantiasis due to Wb infection there was an association between HLA-B15 and the presence of chronic lymphatic obstruction (Chan et al., 1984). When a large Polynesian population living in an endemic area for bancroftian filariasis was studied, however, familial clustering of infected individuals was found but failed to link this with particular genetic determinants (Ottesen et al., 1981). Currently, there are several large-scale studies underway to attempt to make more compelling the argument of an underlying genetic susceptibility for disease outcome in filarial infection. Indeed, in a study of individuals from a brugian-infected area of Indonesia, individuals with a particular serologically defined HLA-DQ locus were shown to be protected from chronic lymphatic obstruction (Yazdanbakhsh et al., unpublished data).

Prenatal Exposure

Because in many ways microfilaremic individuals appear to be 'tolerant' to the parasite (based on antigen-specific T-cell responses [proliferation, Th1 cytokine production, precursor frequencies]) and because the immune responses and clinical findings of temporary visitors to endemic regions differ markedly from those native to endemic regions (Klion et al., 1991), in utero sensitization to parasite antigen has been used as an explanation for these findings (Weil et al., 1983). Indeed, in experimental infections of jirds and dogs with brugian parasites, it has been demonstrated that offspring of microfilaremic mothers and were less likely to develop lymphatic pathology (Klei et al., 1986; Miller et al., 1990). In human populations, it has also been shown that maternal microfilarial status is a major determinant of the microfilarial status of the offspring once infected postnatally (Lammie et al., 1991). In a less epidemiological approach, it has been found that antifilarial antibodies of isotypes that do not cross the placenta (e.g., IgE, IgM) have been found in the cord blood of approximately half of the babies born of infected mothers (Weil et al., 1983) or in the sera of several babies born in a region endemic for *W. bancrofti* (Dissanayake et al., 1980). Thus, for at least a group of individuals, the environmental factors surrounding their birth may be important in determining how they subsequently respond to this particular helminth infection.

Nature of Antigen or Chronicity of Antigen Exposure

The finding that T cells from the same individual when stimulated with an allergen or a parasite antigen expand T cells capable of producing IL-4, IL-5, and IL-10 and when stimulated with a different type of soluble antigen expand IL-2 and IFN-γ producing cells suggests that the structural properties of a given antigen may be the determinant that causes the preferential activation of a particular T-cell subset (Romagnani, 1992). Nevertheless, comparison of primary structures of recombinant antigens capable of inducing particular types of T-cell responses have failed to reveal any common structural motif to suggest that a particular epitope was associated with a bias toward a given T-cell response. Thus, the role of chronic low-dose antigenic stimulation, a process that is found commonly in helminth infections (and particularly the filarial infections), must be considered as a major determinant in the skewing of the immune response away from a Th1-like response and toward a downregulatory Th2-like response. Although direct immunological evidence is lacking, data from cats experimentally infected with *Brugia pahangi* has shown that both the frequency and the intensity of exposure affect the parasitological outcome

(Denham and Fletcher, 1987; Grenfell et al., 1991). Although the immunological reagents to examine T-cell–derived cytokines are not yet available to address the immunological control of the parasitological outcome, this model system should provide insight into whether low-dose, chronically administered antigen shifts the immune response away from a Th1 response and toward a Th2 response.

PROTECTIVE IMMUNITY

There appears to be differential susceptibilities to infection with filarial parasites. In the animal model systems for lymphatic filariasis, there is a range of "permissiveness" for the various stages of the parasite that ranges from fully permissive (e.g., jirds, cats, nude mice for *Brugia*) to the semipermissive (Balb/c mice) to the nonpermissive. Additional complications include differing susceptibilities between sexes within a single animal species or strain as well as differing responses in individuals of the same sex within an inbred strain (Gusmäo et al., 1981). In humans, epidemiological studies in areas where filariasis is endemic have also revealed differential susceptibilities to infection (Subrahmanyam et al., 1978). Finally, there is the generally constant finding that females (both human [Ward et al., 1988; Freedman et al., 1989; Brabin, 1990] and animal [Ash, 1971]) tend to resist infection by filarial parasites better than males.

Animal Models of Protective Immunity

The most efficient form of protective immunity would be that directed against the infective or early developing larval stages of the parasite. Successful vaccination against these stages has been achieved using live, radiation-attenuated, infective third stage larvae of several filarial species; of most relevance to the study of lymphatic filariasis are the experiments with *Brugia* spp. in permissive hosts such as dogs, cats, jirds, and monkeys, as well as in semipermissive hosts such as the Balb/c mouse. Chemically abbreviated infections have also been highly effective in stimulating resistance (reviewed by Philipp et al., 1988). There is also some recent evidence that soluble parasite products or recombinants can confer partial immunity in permissive hosts (Table 1).

Immunity to the microfilarial form of the parasite, while useful for blocking transmission to or development within the intermediate host as well as for diminishing microfilarial-induced pathology, has received less attention than other approaches. Nevertheless, resistance to this stage of the parasite has been achieved with both whole organisms and parasite extracts (see Philipp et al., 1988, for review). Also, a microfilarial-derived antigen has been shown to induce partial protection against the adult stage of the parasite (Kazura et al., 1986).

TABLE 1. Parasite Extracts or Recombinant-Induced Protection in Animal Models

Immunogen	Outcome	Reference
B. malayi microfilarial extracts	Microfilarial clearance	Kazura et al. (1986)
B. malayi λW6	Microfilarial clearance	Kazura et al. (1990)
B. malayi paramyosin	Partial resistance to L3 challenge	Li et al. (1993)
B. malayi chitinase	?	

Protective Immunity in Humans

The presence in all areas endemic for *W. bancrofti* and *B. malayi* of a variable proportion of the adult population that is amicrofilaremic and without clinical evidence of disease (variously described as infection-free, endemic normals, "putatively immune" [Freedman et al., 1989]) and the observation in cross-sectional studies showing that microfilaria rates (i.e., patent infection) usually increase until the age of 20–30 years but then remain constant or decreases in later life (Partono, 1984) provide the best evidence available for naturally developing immunity in humans. However, the study of protective immunity in human populations infected with lymphatic filariasis has been retarded by 1) the difficulty in distinguishing among the uninfected individuals who are truly immune and those harboring occult infection and 2) an inability to evaluate resistance to *reinfection* among those individuals with obvious clinical disease (concomitant immunity).

Cross-Sectional Approach to Immunity

By using rigorously definable groups, one clearly not immune (microfilaremics) and one not infected ("putatively immune"), individuals in hyperendemic areas can be examined for potential immunologic determinants of protective immunity to those parasites responsible for lymphatic filarial disease. In examining such polar clinical groups, it has been found that those nonimmune individuals with circulating microfilariae generally manifested a profound and specific humoral and cellular hyporesponsiveness to parasite antigens; in contrast, those individuals who, by all relevant clinical and laboratory criteria (including assays for circulating parasite antigen and responses to diethylcarbamazine), were free of infection mounted significantly greater responses (both cellular and humoral) to parasite antigens (Ottesen, 1992). Furthermore, in a recent study using immunoblotting of sera from these two groups, those infection-free individuals preferentially recognized a 43 kD antigen derived from infective larvae; when antigens from microfilariae or adults were examined in a similar manner, there were no clear-cut differences in the antigen recognition patterns between these groups of individuals (Freedman et al., 1989). This molecule has recently been cloned and expressed and shown to be present primarily in the larval stage of the parasite (Raghavan et al., 1984). Such studies suggest, but do not prove, that larval antigens may be of paramount importance in the induction of an immune state to filarial infection in humans.

Immunoepidemiological Approach to the Definition of Immunity

Recently, an alternative approach to the definition of filarial immunity was proposed, taking into account the "dynamics" of worm acquisition and loss and the possibility that the acquisition of immunity is age related (Day, 1991; Day et al., 1991a,b). Because there is evidence in other helminth infections to suggest that with increasing age comes increasing immunity to infection and because, in studies of intestinal nematode reacquisition after definitive chemotherapy, estimates of worm acquisition and loss can be made using mathematical modeling, it has been suggested that similar models can be applied to the lymphatic-dwelling filarial parasites (Maizels et al., 1993). Using such an approach in which worm burdens were estimated based on circulating parasite antigen (probably a reflection of adult worm number) and microfilarial levels, the data suggested that resistance was independent of adult worm burdens and was indeed age related. Based on these data, it has been proposed that the majority of adults in filarial endemic regions of the world have acquired immunity to reinfection despite having patent infection (concomitant immunity). While this concept provides a provocative framework to understand resistance to reinfection, it is very difficult to test in human populations because the tools to assess adult worm burden definitively and/or what constitutes immunity (in human populations) are not yet available.

CONCLUSION

The outcome following filarial infection with either *W. bancrofti* or the *Brugia* spp. is certainly related to the nature of the host immune response to these filarial parasites. While it has become increasingly clear that the parasite itself can induce lymphatic abnormalities in the absence of a demonstrable T- and B-cell compartment, it is also clear that with a vigorous immune-mediated inflammatory response comes significant pathology. Furthermore, if one can modulate (or downregulate) this immune response, a state of parasite-specific anergy is induced that results in the lack of clinically apparent pathology (asymptomatic microfilaremia). How this immunologic hyporesponsiveness is mediated is of extreme importance and must reflect a number of factors including genetic predisposition, the nature of the antigen presentation to the immune system, in utero experience with the parasite, and many that remain undefined. Furthermore, how this hyporesponsiveness is overcome determines whether the subsequent acquisition of responsiveness results in serious pathology of protective immunity.

REFERENCES

Ash LR (1971): Preferential susceptibility of male jirds (*Meriones unguiculatus*) to infection with *Brugia pahangi*. J Parasitol 57:777–780.

Brabin L (1990): Sex differentials in susceptibility to lymphatic filariasis and implications for maternal child immunity. Epidemiol Infect 105:335–353.

Case TC, Witte CL, Witte MH, Unger EC, Williams WH (1992): Magnetic resonance imaging in human lymphedema: Comparison with lymphangioscintigraphy. Magn Reson Imaging 10:549–558.

Chan SH, Dissanayake S, Mak JW, Ismail MM, Wee GB, Srinivasan N, Soo BH, Zaman V (1984): HLA and filariasis in Sri Lankans and Indians. Southeast Asian J Trop Med Public Health 15:281–286.

Day KP (1991): The endemic normal in lymphatic filariasis: A static concept. Parasitol Today 7:293–296.

Day KP, Gregory WF, Maizels RM (1991a): Age-specific acquisition of immunity to infective larvae in a bancroftian filariasis endemic area of Papua New Guinea. Parasite Immunol 13:277–290.

Day KP, Grenfell B, Spark R, Kazura JW, Alpers MP (1991b): Age specific patterns of change in the dynamics of *Wunchereria bancrofti* infection Papua New Guinea. Am J Trop Med Hyg 44:518–527.

Denham DA, Fletcher C (1987): The cat infected with *Brugia pahangi* as a model of human filariasis. Ciba Found Symp 127:225–235.

Dissanayake S, DeSilva L, Ismail M (1980): IgM antibodies to filarial antigens in human cord blood: Possibility of transplancental infection. Trans R Soc Trop Med Hyg 74:541–547.

Dreyer G, et al. (1992): Renal abnormalities in microfilaremic patients with Bancroftian filariasis. Am J Trop Med Hyg 46:745–751.

Freedman DO, Nutman TB, Ottesen EA (1989): Protective immunity in bancroftian filariasis. Selective recognition of a 43-kD larval stage antigen by infection-free individuals in an endemic area. J Clin Invest 83:14–22.

Grenfell B, Michael E, Denham D (1991): A model for the dynamics of human lymphatic filariasis. Parasitol Today 12:318–323.

Gusmäo RD, Stanley AM, Ottesen EA (1981): *Brugia pahangi:* Immunologic evaluation of the differential susceptibility of filarial infection in inbred Lewis rats. Exp Parasitol 52:147–159.

Jungmann P, Figueredo-Silva J, Dreyer G (1992): Bancroftian lymphangitis in northeastern Brazil: A histopathological study of 17 cases. J Trop Med Hyg 95:114–118.

Kazura JW, Cicirello H, McCall JW (1986): Induction of protection against *Brugia malayi* infection in jirds by microfilarial antigens. J Immunol 136:1422–1426.

Kazura JW, Maroney PA, Pearlman E, Nilsen TW (1990): Protective efficacy of a cloned Brugia malayi antigen in a mouse model of microfilaremia. J Immunol 145:2260–2264.

King CL, Kumaraswami V, Poindexter RW, Kumari S, Jayaraman K, Alling DW, Ottesen EA, Nutman TB (1992): Immunologic tolerance in lymphatic filariasis. Diminished parasite-specific T and B lymphocyte precursor frequency in the microfilaremic state. J Clin Invest 89:1403–1410.

King C, Mahanty S, Kumaraswami V, Abrams J, Raganathan J, Jayaraman K, Ottesen E, Nutman T (1993): Cytokine control of parasite specific anergy in human lymphatic filariasis:

Preferential induction of a regulatory Th2 lymphocyte subset. J Clin Invest 92:1667–1673.

King CL, Nutman TB (1991): Regulation of the immune response in lymphatic filariasis and onchocerciasis. Immunol Today 12:A54–A548.

Klei TR, Blanchard DP, Coleman SU (1986): Development of *Brugia pahangi* infections and lymphatic lesions in male offspring of female jirds with homologous infections. Trans R Soc Trop Med Hyg 80:214–216.

Klion AD, Massougbodji A, Sadeler BC, Ottesen EA, Nutman TB (1991): Loiasis in endemic and nonendemic populations: Immunologically mediated differences in clinical presentation. J Infect Dis 163:1318–1325.

Lammie PJ, Addiss DG, Leonard G, Hightower AW, Eberhard ML (1993): Heterogeneity in filarial-specific immune responsiveness among patients with lymphatic obstruction. J Infect Dis 167:1178–1183.

Lammie PJ, Hitch WL, Walker Allen EM, Hightower W, Eberhard ML (1991): Maternal filarial infection as risk factor for infection in children. Lancet 337:1005–1006.

Lammie PJ, Leiva LE, Ruff AJ, Eberhard ML, Lowrie R Jr, Katz SP (1988): Bancroftian filariasis in Haiti: Preliminary characterization of the immunological responsiveness of microfilaremic individuals. Am J Trop Med Hyg 38:125–129.

Li BW, Chandrashekar R, Weil GJ (1993): Vaccination with recombination filarial paramyosin induces partial immunity to *Brugia malayi* infection in jirds. J Immunol 150:1881–1885.

Maizels RM, Bundy DA, Selkirk ME, Smith DF, Anderson RM (1993): Immunological modulation and evasion by helminth parasites in human populations. Nature 365:797–805.

Miller S, Snowden K, Schreuer D, Hammerberg B (1990): Selective breeding of dogs for segregation of limb edema from microfilaremia as clinical manifestations of *Brugia* infections. Am J Trop Med Hyg 489:497.

Nelson FK, Greiner DL, Shultz LD, Rajan TV (1991): The immunodeficient scid mouse as a model for human lymphatic filariasis. J Exp Med 173:659–663.

Nutman TB, Kumaraswami V, Ottesen EA (1987a): Parasite-specific anergy in human filariasis. Insights after analysis of parasite antigen-driven lymphokine production. J Clin Invest 79:1516–1523.

Nutman TB, Kumaraswami V, Pao L, Narayanan PR, Ottesen EA (1987b): An analysis of in vitro B cell immune responsiveness in human lymphatic filariasis. J Immunol 138:3954–3959.

Ottesen EA (1992): The Wellcome Trust Lecture. Infection and disease in lymphatic filariasis: An immunological perspective. Parasitology 104:S71–S79.

Ottesen EA, Mendell NR, MacQueen JM, Weller PF, Amos DB, Ward FE (1981): Familial predisposition to filarial infection—Not linked to HLA-A or -B locus specificities. Acta Trop 38:205–216.

Ottesen EA, Nutman TB (1992): Tropical pulmonary eosinophilia. Annu Rev Med 43:417–424.

Ottesen EA, Weller PF, Heck L (1977): Specific cellular immune unresponsiveness in human filariasis. Immunology 33:413–421.

Ottesen EA, Weller PF, Lunde M, Hussain R (1982): Endemic filariasis on a Pacific Island. II. Immunological aspects: Immunoglobulin, complement, and specific antifilarial IgG, IgM and IgE antibodies. Am J Trop Med Hyg 31:953–961.

Partono F (1984): Filariasis in Indonesia: Clinical manifestations and basic concepts of treatment and control. Trans R Soc Trop Med Hyg 78:9–12.

Philipp M, Davis TB, Storey N, Carlow CK (1988): Immunity in filariasis: perspectives for vaccine development. Annu Rev Microbiol 42:685–716.

Piessens WF, McGreevy PB, Piessens PW, McGreevy M, Koiman I, Saroso HS, Dennis DT (1980): Immune responses in human infections with *Brugia malayi*. Specific cellular unresponsiveness to filarial antigens. J Clin Invest 65:172–179.

Raghavan N, Freedman DO, Fitzgerald PL, Unnasch TR, Ottesen EA, Nutman TB (1994): Cloning and characterization of a potentially protective chitinase-like recombinant antigen from *Wuchereria bancrofti*. Infect Immun 62:1901–1908.

Romagnani S (1992): Human TH1 and TH2 subsets: Regulation of differentiation and role in protection and immunopathology. Int Arch Allergy Immunol 98:279–285.

Subrahmanyam D, Mehta K, Nelson DS, Rao YV, Rao CK (1978): Immune reactions in human filariasis. J Clin Microbiol 8:228–232.

Vickery AC, Albertine KH, Nayar JK, Kwa BH (1991): Histopathology of *Brugia malayi*-infected nude mice after immune-reconstitution. Acta Trop 49:45–55.

Vincent AL, Vickery AC, Lotz MJ, Desai U (1984): The lymphatic pathology of *Brugia pahangi* in nude (athymic) and thymic mice C3H/HeN. J Parasitol 70:48–56.

von Lichtenberg F (1987): The Wellcome Trust lecture. Inflammatory responses to filarial connective tissue parasites. Parasitology 94:S101–S122.

Ward DJ, Nutman TB, Zea FG, Portocarrero C, Lujan A, Ottesen EA (1988): Onchocerciasis and immunity in humans: Enhanced T cell responsiveness to parasite antigen in putatively immune individuals. J Infect Dis 157:536–543.

Weil GJ, Hussain R, Kumaraswami V, Tripathy SP, Phillips KS, Ottesen EA (1983): Prenatal allergic sensitization to helminth antigens in offspring of parasite-infected mothers. J Clin Invest 71:1124–1129.

Weller PF, Ottesen EA, Heck L (1980): Immediate and delayed hypersensitivity skin test responses to the *Dirofilaria immitis* filarial skin test (Sawada) antigen in Wuchereria bancrofti filariasis. Am J Trop Med Hyg 29:809–814.

Witte MH, Jamal S, Williams WH, Witte CL, Kumaraswami V, McNeill GC, Case TC, Panicker TM (1993): Lymphatic abnormalities in human filariasis as depicted by lymphangioscintigraphy. Arch Intern Med 153:737–744.

APPENDIX

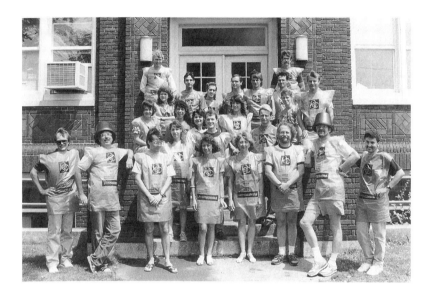

Participants in the Biology of Parasitism course, 1988. **Students:** Myrna Bonaldo, Clotilde Carlow, Glenn Frank, Ricardo Gazzinelli, H.U. Goringer, Jean-Murie Grzych, Maria Guther, Eric James, Jamil Kanaani, Michel Ledizet, Anna Lyles, Rona Mogil, Jeffrey Moore, Silvia Moreno, Peter Sayles, Marianne Stefani; **Faculty and assistants** (*in photo*): Steve Anderson, Steve Beverley, Jennefer Blackwell, Paul Englund (Director), Patrick Farley, Carole Long, Wayne Masterson, Alan Sher (Director); (*not in photo*): Steve Hajduk, Gerald Hart, Paul Knopf, Ed Pearce, David Sacks, Phil Scott, Don Wassom.

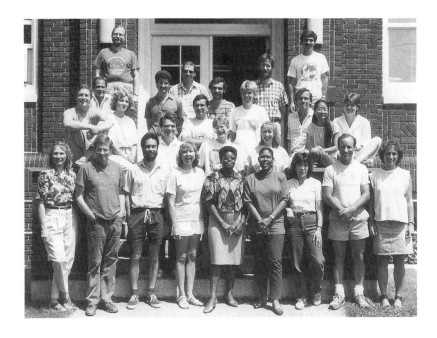

Participants in the Biology of Parasitism course, 1989. **Students:** Tamara Aboagye-Kwarteng, Paulo Andrade, Brenda Beerntsen, Vladimir Correado, Philip Effron, Najib El-Sayed, Phyllis Freeman-Junior, Mary Gonzatti, Christopher Karp, Marika Kullberg, Lynn Morris, Dania Richter, David Siegel, Walter Weiss, David Williams, Lilian Yepez-Mulia; **Faculty and assistants** (*in photo*): Steve Anderson, Steve Beverley, Ted Bianco, John Donelson (Director), Linda Donelson, Chris Donelson, Carole Long (Director), Sam Turco, Wen-lin Zeng; (*not in photo*): Bruce Christensen, Steve Hajduk, Larry Simpson, Mervyn Turner.

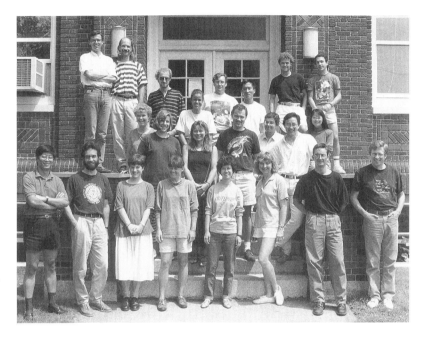

Participants in the Biology of Parasitism course, 1990. **Students:** Wanida Asawamahasakda, Fernanda Gadelha, Eileen Gruszinski, Michael Howard, Christopher Hunter, Gregory Jennings, Christopher Leptak, Congjun Li, Leo Liu, James McCoy, Gloria Palma, Laura Rocco, Nicola Schweitzer, Frank Seeber, Philippe Vandekerckhove, Gayl Wall; **Faculty and assistants** (*in photo*): Ted Bianco, John Donelson (Director), Steve Hajduk, Kwang Kim, Carole Long (Director), Elonne Petrin, Sam Turco, Wen-lin Zeng.

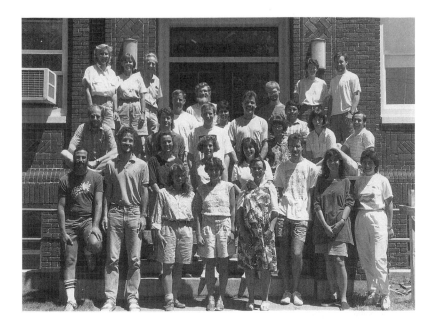

Participants in the Biology of Parasitism course, 1991. **Students:** (*in photo*): Dwight Bowman, Iris Bruchhaus, Larry Buxbaum, Hilary Cadman, Laurie Ellis, Martha Espinosa-Cantella, Kristin Hager, Sandra Halonen, Thomas Ilg, Rebecca Kollberg, Morgana Lima, Patrick Lorenz, John McNally, Ricardo Mondragon, Rupert Quinnell, Andreas Seyfang, Keith Wilson, Nancy Wisnewski, Yun Zhang; (*not in photo*): Pedro Clavijo, Lidya Sanchez; **Faculty and assistants** (*in photo*): Norma Andrews, John Boothroyd (Director), Jean-Francois Dubremetz, Heidi Elmendorf, Alan Fairlamb, Kasturi Haldar, Patsy Komuniecki, Rick Komuniecki, Steve Singer; (*not in photo*): Francisca (Ponchi) Diaz, Emilio Duran, Fred Finkelman, Steve Hajduk, Fred Heinzel, Rich Locksley, Pat Maroney, Tim Nilsen, Vicki Pollard, Joe Urban.

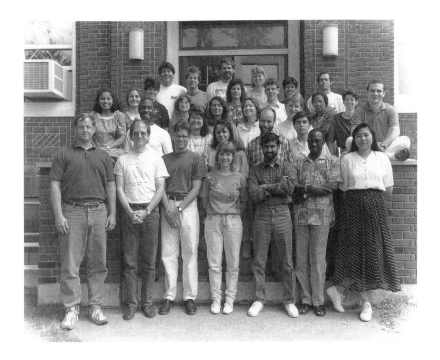

Participants in the Biology of Parasitism course, 1992. **Students:** Tom Allen, Prasanta Chakraborty, Claire Chougnet, Johanna Daily, Hans Hagen, Norton Heise, Hans-Jurgen Hoppe, Kuo-Yuan Hwa, Aslog Jansson, Assan Jaye, Adrian Lawrence, J. Hermenio Cavalcante Lima Filho, Kati Loeffler, Mike McIntosh, Fernando Monroy, C. Alberto Moreno, Sharon Moschitch, Hagir Suliman, Lakshmi Venkatakrishnaiah, Ying-Zi Yang; **Faculty and assistants** (*in photo*): John Boothroyd (Director), Jean-Francois Dubremetz, Heidi Elmendorf, Kasturi Haldar, Michele Klingbeil, Rick Komuniecki (Director), Michelle Rathman, Martine Soete, Michel Tibayrenc; (*not in photo*): Dick Davis, Francisca (Ponchi) Diaz, Patty Dorn, Emilio Duran, Alan Fairlamb, Ashraf El Meanawy, Fred Finkelman, Patsy Komuniecki, Rich Locksley, Suzanne Morris, Steve Reiner, Kevin Smith, Joe Urban.

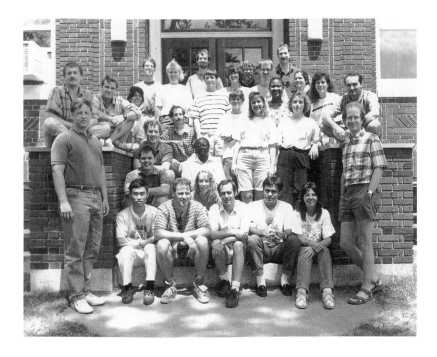

Participants in the Biology of Parasitism course, 1993. **Students:** Niklas Ahlborg, Lisa Barthel, Paul Bloch, Marcelo Briones, Fidel de la Cruz Hernandez, Wolfgang Hoffman, David Horn, Jorge Huete-Perez, Catharine Johnson, Maxine Kellman, Johannes (Hans) Koeller, Fatima Noronha, Claudi Ochatt, Archangel (Levi) Omara-Opyene, Simon Paul, Barbara Rick, Paul Selzer, Tim Stedman, Jan Tachezy, Jianming (James) Tang; **Faculty and assistants** (*in photo*): John Boothroyd (Director), Dick Davis, Jean-Francois Dubremetz, Patricia Johnson, Michele Klingbeil, Rick Komuniecki (Director), Kersten Moorehead, Sally Riddles, Martine Soete; (*not in photo*): Peter Bradley, Emilio Duran, Fred Finkelman, Peter Hotez, Patsy Komuniecki, Rich Locksley, Suzanne Morris, Melissa Perregaux, Steve Reiner, Dominique Soldati, Joe Urban, Keith Wilson.

Index

metalloprotease, 24
Caenorhabditis elegans, 26
nematode metabolism, 109–115, 116–118
Schistosoma mansoni, 23
Latency-associated peptide, 447
Latent TGF-ß, 447
Leishmania donovani, 127
hypoxanthine–guanine
phosphoribosyltransferase, 131–138
Leishmania major
antigen presentation, 455–456
cytokines, 462
IFN-γ, 467
IL-4, 467
IL-12, 438–439
immunomodulation, 440–441
macrophages, 461
therapeutic implications, 462–463
Th1 vs. Th2 response, 456–461
Leishmaniasis. *See Leishmania* spp.
Leishmania spp.
immune response
GM-CSF, 445–446
IFN-γ, 445–446, 449–450
IL-10, 449–450
LTGF-ß, 445–446
macrophage stimulation and inhibition,
443
strategies, 432
TGF-ß, 446–449
therapeutics, 450–452
purine metabolism, 127–128
pyrazolopyrimidines, 128–130
symptoms, 444
transient transfection system, 235,
238–239
Leishmania tarentolae
guide RNA, 248
kinetoplast DNA, 247, 251
Leishmania virus (LRV), 184–185
Leptomonas collosoma, 264
Leptomonas collosum, 311
let-545 mutation, 335, 337
Leucine, 417–419
Leucovorin, 124
Levamisole
mechanism, 70–71, 96
transcuticular diffusion, 59
lgps (lysosomal membrane glycoproteins),
364–365

Ligands
Ancylostoma spp., 26
Theileria spp., 44
lin-15 gene, 291, 296
Lipid biosynthesis, 414
Lipid layer, 59–60
Lipids
Plasmodium falciparum
sphingomyelin, 377–379
tubovesicular membranes, 383–388
Toxoplasma gondii, 348–349
Lipid transport, 389–391
Lipopolysaccharide (LPS), 439, 473
Loa loa, 77
LouTat serodeme, 478–483, 484, 490
LPS (lipopolysaccharide), 439, 473
LRV (Leishmania virus), 184–185
LTGF-ß, 447
Luciferase gene
Plasmodium gallinaceum system, 235–239
Trypanosoma brucei, 415–419
1LUC plasmid, 237
Lymph node cells, 483–486
Lymphocytes. *See* B cells; T cells
Lymphokines. *See* Cytokines; specific
lymphokines
Lymphotoxin, 433
Lysosomal membrane glycoproteins (lgps),
364–365
Lysosomes, mammalian, 360–363

Macrophages
cytokines
stimulation and inhibition, 434, 443
Leishmania major, 461
Trypanosoma brucei rhodesiense, 485–493
mai-1 gene, 292–293, 296
Major histocompatibility (MHC) class II
antigens, 455–456, 484–485, 516–517
Malaria. *See Plasmodium* spp.
Malate metabolism, 110
Malonate, 116
Mammalian tissue factor pathway inhibitor
(mTFPI), 24–25
Mapping. *See* Genetic mapping
Mast cells, 460, 470
maternal effect sterile (mes) mutations, 326
Maurer's clefts, 372, 387–389
Maxicircles in kinetoplast DNA
replication, 156–158